Rabies

Rabies

Edited by

Alan C. Jackson
Queen's University, Kingston, Ontario, Canada

William H. Wunner
The Wistar Institute, Philadelphia, Pennsylvania

ACADEMIC PRESS

An Elsevier Science Imprint

Amsterdam   Boston   London   New York   Oxford   Paris
San Diego   San Francisco   Singapore   Sydney   Tokyo

Cover illustration by George Moogk/London Health Sciences Centre

The following articles are U.S. government works in the public domain:

"Molecular Epidemiology" by Jean S. Smith
"Epidemiology" by James E. Childs
"Animal Rabies" by Michael Niezgoda, Cathleen A. Hanlon, and Charles E. Rupprecht

Academic Press
An Elsevier Science Imprint
525 B Street, Suite 1900, San Diego, CA 92101-4495, USA
http://www.academicpress.com

Academic Press
Harcourt Place, 32 Jamestown Road, London NW1 7BY, UK
http://www.hbuk.co.uk/ap/

Library of Congress Catalog Card Number: 2002102062

International Standard Book Number: 0-12-379077-8

Printed in the United States of America

02 03 04 05 06 SB 9 8 7 6 5 4 3 2 1

Contents

8   Pathology

Yuzo Iwasaki and Muneshige Tobita

9   Diagnostic Evaluation

Charles V. Trimarchi and Jean S. Smith

10   Immunology

Monique Lafon

11   Vaccines

Deborah J. Briggs, David W. Dreesen, and William H. Wunner

12   Public Health Management of Humans at Risk

Deborah J. Briggs

13   Control of Dog Rabies

Konrad Bögel

14   Rabies Control in Wildlife

David H. Johnston and Rowland R. Tinline

15   Future Developments and Challenges

Alan C. Jackson

Contributors

Numbers in parentheses indicate the pages on which the authors' contributions begin.

Konrad Bögel (429) Veterinary Public Health Division of Communicable Diseases, World Health Organization, CH-1211, Geneva 19, Switzerland

Deborah J. Briggs (371, 401) College of Veterinary Medicine, Kansas State University, Manhattan, Kansas 66506

James E. Childs (113) Viral Rickettsial Zoonoses Branch, Centers for Disease Control and Prevention, Atlanta, Georgia 30333

David W. Dreesen (371) Lida Corporation, Winterville, Georgia 30683

Cathleen A. Hanlon (163) Rabies Section, Centers for Disease Control and Prevention, Atlanta, Georgia 30333

Yuzo Iwasaki (283) Miyagi National Hospital, Yamamoto-cho, Watari-gun, Miyagi 989-2202, Japan

Alan C. Jackson (219, 245, 473) Departments of Medicine (Neurology) and Microbiology and Immunology, Queen's University, Kingston, Ontario K7L 3N6, Canada

David H. Johnston (445) Johnston Biotech, Sarnia, Ontario N7V 3B5, Canada

Monique Lafon (351) Institut Pasteur, Unité de Neuro-Immunologie Virale, 75724 Paris Cedex 15, France

Michael Niezgoda (163) Rabies Section, Centers for Disease Control and Prevention, Atlanta, Georgia 30333

Charles E. Rupprecht (163) Rabies Section, Centers for Disease Control and Prevention, Atlanta, Georgia 30333

Jean S. Smith (79, 307) Rabies Section, Centers for Disease Control and Prevention, Atlanta, Georgia 30333

Rowland R. Tinline (445) Queen's GIS Laboratory, Queen's University, Kingston, Ontario K7L 3N6, Canada

Charles V. Trimarchi (307) Rabies Laboratory, Wadsworth Center, New York State Department of Health, Albany, New York 12201-0509

Muneshige Tobita (283) Miyagi National Hospital, Yamamoto-cho, Watari-gun, Miyagi 989-2202, Japan

Lise Wilkinson (1) The Wellcome Trust Centre for the History of Medicine, University College London, London NW1 1AD, United Kingdom

William H. Wunner (23, 371) The Wistar Institute, Philadelphia, Pennsylvania 19104-4268

Foreword

Pasteur's development of the first rabies vaccine is, of course, the stuff of legend, all the more remarkable because the agent of the disease — the "virus" — was unknown at the time.

(From Chapter 1, Lise Wilkinson)

It seems to me that any book on rabies should start with mention of Louis Pasteur. I never get tired of remembering him, his work on rabies, and his role in the evolution of the microbiologic, virologic, and infectious disease sciences; I hope no one else ever does either. As I reflect on the early days, the days that became the *stuff of legend*, I find it fitting that rabies was at the heart of it all — not fowl cholera, not anthrax, Pasteur's other favorites, but rabies. I have always been struck by Pasteur's immediate extension from studies aimed at discovering the causative agent of the disease at hand to the development of specific interventions. In the case of rabies, as Lise Wilkinson reminds us in Chapter 1, even without discovering the causative agent, Pasteur carried through with his usual extension into the then mysterious world of vaccinology. In 1885, when Pasteur gave the first rabies vaccine to the boy, Joseph Meister, bitten severely a few days before by a rabid dog, the infectious disease sciences moved into the modern era, the era that we still inhabit.

From that moment forward, the history of the infectious disease sciences has been crowded with wonderful discoveries and practical applications. The history centers on the replacement of centuries-old beliefs, conceptions, and theories with scientific proofs. Scientific proofs established the concept of *specificity of disease causation*; that is, particular infectious diseases are caused not by some common miasma but rather by specific infectious agents. This concept was Pasteur's key to the search for specific interventions and is the key to the concepts that we use to underpin prevention and control strategies, specific diagnostic tests, and specific therapeutic approaches. In a larger sense, built on Pasteur's vision, the infectious disease sciences have played a paramount role in the reformation of all medical thought — the requirement for verifiable scientific proofs has been extended universally throughout all medical and veterinary sciences. At the same time, the practical application of the infectious disease sciences has led to improvements in human and animal health and well-being that have exceeded the contribution of any other branch of science. This all started because Pasteur targeted rabies!

If we think of the years since Pasteur first investigated rabies (1877), we see many of the great epidemic infectious diseases reaching peaks in prevalence and then declining. Most of the great epidemic pediatric diseases, such as diphtheria, pertussis, measles, rubella, and polio, have fallen like duckpins. Many of the great epidemic diseases of animals, such as rinderpest, classic swine fever, Newcastle disease, and canine distemper, have gone the same way (at least in developed countries). This has occurred because of the development of vaccines and the development of the scientific base on which vaccinology rests. I find it intriguing, or perhaps better, disturbing, that while so many infectious diseases have come and gone, rabies represents a checkered chronicle, an ever-threatening reality. Several thoughts come to mind here.

First, efficacious rabies vaccines, perhaps not the best in terms of purity, potency, and reactogenicity, but good enough, have been around for a long time. When combined with stray animal control, a diagnostics system, and a public health infrastructure, most of the risk posed by terrestrial animals (e.g., dog rabies) can be minimized. When combined with good clinical evaluation of exposure, most of the risk to humans can be minimized. Yet here in the twenty-first century, in so many places in the world where diphtheria and measles have been minimized and where smallpox and polio have been eradicated, rabies goes on and on. I still hear from colleagues who work in places where rabies presents a substantial risk to humans the old saw, "Rabies has always been with us, and it always will be with us... ." I recall investigating a case in a Latin American country, a case diagnosed *ex post facto* by histopathology, and being told, "Oh, the strain of rabies we have here is not very pathogenic; it is not a significant risk." Given the terror that the word *rabies* connotes in all societies, this is hard to understand. Perhaps it is time for more sociologic and motivational research to be added to the kind of modern research that has become the standard of the day, the kind of modern research that fills this volume. Surely, as the eleventh cause of infectious disease deaths in humans globally [Haupt (1999): Rabies-risks of exposure and current trends in prevention of human cases. *Vaccine* **17**, 1742–1749] rabies can be added to the public mindset that has driven the control of so many other infectious diseases. Somehow the public compartmentalization of rabies, the sense that it is a separate, unique problem, must be put to rest. I think that this volume, taken as whole, helps in this regard.

Second, the notion that rabies is zoonotic, with reservoir hosts occupying diverse, worthy econiches, has been understood for a long time. Rabies is not about to be eradicated from large, diverse ecosystems with the kind of resources that are likely to be available. For many years this point was understood, and research was aimed at "being smarter than the virus." Wildlife vaccination represents one concept that seemed to fit this reality. Elimination of rabies from Switzerland and then France and southern Germany seemed to confirm the notion. I recall that at a Carter Center meeting on the concept of global eradication, where the success with smallpox and polio was used to search for other targets, the question of global rabies eradication was studied. It was as if the reality of India, the Philippines, and West Africa was forgotten. It is as if the reality of bat rabies can been forgotten. It is as if the key sciences of mammalogy, wildlife biology, reservoir host ecology, etc. can been dissociated from the sciences of virology, epidemiology, clinical medicine, clinical veterinary medicine, and public health. I think that several chapters in this volume will help to reestablish the association and will help to remind everyone that understanding rabies in its reservoir host populations around the world is essential if we are to move forward from here. In this lies the key to the dream that rabies perhaps may be eliminated regionally or even eradicated globally.

Third and last, the ever-threatening reality of rabies as a global health problem (and in some places in the world a domestic animal health problem) should be enough to bring into the fold a new generation of scientists. The ghost of Pasteur, the nature of the work to be done — what a romantic call to young people who want fulfilling careers! The romance that brings young people into my office every month may have to be shared with Ebola hemorrhagic fever, West Nile virus encephalitis, hantavirus pulmonary syndrome, and other zoonoses that are mentioned as "new, emerging and reemerging infectious diseases," but in the context of exciting careers, rabies easily holds its own. I think that this volume, reflecting the state of the art, is full of "hooks" that will influence career decisions of the next generation of would-be scientists.

I would, in closing, like to congratulate the editors for their vision in seeing the need for this book and for their hard work in bringing their vision to reality. I would like to congratulate the authors for contributing such excellent chapters. I sense their love of the work, their fidelity to Pasteur's foresight. I sense in the authors the same kind of feeling I had when I worked on the virus and the disease: It is a thing of beauty, but it is "a terrible beauty." As I think of the editors and authors, I conclude that the scientific base for rabies prevention and control, globally, is in good hands.

Frederick A. Murphy
University of California, Davis

Preface

Although this comprehensive book was written primarily with a clinical audience in mind, it will be of interest to public health advisors, epidemiologists, and basic research scientists who have an interest in rabies. The basic biology and molecular virology of rabies are emphasized because an understanding of the underlying mechanisms involved in the disease is essential for diagnosis and strategies for disease prevention by veterinarians and physicians in a variety of specialties, including family medicine, emergency medicine, internal medicine, infectious diseases, and neurology.

Many important developments have occurred over the past century to counteract this ancient disease. Among the most significant areas, the development of methods for pre- and postexposure prophylaxis of human rabies and the control of wildlife rabies have resulted from the efforts of many with medical and basic science expertise in the field. During the past decade, in particular, several major advances in the rabies field have contributed to our understanding of the basic virology, pathogenesis, and molecular epidemiology of the disease, and also to the development of effective programs for the control of rabies in wildlife. However, despite these efforts, rabies remains a global problem of major importance. Unfortunately, human rabies remains an important public health problem in developing countries due to uncontrolled dog rabies. In addition, there has been a reemergence of rabies in the United States in the 1990s due to bat rabies virus variants that pose an ongoing threat to humans.

The field of specialists dealing with the rabies problem is changing and includes people in many diverse disciplines. This book is a truly multidisciplinary effort by contributors with expertise in medicine (neurology and pathology), verterinary medicine, virology, immunology, biology, epidemiology, geography, and history. We are very grateful for their efforts. It is our hope that this book will be helpful to medical and veterinary clinicians, public health officials, research scientists, and students involved in understanding, diagnosing, and preventing rabies worldwide.

Alan C. Jackson
William H. Wunner

xvii

1

History

LISE WILKINSON

The Wellcome Trust Centre for the History of Medicine
University College London
London NW1 1AD, United Kingdom

The dictionary tells us that *rabies* is derived from the Latin *rabere*, "to rage or to rave," as is the corresponding adjective *rabid*; *rabere* possibly may have earlier origins in the Sanskrit *rabhas*, for "violence." The Greeks adopted their own word, *lyssa*, meaning "madness," for rabies; this in turn is still reflected in English in *lyssophobia*, described in the *Oxford English Dictionary* as "a morbid dread of hydrophobia, the symptoms of which sometimes simulate those of the actual disease." Not surprisingly, then, it is the image of the mad dog that has for centuries past come to symbolize humankind's fear of the disease as expressed by writers, legislators, and medical practitioners and philosophers (Fig. 1). "Mad" or "vicious" dogs began to appear in legal documents in Mesopotamia as early as 2300 B.C., when owners of such animals were held responsible for any deaths resulting from their bites: "If a dog is mad, and if the authorities have made its owner aware of this fact; if then the latter does not keep the dog under guard at home and it bites a man and causes his death, the owner must pay two thirds of a *mina* (40 shekels). If it causes the death of a slave, he must pay 15 shekels," as cited by Théodoridès (1986) from the *Eshunna* code. Comparison of the amounts to be paid cast a chilling reflection on relative values of lives in Mesopotamian society then. Three millenia later, the code of medieval Welsh laws credited to Hywell Dha (Howel the Good), King of Wales (Probert, 1823), still struggled with the legal problems relating to bites by such dogs.

During the intervening centuries, there was an increase in the general understanding of the nature and development of diseases. According to Nutton (1983) the "atomic theory" of Democritus (fl. 460–370 B.C.) and the pre-Socratic philosophers in the fifth century B.C. may have influenced the development of subsequent ideas of "seeds" of disease, reflected in the more specific writings on

1

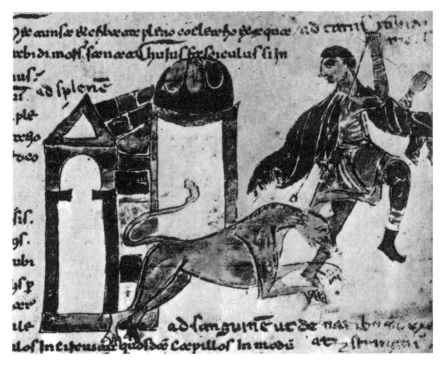

Fig. 1. Italian miniature, twelfth century, showing a man being bitten by a mad dog. (*Wellcome Library, London.*)

rabies by Aristotle in the fourth century B.C. and Celsus in the first and Galen in the second centuries A.D. Aristotle wrote briefly, when describing diseases of dogs, "Rabies drives the animal mad, and any animal whatever, excepting man, will take the disease if bitten by a mad dog so afflicted; the disease is fatal to the dog itself and to any animal it may bite, man excepted" (Aristotle, fourth century B.C.). His reference to man is puzzling and led some nineteenth-century commentators to suggest a possible change in the syndrome over the centuries. A more likely explanation had been offered in mid-sixteenth century by Fracastoro, who believed that Aristotle intended merely to draw a distinction between animals, which were thought to develop frank disease inevitably when bitten by a rabid dog, and humans, who may or may not develop clinical disease (Fracastoro, translated by W. C. Wright, 1930).

Celsus, the Roman doctor, was more concerned with disease in humans, with prophylaxis, and with what could be done once hydrophobia had become manifest. He wrote of the essential primary measure of cauterization and subsequent necessity of keeping the wound open to allow the "virus" to run out freely, even when first having been "drawn out with a cupping glass" — *virus* in the Latin of Celsus' day meant "poison" or "slimy liquid," an apt enough description of rabid saliva. *Virus* in the sense of "poison" was to survive as a general term for disease-causing agents in French as late as the time of Pasteur and his school and until developments in the twentieth century allowed more specific definitions. Celsus had no illusions regarding therapies and only briefly mentioned "antidotes," but he described at length the treatment, which remained the only generally accepted weapon against hydrophobia until the appearance of Pasteur's vaccine in the 1880s. Admitting to "very little hope for the sufferer" once the frank and deeply distressing symptoms with simultaneous thirst and fear of water were manifest, Celsus described "just one remedy, to throw the patient unawares into a water tank which he has not seen beforehand. If he cannot swim, let him sink under and drink, then lift him out; if he can swim, push him under at intervals so that he drinks his fill of water even against his will; for so his thirst and dread of water are removed at the same time. Yet this procedure incurs a further danger, that a spasm of sinews, provoked by the cold water, may carry off the weakened body. Lest this should happen, he must be taken straight from the tank and plunged into a bath of hot oil." (Celsus, translated by W. G. Spender, 1938). It is not specified how hot the oil should be, nor is Celsus' warning of further danger easy to interpret in terms used today. Many later versions of this rather desperate treatment recommended seawater if nearby beaches were available. On the whole, either choice of therapy seems gruesome for what later knowledge has identified as rabies encephalitis. The therapies may have worked, of course, in cases of hysterical, and hence curable, reactions that were not true rabies.

The use of the term *sinews* in relevant translations is questioned by today's authorities, and this emphasizes the difficulties faced by translators of classical Greek and Latin texts searching for meaningful current equivalents of their classical terms. The best we can do today is perhaps to read *tendon* for *sinew*, but even this leaves the usage unclear. Translations of Caelius' fifth-century Latin version of a treatise on acute and chronic diseases in Greek by Soranus of Ephesus (fl. first–second century A.D.), which in turn leaned on texts by Democritus (fl. 460–370 B.C.), underline the difficulties, and the loss of Democritus' original manuscripts in the destruction of the great library at Alexandria further complicates the issue (Caelius Aurelianus, translated by I. E. Drabkin, 1950). In 1950, Drabkin refuted claims by certain nineteenth-century writers that use of the terms *nervus* in Latin and *neuron* in Greek suggested an early awareness of involvement of the nervous system in the disease; Drabkin also settled for *sinews* as a more likely translation. Whatever the status of sinews (or tendons, nervus, or neuron) today, the fact remains that even an elementary understanding of the anatomy of the brain and nervous system only began to develop with Herophilus' dissections of human cadavers more than a century after the death of Democritus.

Pliny the Elder (23–79 A.D.), a near-contemporary of Celsus, reviewed in his *Natural History* prevailing ideas of his time on the nature of the disease and possible therapies. The long-held belief in its spontaneous occurrence as caused by extreme conditions of heat, drought, sexual frustration, and other forms of stress was included and was to survive at least until the nineteenth century, into a period of time when transmission by "foaming saliva" also was becoming accepted as a distinct possibility (Fig. 2). Instead of the straightforward cauterization recommended by Celsus, Pliny offered a variety of therapeutic measures that included applying axle grease pounded with lime to the wound or ash from the burnt head of a dog, as well as, optimistically, as a long-term preventive measure, removal of the "worm" from the tongues of puppies: "Dogs have on their tongue a small worm, called by the Greeks *lytta*; if it is removed from young puppies, they are protected against rabies and never lose their appetite." Belief in the benefit of this practice, as in many other remedies, continued well into the nineteenth century (Fig. 3). Other recommendations by Pliny included decoctions (a Middle English term, preserved in pharmaceutical Latin, for extracts of one or more substances prepared by boiling down of suspensions) of dung of badger, cuckoo, and swallow, which were believed to provide relief (Fig. 4), as was the "cast slough" of snakes when pounded in wine with a male crab. Perhaps less

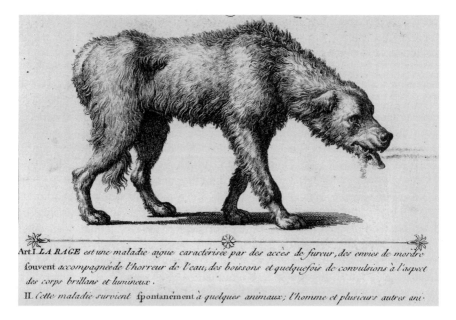

Art.I. *LA RAGE est une maladie aigue caractérisée par des accès de fureur, des envies de mordre* souvent *accompagnée de l'horreur de l'eau, des boissons et quelquefois de convulsions à l'aspect des corps brillans et lumineux.*

II. *Cette maladie survient* spontanément *à quelques animaux; l'homme et plusieurs autres ani-*

Fig. 2. Bedraggled dog suffering from rabies. Detail of French line engraving, Dijon 1785. (*Wellcome Library, London.*)

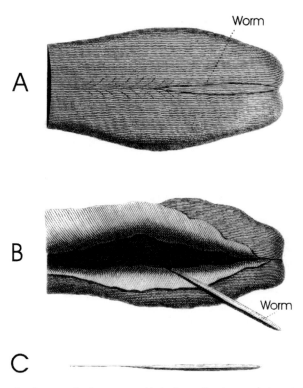

Fig. 3. Plate showing part of a dog tongue with the "worm" as it appears through the cuticle (*A*); the cuticle separated and laid back showing the "worm" and its attachment to muscle (*B*); and the detached "worm" (*C*). (*Adapted from W. Daniel, "Rural Sports," 1813; courtesy A. C. Jackson.*)

objectionable and "recently revealed by an oracle" was a decoction prepared from the root of the dog rose (*Rosa canina*).

A century later, Galen reached the conclusion that only dogs were natural hosts to rabies and that a mere drop of saliva from a rabid dog on human skin could cause hydrophobia in humans (Nutton, 1983). From the time of Galen onward through the dark ages and the Arab interpretations of the classical texts, little was added to the still-cursory understanding of rabies in dogs and in humans (usually referred to as *hydrophobia*). Then, in 1546, Girolamo Fracastoro (1478–1553) published in Venice the first known treatise dealing exclusively with contagious diseases. Fracastoro's concepts of contagion and of "seeds of disease" have been much lauded by later generations, but Nutton has pointed to earlier sources not acknowledged by Fracastoro, such as Lucretius's disease-causing "seeds" and Galen's reference to "seeds of disease," which may have been inspired by the thoughts of pre-Socratic atomists (Nutton, 1983). Received ideas they may have

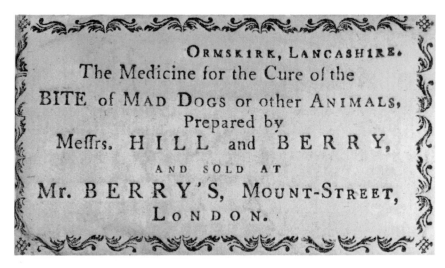

Fig. 4. Label for one of many recommended rabies "cures," *circa* 1800. (*Wellcome Library, London.*)

been, but Fracastoro was able to develop them convincingly, and his chapters on specific diseases stand out for clarity of thought and the felicity of his writing.

Fracastoro's chapter on rabies certainly can be seen as a significant step on the way from the classics to the final conclusive nineteenth century developments in true understanding of the nature of the disease. He left his readers in no doubt that it could not be transmitted to humans by simple "contact, or by fomes, or at a distance, but only when the skin is so torn by the bite of a dog that blood is drawn, as though contagion takes place in the blood itself through contact with the teeth and foam from the mouth of the rabid animal" (Fig. 5). Writing more than a century before Leeuwenhoek (1632–1723) even began grinding his lenses, when Fracastoro mentioned "germs" or "seeds of disease," with the power "to propagate and engender what is similar to themselves," he certainly did not see them as living organisms, let alone *animalculae*, although he did add that animals dead of the disease no longer "preserved the contagion" because "germs of the contagion have perished together with the innate heat." [If read by pathologists about to perform post mortems, this might just be advice better ignored (Fracastoro, translated by W. C. Wright, 1930).]

For all the clarity of his thought, Fracastoro's ideas were not immediately of particular influence at a time when science relied on philosophy rather than experiment to prove its points, or as Nutton has memorably put it, "the hypothesis of causative seeds was a philosophical luxury for the intellectual practitioner" (Nutton, 1983). The nature of contagion, let alone of virus diseases in general and of rabies in particular, would continue to defeat the best efforts of medical practitioners and scientists for more than another three centuries. In the case of rabies,

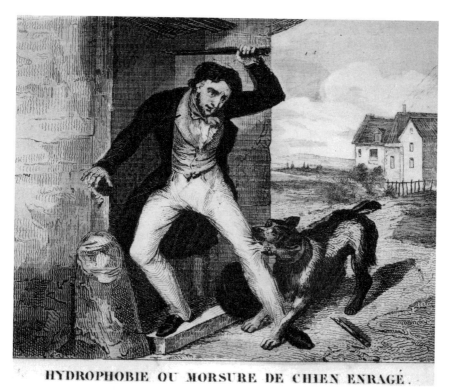

HYDROPHOBIE OU MORSURE DE CHIEN ENRAGÉ.

Fig. 5. Man attempting to fend off a rabid dog. Details of French broadsheet, Paris, nineteenth century. (*Wellcome Library, London.*)

development of Pasteur's postexposure prophylaxis predated any real understanding of its etiology by decades. In an exemplary translation, Wilmer Cave Wright (1930) allows Fracastoro to discuss the possibility of "immunization" against pestilence; this may be an overenthusiastic use of translator's poetic licence, since neither the context nor the Latin verbs used seem to suggest anything more than achieving a certain tolerance for the "germs" in question as in the case of some poisons such as arsenic.

Over subsequent centuries there was little progress in knowledge of either the clinical disease in humans or possible therapies, nor of how to protect human populations against roaming rabid dogs or wolves. However, there was no letup in the flow of literature on the subject; in addition to largely repetitive reports on remedies against the disease, there was a growing volume of papers detailing outbreaks of canine rabies throughout Europe and the Americas with numbers of recorded cases in epizootics and resulting human fatalities, as listed by George Fleming in 1872 and, more recently, by James H. Steele (1975 and 1991). A few descriptions of outbreaks through the centuries in greater detail can be found in Théodoridès's account in his definitive *Histoire de la Rage* (1986). There must, of course, remain doubts on the accuracy of early "statistics." The relatively small numbers of human victims dying after mad dog bites on the whole may be accepted; the considerable numbers of animal deaths recorded in individual outbreaks, whether of dogs, foxes, wolves, cattle, etc., could have been overestimated or, perhaps more likely, underestimated. Not surprisingly, few attempts were made to estimate numbers of animals affected in epizootics before 1700, even if they were reported. This has led some authors to assume that epizootics were rare until the Middle Ages; in any case, reports usually were restricted to single-animal attacks resulting in human fatalities that were duly counted and published: Around 900 A.D., a rabid bear bit 20 persons who attempted to kill it, of whom 6 unfortunates developed the disease and consequently were smothered to death over a 27-day period (Fleming, 1872; Steele, 1975, 1991) — a "treatment" still in use by the early eighteenth century when it was deplored and criticized in print by the father of Honoré de Balzac (discussed below).

In 1271, flocks of rabid wolves attacked herds of domestic animals in what was then Franconia; 30 human fatalities caused by bites were recorded. Epizootics of rabies were registered elsewhere in Europe in the sixteenth century; by 1604, there was a major outbreak of canine rabies in Paris, and from then on, European records show rabies to be present in frequent outbreaks among dogs, foxes, and wolves. It was known in England at least from the time of Edward, Second Duke of York (1373?–1415), who wrote an account of the disease.

In *Rabbis and Rabies*, G. M. Baer *et al.* (1996) have claimed — without documentation — that Edward, Second Duke of York, "clearly described rabies in hounds and the manner of transmission" in 1420. Since this Second Duke is known to have died on the battlefield of Agincourt in 1415, this seemed to stretch credulity and warrant further investigation. Scrutiny of library catalogues has revealed that this colorful duke did indeed write the oldest English book on hunting, most of which was based on a translation of the *Livre de la Chasse* by Gaston III Phoebes, Comte de Foix, with an added five chapters by the duke himself, all written between 1406 and 1413. Chapter 13, written by the Duke, is entitled "Of the Sicknesses of Hounds and of [Their] Corrupcions [*sic*]." Here he described both "furious madness," in which the hounds howl and cry, escaping in their fury to "go everywhere, biting both men and women and all that they find before them…if they draw blood it shall go mad whatever thing it be…." He also describes dumb madness, which in the language of his time he calls *ragemuet*, in which "…they neither bite nor run…and so they die…." The duke also mentions "remedies for men or for beast, including going to the sea and making nine waves, widening the wounds inflicted and letting a cock's vent suck all the venom of the biting," as well as the usual range of herbal remedies and decoctions. Long copied and circulated in manuscript form, the duke's book was printed in 1904, with a foreword by Theodore Roosevelt, who also took a particular interest in hunting.

By the mid-eighteenth century, reports of the presence of rabies appeared not only from the old world but also from locations throughout the new world; the practice of shooting all suspect dogs on sight and the introduction of quarantine arrangements began to spread from the 1752 outbreak in St. James, London, to rapidly growing colonial outposts (Fleming, 1872). According to Fleming, rabies was introduced into Argentina by the "sporting dogs" brought by English officers; it has remained enzootic there since. By then, canine rabies had been well established in colonial North America for more than 20 years, with serious outbreaks between 1785 and 1789, when a man having skinned a cow that died of rabies subsequently himself died of hydrophobia (Steele, 1975, 1991). From then on, and well into the following century, there were widespread outbreaks throughout Europe and other parts of the world, including the Americas and China and for the first time in Hong Kong in 1857, with both animal and human cases of rabies and hydrophobia.

One case abroad was reported by Fleming and later Steele and others: the death of Charles Lennox, Fourth Duke of Richmond (1764–1819), at the time governor-general of Canada, of hydrophobia, having been bitten 2 months earlier by a tame fox worried by dogs. J. D. Blaisdell (1992) questioned the diagnosis of hydrophobia, suggesting instead "hysterical rabies" brought on by an initial "mild cerebro-vascular accident," but his comments are not accepted by others with expertise in neurologic disorders, including rabies, as well as an interest in its history. Jackson, who in addition to his own expert knowledge of the disease has had access to contemporary case reports and papers held in the Public Archives of Canada, came to a different conclusion (Jackson, 1994). The records support and extend the nineteenth-century opinions: the 2-month incubation period following the fox bite and the details of the duke's clinical illness as recorded in the journals of the military officers who accompanied him. Jackson is convinced that it was a case of true rabies rather than the combination of an atypical presentation of two separate diagnoses (stroke and rabies hysteria) suggested by Blaisdell (1992) (A. C. Jackson, personal communication). After nearly two centuries, the diagnosis is confirmed: The duke died of hydrophobia and had not suffered from "hysterical rabies."

Occasional descriptions of episodes of hysterical rabies serve to underline the warnings of Bernard-François Balzac (1746–1826), father of the novelist, who was a hospital administrator at Tours. In a volume on the history and prevention of rabies, he — a stern critic of dogs, described as enemies of the public and of an "*immoralité incurable*" — recommended introduction of a tax on dogs, the amounts to depend on whether working dogs or mere pets (the tax was implemented 45 years later, long after his death). His main concern, however, was with those unfortunates who might be suffering only from imagined hydrophobia.

Balzac was anxious to protect such patients from the long-practiced form of euthanasia intended to end the distressing sufferings of victims of true rabies/ hydrophobia: strangling or suffocation, using the patient's own sheets and pillows, respectively (Balzac, 1810). Good intentions aside, Balzac feared that it might, in the wrong hands, prove "too tempting to the heirs or enemies of the patient."

While such episodes in Europe and North America show increasing concern with prevention and avoidance of unnecessary suffering, in Russia, serious outbreaks of rabies with inevitable hydrophobia casualties in poor and remote village communities in that vast country were recorded by Michele Marochetti, one of many European professionals working there during the nineteenth century. Personal physician to one Count Moszezensky, Marochetti spent years in the Ukraine and witnessed the consequences of "large hydrophobic dogs" terrorizing villagers. He wrote later: "On several occasions I was devastated when victims perished under my very eyes." His only suggestions for therapy were repetitions of the decoctions recommended through previous centuries (Marochetti, 1849).

In fact, both the case of the Duke of Richmond and Marochetti's notes serve to demonstrate how little progress had been made since the seventeenth century, despite the growing medical and scientific awareness of the century of enlightenment. For two centuries, research on rabies had been limited to attempts to reexamine recommended therapies of old, which in the case of rabies had by then held sway for so many centuries without being challenged. Already reports in the very first volume (1665–1666) of the *Philosophical Transactions* of the Royal Society, back in London after the disastrous year of the great plague, had touched briefly on age-old seawater treatment recommended for rabies (see above). The society had asked Robert Boyle (1627–1691) for answers to questions on a number of problems connected with seawater, among them, "What are the Medical Virtues of the sea, especially against *Hydrophobia?*" Despite his own later extensive writings on aspects of seawater, its saltiness at different depths, temperatures, and locations, even attempts to "sweeten" it — he never tried to answer this particular question.

However, elsewhere in his writings, where he considered "true and medical virtues" of other recommended therapies, Boyle was reluctant entirely to dismiss possible medicinal benefits of other time-honoured remedies. Some, valued for both prophylactic and possible curative properties since antiquity, were a variety of gemstones — "bezoars" or "madstones" — reputedly helpful against both plague and hydrophobia (Boyle, 1672). Boyle's contemporary, Nathaniel Hodges (1629–1688), a physician who remained in London bravely caring for his patients during the great plague of 1665 while others fled, was doubtful, considering the "Oriental Bezoar" overpriced and overrated (Holland, 2000). Sadly, after an impressive career and wide recognition, Hodges died in a debtors' prison. As far as the Royal Society was concerned, the belief in beneficial effects of "Bezoar-Stones" was laid to rest after Boyle's death by Frederick Slare (1647?–1727) in his *Experiments and Observations upon Oriental and Other BEZOAR-Stones,* with the telling subtitle, "which prove them to be of no Use in *Physic*" (against hydrophobia or anything else) (Slare, 1715). Elsewhere, notably in the United States, belief in curative powers of "madstones" continued among Native Americans and others until modern times (Baer *et al.*, 1996).

In the later seventeenth century there were signs of a growing realization that the *animalculae* observed by Antony van Leeuwenhoek (1632–1723) in his improved microscopes were indeed, as he claimed, "living creatures" and possibly could cause disease. Such ideas were reflected in the work of Francesco Redi (1626–1697), who in the late 1680s was the first to refute experimentally the long-held belief in spontaneous generation (Redi, 1688). His associates, Bonomo (d.1696) and Cestoni (1637–1718), then were able to implicate the mite *acarus* as the agent of scabies in humans. On the other hand, at this stage, the works of Leeuwenhoek and Redi had little impact on the literature on rabies. Terrifying as its manifestations were, rabies affected so few humans, or even their animals, when compared with the ravages of major scourges of the seventeenth and eighteenth centuries such as smallpox and bubonic plague in humans and cattle plague in their animals, that it could not be counted among the major problems of the age.

Curiously, one isolated example of an influence of the new ideas appeared in London in 1735 in the *London Magazine*, not a scientific publication. The anonymous author agreed with the general opinion that the rabid dog's saliva must be the seat of the disease but believed that the infection was caused by "minute particles or animalcules, mixt with saliva" that affected the brains of victims by incorporation into their "nervous juices." It was a bold statement for its time, which may perhaps account for its anonymity (Mullett, 1945).

Further advances in knowledge and understanding of the pathogenesis of rabies in humans and in animals progressed slowly, accelerating only in the nineteenth century in the wake of animal experiments and growing acceptance of the "germ theory." During the last decade of the nineteenth century, interest in research activities was increasing in medical and scientific societies everywhere. In England, the Literary and Philosophical Society of Manchester and the Society for the Improvement of Medical and Chirurgical Knowledge were founded in London in 1783 by John Hunter (1728–1793), surgeon and anatomist *par excellence*, and George Fordyce (1736–1802). In 1793, by happy coincidence, Samuel Argent Bardsley (1764–1851) in Manchester and Hunter's younger namesake and protégé, John Hunter, M.D. (1754–1809), each published papers that were to be seminal for work in the early nineteenth century. Bardsley had been appointed physician to the Manchester Infirmary in 1790; he remained there, as "the very model of a hospital physician" (*Dictionary of National Biography*, hence forth *DNB*, 1885), until he retired in 1823, continuing to contribute papers to the *Memoirs* of the Literary and Philosophical Society there. His 1793 observations on rabies and hydrophobia anticipated what was to follow in the next century by their clarity and confidence in disposing of age-old superstitions and replacing them with reason, facts, and common sense. He was convinced that neither rabies in dogs ("canine madness") nor hydrophobia in humans could occur spontaneously and ascribed apparent cases of the latter unconnected with animal bites to other diseases and "sometimes hysteria" (Bardsley, 1793).

John Hunter's paper had been published in 1793 in the *Transactions* of the London Society (Hunter, 1793). John Hunter, M.D., appeared as sole author, although his entry in the *DNB*, written by Charles Creighton (1847–1927), notes that it was "drawn up at the Society's request" — presumably other members of the society's total of 12 had been consulted. On the other hand, it *was* based largely on the younger John Hunter's own experiences in Jamaica, where he had been superintendent of military hospitals from 1781 to 1783, before settling down to practice in London. It also reflects Hunter's reputation, from the days of his Edinburgh thesis, for "correct reasoning" (*DNB*, 1819). His experiences in Jamaica had fired his interest in epidemiology and prevention of contagious diseases; he had written papers on outbreaks of typhus fever among poor London families before publishing, in 1788, *Observations on the Diseases of the Army in Jamaica* (Wilkinson, 1982). The latter contained important notes on remittent fever in the army but missed, as so many other observers did at the time, the role of mosquitoes in transmission, despite critical mention of the nuisance of their presence on the island.

Although in the paper on canine madness Hunter admitted having no direct proof that the disease could never occur spontaneously, his records from Jamaica at least provided circumstantial evidence: On that island full of dogs, in a hot climate, up to 40 years had elapsed with no occurrence of rabies. Before that, any outbreaks could be traced to dogs introduced from North America. On this basis, Hunter formed his conclusions, which contain suggestions pointing the way to the kind of animal experiments soon to become the mainstay of infectious disease research in the following century: experiments to be made "upon the poison," in this case of rabies, to determine its nature and path of transmission, including inoculating dogs and other species of animals with saliva from dogs suffering from canine rabies or even from "an hydrophobic patient." The inoculated animals were then to be observed, recording progress of the disease. Other suggestions included attempts to establish possible effects of "counter poisons" and of the length of time beyond which excision of the tissue around the inoculation site could not longer prevent development of the disease.

Nobody within the society, or elsewhere in the country, attempted to test the recommendations. Perhaps no suitable cases were available, or again, the death of their mentor, *the* John Hunter, in the same year may have removed their inspiration. The challenge was taken up 10 years later in Germany by Georg Gottfried Zinke (d. 1813), who carried out all the experiments suggested with one exception, the one involving saliva from a human patient. Zinke recorded his results in a volume published at Jena in 1804, the first description of experiments specifically intended to follow the path of transmission of the unknown agent of rabies. Zinke successfully produced rabies in healthy dogs, cats, rabbits, and fowl using a small brush to transfer saliva into incisions (Hunter had suggested the point of a lancet). With Hunter's suggestions and Zinke's experiments began the era of animal experiments and of the rapid development of comparative medicine and pathology (at the time referred to as "pathological physiology" or *pathologie expérimentale*") in France and Germany in the nineteenth century (Wilkinson, 1992).

The missing experiment with saliva from a human case was carried out barely 10 years later in the year of Zinke's death in France by François Magendie (1783–1855), who published his results in 1821 in a paper that with gallic abandon and almost relish described a series of dramatic and dramatically presented experiments in a Parisian establishment for fighting dogs carried out between 1810 and 1820 with the assistance of medical students chosen for their "courage and *sang-froid*": The experiments involved transmission of rabies to mastiffs via saliva from a human case (Magendie, 1821). Others warned of the moral implications of such experiments; in London, Benjamin Mosely had written as early as 1808: "I have no doubt but deadly inoculation [with rabid saliva] might be performed in a way, which I do not think prudence would justify the mentioning — there is mischief enough already in the world" (Moseley, 1808). By the 1820s, however, rabies was well established as the first zoonosis to become a focus for research in comparative medicine.

In Berlin in the later 1820s, K. H. Hertwig (1798–1881) attempted, but failed, to induce rabies in healthy dogs by implantation of nervous tissue from rabid dogs (Hertwig, 1828), although like others before him he had some success with rabid saliva. It is the background and career of Hertwig, as of Magendie earlier, that point the way to further developments during the nineteenth century. Magendie was a pioneer neurophysiologist, architect with Sir Charles Bell (1774–1842), neuroanatomist, of the Bell-Magendie law (ventral spinal roots carry motor fibers and dorsal roots carry sensory fibers), and his involvement in rabies research at this stage reflects a new awareness of the neurotropic character of the disease. Hertwig, on the other hand, having qualified in medicine at Breslau in 1819, had gone on to supplement his medical degree with veterinary studies in Vienna, Munich, and Berlin, preparing himself for the opportunities now opening up for studies in comparative medicine and pathology. For the rest of his working life, Hertwig combined medical practice and research with teaching at the Berlin veterinary school. In this capacity he came to be an outstanding representative of the kind of cooperation between medical and veterinary science that was to carry comparative medicine into the future. It was made possible by the fact that education in medical schools could now be supplemented by courses at veterinary schools and colleges opening throughout Europe in rapid succession to the original French ones at Lyons in 1761–1762 and at Alfort in 1766 (Wilkinson, 1992).

As outbreaks of rabies became more common in Britain and the rest of Europe during the nineteenth century, the voice of the new veterinary profession also began to be heard. In London, William Youatt (1776–1847) took a particular interest in the disease and gave a course of lectures on "canine madness" in the 1830s. Toward the end of his life he wrote a manual on dogs, published posthumously, in which he included a chapter on rabies. Here he quotes Bardsley, agreeing absolutely that rabies is transmissible and never occurs spontaneously. Consequently, he also followed Bardsley's views on prevention. He wrote, "...if a species of quarantine could be established, and every dog confined separately for eight months, the disease would be annihilated in our country or could only reappear in consequence of the importation of some infected animal" (Youatt, 1851). Perhaps curiously for a veterinarian but showing a healthy respect for reality, he even shared the views of Balzac père in his critical attitude to prevailing numbers of "useless and dangerous dogs" and in particular to the practice of keeping "fighting-dogs" for "most brutal purposes." He referred to the "rabid virus" but only to admit that little was known of it and that at present it would be a "difficult process to analyse it." He was, however, the first to make a suggestion for further experiments that would prove to be of definitive importance for rabies research and the development of vaccines in France later in the century. Youatt's final words on the subject were, "I very much regret that I never instituted a course of experiments on the production and treatment of rabies in [the rabbit]. It would have been attended with little expense or danger, and some important discoveries might have been made."

Three decades later, the rabbit began its rapid rise to a position as the animal of choice in experiments on rabies in France. As Youatt knew, the rabbit develops the predominantly paralytic form of rabies and so could serve as a less dangerous and more convenient object for experiments than the dog with the furious form of the disease. Thirty years after the death of Youatt, it fell to Pierre-Victor Galtier (1846–1908), professor at the Lyons Veterinary School, to reintroduce Youatt's rabbit to the general world of science and veterinary medicine in Paris in 1879 (Galtier, 1879). Galtier had been educated at the Lyons school and subsequently spent all his working life there. Carrying out experiments on rabies, he emphasized the advantage of using rabbits a whole year before Louis Pasteur (1822–1895) began work on the subject. By then he was aware of the work of Galtier and had visited Lyons, where Chauveau had introduced him to the full volume of Galtier's publications. In December 1880 he was ready to begin his own experiments (Guiart, 1922).

Whatever the final verdict on Galtier's influence on Pasteur may be, there can be no doubt about the seminal influence of his original experiments with rabbits on all the work that followed after 1880 (Fig. 6). Théodoridès has given an extensive and definitive analysis of Galtier's contributions in 1986, unfortunately too late for Steele in 1975 (and repeated in 1991) to correct his misapprehensions

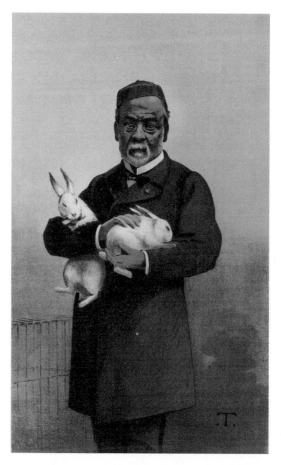

Fig. 6. Louis Pasteur holding two white laboratory rabbits. From *Vanity Fair*, 1887. (*Wellcome Library, London.*)

about the experiments of Galtier, whom he dismissed in a few lines, citing only his two pages of summary report delivered at the *Académie des Sciences* in 1879. On this basis, Steele remarked briefly that Galtier reported transmission of rabies to rabbits and from rabbit to rabbit "unfortunately without much needed detail." The details could have been found in the two original papers, published in separate veterinary journals, on which the report was based. There, in a total of 22 pages, Galtier provided all the information needed to evaluate his results, including his method of inoculating canine rabid saliva on the point of a lancet or directly by bite, introducing the ear of the live rabbit into the jaws of the rabid dog (Galtier, 1879).

Earlier in his chapter Steele had introduced "Bouchardat" (Apollinaire Bouchardat, 1806–1886) as being "among the first to think about inoculations against rabies and had an early influence on Pasteur. He attempted many experiments at the Lyon veterinary faculty." Since he had never worked at Lyons but was a pharmaceutical chemist attached to the Paris medical faculty and *Hotel-Dieu*, this is unlikely. In fact, the two papers by Bouchardat cited by Steele were written in response to a request for information during a serious outbreak of the disease — one of many in France in the nineteenth century — in the early 1850s. They contain evaluations of all the countless remedies against hydrophobia, mostly spurious, recommended over the centuries; Bouchardat made it clear that he had no reservations about the uselessness of any of them. Steele may have confused the texts and personalities of Galtier and Bouchardat (Bouchardat, 1852–1853, 1854–1855; Julien, 1977). The confusion is carried over, unchanged, into the updated chapter by Steele and Fernandez in the 1991 second edition of *The Natural History of Rabies*.

By the time Pasteur became aware of Galtier's contributions, he himself had already established the value and possibilities of prophylactic inoculation with attenuated material. It was a milestone not just in the history of rabies but in that of virus research in general and vaccine development in particular. Yet it was based on a chance observation, a case of serendipity to match Fleming's discovery of penicillin half a century later. But where Fleming did not quite have the courage of his convictions to take his discovery further at the time, Pasteur recognized the potential of his and immediately applied himself to its realization. Pasteur's fortuitous observation concerned a forgotten sealed flask of chicken cholera culture by mistake left undisturbed for a few weeks instead of the routine 24 hours. The observed attenuation of the agent responsible led, through the work of Toussaint (1847–1890) on defibrinated anthrax blood to the production of the first anthrax vaccine. The following year Pasteur addressed the International Medical Congress in London on vaccination, where he explained his use of the terms *vaccination* and *vaccine*, acknowledging Jenner's contribution (Pasteur, 1881).

Pasteur's development of the first rabies vaccine is, of course, the stuff of legend, all the more remarkable because the agent of the disease — the "virus" — was unknown at the time, unlike the bacillus of anthrax. However, this did not shake his determination to develop a vaccine, nor that of his colleagues, Émile Roux (1853–1933), who as the only man with a medical degree in the group was essential to Pasteur the chemist, Charles Chamberland (1851–1908), physiological chemist, Edmond Nocard (1850–1903), veterinarian, director of the Veterinary School at Alfort from 1889, and Louis Thuillier (1856–1883), who sadly died before he was 30, in pursuit of his duties, of cholera in the epidemic in Egypt that he had gone to investigate with Émile Roux and other members of the group. Pasteur pursued the work on rabies and decided that a vaccine against the disease should be the next major achievement in his laboratories.

In the case of rabies, Pasteur was faced with a disease agent about which, unlike the recently described anthrax bacillus, little, if anything, was known. Neither he nor anyone else had been able to see it in the microscope, let alone grow it in culture on artificial medium. Pasteur refused to give up; with characteristic ingenuity and determination, he bypassed established methods of culture and attenuation and turned to what he knew to be the natural habitat of the elusive "invisible virus": the spinal cords of his laboratory rabbits. Even then, he had first to confirm two necessary preconceptions: the neurotropic character of the virus, suspected certainly since the time of Magendie, and equally important and a concept totally his own, production of a "*virus fixe*." Working with Chamberland and Roux, he delivered the necessary proof of the neurotropic character of the virus; they also could show that the agent was present not only in the saliva of the rabid animal but also throughout its nervous system. The second important point was the production of a standardized form of the virus with a fixed incubation period. Initially, street virus was inoculated directly under the *dura mater* of dogs and then serially passed through rabbits until the length of the incubation period was shortened to a final limit of 6 to 7 days. Pasteur had achieved his goal: a fixed virus on which to base a vaccine (Fig. 7) (Pasteur *et al.*, 1884; Pasteur, 1885).

After much additional laborious work, the vaccine in its final form was tried out on dogs and rabbits with encouraging results announced at the *Académie des Sciences* in 1885. Even then, Pasteur himself dreaded the first trial on a human patient, as he wrote to the Emperor of Brazil: "…however much I multiply my cases of protection in dogs I think my hand will tremble when I go on to mankind" (Vallery-Radot, 1900). This pained remark may to some extent also reflect Pasteur's experiences in May–June 1885, never published and only known now, more than 100 years later, when G. L. Geison was able to examine Pasteur's private laboratory notebooks and his correspondence with Dujardin-Beaumetz. The episode concerned two patients admitted to hospital as suspected rabies cases. The hospitals appealed to Pasteur as a last resort. One M. Girard was treated in May 1885 with "attenuated rabies virus." It was a curious case of on-and-off apparent recovery followed by repeated relapses, but after 3 weeks Girard was discharged, supposedly cured, from the Necker Hospital. His later fate is not known.

Within a month, 11-year-old Julie-Antoinette Poughon was admitted to the St. Denis Hospital. Bitten on the upper lip by her puppy sometime in May and admitted on June 22, 1885, after 2 days of "severe headache," a diagnosis of rabies was confirmed. The girl was given one injection of an attenuated preparation immediately and a second at midnight, sadly to no avail. She died at 10:30 the following morning (Geison, 1995). A month later, Pasteur's hand was finally forced in the glare of publicity. A 9-year-old boy, Joesph Meister, was brought from Alsace with severe wounds from the bites of a mad dog, almost certainly fatal. Pasteur agonized, discussed ethical aspects of the case with trusted medical advisers, and finally decided that the only hope of saving the boy was a course of

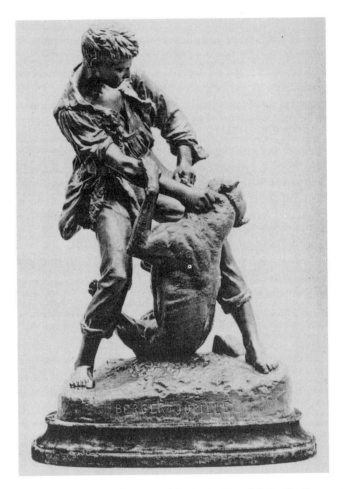

Fig. 7.   Statue in Paris celebrating the case of the shepherd boy J.-B. Jupille, the second survivor
of rabies bites following treatment with Pasteur's vaccine in 1885. (*Wellcome Library, London.*)

postexposure prophylaxis. It was successful; the boy, despite his injuries, failed
to develop rabies, and the vaccine was established. There were to be setbacks as
well as many lives saved, but the principle of postexposure prophylaxis in rabies
had been established (see Fig. 7), ready for the improvements and developments
of the twentieth century (Paget, 1914).

The question of the nature of rabies virus was still, during the lifetime of
Pasteur, left wide open. At the turn of the century, work on tobacco mosaic virus
and foot-and-mouth disease opened the floodgates to a new era where "invisible,"
"filterable" viruses, including the virus of rabies, eventually would come into

their own and play their role in molecular biology (Waterson and Wilkinson, 1978). Before that, the importance of Pasteur's work already was beginning to be reflected in developments at home and abroad. The Pasteur Institute (Fig. 8), funded by public subscriptions in Paris between 1886 and 1888, primarily to develop rabies vaccine, soon widened its horizons and was followed by a number of sister institutes with similar aims of vaccine production and research abroad [at Saigon (Cochin China) 1890, Tunis 1894, Indo-China 1895, and Algiers 1910] and at home (Lille 1895 and Nancy 1898) (Dedonder, 1985). In London, the British Institute of Preventive Medicine was incorporated in 1891, modeled on the Pasteur Institute with its commitments to both research and vaccine production.

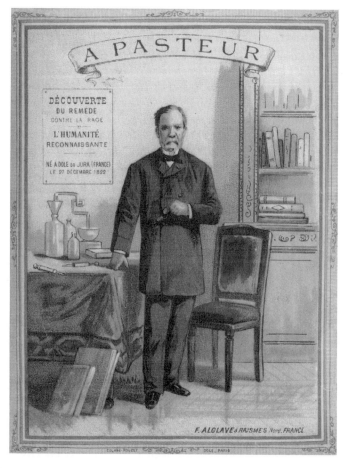

Fig. 8. Chromolithograph celebrating Pasteur's work and discoveries. Paris, *circa* 1890. (*Wellcome Library, London.*)

Initially, rabies was not mentioned specifically among its aims, although Victor Horsley (1857–1916), among the experts consulted and an adherent of Pasteur's methods, must have been in favor of rabies vaccine production at home to avoid unnecessary and possibly fatal delays when patients were sent to Paris. He did, in fact, lose a laboratory assistant, bitten by a rabid cat, who died in spite of prophylactic treatment by Pasteur, having arrived in Paris too late (Bristowe and Horsley, 1889). In the event, rabies vaccine production at the institute in London did not begin until after the disease had been eradicated for the first time in 1902 (Wilkinson, 1992).

The early years of the twentieth century, before the outbreak of the Great War in 1914, were dominated by attempts in many laboratories to clarify the concepts of invisibility and filterability in the new type of infectious "microbes." In 1903, Paul Remlinger (1871–1964) was able to demonstrate, not without difficulty, the filterability of rabies virus, but like most of his colleagues in and out of the Pasteur Institutes at home and abroad, he was to remain reluctant to accept M. W. Beijerinck's theory of the *contagium vivium fluidum* (Remlinger, 1903). In the same year, Negri in Pavia contributed to the general confusion in early virus research when he described the eosinophilic inclusion bodies and identified them as protozoa causing the disease; he eventually named the putative organism *Neurocytes hydrophobiae*. On the other hand, over the years, Negri bodies, like Koch's tuberculin, have come into their own as an important diagnostic tool (Negri, 1903, 1909; Kristensson *et al.*, 1996). Real progress in factual knowledge of morphology of the filterable viruses began with the introduction of the ultracentrifuge by The Svedberg and R. Fåhraeus in 1926, of electron microscopes in the 1930s, and with W. J. Elford's work on ultrafiltration beginning in 1928 (Waterson and Wilkinson, 1978). Helped by such techniques, perfected over the years, virologists had, by the 1960s and 1970s, for the first time a clear picture of the morphology, chemical composition, antigenic properties, and possibilities for cultivation. The virus of rabies finally could be defined as an RNA core contained in an envelope necessary for its infectivity with average overall dimensions of 180×75 mm and typically bullet-shaped (Topley and Wilson, 1984). Here the historian must come to a halt and leave the present and future to the authors of the following chapters, who are at the cutting edges of today's research. Except perhaps for a few concluding reflections on the continuing saga of outbreaks of rabies still occurring not only in endemic and underreported areas in Asia, the Middle East, Africa, and South America but also in countries in the Western world with access to the latest vaccines, such as the bioengineered V-RG (vaccinia-recombinant glycoprotein vaccine), developed by teams at the Wistar Institute in Philadelphia and the National Institutes of Health, cooperating with a French biotechnology firm. In 1984 this glycoprotein was found to be effective as an oral vaccine after outbreaks in racoons in the "Wistar's backyard" that began in 1982 (Findley, 1998).

REFERENCES

Aristotle, "Historia Animalium," Vol. IV, Book VIII, p. 604a.

Baer, G. M., Neville, J., and Turner, G. S. (1996). *Rabbis and Rabies: A Pictorial History of Rabies Through the Ages*. Laboratorios Baer, Mexico.

Balzac, B.-F. (1810). "*Histoire de la rage et moyen d'en preserver, comme autrefois, les hommes et de les délivrer de plusierus autres malheurs attaquant leur existence*," Tours.

Bardsley, S. A. (1793). Miscellaneous observations on canine and spontaneous hydrophobia. *Mem. Lit. Phil. Soc. Manch.* **4**, 431–488.

Blaisdell, J. D. (1992). Rabies and the Governor-General of Canada. *Vet. Hist., n.s.* **7**, 19–26.

Boyle, R. (1672). *An Essay about the Origine and Virtues of GEMS*, William Godbid, London.

Bristowe, J. S., and Horsley, V. (1889). A case of paralytic rabies in man, with remarks. *Trans. Clin. Soc. Lond.* **22**, 38–47.

Bouchardat, A. (1852–1853 and 1854–1855). Rapport…sur divers remèdes proposés pour prévenir ou combattre la rage. *Bull. Acad. Nat. Med.* **18**, 6–30; **20**, 714–727.

Celsus, with an English translation by W. G. Spencer (1938). *De Medicina*. Heineman, London.

Caelius Aurelianus (Soranus of Ephesus), edited and translated by I. E. Drabkin (1950). *On Acute Diseases and on Chronic Diseases*. University of Chicago Press, Chicago.

Dedonder, R. (1985). Worldwide impact of Pasteur's discoveries and the overseas Pasteur Institutes. In *World's Debt to Pasteur* (Wistar Symposium Series), Vol. 3, pp. 131–140. A. R. Liss, New York.

Edward, Duke of York (1904). In *The Master of Game*, W. A. & F. Baillie-Grohman (eds.), Chap. XIII, pp. 47–49. Ballantyne, Hanson & Co., London.

Findley, D. (1998). *Mad Dogs: The New Rabies Plague*. Texas A&M University Press, College Station, TX.

Fleming, G. (1872). *Rabies and Hydrophobia*. Chapman and Hall, London.

Fracastoro, H., translation and notes by Wilmer Cave Wright (1930). *De Contagione et Contagiosis Morbis et Eorum Curatione*, Book II, Chap. X, "*Rabies*," **1546**, pp. 124–133.

Galtier, V. (1879). *Études sur la rage*. *Rec. Med. Vet.* **6**, 857–867; *Ann. Med. Vet.* **28**, 627–639.

Geison, G. L. (1995). *The Private Science of Louis Pasteur*. Princeton University Press, Princeton, NJ.

Guiart, J. (1992). Homage à Pasteur. *Paris Med.* **46**, 426–441.

Hertwig, K. H. (1828). Beiträge zur nähern Kenntnis der Wuthkrankheit oder Tollheit der Hunde. *Hufeland's Journal der Practischen Arzneykunde und Wundarzneykunst* **67**, 3–173.

Holland, B. K. (2000). Treatments for bubonic plague: Reports from seventeenth century British epidemics. *J. R. Soc. Med.* **93**, 322–324.

Hunter, J. (1793). Observations, and heads of inquiry, on canine madness, drawn from the cases and materials collected by the society, respecting that disease. *Trans. Soc. Improv. Med. Chir. Knowl.* **1**, 294–329.

Jackson, A. C. (1994). The fatal neurologic illness of the Fourth Duke of Richmond in Canada: Rabies. *Ann. R. Coll. Phys. Surg. Can.* **27**, 40–41.

Julien, P. (1977). Apollinaire Bouchardat. *Rev. Hist. Pharm.* **24**, 300.

Kristensson, K., Dasturt, D. K., Manghanit, D. K., and Tsiang, H. (1996). Rabies: Interactions between neurons and viruses. A review of the history of Negri inclusion bodies. *Neuropathol. Appl. Neurobiol.* **22**, 179–187.

Magendie, F. (1821). Expérience sur la rage. *J. Physiol. Exp.* **1**, 40–46.

Marochetti, M. (1849). Observations sur l'hydrophobie. In *Opuscoli Medici*. Milano.

Moseley, B. (1808). *On Hydrophobia, Its Prevention and Cure, with a Dissertation on Canine Madness.* Longman, London.

Mullett, C. F. (1945). Hydrophobia: Its history in England to 1800. *Bull. Hist. Med.* **18**, 44–65.

Negri, A. (1903). *Zur Aetiologie der Tollwuth: Die Diagnose der Tollwuth auf Grund der neueren Befunde. Z. Hyg. Infektkrankh.* **44**, 519–540.

Negri, A. (1909). *Über die Morphologie und der Entwicklungszyklus des Parasiten der Tollwuth (Neurocytes hydrophobiae Calkins). Z. Hyg. Infektkrankh.* **63**, 421–440.

Paget, S. (1914). *Pasteur and After Pasteur.* Adam and Charles Black, London.

Pasteur, L. (1881). Vaccination in relation to chicken cholera and splenic fever. *Lancet* **ii**, 271–272.

Pasteur, L., Chamberland, C., and Roux, E. (1884). *Sur la rage. Bull. Acad. Med.* **13**, 661–664.

Pasteur, L. (1885). *Méthode pour prévenir la rage après morsure. C. r. hebd. Séanc. Acad. Sci. Paris* **101**, 765–774.

Redi, F. (1688). Esperienze intorno alla generatione *degl'insetti.* Firenze.

Remlinger, P. (1903). *Le passage du virus rabique à travers les filtres. Ann. Inst. Pasteur Paris* **17**, 834–849.

Slare, F. (1715). *Experiments and Observations upon Oriental and Other BEZOAR-Stones, which Prove Them to Be of No Use in Physick.* Tim.Goodwin, London.

Steele, J. H. (1975). History of rabies. In *The Natural History of Rabies*, G. M. Baer (ed.), Vol. 1, pp. 1–32. Academic Press, New York.

Steele, J. H., and Fernandez, P. J. (1991). History of rabies and its global aspects. In *The Natural History of Rabies*, G. M. Baer (ed.), 2nd ed., Vol. 1, pp. 1–24. CRC Press, Boca Raton, FL.

Théodoridès, J. (1986). *Histoire de la Rage.* Masson, Paris.

Topley and Wilson (1984). *Principles of Bacteriology, Virology and Immunity*, Vol. 4, pp. 472–486.

Vallery-Radot, R. (1900). *La vie de Pasteur.* Librairie Hachette, Paris.

Waterson, A., and Wilkinson, L. (1978). *An Introduction to the History of Virology.* Cambridge University Press, Cambridge, England.

Wilkinson, L. (1982). The other John Hunter, MD, FRS (1754–1809): His contributions to the medical literature, and to the introduction of animal experiments into infectious disease research. *Notes and Records R. Soc. Lond.* **36**, 227–241.

Wilkinson, L. (1992). *Animals and Disease.* Cambridge University Press, Cambridge, England.

Youatt, W. (1851). *The Dog.* Longman, London.

Zinke, G. G. (1804). *Neue Ansichten der Hundswuth, ihrer Ursachen und Folgen, nebst einer sichern Behandlungsart der von tollen Tieren gebissenen Menschen.* C. E. Gabler, Jena.

2

Rabies Virus

WILLIAM H. WUNNER

The Wistar Institute
Philadelphia, Pennsylvania 19104-4268

I. INTRODUCTION

Rabies virus is the prototype species of the genus *Lyssavirus* (from the Greek *lyssa*, meaning "rage") in the family *Rhabdoviridae* (from the Greek *rhabdos*, meaning "rod"). It is in many ways considered a close relative of the prototype species vesicular stomatitis virus (VSV) of the genus *Vesiculovirus*, in the same family, since it shares a similar morphology, chemical structure, and life cycle,

23

and it can infect mammalian (animal and human) hosts. However, because the rabies virus is highly neurotropic in the infected host, invariably causing a fatal encephalomyelitis, rabies virus and the rabies-related viruses belong to a separate genus (Murphy *et al.*, 1995). The family *Rhabdoviridae* together with the families *Paramyxoviridae, Filoviridae*, and *Bornaviridae* constitute the "superfamily" taxon, order *Mononegavirales*, because all members of the order are RNA viruses that contain nonsegmented, negative-sense, single-strand RNA genomes (Mayo and Pringle, 1997). The genus *Lyssavirus* presently contains seven virus genotypes (Bourhy *et al.*, 1992, 1993a,b; Kissi *et al.*, 1995; Gould *et al.*, 1998). One of these defines rabies virus (RABV) (genotype 1, serotype 1), whereas the other six represent specific rabies-related lyssaviruses, reflecting the genetic diversity of viruses that share with rabies virus, the primary etiologic agent of rabies, the unique capability to produce a rabies-like encephalomyelitis. The rabies-related lyssaviruses include Lagos bat virus (LBV, genotype 2, serotype 2), Mokola virus (MOKV, genotype 3, serotype 3), Duvenhage virus (DUVV, genotype 4, serotype 4), European bat lyssavirus type 1 (EBL-1, genotype 5), European bat lyssavirus type 2 (EBL-2, genotype 6), and Australian bat lyssavirus (ABLV, genotype 7). Three other viruses included in the genus *Lyssavirus*, Kotonkon (KOTV), Obodhiang (OBOV), and Rochambeau (RBUV), which have a serologic (antigenic) relationship distant from all other genus members and have not been involved in rabies-like infections of mammals, will not be considered further in this chapter. All lyssaviruses share many biologic and physico chemical features as well as amino acid sequence characteristics that classify them with other rhabdoviruses. These include the bullet-shaped morphology, helical nucleocapsid (NC) or ribonucleoprotein (RNP) core, RNA genome structure and organization, and structural proteins of the virus. The five structural proteins of the virion include a nucleocapsid protein (N), phosphoprotein (P, M1 or NS), matrix protein (M or M2), glycoprotein (G), and RNA-dependent RNA polymerase or large protein (L). Lyssaviruses, like other rhabdoviruses, use similar mechanisms to penetrate susceptible cells, express and replicate their genome RNA, and release mature virus particles from the plasma membrane of infected cells. The structural proteins of lyssaviruses can differ significantly between serotypes and genotypes by their antigenic properties, and some of the proteins have different posttranslational modifications and properties that distinguish them from the proteins of other rhabdoviruses. Nevertheless, they share many of the biologic functions that the same viral proteins have in other rhabdoviruses. In this chapter the focus is on the rabies virus structure, its molecular composition and morphology, genome organization, and genetic relationship to the structural proteins of the virus. This chapter also reviews the current knowledge of the virus's life cycle (attachment, penetration, replication, assembly, and egress) in susceptible host cells, along with mechanisms of virus spread, defective viruses, and the molecular biology of the rabies virus proteins in relation to their structure and function.

II. RABIES VIRUS STRUCTURE

A. Molecular Composition and Chemical Architecture

Lyssaviruses, like other rhabdoviruses, consist mainly of RNA (2–3%), protein (67–74%), lipid (20–26%), and carbohydrate (3%) as integral components of their structure (reviewed in Wunner, 1991). At the center of the bullet-shaped virus particle is a core of helical RNA (the viral genome) and protein, the RNP core, that extends along its longitudinal axis and is surrounded by a lipid-protein envelope. The RNA is single-stranded, nonsegmented, and has negative-sense or minus-strand polarity (Sokol *et al.*, 1969). This implies that isolated (naked) minus-strand genome RNA is not infectious. In the cell, the viral RNA must be transcribed (copied) first to produce complementary mRNA transcripts of the individual genes, and the mRNAs must be translated into viral proteins before the virus RNA is replicated and the virus infection can spread from cell to cell. The complete sequence and total length of three lyssavirus RNA genomes have been reported to date. Two of these are rabies virus genomes of the Pasteur virus (PV) strain (Tordo *et al.*, 1986b, 1988) and Street Alabama Dufferin (SAD)–B19 strain (Conzelmann *et al.*, 1990), which contain 11,932 and 11,928 nucleotides, respectively. The third is the rabies-related Mokola virus genome (Bourhy *et al.*, 1989, 1993a; Le Mercier *et al.*, 1997) originally isolated from shrews in Nigeria (Shope *et al.*, 1970; Kemp *et al.*, 1972). Its 11,939 nucleotides are less well conserved than the PV and SAD-B19 rabies virus genomes in many regions throughout the genome, particularly in the noncoding regions and in the coding sequences of the P and G proteins (Le Mercier *et al.*, 1997). Possibly the next complete genome sequence to be determined will be that of the Australian bat lyssavirus. The 3' half of this viral genome, which includes the first four genes of the genome and their respective open reading frames (ORFs), has been determined (Gould *et al.*, 1998). Comparisons of the deduced amino acid sequences for the four ORFs (N, P, M, and G) encoded in the 3' half of the Australian bat lyssavirus genome showed that the virus is more closely related to the genotype 1 rabies virus than to the other rabies-related virus genotypes. We learn from the sequences of all four viral genomes that even for the most divergent rabies-related lyssavirus (MOKV), the general organization of the genome is the same and that only slight differences are observed in the length of the genome and in the intergenic sequences between rabies and the rabies-related viruses. For example, the 3' half of the Mokola virus genome, which includes the first four nonoverlapping ORFs that code for the structural viral proteins (N, P, M, and G), is slightly longer than the PV and SAD-B19 genomes by 25 and 29 nucleotides, respectively (Bourhy *et al.*, 1993a). Both the second ORF (P gene) and the fourth ORF (G gene) of the Mokola virus genome encode proteins that are six amino acids longer and three amino acids shorter, respectively, than the corresponding ORFs in the rabies virus genome.

On examination of the 3′ half of the Ballina isolate of the Australian bat lyssavirus, the first four ORFs correspond in length precisely with the corresponding ORFs of the rabies virus genome (Gould *et al.*, 1998). This does not take into account, however, the genetic diversity that occurs within the ORFs between the different genotypes.

The five unique proteins of rabies virus comprise the bulk of the virion by weight. Initially, estimates of protein size, stoichiometric proportions, and spatial relationships in purified rabies virions were based on chemical dissociation of virions and determination of relative concentrations of the viral proteins resolved by sodium dodecyl sulfate–polyacrylamide gel electrophoresis (SDS-PAGE) (Sokol *et al.*, 1971; Madore and England, 1977; Delagneau *et al.*, 1981). Now the protein molecular weights are determined from the nucleotide sequences that encode the viral proteins. From the nucleotide sequences, the amino acid composition of the viral proteins is deduced (Anilionis *et al.*, 1981; Rayssiguier *et al.*, 1986; Tordo *et al.*, 1986a,b, 1988). Three of the viral proteins are located in the RNP core. They are the N, the noncatalytic polymerase-associated P, and the catalytic L (RNA polymerase). All three proteins are involved in the RNA polymerase activity of the virion. Both the N and P are phosphorylated in rabies virus, unlike in other rhabdoviruses, including VSV, in which only the P is phosphorylated (Sokol and Clark, 1973; Dietzschold *et al.*, 1979, 1987a; Bourhy *et al.*, 1993a). The P in rabies virus is phosphorylated by a unique cellular protein kinase and specific isomers of protein kinase C (Gupta *et al.*, 2000). The number of molecules of each protein per virion has been estimated in different laboratories with somewhat variable results (reviewed in Tordo and Poch, 1988). One laboratory has reported 1325 molecules of N, 691 molecules of P, and 72 molecules of L in the RNP complex of the rabies virion (Flamand *et al.*, 1993). This is slightly different from the 1800 molecules of N, 950 molecules of P, and 25 molecules of L reported from another laboratory (Madore and England, 1977). It can be argued reasonably that these differences in estimates of protein molecules per virion simply may be a reflection of variables associated with the way the studies were conducted in the different laboratories. Nevertheless, one stoichiometric relationship that emerges from these estimates with respect to the RNP composition that appears to be valid is the 2:1 ratio of the N and P molecules per virion. During nascent protein synthesis and replication of viral progeny RNA, these two proteins interact in the same 2:1 ratio to bind to the newly synthesized progeny RNA (see below for further discussion). Also, the L is typically the protein produced in least amount. The remaining two structural proteins of the rabies virion, the G and M, are associated with the lipid-bilayer envelope that surrounds the RNP core. The M lines the viral envelope, forming an inner leaflet between the envelope and RNP core, whereas the G produces the spikelike projections or peplomers on the surface of the viral envelope (Gaudin *et al.*, 1992). The number of G and M molecules per virion is estimated to be 1205 and 1148 (Flamand *et al.*, 1993), respectively, or 1800 and 1547 (Madore and England, 1977), respectively. Rabies virions also have been found to contain such cellular proteins as actin and heat shock proteins of the hsp70 type, similar to other negative-strand RNA viruses (Naito and Matsumoto, 1978; Sagara and Kawai, 1992; Sagara *et al.*, 1995). Although the explanation for cellular proteins in mature virions is not entirely clear, it is possible that the molecular chaperones, such as the heat shock protein calnexin, that associate with the viral proteins during synthesis are incorporated into virions after binding to and assisting in G folding (Gaudin, 1997). Also, a small fraction of calnexin and possibly other chaperone proteins may escape from the endoplasmic reticulum (ER), where they function to ensure proper protein folding before being expressed on the cell surface where virus budding occurs (Okazaki *et al.*, 2000). In a similar manner, cytoskeleton proteins normally expressed on the cell surface may be incorporated into virions as a consequence of their proximal location and function in virus budding (Sagara *et al.*, 1995, 1998). Other cytoskeletal proteins may ensure intracellular transport of viral RNP (Raux *et al.*, 2000; Jacob *et al.*, 2000). Cellular kinases that activate the transcriptional function of P in rabies virus also may be packaged into rabies virions (Gupta *et al.*, 2000).

   The viral G molecule is glycosylated with branched-chain oligosaccharides, which account for 10–12% of the total mass of the protein (Reading *et al.*, 1978) and the 3% carbohydrate mass of the virion (reviewed in Wunner, 1991). The oligosaccharides are linked to asparagine (N, in single-letter code) residues in the tripeptide sequon asparagine-X-serine or threonine, where X is any amino acid other than proline. Rabies virus G molecules may contain one, two, or three (and sometimes four) N-linked oligosaccharides or N-glycans per molecule depending on the virus strain. G molecules in some virus strains are variously glycosylated, which introduces a detectable microheterogeneity in the population of G molecules per virion (Dietzschold *et al.*, 1983a; Wunner *et al.*, 1985; Shakin-Eshleman *et al.*, 1992; Shakin-Eshleman *et al.*, 1993; Coll, 1995; Kasturi *et al.*, 1995). The structure of each N-linked oligosaccharide on the rabies virus G has not been determined by direct carbohydrate analysis to establish whether every branch chain is identical, although each N-glycan is presumed to be of the "complex type" (Burger *et al.*, 1991; Shakin-Eshleman *et al.*, 1992). The sugar residues of the N-glycan are presynthesized in the cell and transferred as a unit ($Glc_3Man_9GlcNAc_2$), known as the *precursor core oligosaccharide*, to the asparagine residue of the asparagine-X-serine or threonine sequons of the nascent G molecule. Typically, the transfer occurs as the protein is synthesized on the membrane-bound ribosomes and during translocation to the cytoplasmic ER membrane. After the precursor core oligosaccharide is transferred, the high-mannose triglucoslylated oligosaccharide is trimmed and processed in the lumen of the rough ER and Golgi stacks to form the "complex type" N-linked monoglucosylated oligosaccharide of the mature G molecule (Kornfeld and Kornfeld, 1985; Kaplan *et al.*, 1987). The molecular chaperone calnexin recognizes the partially trimmed monoglucosylated glycan and binds to it, assisting the G to fold correctly and completely in order to achieve its biologic activity, stability, and antigenicity (Shakin-Eshleman *et al.*, 1992; Hebert *et al.*, 1995; Gaudin, 1997). This dependence of the rabies virus G on molecular interaction with calnexin explains why it is critical that at least one of the asparagine residues (i.e., N319) in the rabies virus G is conserved in all virus genotypes. It appears that N319 is essential for correct and complete folding of the nascent rabies virus G and subsequent transport to the cell surface (Shakin-Eshleman *et al.*, 1992).

Lipids constitute 50% of the lipoprotein bilayer that forms the viral envelope (or membrane matrix) surrounding the helical NC or RNP core. The major protein constituent of the lipoprotein envelope is the externally oriented rabies virus G, which is anchored in the membrane by the 22-amino-acid hydrophobic transmembrane domain that spans the viral envelope. The lipids of the viral envelope are derived entirely from the host cell, and depending on where the virus buds through the cellular membrane, concentrations of certain lipids may be higher in the viral envelope than in the plasma membrane (Schlesinger *et al.*, 1973; Patzer *et al.*, 1978). In general, the rabies virus membrane contains a mixture of lipids that include phospholipids (mainly sphingomyelin, phosphatidylethanolamine, and phosphatidylcholine, 42%), neutral lipids (mainly triglycerides and cholesterol, 58%), and glycolipids (Schlesinger *et al.*, 1973; Schneider and Diringer, 1976; Blough *et al.*, 1977). The rabies virus G is also modified by the addition of palmitic acid (referred to as *fatty acid acylation* or *palmitoylation*) at Cys-461, located in the intracytoplasmic domain on the C-terminal side of its transmembrane region (Gaudin *et al.*, 1991a). Although the functional significance of palmitoylation is not entirely clear, it is presumed to have a stabilizing effect on the trimeric G spike anchored in the membrane. Palmitoylation also may play a role in the virus budding process by facilitating the interaction between the cytoplasmic "tail" of the G and the M in the RNP-M complex at the cell membrane.

B. Morphology and Architectural Features of Rabies Virus Particles

Illustrations of the rabies virus particle (or virion) typically depict the bullet-shaped or bacilliform morphology that is the structural hallmark of all rhabdoviruses (Fig. 1). The physical appearance of this rigid, rodlike, often cone-shaped or bullet-shaped structure of the rabies virion, with one end flattened (planar) and the other rounded (hemispherical), was first described in the early 1960s with the aid of the electron microscope (EM) (Matsumoto, 1962, 1963; Davies *et al.*, 1963). Subsequently, EM studies have shown rabies virions attached to cells, gaining entry into cells, and budding from cellular membranes (Hummeler *et al.*, 1967; Murphy *et al.*, 1973b, 1980; Iwasaki *et al.*, 1973, 1975; Iwasaki and Clark, 1975; Matsumoto, 1975). Schematic illustrations of the rabies virus that depict

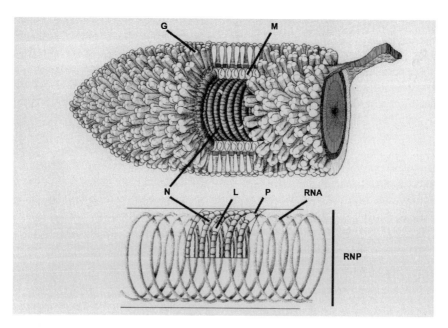

Fig. 1. Schematic representation of the rabies virion showing the internal ribonucleoprotein (RNP) core consisting of the single-strand, negative-sense genome RNA encapsidated with nucleocapsid protein (N), the virion-associated RNA polymerase (L), and polymerase cofactor phosphoprotein (P). The RNP core in association with the matrix protein (M) is condensed into the typical bullet-shaped particle that is characteristic of rhabdoviruses. The RNP–M structure is surrounded by a lipid-bilayer envelope (or membrane) in which the surface trimeric glycoprotein (G) spikes are anchored. The membrane tail depicted in the drawing represents the trailing piece of envelope that is frequently observed in the electron microscope attached to the virus as it buds from the plasma membrane of the infected cell. (*Reproduced from Wunner, W. H., Larson, J. K., Dietzschold, B., and Smith, C. L., Fig. 1 in Rev. Infect. Dis. 10, Suppl. 4, S771–S784, 1988, with permission from The University of Chicago Press.*)

this unique rhabdovirus structure in both surface views and cross sections are based on these morphologic perceptions (Ackerman and Berthianume, 1995). They typically show the helical RNP core, seen as cross-striations in the EM, and a double membrane layer with an outer-surface fringe of finger-like projections (Murphy and Harrison, 1979). The G surface projections appear to cover all but the flat end of the particle. The molecular architecture of the virion, from the outer membrane to the inner core, has been further defined with the help of biochemical studies of virus particles grown and purified from cell culture (Wiktor *et al.*, 1973; Sokol, 1975; Schneider and Diringer, 1976).

The Negri body is perhaps the best structural characterization of rabies virus infection. It is sometimes more prominent than the morphologic appearance of virions in the infected cell. The Negri body, seen as an accumulation of intracellular inclusions or "matrix" formations, represents the unique gross pathologic change in rabies virus-infected neuronal cells *in vivo* (Miyomoto and Matsumoto, 1965; Hummeler *et al.*, 1968; reviewed in Wunner, 1987, see Chap. 8). These intracellular matrices are regarded as a significant diagnostic marker of rabies virus infection because they usually do not occur in other diseases (Hummeler *et al.*, 1968; see Chap. 9). They are seen as filamentous structures formed by the accumulation of an excess amount of RNA–protein complex, a product of viral replication in the cell (Hummeler *et al.*, 1967; Schneider *et al.*, 1973).

The average length of standard size infectious virions is 180 nm (130–250 nm), and the average diameter is 75 nm (60–110 nm) (Davies *et al.*, 1963; Hummeler *et al.*, 1967; Sokol, 1975). Standard size (B) virions are typically rigid, bullet-shaped particles. The term *B virions*, which refers to the bullet-shaped morphology, also can refer to the sedimentation position ("bottom" band) that standard virions occupy in a sucrose density gradient after gradient centrifugation (Fig. 2). Other shorter, often cone-shaped virions coproduced with B virions are physically distinguishable from B virions both in the EM and by certain structural features. They are noninfectious, incomplete (substandard size) "defective" virions that, by definition, contain RNA genomes that typically are shorter than the standard-sized genomes as a result of internal deletions (Holland, 1987). Because defective virions most often are shorter and therefore lighter than the B virions due to their defective genomes, they can be separated physically from B virions by velocity centrifugation in a sucrose density gradient. The substandard size defective virions sediment more slowly than the B virions in a density gradient, and consequently, defective virions can be isolated in the uppermost virion band(s) after centrifugation in a sucrose density gradient. These defective virions are referred to as *T virions* (for "truncated" or "top" band). They

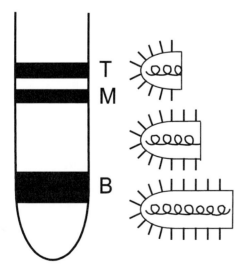

Fig. 2. Schematic drawing of infectious and defective interfering (DI) rabies virus particles propagated in cell culture and separated by velocity sedimentation in a sucrose density gradient. The shorter, cone-shaped DI virus particles in the top (*T*) band sediment more slowly than the thimble-like DI virus particles in the middle (*M*) band due to their relative size. The standard infectious bullet-shaped virus particles in the bottom (*B*) band sediment fastest due to their full-length size. (*Adapted from Clark, H. F., Parks, N. F., and Wunner, W. H., J. Gen. Virol.* **52,** *245–258, 1981, with permission.*)

appear cone-shaped because the cylindrical region between the rounded end and flat end is reduced (truncated) to a minimal length. The cone-shaped T virions have genomes approximately one-third to one-half the size of the full-length genome of standard size B virions. Other defective virions can have slightly longer cylindrical regions ("thimble shape") that correspond to a partially deleted genome one-half to two-thirds the size of the standard B virion genome. These slightly longer particles tend to sediment to a banding position in a sucrose density gradient that lies between the T and B particle bands due to their slightly faster sedimentation velocity. These are referred to as the *M* (or "middle" band) *particles* when both T and B particles are also present in a mixed population of virion sizes. All truncated RNA genomes form RNP complexes that determine the length and characteristic symmetry of defective virions.

Defective virions of rabies viruses, like other rhabdoviruses and other RNA viruses, have been important particles to examine from both structural and biologic points of view because of their defective genomes. They contain all the virus structural proteins, and they replicate at the expense of standard "helper" virus, which is essential for their replication. Thus the defective virus can become the dominant particle in the infected cell by interfering with production of standard infectious virus. Consequently, defective particles are known as *defective-interfering* (DI) *virions* (Huang, 1973; Wiktor *et al.*, 1977; Clark *et al.*, 1981; Holland, 1987). DI virions of rabies virus are generated easily and produced readily for study in standard cell cultures infected with laboratory-adapted (fixed) strains of rabies virus (Wunner and Clark, 1980; Clark *et al.*, 1981). They have not been described in rabies virus infections *in vivo*, however, although their role in controlling production of infectious B virions *in vivo* has been implicated (see Holland, 1987).

The RNP that becomes the tightly coiled core of all virions is produced from a flexible right-handed helix structure that has a periodicity of approximately 7.5 nm per turn. The RNP core in standard size infectious virions measures approximately 165×50 nm (Murphy, 1975; Murphy and Harrison, 1979) but measures between 4.2 and 4.6 mm in length when relaxed and fully extended, like a thread, outside the virion (Murphy and Harrison, 1979; Sokol *et al.*, 1969). During virus assembly, the RNP core is surrounded by M, one of the two membrane proteins of the virus, to form the "skeleton" structure of the virus (Mebatsion *et al.*, 1999). As virus particles mature and bud through the cellular membrane, the skeleton structure acquires the lipid bilayer envelope that is 7.5 to 10 nm thick surrounding the mature virion. Located on the external surface of the viral envelope are the surface projections that measure 8.3–10 nm in length, each projection or spike containing three molecules (a trimer) of the viral G (Gaudin *et al.*, 1992) (see Fig. 1). These have been described when viewed in the EM as the "short spikes extending outward with the appearance of hollow knobs at their distal ends" (Murphy and Harrison, 1979). It is estimated that the height of the "hollow knobs" or "heads" of the spike is about 4.8 nm; the rest of the spike is made up of the thin "stalk" on which the head rests (Gaudin *et al.*, 1992).

C. Dissociation of Virion Molecular Components

Because the membrane envelope of virus particles is made up of phospho-lipids, neutral lipids, and glycolipids, virions are easily dissociated by treatment with organic solvents or surface-active agents. Selective dissociation of virions and subsequent isolation of the viral components have made it possible to attribute functions to the various molecular structures. For example, treatment of rabies virions with sodium deoxycholate, an ionic detergent, dissociates the virion envelope and releases the viral RNP from the membrane components (Sokol *et al.*, 1969). Treatment of virions with nonionic detergents NP-40, Triton X-100, *n*-octylglucoside, and tri-(*n*-butyl)phosphate in the presence of Tween 80 also dissociates the viral protein-lipid envelope by emulsifying the lipids, selec-tively releasing the surface G molecules, and leaving skeleton particles (Gyorgi *et al.*, 1971; Sokol *et al.*, 1971; Neurath *et al.*, 1972; Cox *et al.*, 1980). When the ionic detergent sodium dodecyl sulfate (SDS) is used to treat intact virus parti-cles, skeleton particles (stripped of their G spikes) or delipidized RNP complexes that formed the dense virion core are liberated as intact substructures. Subsequent treatment of the RNP complex with an ionic detergent such as sodium deoxy-cholate releases the P and L but does not affect the tight association between the N and genome RNA. Heating at 95°C in addition to SDS treatment completely denatures the viral proteins such that some are no longer antigenically recogniz-able by conformation-dependent monoclonal antibodies.

D. Genome Organization

The rabies virus genome is a nonsegmented (monopartite) single-strand RNA with negative-sense polarity, which implies that the genome RNA is not infec-tious and that it cannot be translated directly into protein. The first event in infec-tion, therefore, is transcription of the genome RNA to produce complementary (positive strand) monocistronic messenger RNA (mRNA) molecules from each of the viral genes or cistrons in the genome. The viral proteins are synthesized from the monocistronic mRNAs. The organization and general features of the rabies virus genome RNA are similar to other negative-strand RNA viruses within the *Mononegavirales* order and, in particular, to other rhabdoviruses (Tordo *et al.*, 1992). At the 3' end (first 58 nucleotides) of the 11,932-nucleotide genome RNA of rabies virus (PV strain) is a noncoding (extragenic) leader (Le) sequence. Immediately downstream of the Le sequence, in sequential order, are the five structural genes (N, P, M, G, and L) followed by a noncoding trailer (Tr) sequence (last 70 nucleotides) at the 5' end (Fig. 3) (Tordo *et al.*, 1986a,b). The genes are separated by relatively short (dinucleotide or pentanucleotide) sequences that rep-resent the intergenic regions (stretch of nucleotides from the 5' end of one gene

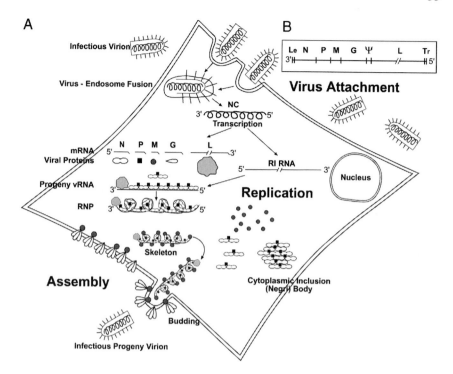

Fig. 3. (*A*) Rabies virus life cycle in the cell. Virus enters the cell through coated pits (viropexis) or via cell surface receptors, mediated by the viral glycoprotein (G) fusing with the cellular membrane (endocytosis). After internalization, the viral G mediates low-pH-dependent fusion with the endosomal membrane, and the virus is uncoated, releasing the helical nucleocapsid (NC) of the ribonucleoprotein (RNP) core. The five structural genes (N, P, M, G, and L) of the genome RNA (see genome organization in panel *B*) in the NC are transcribed into five positive-strand monocistronic messenger RNAs and a full-length positive-strand (antigenome) replicative intermediate (RI) RNA. The antigenome RNA serves as the template for replication of progeny genome (negative-strand) RNA. The proteins (N, P, M, and L) are synthesized from their respective mRNAs on the free ribosomes in the cytoplasm, and the G is synthesized from the G–mRNA on membrane-bound ribosomes (rough endoplasmic reticulum). Some of the N–P molecular complexes produce cytoplasmic inclusion bodies (Negri bodies *in vivo*), and some N–P complexes encapsidate the positive-strand and negative-strand viral RNAs. After progeny genome RNA is encapsidated by N + P proteins and L protein is incorporated to form progeny RNP (both full-length standard and shorter defective) structures, the M protein binds to the RNP and condenses the RNP into the skeleton structures. The skeleton structures interact with the trimeric G protein structures anchored in the plasma membrane and assemble into virus particles that bud from the plasma membrane of the infected cell into adjacent extracellular or interstitial space. (*B*) Organization of the rabies virus genome. A leader (Le) and trailer (Tr) noncoding sequences at the 3′ and 5′ ends of the genome, respectively, flank the structural genes that code for the nucleoprotein (N), phosphoprotein (P), matrix protein (M), glycoprotein (G), and RNA transcriptase (L). The genes are separated by a dinucleotide (N–P), two pentanucleotide (P–M and M–G), and one 423-nucleotide (G–L) noncoding intergenic regions. The long intergenic sequence (G–L) is called a pseudogene (Ψ) in recognition of a sequence of suitable length but lacking an open reading frame, to code for a detectable protein.

to the 3′ start of the next gene) of the genome. These short intergenic regions are located between the N and P genes (2 nucleotides) and between the P and M genes and the M and G genes (each 5 nucleotides long). The remaining intergenic region between the G and L genes contains a long stretch of 423 nucleotides in the rabies virus genome, 504 nucleotides in the Mokola virus genome (LeMercier *et al.*, 1997), and 475 nucleotides in the Australian bat lyssavirus genome (Gould *et al.*, 1998). The G–L intergenic region is sufficiently long to represent a potential gene but lacks an ORF for a detectable protein. It has been given the designation of *remnant gene* or *pseudogene* (Ψ), recognizing that it once represented an ORF of sufficient size to code for a recoverable protein (Tordo *et al.*, 1986b). Interestingly, in this long intergenic region, two sequences stand out that appear to give credence to its former function. One is a sequence motif that resembles the rabies consensus mRNA start signal (UUAU), which is located 10 nucleotides downstream (or UUGU in MOKV, 20 nucleotides downstream) from the stop signal for the mRNA of the G gene in the rabies virus genome. The other is a stretch of 25 nucleotides located upstream from the L gene, which resembles a polyadenylation (polyA) signal located at the end of mRNA molecules. These signals suggest that the virus may have inherited and since lost a protein ORF in its evolution, analogous to the nonviral protein of the infectious hematopoietic necrosis virus, a fish rhabdovirus (Tordo *et al.*, 1992). Strangely, the Ψ region represents the most divergent area of the genome (Sacramento *et al.*, 1991). To understand the relevance of this highly mutable region of the genome for monitoring epidemiologic changes in the evolution of rabies viruses, the sequences of 7 laboratory (vaccine) strains and 12 street (wild) rabies viruses isolated from different host species were compared (Sacramento *et al.*, 1992). Interestingly, this study has raised the question of whether the viral sequences that show a marked divergence from vaccine strains, in contrast to sequences of relative intrinsic homology, as for the viral gene sequences, should be required for analysis in epidemiologic studies.

The Le sequence at the 3′ end of the genome RNA serves a multifunctional purpose in rabies virus as it does in VSV and Sendai virus (family *Paramyxoviridae*). Within the 3′ terminal Le sequence, a specific *cis*-acting signal (a specific nucleotide sequence "acting within" the genome RNA) functions as a signal (or promoter) for template recognition by the viral RNA transcriptase (L alone) or RNA polymerase complex (L and P). This particular signal initiates genome RNA transcription (Conzelmann and Schnell, 1994; Wertz *et al.*, 1994; Calain and Roux, 1995; Whelan and Wertz, 1999a). Within the first 10 to 20 nucleotides at the 3′ and 5′ ends of the rabies virus RNA genome there is a high level of sequence complementarity, including an exact base complementarity between the first and the last 11 nucleotides at the 3′ and 5′ ends of the genome RNA, respectively. This is compelling evidence that the promoter sequences, which are shared in the Le and TrC (3′ end of the antigenome RNA that is complementary to the 5′ end of the genome) regions, provide a common function in transcription and replication.

III. INTRACELLULAR LIFE CYCLE OF RABIES VIRUS

The sequence of events in rabies virus replication *in vivo* can be divided into three phases. The first, or early, phase includes virus attachment to receptors on susceptible host cells, entry via direct virus fusion externally with the plasma membrane and internally with endosomal membranes of the cell, and uncoating of virus particles and liberation of the helical RNP in the cytoplasm. The second, or middle, phase includes transcription and replication of the viral genome, and the third, or late, phase includes virus assembly and egress from the infected cell. The early phase of the rabies virus life cycle, often regarded as the most difficult of the events in rabies virus infection to fully understand, has been studied in many different cell culture systems. These include neuronal and nonneuronal cell lines and primary dissociated cell cultures derived from dissected pieces of nervous tissue. One caveat that overshadows the use of experimental cell culture systems is that the cells may behave differently *ex vivo* in their susceptibility for rabies virus infection compared with their susceptibility to infection *in vivo*. That is, once cells are removed from their *in vivo* environment, particularly neuronal cells, they lose their natural control over susceptibility (or resistance) to rabies virus infection. Nevertheless, many studies using *in vitro* cell culture systems describe how virus enters the host cell by direct membrane fusion (Iwasaki *et al.*, 1973; Perrin *et al.*, 1982) or by receptor-mediated endocytosis (Hummeler *et al.*, 1967; Iwasaki *et al.*, 1973; Superti *et al.*, 1984; Tsiang *et al.*, 1986; Lycke and Tsiang, 1987). No *in vitro* system has yet provided a detailed explanation of how rabies virus enters muscle cells *in vivo* to support the experimental infections in hamster (Murphy *et al.*, 1973a; Murphy and Bauer, 1974) and skunk (Charlton and Casey, 1979) that show virus replication in striated muscle cells near the site of inoculation.

A. Early-Phase Events (The Rabies Virus Receptor)

Infection starts with rabies virus attachment to a target cell surface and uptake most likely by a receptor or cellular receptor unit (CRU) that permits virus entry into susceptible cells in culture (*in vitro*) or specific target cells at the site of inoculation (*in vivo*). Several studies using various cell culture systems have implicated lipids, gangliosides, carbohydrate, and protein of the plasma membrane in rabies virus binding to cells in culture (Perrin *et al.*, 1982; Superti *et al.*, 1984b; Wunner *et al.*, 1984; Superti *et al.*, 1986; Conti *et al.*, 1986, 1988; Broughan and

Wunner, 1995). Others have focused on specific cellular receptor molecules or CRUs *in vivo* that appear to correlate with the defined neurotropism of the virus. The first of such receptor candidates to be investigated was the nicotinic acetyl-choline receptor (AChR) found at the neuromuscular junctions, where rabies virus also can be found *in situ* (Burrage *et al.*, 1982). The model systems chosen to investigate the interaction of rabies virus with the AChR were nerve-enervated mouse diaphragm tissue and cultured chick myotubes (Lentz *et al.*, 1982; Burrage *et al.*, 1985). These studies showed that rabies virus colocalizes with AChRs at neuromuscular junctions in the diaphragm model and in high-density clusters in chick myotubes. Pretreatment of myotubes with α-bungerotoxin or *d*-tubocu-rarine, two nicotinic cholinergic antagonists that bind to AChRs, decreased the number of rabies virus–infected myotubes. Additionally, competition-binding experiments with α-bungerotoxin and synthetic peptides corresponding to the AChR binding site (residues 190–203) have suggested that the AChR was used by rabies virus to infect these cells (Lentz *et al.*, 1982, 1987; Tsiang, 1988; Bracci *et al.*, 1988). Further support for the hypothesis that the AChR may be biologi-cally important in rabies virus infection *in vivo* comes from studies with an anti-idiotypic antibody (Hanham *et al.*, 1993). An antibody that mimics a neutralizing epitope on the rabies virus attachment protein (the G molecule) and competes with rabies virus binding to cell lines expressing the AChR, but not to cells lack-ing the receptor effectively links rabies virus to the nicotinic AChR. Not all cell lines that are susceptible to rabies virus infection *in vitro*, however, express the AChR (Reagan and Wunner, 1985; Tsiang *et al.*, 1986; Tsiang, 1993). Furthermore, some neuronal cells infected with rabies virus *in vivo* may not express the AChR (Tsiang *et al.*, 1986; Kucera *et al.*, 1985; Lafay *et al.*, 1991). Therefore, it is still debatable whether the nicotinic AChR is sufficient for rabies virus entry into cells. This raises the question of whether rabies virus uses more than one type of cell surface receptor, supporting the concept of multivalency in the cellular receptor site (Lonberg-Holm, 1981), or whether different receptors might act in a sequential manner to facilitate initial attachment and subsequent virus uptake (penetration). That is, does one receptor bind the virus before a sec-ond receptor is able to bind virus, or in a cooperative manner, do both receptor types bind virus simultaneously (Lentz, 1990; Haywood, 1994)? The answer to this perplexing possibility still needs to be resolved.

Research to identify an alternative rabies virus receptor(s) continues, with the goal of the search being to identify a candidate receptor for rabies virus that would be as effective and specific *in vivo* as *in vitro* and as biologically signifi-cant as the AChR is for rabies virus. Regardless of the broad rabies virus–sus-ceptible host range that exists *in vitro*, including practically every neuronal and nonneuronal cell line tested (Superti *et al.*, 1984a; Reagan and Wunner, 1985; Seganti *et al.*, 1990), the highly restricted neuronal tropism of rabies virus *in vivo* makes this effort a particularly unusual and daunting challenge. Recently, the neural cell adhesion molecule (NCAM) CD56 on the cell surface of rabies virus–susceptible cell lines (Thoulouze *et al.*, 1998) and the low-affinity neurotrophin (NT) receptor p75NTR (a nerve growth factor) expressed on the surface of cultured BSR cells (Tuffereau *et al.*, 1998) were shown to be receptors for rabies virus. Some doubt, however, has been cast already on the importance of p75NTR as an obligatory rabies virus receptor because virus [challenge virus standard (CVS strain)] infects p75NTR-deficient mice (Jackson and Park, 1999). Is it possible that the virus chooses alternative receptors in neuronal cells when the cells are deprived of one type of receptor in order to complete the virus life cycle in the infected animal? To determine whether either of these putative rabies virus receptors or other candidate molecules will be specific biologically active receptors, more effort and additional animal models will be needed in which to study rabies virus infection of the central nervous system (CNS).

After rabies virus binds to its cellular receptor, viral entry (internalization) proceeds by fusion of the viral envelope with the cellular membrane (Superti *et al.*, 1984a). Rabies virus, like VSV, also may enter the cell through coated pits and uncoated vesicles (viropexis or pinocytosis), which often incorporate several (two to five) virions per vesicle (Tsiang *et al.*, 1983a). After internalization, whether by receptor-mediated endocytosis (via the endocytic pathway) or through coated pits, the viral G mediates fusion of the viral envelope with the endosomal membrane (Marsh and Helenius, 1989; Whitt *et al.*, 1991; Gaudin *et al.*, 1992). The capacity of rabies virus to enter the cell via fusion with the endosomal membrane depends on the low pH within the endosomal compartment. The threshold pH for fusion activation for rabies virus is about pH 6.3 and involves a series of specific and discrete conformational changes in G (Gaudin *et al.*, 1993, 1995; Gaudin, 1997). These conformational changes are described below (see Sect. VI.E). At the same time, changes may occur in the cellular membrane to facilitate virus uptake, which include the formation of membrane fusion pores (Gaudin, 2000).

B. Genome RNA Transcription

In the second phase of the virus life cycle, transcription of the virus RNA genome is initiated in the cytoplasm of the infected cell once the tightly coiled, transcriptionally active RNP core is released from endosomal vesicles. The tightly coiled NC of the RNP structure relaxes to form a loosely coiled helix, conceivably to facilitate the ensuing viral replication events in the cell (Iseni *et al.*, 1998). The transcription process in virus replication is carried out on the genome RNA–N protein complex by the virion-associated RNA polymerase complex (L plus the P cofactor) and is independent of host-cell functions. The virion-associated polymerase complex either initiates transcription at the 3′ end of the genome RNA or resumes transcription at the next downstream internal mRNA start site on the viral genome, close to where the polymerase complex was "frozen" in place during progeny virus assembly in a previously infected cell. This part of the replication process has been termed *primary transcription* because it takes place on the parental nucleocapsids released into the cytoplasm from the input virus and does not require concomitant host or viral protein synthesis (Huang and Manders, 1972). Each of the five genes produces in sequential order a monocistronic mRNA transcript that eventually is translated into one of the five viral proteins (Flamand and Delagneau, 1978; Holloway and Obejeski, 1980). At each intergenic junction, however, the polymerase pauses before continuing the downstream mRNA transcription process, and an estimated 20–30% of the polymerase complexes that reach the gene junction dissociate from the nucleocapsid. As a result, fewer polymerase molecules remain associated with the genome RNA–N template after each gene junction to resume the transcription process. Thus the number of mRNAs synthesized from the remaining genes downstream in the genome gradually decreases in proportion to the number of polymerases that fall off. This phenomenon of self-regulating viral gene expression is a form of "localized" attenuation (Iverson and Rose, 1981).

1. Le RNA Transcripts

The first RNA transcripts produced in the process of transcribing and reproducing the genome RNA are the small 55- to 58-nucleotide-long complementary, positive-strand, nontranslated leader RNA (Le$^+$) transcripts. The Le$^+$ transcripts are neither capped nor polyadenylated, in contrast to the mRNA transcripts (Colonno and Banerjee, 1978; Leppert *et al.*, 1979). In rabies virus–infected cells and in VSV-infected cells, the Le$^+$ transcripts interact with the host cellular protein La, which normally associates with cellular RNA polymerase III precursor transcripts (Kurilla *et al.*, 1984). In VSV-infected cells, the association between Le$^+$ transcripts and La protein has been implicated in the shutoff mechanism of host-cell RNA and protein synthesis. The association of these two elements in rabies virus–infected cells does not affect host macromolecular synthesis in rabies virus–infected cells (Tuffereau *et al.*, 1985). Le$^+$ transcripts also may interact with conserved *cis*-acting signals that act as transcription promoters (L protein binding sites) at the start of each gene. These transcription-promoting Le$^+$ transcripts would appear to initiate mRNA synthesis in a "stop–start" mechanism of genome transcription as the RNA polymerase moves along the genome (see references in Banerjee and Barik, 1992; Schnell *et al.*, 1996; Yang *et al.*, 1999). Accordingly, a conserved *cis*-acting sequence would be required to signal termination of transcription and polyadenylation of the upstream mRNA, whereas another is required to signal reinitiation of the next downstream mRNA transcript (Barr *et al.*, 1997a; Schnell *et al.*, 1996; Stillman and Whitt, 1997). Furthermore, there must be a Le termination signal for the switch from transcription of mRNAs to synthesis of full-length antigenomic RNA (Banerjee *et al.*, 1977; Ball and Wertz, 1981). Precisely how the Le$^+$ transcripts function in transcriptional regulation of the mRNAs and in virus RNA replication (i.e., synthesis of full-length antigenome and progeny genome RNA) is not entirely clear. It is apparent, however, that after release of the Le$^+$ transcripts, the RNA–polymerase complex is fixed in the transcription mode, in which a downstream transcription signal present at the 3′ end of each gene is recognized, and transcription proceeds until the switch from transcription to replication occurs. One way this switch may occur is if the Le$^+$ transcripts become encapsidated by N (see discussion below), preventing them from acting further as initiators of genomic RNA transcription (Yang *et al.*, 1998, 1999).

Just as the extreme 3′ end of the genome RNA provides a specific *cis*-acting signal for transcription of the viral genome, the 3′ end of the antigenome RNA (TrC) provides a specific *cis*-acting signal for replication (copy-back) of antigenome RNA, which acts as the template for progeny genome RNA synthesis. These signals have been demonstrated for rabies virus (Finke and Conzelmann, 1997) and for VSV (Whelan and Wertz, 1999a). In the replication phase, the promoter at the 3′ end of the "replicative intermediate" antigenome RNA is rendered replication-competent for a full-length copy-back of the antigenome RNA to be produced as the progeny genome RNA. Thus conservation of the extremities, the 3′ and 5′ ends, of the genome (and antigenome) RNA is crucial for successful viral genome RNA transcription and antigenome replication to maintain virus infection.

Another function of the Le$^+$ transcripts from the 3′ Le sequence in the genomic RNA is to provide specific *cis*-acting signals for RNA encapsidation by soluble N (Blumberg *et al.*, 1983; Yang *et al.*, 1998). Identical *cis*-acting signals also are found in the Le$^-$ (minus strand) transcripts that are produced from the 3′ TrC sequence of the antigenome RNA, which is complementary to the genome Tr sequence in the genome RNA. These encapsidation signals (N binding site on RNA) are present at or close to the 5′ end of the antigenome RNA (mimicking the location of the Le$^+$ transcripts) and at or near the 5′ end of the progeny genome RNA (mimicking the location of the Le$^-$ transcripts). They act as nucleation sites for genome and antigenome RNA encapsidation by N and assembly of RNP complexes. Using synthetic RNA probes that mimic the Le$^+$ transcripts (and sometimes the natural Le$^+$ transcripts) corresponding to the 5′ end of the rabies virus antigenome RNA, researchers have begun to identify the specificity of RNA encapsidation by N (Yang *et al.*, 1998). The RNA probes are also useful in locating the RNA binding site on the rabies virus N protein (Kouznetzoff *et al.*, 1998). Together the studies indicate that amino acid residues 298–352 in a highly conserved region of rabies virus N bind specifically to a site within nucleotides 20–30 of Le$^+$ transcript, which would be equivalent to nucleotides 20–30 of the 5′ end of antigenome RNA.

2. mRNA Transcripts

The RNA transcripts produced from the negative-strand genome RNA immediately after the Le^+ transcripts are the five gene-encoded monocistronic mRNAs. The invariant sequence 3′–UUGU–5′ in the genome RNA at the 3′ end of each gene (5′–AACA–3′ at the 5′ end of each complementary mRNA) identifies the start of mRNA transcription. During synthesis of the nascent mRNAs, the L protein caps the 5′ end of each mRNA by attaching a 7-methyl guanosine (5′–m^7Gppp–) to the 5′ nucleotide of the mRNA (Testa et al., 1980). In the rabies virus and Mokola virus genomes, the invariant sequence 3′–AC(U)$_{7-8}$–5′ at the 5′ end of each gene (upstream of the intergenic sequence) signals the termination and polyadenylation of the mRNA (5′–TGAAAAAAA–3′ at the 3′ end of each complementary mRNA) (Tordo et al., 1986a). In the Australian bat virus genome, the signal to start mRNA transcription is the same as in the rabies virus genome, but the signal to terminate and polyadenylate the mRNA is either 3′–TTC(U)$_6$–5′ for N–mRNA or 3′–AC(U)$_7$–5′ for P–mRNA, M–mRNA, and G–mRNA. The latter mRNA includes the ORF sequence for G plus the nontranslated Ψ sequence (Gould et al., 1998). When the viral polymerase operating in the transcription mode reaches the string of 7 (or 8) U's in the genome, it pauses and begins to stutter or slip as it reiteratively copies the U's. This slows up the transcription process while a poly(A) tract of variable length (up to 200 A's) is produced at the 3′ end of the mRNA. The mRNA, which is capped and polyadenylated, is released, and the transcriptase, after skipping the next intergenic nucleotides, initiates transcription of the next mRNA.

In the rabies virus genomes of the PV and Evelyn-Rokitnicki-Abelseth (ERA) strains, two functional polyadenylation [poly(A)] or transcriptional stop signals exist that terminate the G–mRNA transcript in comparison with one poly(A) signal in other virus strains such as the Flury high egg passage (HEP), CVS, Pitman Moore (PM), SAD-B19, and Nishigahara strains (Tordo et al., 1986b; Morimoto et al., 1989; Conzelmann et al., 1990; Sakamoto et al., 1994) and in MOKV (Bourhy et al., 1993). In those genomes where two functional poly(A) signals exist, the first is located at the end of the G gene and beginning of the Ψ sequence, and the second is at the end of the Ψ sequence. As a result of these respective locations, the poly(A) signals produce either a short G–mRNA transcript or a long G–mRNA transcript, respectively (Tordo and Poch, 1988; Morimoto et al., 1989; Sakamoto et al., 1994). Although the signal before the Ψ is functional in the ERA strain, it is leaky, and consequently, the Ψ region is included in approximately 50% of the G–mRNA transcripts produced (Morimoto et al., 1989). In most of the other rabies virus strains, Mokola virus, and several street rabies virus strains, the transcriptional stop signal before the Ψ is either degenerate or absent, leaving only the poly(A) signal at the end of the Ψ sequence (Morimoto et al., 1989; Sacramento et al., 1992; Sakamoto et al., 1994). Again, a long G–mRNA transcript is produced that includes the coding sequence for G plus the noncoding Ψ sequence.

All but one of the monocistronic mRNAs produces a single protein from a single ORF. For these mRNAs, translation starts with the first initiation codon AUG (coding for methionine) from the 5' end of the mRNA and terminates near the 3' end with the stop codon UAA or UGA. An exception to this rule is the three or four proteins derived from the P gene of rabies virus, which are initiated from secondary downstream in-frame AUG initiation codons (Chenik *et al.*, 1995). These smaller amino-terminal truncated products that are translated from the P–mRNA have been found in purified virions, in infected cells, and in cells transfected with a plasmid encoding the complete P sequence. It is thought that a leaky scanning mechanism is responsible for translation of the P gene at several of the internal in-frame AUG initiation sites. The function(s) of these shorter P-related proteins, given the "anomalous" nature of their derivation and that some of the shorter products end up in the nucleus and the two largest P products remain in the cytoplasm, is unknown (Chenik *et al.*, 1995). The major ORFs of the five mRNAs encode proteins of approximately 450 (N–mRNA), 297 (P–mRNA), 202 (M–mRNA), 524 (G–mRNA), and 2,142 (L–mRNA) amino acids. Some of the lyssavirus mRNAs contain a few more or a few less codons (and hence produce proteins that will contain a few more or a few less amino acids) depending on the genotype of the virus.

C. Virus Replication (Synthesis of Antigenome and Progeny Genome RNA)

Viral RNA replication (production of progeny genome RNA) becomes the dominant event following primary transcription in the late phase of virus growth. As rapidly as nascent soluble N is produced in the cytoplasm from the primary mRNA transcripts, some of the N encapsidates the Le^+ RNA transcripts. Protein encapsidation of the Le^+ RNA transcripts either prevents termination of Le^+ RNA transcription at the Le–N gene junction or prevents Le^+ RNA transcripts from initiating the transcription of individual downstream mRNAs. As a result, RNA transcription continues to produce full-length complementary (positive strand) copy of the genome RNA (Blumberg *et al.*, 1983; Banerjee and Barik, 1992; Yang *et al.*, 1998, 1999). Although the precise mechanism of switching from transcription to replication remains unclear at this time, it is understood that viral protein synthesis is essential and that the polymerase complex no longer recognizes subsequent intergenic events that cause transcript termination and initiation at the gene junctions (Banerjee and Barik, 1992). Thus the start of viral genome replication is synthesis of a full-length complementary copy of the genome RNA known as the *antigenome* or *replicative intermediate RNA*. The replicative intermediate (RI) RNA serves as the template for progeny (negative strand) genome RNA replication. After the antigenome and progeny genome RNAs are synthesized, they too are cotranscriptionally encapsidated by soluble N in the cytoplasm. The 5′-terminal *cis*-acting encapsidation signal in the antigenome and genome RNAs acts as a nucleation signal for the nascent soluble N to interact with the viral + strand and − strand RNAs. After the specific nucleation signal for encapsidation has been recognized by N, encapsidation is believed to proceed rapidly in the 5′ to 3′ direction on the RNA, independent of the viral RNA sequence (Banerjee and Barik, 1992). During infection, however, the two full-length RNAs are produced in disproportionate amounts. The stoichiometric relationship of the genome and antigenome RNAs is 50:1 (Finke and Conzelmann, 1997). The bias for the excessive production of genome RNA over antigenome RNA in the rabies virus–infected cell is attributed to the activity of their *cis*-acting sequences. These so-called genome and antigenome promoters at the 3′ end of the respective genome and antigenome RNAs are required to direct both replication and encapsidation (Calain and Roux, 1995).

D. Viral Protein Synthesis

The proteins of the virus are synthesized using the protein synthesis machinery (polyribosomes) of the host cell. Four of the viral mRNAs, N–, P–, M–, and L–mRNA are translated on free (unbound) ribosomes, whereas the G–mRNA is translated on membrane-bound ribosomes. The nascent G is inserted cotranslationally into the lumen of the ER, where disulfide bond formation occurs and the folding enzymes and molecular chaperones are available to assist in the folding of G before the molecule is transported out of the ER (Gaudin, 1997). While in the lumen of the ER, the G monomers undergo modification at specific asparagine (N in single-letter code) residues by core glycosylation and N-glycan processing (Shakin-Eshleman *et al.*, 1992), and they form homotrimers (Whitt *et al.*, 1991; Gaudin *et al.*, 1992). The final processing of the N-linked carbohydrate side chains takes place in the Golgi apparatus of the intracellular membrane network. This is accomplished with the sequential removal and then addition of monosaccharides by glycosidases and glycosyltransferases (Kornfeld and Kornfeld, 1985) before the viral G trimers appear on the surface of the infected cell.

E. Virus Assembly (Morphogenesis and Budding)

Once sufficient pools of viral progeny (negative strand) RNA and the viral N, P, and L have accumulated in the infected cell, rabies viral nucleocapsids are formed, and virus assembly begins and continues as long as the cells remain metabolically competent. Rabies virus morphogenesis is associated with the formation of an intracytoplasmic ground substance or "matrix" commonly found in brain tissue as well as in tissue culture (Hummeler *et al.*, 1968). This filamentous matrix substance constitutes the Negri bodies found in neurons of the infected brain (Matsumoto, 1962; Matsumoto and Miyamoto, 1966), a development that precedes the formation of virus particles (Hummeler *et al.*, 1967). The process of virus assembly really begins with encapsidation of viral progeny RNA, i.e., the addition of N to the 5' end of the nascent RNA, and the formation of genome RNA–N complexes. When N binds to the phosphate–sugar backbone (exposing the nucleotide bases), the RNA becomes fully protected from degradation by cellular ribonucleases (Kouznetzoff *et al.*, 1998; Iseni *et al.*, 2000). As nascent N and P molecules accumulate in the cytoplasm of the rabies virus–infected cell, as in VSV infection, they form both homologous and heterologous (N–P) complexes. On the one hand, in high concentrations, N protein may aggregate with itself $(N-N)_n$ to form the large intracytoplasmic "matrix" bodies found in brain tissue, whereas the P oligomerizes aggregates to form trimers or tetramers that seem to be necessary for the transcriptional activity of the protein, whereby it forms specific complexes with the genome-associated N and L (Gigant *et al.*, 2000). On the other hand, with an equilibrium shift in concentration of monomers of soluble N and P, heterologous complexes may form between the two proteins (Chenik *et al.*, 1994; Fu *et al.*, 1994; Gigant *et al.*, 2000). When P interacts with N, it prevents soluble N from self-aggregating, and it also maintains N in a soluble form for efficient RNA encapsidation during replication (Davis *et al.*, 1986; Prehaud *et al.*, 1992; Fu *et al.*, 1994). In some of these N–P complexes, the N-to-P ratio is 2:1, similar to that found in rabies virions. It has been suggested that these complexes are responsible for the specificity of viral RNA encapsidation by N and for preventing encapsidation of nonviral RNA species (Masters and Banerjee, 1988). Despite current knowledge of the virus assembly process, little is known about how the L is added to the NC complex. It is thought that the P in the RNA–N–P complex mediates L binding (Mellon and Emerson, 1978) to complete the transcriptionally active virion RNP core (Buchholz *et al.*, 1994). More recent studies describe the formation of ring structures by recombinant RNA–N complexes, which have biochemical and biophysical properties that appear to be indistinguishable from rabies virus nucleocapsids. These structures define the spatial relationships between the core proteins and RNA in the assembled rabies virus NC structure (Schoehn *et al.*, 2001). Clearly, further studies on these and other recombinant NC-like structures likely will clarify the role of specific amino acid residues or motifs in the molecular mechanisms controlling nucleocapsid (RNP) assembly.

The next protein to become associated with RNP complexes is the M as the complexes migrate toward the cellular membranes and before they become enveloped by the cellular membrane and enter the virus budding process. From the time M enters the virus assembly pathway as a soluble protein in the cytoplasm, it is involved in all the steps that lead to viral budding. This is based on the observation that assembly and budding of bullet-shaped particles can occur in the absence of the transmembrane G spikes that normally are associated with infectious particles (Mebatsion et al., 1996; Robinson et al., 2000). The first thing the M does is bind to the RNP and condense the RNP coil from the out-side, a step that is sufficient to initiate virus budding (Mebatsion et al., 1996; Lyles and McKenzie, 1998). The M will then localize the RNP coil at the cel-lular membrane, where the nascent viral G is concentrated and where the M is able to interact with G (Simons and Garoff, 1980; Mebatsion et al., 1999). In the mature rabies virion, i.e., that which buds from the cell membrane, the M lies between the lipid bilayer envelope (formed by interaction with the host cell membrane) and the helical RNP that it covers (Mebatsion et al., 1999). This is in contrast to one VSV model that has been described in which the M appears to be inside, at the core of the RNP coil. This is shown in isolated "skeletons" prepared by stripping off the external G spikes on the surface of infectious VS virions (Barge et al., 1993). It was proposed, in the VSV model, that the M becomes the core that fills the "axial channel" created by RNP coil and that the only place of contact between the M and the lipid envelope is at the extreme ends of the skeleton. In rabies virus, the M covering and condensing the heli-cal RNP is thought to play an important role in virion morphogenesis, i.e., giv-ing the particle its bullet-shaped morphology (Mebatsion et al., 1999). If the M is missing from VSV particles, spherical particles are released from cells, or if nucleocapsids contain a temperature-sensitive mutant of M (demonstrated with VSV), spherical particles are released at the nonpermissive temperature instead of the expected filamentous or bullet-shaped particles (Lyles et al., 1996). Similarly, for rabies virus particles that contain G spikes on the outer surface but lack M, a morphologic variation in budded particles is observed that sug-gests that the particles contain uncondensed RNP (Mebatsion et al., 1999). M-deficient rabies virus also causes increased cell–cell fusion and enhanced cell death, in contrast to the relatively benign cytopathic effect that is observed with wild-type virus. Also, virus budding is much less efficient in the absence of M, demonstrating again the multifunctional role of M in virus assembly and budding.

Another role of the M in rabies virus, as in VSV, that relates to virus assembly is in the downregulation of the viral-associated polymerase that occurs during infection, causing complete suppression of transcriptase activity during virion egress (Clinton et al., 1978; Carroll et al., 1979; De et al., 1982; Ito et al., 1996; Flood et al., 2000). Perhaps as a consequence of the interaction between M and the RNP core, the suppressive effect on the virion-associated polymerase preserves the potential of remaining active viral-associated polymerase complexes in the RNP core to resume transcription activity when progeny virions infect a second host cell. After the virus in secondary infection is uncoated and the nucleocapsid relaxes its tight coil, the virion-associated polymerase can resume activity by reinitiating transcription of the next gene or inducing initiation of other polymerase molecules bound at a promoter (Emerson, 1987).

In the final stages of rabies virus assembly, the mature virions acquire their lipid bilayer envelope as the assembled skeleton (RNP–M) structure buds through the host cell plasma membrane. Mature viruses budding through the plasma membrane into the extracellular space are observed frequently in extraneural tissue cells *in vivo* (Murhpy *et al.*, 1973a) and in a variety of *in vitro* tissue culture systems (Davies *et al.*, 1963; Hummeler *et al.*, 1967; Matsumoto and Kawai, 1969; Iwasaki *et al.*, 1973; Matsumoto *et al.*, 1974; Tsiang *et al.*, 1983a). Occasionally, virions mature intracellularly by budding through the cytoplasmic ER or Golgi apparatus. Cytoplasmic maturation within infected neuronal cells of brain commonly appeared to occur by budding on the intracytoplasmic membranes of the ER; Golgi membranes occasionally were involved (Murphy *et al.*, 1973b; Matsumoto *et al.*, 1974; Matsumoto, 1975; Gosztonyi, 1994). If budding occurs at a site in the cell membrane where the nascent rabies virus transmembrane glycoprotein (G) is also targeted, then infectious virions will be produced bearing the G molecules arranged as trimeric spikelike structures tightly packed and anchored in the viral envelope. Given the way the spikes are oriented in the viral membrane, more than 80% of G molecule (the ectodomain) is exposed on the surface of the virion, and the cytoplasmic tail C-terminal to the transmembrane domain of the G extends beneath the lipid bilayer envelope. The C-terminal tail of the G molecule is then free to interact with the M that surrounds the RNP core (i.e., the skeleton structure). Interaction of G with M is essential for stabilization of the G in trimers on the virion surface and for efficient budding of rabies virus (Lyles *et al.*, 1992; Mebatsion *et al.*, 1996, 1999). This does not preclude the possibility that skeleton structures may bud from membrane regions where no G exists. In this case, budding would be inefficient, producing low levels, and the bullet-shaped particles produced would be spikeless (free of G) and noninfectious (Mebatsion *et al.*, 1996). If skeletons bud through ER or Golgi membranes, they bud into the lumina of vesicles produced from these membranes and may be secreted out of the cell through the normal secretory pathway.

IV. GENOME VARIABILITY

In the rabies virus life cycle, the genome RNA is subject to limited replication fidelity due to an absence of RNA proofreading/repair and postreplication error-correction mechanisms. Consequently, mutations that are introduced at a relatively high frequency, by the "error-prone" virion-associated RNA polymerase as the enzyme replicates the genome RNA, remain in the genome RNA. This produces a population of different viral genomes that share a common origin; i.e., they are related but distinct (Kissi *et al.*, 1999). Genome RNA mutations (misincorporation of nucleotides) occur at different rates, on the order of 10^{-4} to 10^{-5} substitutions per nucleotide per cycle, depending on the region of the genome RNA considered (Domingo and Holland, 1997; Bracho *et al.*, 1998; Kissi *et al.*, 1999). On the one hand, the genetic variation in complex mixtures of related genomes has resulted in such major comprehensive differences that viruses could be sorted taxonomically into different families, genera, and species. In other cases of less marked differences, genetic variations have provided the basis for grouping viruses into serotypes, genotypes, or phenotypes within a genus or virus species. Several other factors that may be involved in generating RNA sequence heterogeneity in rabies virus include duration of infection, route of transmission, virus load, host immune response, and virus–host protein cooperation (Kissi *et al.*, 1999). Despite these other influences, the infidelity of the RNA polymerase of negative-strand RNA viruses remains the single major factor responsible for the nucleotide misincorporation in the genome RNA. Assuming a random distribution of mutations among the population of replicating genomes, the variant genomes form complex "quasi-species" populations that increase very rapidly within infection cycles over time (reviewed in Holland *et al.*, 1992; Smith *et al.*, 1997; Domingo and Holland, 1997). As a result of this extreme form of genetic instability, out of a quasi-species population of rabies viral RNA genomes, a true rabies virus variant may evolve that harbors a specific mutation or set of specific mutations capable of imparting to the virus a distinctive phenotypic or unique virus–host relationship. For example, several mutations have been identified in protein coding regions of the genome of virus variants that correlate with a selective tropism for neurons or for an avirulent phenotype of the virus in a particular animal host (Murphy and Nathanson, 1984; Domingo *et al.*, 1998; Morimoto *et al.*, 1998). Mutations in noncoding regions of the genome also may affect the balance between replication of standard versus defective genomes and possibly increasing or decreasing survival of the infected cell or animal host. Or they may influence long-term survival (persistence) of the virus in its host as a result of specific interactions between viral and host determinants (Domingo *et al.*, 1998). The quasi-species model of mixed RNA virus populations provides a plausible explanation for the rapid selection of mutants that fit into any new environmental condition (Morimoto *et al.*, 1998). This selection process may occur in any of the viral genes whose proteins influence the particular structure, function, or phenotype of the virus.

V. VIRUS SPREAD

Progeny rabies virions that bud from infected cells are able to spread from cell to cell in cell or tissue culture (*in vitro*) presumably as they do *in vivo*. They have the option of spreading to contiguous cells (direct cell-to-cell spread) or to noncontiguous cells, which are surrounded by interstitial space. In the case of direct cell-to-cell spread, rabies virus spreads despite a continuous presence of serum virus-neutralizing antibody (VNA). Alternatively, virus that buds from an infected cell into the surrounding interstitial space must find another cell to infect. In this case, the spread of virus is limited by the presence, *in vitro* and *in vivo*, of VNA that blocks virus attachment to cellular receptors and subsequent virus entry into a susceptible cell (Dietzschold *et al.*, 1985; Flamand *et al.*, 1993). *In vivo*, rabies virus also can spread in the cell, particularly cells of peripheral nerves and neuronal cells of the CNS, through intraaxonal transport in a microtubule net-work–dependent process. Virus that moves intraaxonally can cover great distances, particularly in bipolar neurons, before reaching and crossing the synapse of one dendritic process into another (Tsiang, 1979; Kucera *et al.*, 1985; Gillet *et al.*, 1986; Ceccaldi *et al.*, 1989; Coulon *et al.*, 1989; Lafay *et al.*, 1991). It was even postulated that naked viral nucleocapsids (RNPs) might be transported in the axoplasmic flow along axons and through the synapse into the postsynaptic neuron, particularly because this provides an alternative mechanism of virus spread along neuronal networks when mature virions cannot be detected at synapses (Gosztonyi, 1994). This hypothesis of transsynaptic transfer of naked nucleocapsids, however, was weakened considerably, if not negated, by recent studies that demonstrate an absolute requirement for the virion G in transsynaptic spread of rabies virus both *in vivo* and *in vitro* (Etessami *et al.*, 2000). Other significant studies of rabies virus spread also point to the nature of the viral tropism and its relationship to the G of the virion. In particular, viruses that are pathogenic or virulent *in vivo* differ in their ability to invade the CNS and spread within the brain in comparison with the apathogenic or avirulent virus phenotype (Coulon *et al.*, 1989; Lafay *et al.*, 1991). This phenotypic difference, which is determined by the surface G (Coulon *et al.*, 1983; Dietzschold *et al.*, 1983b), is discussed further in Sect. VI.E.

VI. MOLECULAR BIOLOGY OF RABIES VIRUS PROTEINS

A. Nucleocapsid Protein (N)

The N, P, and L proteins, which form the RNP core of the virus, will be discussed first, and then M and G proteins will be discussed as they interact with the RNP to form the assembled virion. The N contains 450 amino acids and has a molecular weight of ~57,000. It is a major component of the virus and the major protein of the internal helical NC (RNP core). It represents the virus group-specific core antigen (Schneider *et al.*, 1973). The N is the most conserved of the viral components in terms of amino acid sequence similarity within genotypes, despite a relatively high degree of genetic diversity within short regions of the N gene between the genotypes (Conzelmann *et al.*, 1990; Bourhy *et al.*, 1993a; Kissi *et al.*, 1995). The highest degree (98–99%) of N amino acid sequence similarity is shared by the different rabies virus "fixed" laboratory strains (genotype 1) (Wunner *et al.*, 1988; Conzelmann *et al.*, 1990). Based on present knowledge, it appears that rabies and rabies-related virus isolates that share less than 80% of nucleotide similarity in the N gene (including noncoding regions) and less than 92% of N amino acid similarity belong to different genotypes (Bourhy *et al.*, 1993; Kissi *et al.*, 1995). These often represent populations of stable, optimally adapted variant virus phenotypes. One of the reasons for the high level of conservation, particularly within specific regions in the N, is that key functions of the N must be retained. For example, the N has specific and absolute requirements for N-specific encapsidation of genome RNA and protection of the RNA template from ribonuclease activity (Sokol *et al.*, 1969; Wunner, 1991). Another example is its role in regulating RNA transcription and modulating viral RNA transcription and replication by promoting read-through of the termination signals (Patton *et al.*, 1984; Yang *et al.*, 1998, 1999). Some of the amino acid differences produce unique, genotype-specific epitopes in the N that can be used to assign viruses to the different serotypes and genotypes on the basis of their reactivity patterns with a panel of anti-N monoclonal antibodies (MAbs) (Flamand *et al.*, 1980a; Dietzschold *et al.*, 1987a; Smith, 1989). This qualitative diversity built into the N that appears to reliably characterize the different lyssaviruses antigenically also has been exploited at the nucleotide level by the polymerase chain reaction (PCR) technology (Sacramento *et al.*, 1991; Bourhy *et al.*, 1993). The so-called molecular or genetic typing technique, which employs reverse transcriptase (RT)–PCR technology and the viral genome RNA as template, is targeted either to a selected short (~200 nucleotide) region of the N gene or to the entire N gene. First used as a fairly simple diagnostic technique, the RT-PCR approach has been used recently to elucidate the epidemiologic and evolutionary relationships between rabies and rabies-related viruses (Smith *et al.*, 1992; Nadine-Davis *et al.*, 1994; Kissi *et al.*, 1995) (see Chap. 3).

Nascent N can be found by immunostaining technique distributed diffusely in the cytoplasm of infected cells. The N is quickly consumed in the formation of homologous (N–N) and heterologous (N–P) complexes and assembled into nascent viral nucleocapsids (RNP complexes). The N also may be concentrated, usually in complexes with P, in one or more cytoplasmic inclusion bodies in the cell (*in vitro*) or in Negri bodies *in vivo* (Chenik *et al.*, 1994; Kawai *et al.*, 1999). The immediate interaction of nascent N with P serves to prevent self-aggregation of N and provide the specificity required for N–viral RNA encapsidation (Masters and Banerjee, 1988; Chenik *et al.*, 1994; Fu *et al.*, 1994; Yang *et al.*, 1998). Interestingly, N interaction with P occurs either at the N or C terminus of N, both of which modulate and enhance N encapsidation of viral RNA. Moreover, the function of P in supporting RNA encapsidation by N depends on the *de novo* interaction between P and N (Yang *et al.*, 1998). The RNA binding site in N appears to lie within the N-terminal domain (first 376 amino acids), possibly between amino acid residues 298 and 352 (Kouznetzoff *et al.*, 1998). After N binds to viral RNA, it undergoes conformational change, acquiring a number of conformation-dependent epitopes, and is phosphorylated at serine 389 (Dietzschold *et al.*, 1987a; Kawai *et al.*, 1999). It is possible that during RNA encapsidation, an encapsidation-associated conformational change exposes serine at position 389, making it accessible for phosphorylation (Kawai *et al.*, 1999). Phosphorylation of N is unique to rabies virus, in contrast to N of VSV and other rhabdoviruses (Sokol *et al.*, 1974; Sokol and Koprowski, 1975), but not to NC proteins of other negative-strand RNA viruses (Lamb and Choppin, 1977; Robbins and Bussell, 1979; Hsu and Kingsbury, 1982). The phosphorylated N of rabies virus raises the interesting question of whether phosphorylation of N in rabies virus causes the N to function differently in viral RNA transcription and replication compared with the unphosphorylated N in VSV. One study that attempts to address this question has expressed unphosphorylated N (one that has substituted serine at position 389 with arginine) in a rabies virus–like particle instead of the wild-type N that is phosphorylated. The result was that the rates of transcription and replication of the rabies-like viral RNA were significantly lower with unphosphorylated N than with expression of phosphorylated N even though the unphosphorylated N bound less strongly to the leader RNA (Yang *et al.*, 1999). Perhaps this, at least in part, explains the slower growth of rabies virus compared with VSV.

When recombinant rabies virus N produced in insect cells was bound to viral RNA, ring structures were generated that were suggestive of the helical structure of rabies virus nucleocapsids (Schoehn *et al.*, 2001). Importantly, the recombinant N that is expressed in insect cells is phosphorylated (Prehaud *et al.*, 1990). These recombinant ring structures are biochemically and biophysically indistinguishable from authentic rabies virus N–RNA complexes, and when observed in the EM, they appear to be identical to rabies virus nucleocapsids (Iseni *et al.*, 1998; Schoehn *et al.*, 2001). In the EM images, the N molecule of the recombinant ring structures bends slightly, giving it a bilobed shape and permitting one N molecule to contact the next N monomer on the viral RNA strand at two nonidentical sites. Such images also reveal that the N subunits are packed closely, every 9 to 11 nucleotides, along the RNA. This is sufficient to protect the viral RNA against ribonuclease activity and to give the recombinant structure the same density as that of authentic viral N–RNA complex (Iseni *et al.*, 1998). As a model for authentic viral nucleocapsids, it is interesting to see how the P binds to the recombinant N in the N–RNA ring. The P, which binds to the unique trypsin-sensitive cleavage site close to the C-terminal end of N (Dietzschold *et al.*, 1987a; Kouznetzoff *et al.*, 1998), ends up in different positions, one bending toward the inside and the other bending toward the outside of the ring (Schoehn *et al.*, 2001). In either position, the interaction of N with P probably causes a further conformational change in N similar to the conformational change that is believed to occur when N first associates with P after N encapsidates the viral RNA (Kawai *et al.*, 1999).

The N is the second most extensively analyzed of the rabies virus proteins (after the G) with respect to its antigenic and immunogenic structure and function. The immunologic interest in N stems from the observation that the RNP core of rabies virus induces protective immunity against a peripheral challenge of lethal rabies virus in animals (Dietzschold *et al.*, 1987b; Tollis *et al.*, 1991). Two distinct immunogenic features associated with the rabies virus N relate to the immunoprotection induced in animals by the internal viral nucleocapsid. First, N is able to protect animals against a peripheral challenge with rabies virus in the absence of detectable VNA (Lodmell *et al.*, 1991; Sumner *et al.*, 1991; Tollis *et al.*, 1991). Second, the N is able to prime the immune system and enhance the production of VNAs following subsequent inoculation of animals with inactivated rabies virus vaccine (Dietzschold *et al.*, 1987b; Tollis *et al.*, 1991; Fu *et al.*, 1991). B- and T-cell-specific epitopes in N were defined initially using MAbs and synthetic peptides in competitive binding assays. These reagents delineated the topography of functional antigenic sites common to rabies and rabies-related viruses (Flamand *et al.*, 1980a; Lafon and Wiktor, 1985; Dietzschold *et al.*, 1987a; Ertl *et al.*, 1989). Subsequently, several linear B- and T-cell epitopes were physically mapped on N (reviewed in Fu *et al.*, 1994; Goto *et al.*, 1995, 2000). Three linear antigenic epitopes (antibody binding sites) on N were mapped to amino acids 358–367 (antigenic site I), and three linear epitopes (antigenic site IV) were mapped to two independent regions, amino acids 359–366 and 375–383 (Minamoto *et al.*, 1994; Goto *et al.*, 2000). Although the region between residues 359 and 366 is shared by the two independent antigenic sites (I and IV), the MAbs that recognize epitopes within these sites do not compete with each other for binding to the N antigen. Thus it would appear that the respective epitopes are detected on different forms of N, one that represents N that is diffuse in the cytoplasm and the other that is associated with cytoplasmic inclusion bodies. The two forms of N might even have different degrees of protein folding or maturation (Goto *et al.*, 2000). The fact that the N that is associated with inclusion bodies may be the more mature form, having gained a greater degree of folding, is suggested by another MAb that is specific for antigenic site II, which only recognizes a conformation-specific epitope on the inclusion body–associated N antigen. The linear epitope (amino acids 373–383) that appears to overlap but may not be identical to another epitope (375–383) in site IV is recognized by a different anti-N MAb (Dietzschold *et al.*, 1987a). Three of the five epitopes from sites I and IV in rabies virus N, which are also shared by rabies-related viruses, represent cross-reactive determinants (Goto *et al.*, 2000). Conformation-dependent epitopes are present in antigenic sites II and III (Minamoto *et al.*, 1994).

The N protein is a major target antigen for T-helper (Th) cells that cross-react among rabies and rabies-related viruses (Celis *et al.*, 1988a,b; Ertl *et al.*, 1989). Several Th cell epitopes in the rabies virus N were identified and mapped using a series of overlapping synthetic peptides corresponding to N sequences of approximately 15 amino acids in length (Ertl *et al.*, 1989). Antigenic peptides (bearing a specific epitope for each subset of Th cells) that were capable of stimulating rabies virus–specific Th cells *in vitro* were selected and subsequently tested for stimulation of rabies virus–specific Th cells *in vivo* (Ertl *et al.*, 1989, 1991). One such peptide, designated 31D, which corresponds to N residues 404–418, was found to be an immunodominant epitope capable of stimulating production of rabies virus–specific Th cells, at least *in vitro*. The same peptide also induced a significant Th cell response *in vivo* and an accelerated VNA response after a booster immunization with inactivated rabies virus *in vivo* (Ertl *et al.*, 1989). Neither the peptide-induced Th cell response nor the increase in VNA titer on vaccine boost induced by this peptide epitope, regardless of the immunodominance, however, was sufficient to protect against a lethal virus challenge dose in mice.

Finally, certain other properties and immune responses that the rabies viral nucleocapsid specifically elicits in humans suggest that the rabies virus N functions as an exogenous superantigen (Lafon *et al.*, 1992). It is perhaps the only viral superantigen that has been identified in humans (Lafon, 1997). Some of the properties and responses found not only in humans but in mice that are attributable to the rabies virus N in the role of superantigen include (1) its potent activation of peripheral blood lymphocytes in human vaccinees (Herzog *et al.*, 1992), (2) its ability to produce a more rapid and heightened VNA response on injection of inactivated rabies vaccines (Dietzschold *et al.*, 1987b; Fu *et al.*, 1991), (3) its induction of early T-cell activation steps and expansion and mobilization of CD4+ Vβ8 T cells to trigger and support production of VNA (Lafon *et al.*, 1992; Martinez-Arends *et al.*, 1995), and (4) its ability to bind to HLA class II antigens expressed on the surface of cells (Lafon *et al.*, 1992).

B. Phosphoprotein (P, M1, or NS)

The P of lyssaviruses, like the P in other *Mononegavirales* viruses, is a multifunctional protein in its interaction with N and a key component of the virion-associated RNA polymerase complex as a regulatory protein in viral genome replication. The P has been identified by other designations in the literature, which may be confusing to anyone entering the field for the first time. The *M1* designation described the earliest interpretative view of the protein as a membrane-associated protein, similar to the *M2* (now designated *M*) (György *et al.*, 1971). The *NS* designation, referring to nonstructural protein, was adopted from the corresponding protein in VSV, so designated because large amounts were found in virus-infected cell extracts and none was detected in purified virions (Kang and Prevec, 1971). The *P* designation, which refers to the protein as the nominal phosphoprotein in rabies virus, is becoming the accepted designation because it conforms to the currently accepted designation for the corresponding protein in VSV and other *Mononegavirales* viruses. It is not, however, the only phosphorylated protein in rabies virus because it shares this posttranslational modification with the N of rabies virus.

The rabies virus P contains 297 amino acids (MOKV P has 303 amino acids) (38–41 kDa), is well conserved (>97%) among genotype 1 lyssaviruses and is found in a variety of phosphorylated forms (Gupta *et al.*, 2000). Among its many functions, the P acts as a chaperone of soluble nascent N, preventing its polymerization (self-assembly) and nonspecific binding to cellular RNA. The P in N–P complexes specifically directs N encapsidation of the viral RNA (Chenik *et al.*, 1994; Fu *et al.*, 1994; Gigant *et al.*, 2000). As a subunit of the RNA polymerase (P–L) complex, the P plays a pivotal role as a cofactor in transcription and replication of the viral genome (Chenik *et al.*, 1994; Fu *et al.*, 1994; Chenik *et al.*, 1998). Essentially, the P serves both to stabilize the L protein (Curran *et al.*, 1994) and to place the polymerase complex on the RNA template, which the L protein alone is unable to do (Mellon and Emerson, 1978).

The P in both rabies virions and virus-infected cells is present in two prominent forms, one that is hyperphosphorylated and the other that is hypophosphorylated. These two forms migrate with different mobilities in SDS-PAGE (Wunner *et al.*, 1985; Gupta *et al.*, 2000). Other forms of P, also detected in SDS-PAGE, may exist in rabies virus–infected cells. These will have fewer amino acids than P, the result of N-terminally truncated products due to translation initiation at internal AUG codons located in-frame within the P mRNA (Conzelmann *et al.*, 1990; Fu *et al.*, 1994; Chenik *et al.*, 1995). The most hydrophilic and conserved region of P is located in the center of the sequence between amino acids 139 and 170, which is where one might predict most of the phosphate acceptor amino acids to be located (Conzelmann *et al.*, 1990). This is in contrast, however, to VSV P, where the highest degree of hydrophilicity and most of the phosphate residues are found in the N-terminal portion (between amino acids 35 and 106) of the protein (Bell and Prevec, 1985; Hsu and Kingsbury, 1985). Interestingly, the center region of the rabies virus P is not the region where most residues are phosphorylated. Recent studies investigating different protein kinases present in a cell extract from rat brain have shown that rabies virus P is phosphorylated in the N-terminal portion by two distinct types of protein kinases, one of which is a unique heparin-sensitive protein kinase (Gupta *et al.*, 2000). This unique 71-kDa kinase, designated *rabies virus protein kinase* (RVPK), phosphorylates recombinant P (36 kDa, expressed in *Escherichia coli*) at serine 63 and serine 64 (CVS strain) and alters its mobility in SDS-PAGE to migrate more slowly, as a protein of 40 kDa. The other phosphorylating enzyme is protein kinase C, which has several isomers (PKCα, β, χ, and δ). In contrast to the RVPK, phosphorylation of P by the PKC isoforms, dominated by PKCγ activity, did not alter the migration of P in SDS-PAGE (Gupta *et al.*, 2000). On analyzing the protein kinase activity in rabies virions for the presence of these two types of enzymes, it was concluded the RVPK is selectively packaged in mature rabies virions along with a smaller amount of the predominant PKCγ isoform as the rabies virion–associated protein kinases (Gupta *et al.*, 2000).

In accordance with the multifunctional role of rabies virus P, like the P molecules in other *Monegavirales* viruses, its cofunction with the N and L is mediated by domains of P that specifically interact with each protein. As mentioned previously, nascent rabies virus P binds to nascent soluble N and maintains N in a competent form for RNA encapsidation. Recent findings indicate that P binds to the C-terminal part of N in the RNA–N complex (Schoehn *et al.*, 2001). Using the method of deletion mutant analysis to map the region(s) of the rabies virus P that binds to N, at least two independent N-binding sites were found on P (Fu *et al.*, 1994; Chenik *et al.*, 1994). One site is located within the C-terminal 30 amino acids of P and another in the N-terminal portion of the protein between amino acids 69 and 177 (Chenik *et al.*, 1994). Depending on whether the two proteins are synthesized simultaneously, mimicking the *in vivo* situation, or synthesized separately and then mixed together, the two proteins interact in a manner that is mutually independent (Fu *et al.*, 1994). For example, when the two proteins are synthesized simultaneously, P mutants with C-terminal deletions of up to 166 amino acids still form complexes with N, indicating that the N-terminal region of P is involved in the interaction. In a contrasting manner, when the two proteins are synthesized individually and then mixed together, deletions of more than 47 amino acids from the C terminus of the P fail to bind to the N (Fu *et al.*, 1994). This demonstrates two points. The first point is that the P molecule has a C-terminal binding site for N (between amino acids 267 and 297) that is used when the two proteins are presynthesized and then mixed together. The second point is that the initial interaction of the two proteins, involving the N-terminal region of P binding to N, is linked directly and immediately to the simultaneous synthesis of the two proteins *in vitro*, mimicking the *in vivo* situation. That is, when P molecules with N-terminal deletions of up to 68 amino acids are synthesized simultaneously with N, binding to N occurs (Chenik *et al.*, 1994), but with less efficiency compared with full-length P binding to N (Fu *et al.*, 1994). When the two proteins are synthesized separately and then mixed, P molecules with N-terminal deletions bind to N with equal efficiency (Fu *et al.*, 1994). This suggests that P molecules with N-terminal deletions are able to bind to N as well as full-length P via the C-terminal binding site on P or via a binding site for N that is located further downstream from amino acid 69, or both. One study has mapped the N-terminal binding site on P between amino acids 69 and 177 (Chenik *et al.*, 1994). Together these findings suggest that P molecules use the two binding sites to interact with N, but at different times and perhaps for different purposes. The interaction involving the N-terminal binding site of P requires that P interacts with N soon after the two proteins are synthesized *in vivo* but that it may compete with another molecule that interacts with N independently. The other interacting molecular species that competes for the binding site on N might be endogenous RNA. This dual-binding-site model that depicts the P associating with N reflects how the P may play a regulatory role in viral RNA transcription and replication.

Once bound to the RNA–N template in progeny RNP formation, the P is required to bind L to produce a virus-encoded RNA–polymerase complex that is fully active (Chenik *et al.*, 1998). The P subunit in the P–L complex has a major binding site for L protein within the first 19 amino acids of P (Chenik *et al.*, 1998). This is in agreement with the model that suggests that the L binding site resides in the negatively charged N terminus of the VSV P, although another region also has been shown to contribute to L binding (Takacs and Banerjee, 1995). Unlike the P of VSV, the rabies virus P does not appear to be required for L stabilization. The P is able to oligomerize (form complexes) with itself, although it is not entirely clear whether trimers or tetramers, or both, are formed and which of these oligomers is necessary for binding to L (Gao *et al.*, 1996; Spadafora *et al.*, 1996; Gigant *et al.*, 2000). The oligomeric forms of rabies virus P coexist in the cytoplasm in equilibrium with the monomer species. Like the P of Sendai virus, a paramyxovirus, oligomerization of rabies virus P does not require phosphorylation nor is the N-terminal domain (first 52 amino acids) necessary for oligomerization or binding to the N–RNA template (Curran *et al.*, 1995; Tarbouriech *et al.*, 2000; Gigant *et al.*, 2000). This is in contrast to the P of VSV, which requires phosphorylation for oligomer formation to be fully active and necessary for binding both to L protein and to the RNA template (Gao *et al.*, 1996).

Mention of other protein–protein interactions that involve the rabies virus P begins to address the question of whether rabies virus proteins specifically interact with cellular factors (i.e., proteins) beside the host cell receptor to influence or help regulate virus tropism and cell-to-cell spread. Using the yeast two-hybrid approach to identify interactive cellular factors, the cytoplasmic dynein light chain (LC8), an 89-amino-acid protein (10 kDa), was found to interact strongly with the P of rabies virus and Mokola virus (Jacob *et al.*, 2000; Raux *et al.*, 2000). In both studies, the P domain that interacts with dynein LC8 was mapped to the N-terminal half of the P; one of them mapped the interactive site to within amino acids 138–172 in the P (Raux *et al.*, 2000). Of particular interest, with regard to the manner in which rabies virus spreads along neurons *in vivo*, often over long distances, is the manner in which dynein LC8 might facilitate this movement. Dynein

LC8, as a part of cytoplasmic dynein and myosin V, participates in the myosin V complex, a microtubule-associated motor protein complex that is implicated in the actin-based motor transport of ER vesicles in brain neurons (Jacob *et al.*, 2000). Thus the retrograde axonal transport of uncoated nucleocapsids along axons to the perikaryon and transport of nascent RNP from the perikaryon along dendrites to the next neuron might be mediated by the P protein–dynein LC8 complex in transporting the viral RNP along the microtubule network (Ceccaldi *et al.*, 1989).

C. Virion-Associated RNA Polymerase or Large Protein (L)

The L in rabies virus is encoded in the fifth gene, which comprises more than half (54%) of the coding potential of the rabies virus genome. The L contains 2142 and 2127 amino acids in the PV and SAD-B19 strains of rabies virus, respectively, and 2127 amino acids in MOKV (244 kDa). The L is the catalytic component of the polymerase complex and along with the noncatalytic cofactor P is responsible for the majority of enzymatic activities involved in viral RNA transcription and replication. Many of the activities of this multifunctional enzyme have been demonstrated in genetic and biochemical studies with VSV, the prototype virus and model for studying the virion-associated RNA polymerase of negative-strand RNA viruses (Banerjee and Chattopadhyay, 1990). The viral RNA–polymerase plays a unique role at the start of infection by initiating the primary transcription of the genome RNA once the NC core is released into the cytoplasm of the infected cell. The enzymatic steps of transcription include initiation and elongation of the Le^+ RNA and mRNA transcripts as well as cotranscriptional modifications of the mRNAs that include 5′ capping, methylation, and 3′ polyadenylation. Comparisons of L sequences from different *Mononegavirales* viruses have helped to map the functionally homologous and unique sequences in attempts to locate the ascribed enzyme activities (Tordo *et al.*, 1988; Poch *et al.*, 1990; Barik *et al.*, 1990). One of the main features of L that comes out of the sequence comparison is that the domains of sequence homology are not distributed randomly along the protein. Some domains are highly conserved, with the high proportion of amino acids either strictly or conservatively maintained in identical positions, whereas other domains are more variable, consistent with the multifunctional nature of L (Tordo *et al.*, 1988; Poch *et al.*, 1990; Banerjee and Chattopadhyay, 1990). Four motifs, labeled A through D, in the central part of the rabies virus L, between residues 530 and 1177 and between residues 532 and 1201 in the VSV L, represent regions of highest similarity (Tordo *et al.*, 1988; Poch *et al.*, 1989; Barik *et al.*, 1990). These motifs, which are thought to constitute the polymerase module of L, maintain the same linear arrangement and location in all viral RNA-dependent RNA and DNA polymerases (Poch *et al.*, 1990; Barik *et al.*, 1990; Delarue *et al.*, 1990). Among the conserved sequences in these four motifs is the tri-amino acid core sequence GDN (standing for glycine, aspartic acid, and asparagine) in motif C, which is extensively conserved in all nonsegmented negative-strand RNA viruses (Poch *et al.*, 1989). A recent study has shown that not only the GDN core sequence but also specific amino acids downstream from the core sequence are crucial for the maintenance of polymerase activity that catalyzes the polymerization of nucleotides (Schnell and Conzelmann, 1995). In addition, at least two other sequences between amino acid residues 754–778 and 1332–1351 in the VSV L have been identified as consensus sites for binding and utilization of ATP, similar to those found in cellular kinases (Barik *et al.*, 1990; Canter *et al.*, 1993). Three essential activities encoded by L are involved in the binding and utilization of ATP. These are (1) the transcriptional activity that requires binding to substrate ribonucleoside triphosphates (rNTPs), (2) polyadenylation, and (3) protein kinase activity for specific phosphorylation of the P in transcriptional activation (Sanchez *et al.*, 1985; Chattopadhyay and Banerjee, 1987). Many of the putative functions of this multifunctional protein, including mRNA capping, methylation, and polyadenylation, remain to be delineated and mapped within the L of rabies virus. The process of mapping active sites in the rabies virus L using the mutational and deletion approach will be helped considerably now that it is feasible to apply the powerful technique of reverse genetics (Conzelmann and Schnell, 1994; Schnell *et al.*, 1994; Schnell and Conzelmann, 1995). With reverse genetics, it is possible to express the rabies virus L with amino acid deletions and point mutations introduced into the cDNA of the L gene to map the locations in L that have functional activities. Similarly, the role of the cofactor P in the RNA–polymerase complex can be better defined using reverse genetics. Since the L protein relies exclusively on its interaction with the phosphorylated P to be fully active, the major question, does the P complement any of the specific enzymatic functions of L or does the P function solely as a regulatory protein in the RNA transcription and replication process? For example, does the cofactor P unwind the RNA–N complex of the NC to facilitate entry as well as movement of L on the genome template (De and Banerjee, 1985)? The cooperative function of the noncatalytic cofactor P and catalytic L in the polymerase complex is clearly intriguing and of critical importance to warrant further examination.

D. Matrix Protein (M)

The M of rabies virus and of MOKV is the smallest of the virion proteins. It contains 202 amino acids (25 kDa) (Rayssiguier *et al.*, 1986; Todo *et al.*, 1986; Conzelmann *et al.*, 1990; Hiramatsu *et al.*, 1993; Bourhy *et al.*, 1993a; Gould *et al.*, 1998). The M forms a sheath around the RNP core in virion assembly, producing the skeleton structure of the virion. It, too, is a multifunctional protein that interacts with viral proteins and protein components of cellular membranes. The functional properties of M include downregulation of viral RNA transcription, condensation of helical NC cores into tight coils, association with membrane bilayers, and involvement in the cytopathogenesis of virus-infected cells (see references in Ito *et al.*, 1996) The N-terminal region of the rabies virus M has a high content of charged amino acids and proline residues (Poch *et al.*, 1988), similar to the M of VSV (Rose and Gallione, 1981) and paramyxoviruses (Chambers *et al.*, 1986). It would appear from anti-M MAb blocking studies that the N terminus of rabies virus M plays a critical role in the regulation of RNA transcription (Ito *et al.*, 1996). The M of VSV is a potent inhibitor of RNA transcription, shutting down transcription of both viral genes and independently cellular genes of the infected cell by inhibiting host RNA polymerase (Ferran and Lucas-Lenard, 1997; Ahmed and Lyles, 1998). The ability of the VSV M to inhibit host transcription correlates with the cell rounding cytopathic effect observed in VSV-infected cells in culture (Blondel *et al.*, 1990; Simon *et al.*, 1990). However, a similar cytopathic effect is not as prominent in rabies virus–infected cultures, suggesting that the rabies virus M may not play the same role or perhaps have the same specificity for cellular factors to inhibit cellular RNA transcription (Lyles and McKenzie, 1997). The central portion contains a hydrophobic domain (residues 89–107) that is presumed to interact with membrane lipids (Capone and Ghosh, 1984; Tordo *et al.*, 1986b). The M of rabies virus is also palmitoylated, although the site(s) of the presumed cysteine residue(s) for palmitoylation has not been identified (Gaudin *et al.*, 1991).

The M binds to and condenses the nascent NC core into a tightly coiled, helical ribonucleocapsid-M protein (the skeleton) complex. Approximately 1200 to 1500 copies of M molecules bind to rabies virus RNP core. At the same time M binds to the RNP structure, it mediates binding of the viral core structure to the host membrane at the marginal region of the cytoplasm, where it initiates rabies virus budding from the cell plasma membrane (Mebatsion *et al.*, 1999). The M gives the virion its characteristic bullet-like shape, regardless of whether its location is within the RNP core or on the external surface of the core (Barge *et al.*, 1993; Lyles *et al.*, 1996). The mechanism by which M mediates the budding of virus off the cell membrane appears to be associated with a proline-rich (PPPY, PP*x*Y or PY) domain located at residues 35–38 within the highly conserved 14-amino-acid sequence near the N terminus of the rabies virus M (Harty *et al.*, 1999). A corresponding proline-rich motif (in the single-letter code, P is proline and Y is tyrosine, and *x* is any amino acid) is found in the M of VSV (Gill and Banerjee, 1986), as well as in the M of Ebola and Marburg viruses (Sanchez *et al.*, 1993). The PY motif is very similar to the late budding domain identified in viral proteins such as the Gag protein p2b of Rous sarcoma virus (Wills *et al.*, 1994) and the p6 Gag protein in human immunodeficiency virus (Gottlinger *et al.*, 1991), both of which are associated with virus budding. The unique function of the PY motif is that it interacts with a WW domain, 38–40 amino acids long with two highly conserved tryptophans (in single-letter code, tryptophan is W) spaced 20–22 amino acids apart, found in a wide range of cellular proteins. Some of the WW domain-containing proteins are involved in cytoskeletal formation, whereas others are involved in signal transduction and gene regulation (Sudol, 1996). It is therefore likely that the rabies virus M involves cellular proteins in the release (exocytosis) of rabies virions from the cell (Harty *et al.*, 1999; Craven *et al.*, 1999; Jayakar *et al.*, 2000). Although the exocytotic release of virus particles requires the M in RNP–M skeletons, the efficiency of virus budding is enhanced greatly by the interaction of the RNP–M complex with the envelope G (Mebatsion *et al.*, 1996). Increased virion production as a result of direct interaction of the cytoplasmic domain of the transmembrane spike G and the viral RNP–M core suggests that a concerted action of both core and spike proteins is necessary for efficient recovery of virions. However, the interaction of M with the cytoplasmic domain of G does not need to be optimal; i.e., the interaction is sufficient if the G of different viruses are substituted for the homologous G in budding virions (Mebatsion *et al.*, 1995; Morimoto *et al.*, 2000).

E. Glycoprotein (G)

The mature G of all rabies virus strains examined is a 505-amino-acid (~65 kDa) type I membrane glycoprotein (there are 503 amino acids in MOKV G) translated from a G–mRNA transcript that encodes 524 amino acids (522 amino acids from MOKV G–mRNA) (Benmansour *et al.*, 1992; Bourhy *et al.*, 1993). The first 19 amino acids represent the signal peptide (SP) that provides the membrane insertion signal, which transports the nascent protein into the membranes of the rough ER–Golgi–plasma membrane pathway before it is cleaved from the N terminus of the G molecule in the Golgi apparatus. The G, which forms the trimeric spikes that extend 8.3 nm from the virus surface, is the only surface protein of the virion. Each G of the spike is anchored in the viral envelope by a 22-amino-acid transmembrane (TM) domain located between residues 439 and 461 (Gaudin *et al.*, 1992). The C-terminal portion of G, the cytoplasmic domain (CD), extends from under the viral envelope to the cytoplasm of the infected cell, where it interacts with M of the skeleton particle to complete the virion assembly. The ectodomain of G (residues 1–439), that portion which extends outward on the virion surface, is the business end of the molecule. It is responsible for virus interaction of rabies virus with its cellular binding sites (receptors) and therefore is important in viral pathogenesis. It is critical to the host immune response to rabies virus infection because it is responsible for the induction of VNA as well as being the target of VNA, and it is a target for virus-specific helper and cytotoxic T cells.

Rabies virus G is a fusion protein that mediates virus entry into host cells. Following binding to its receptor(s) on target host cells, the virus is internalized, and the G spike fuses in a low-pH-dependent process with the endosomal membranes as it enters the endosome. In this process, the G goes through significant and critical conformational change whereby it assumes at least three structurally distinct conformational states (Gaudin *et al.*, 1991b, 1993, 1995a, 1999). Prior to virus binding to the cellular receptor, the G on the virion surface is in its native state. After the virus attaches to the receptor and the virus is internalized, the G is activated to a hydrophobic state, enabling it to interact with the hydrophobic endosomal membrane. On entering the endosomal compartment and low-pH environment of the cellular compartment, the fusion capacity of the G is activated via a major structural change in the G that exposes the fusion domain, which interacts with and destabilizes one or both of the participating membranes (Gaudin *et al.*, 1995a). The low-pH-induced fusion domain, which is thought to lie between amino acids 102 and 179 (Gaudin *et al.*, 1995a), is not to be confused with the proposed fusogenic domain on the rabies virus G that appears to be involved in pH-independent (neutral pH) cell fusion (Morimoto *et al.*, 1992). The pH for endosomal membrane fusion in the viral entry process is 6.2–6.3. After fusion, the G assumes a reversible fusion-inactive conformation, which makes the G monomer appear longer than the native conformation and assume selective antigenic distinctions (Gaudin *et al.*, 1993). The fusion-inactivated G, which is no longer relevant to the fusion process, is highly sensitive to cellular proteases and appears to be in a dynamic equilibrium with the native G that is regulated by lowering and raising the pH (Gaudin *et al.*, 1991b, 1996). Interestingly, the fusion-inactive conformation serves the G in another capacity. During nascent viral protein synthesis, the G assumes an inactive state–like conformation, which protects the G posttranslationally from fusing with the acid nature of Golgi vesicles while it is transported through the Golgi stacks to the cell surface, where it acquires its native conformation and structure (Gaudin *et al.*, 1995b).

Mutations in the rabies virus G play a critical role in viral pathogenesis. Amino acid Arg-333 (or Lys-333) in the wild-type (normal) G is responsible for the virulence phenotype of rabies virus. Virus variants that have a glutamine (Gln), isoleucine (Ile), glycine (Gly), methionine (Met), or serine (Ser) substituted for Arg-333 in the G express a phenotype that is either less pathogenic or avirulent in comparison with the parental wild-type virus when inoculated intracerebrally into adult immunocompetent mice (Dietzschold *et al.*, 1983b; Seif *et al.*, 1985; Tuffereau *et al.*, 1989). It is remarkable that this single amino acid substitution (e.g., Gln for Arg-333) can affect the rate of virus spread from cell to cell (Dietzschold *et al.*, 1985) as well as the neuronal pathway(s) that the virus takes to reach the CNS (Kucera *et al.*, 1985). Interestingly, even the transsynaptic spread of the virus requires the envelope spike G, again showing the critical role of the G in viral pathogenesis (Etessami *et al.*, 2000).

It is to the advantage of rabies virus that it is capable of spreading from cell to cell in tissue culture without budding into the culture medium, where it would be neutralized in the presence of antirabies VNA (Dietzschold *et al.*, 1985). While the precise mechanism of direct cell-to-cell spread of virus is not clear, the observation that virus is internalized by a cell without being compromised, i.e., prevented from attaching to the cell surface receptor, points to importance of the fusion function of the G in virus spread. When rabies virus of the virulent phenotype was used to infect cultures of neuroblastoma (NA) cells and baby hamster kidney (BHK) cells in the presence of antirabies VNA, the virus spread throughout the NA cell culture, whereas the avirulent virus failed to spread. The two viruses spread cell to cell equally well in the BHK cell culture (Dietzschold *et al.*, 1985). In many ways, the pathogenic and avirulent viruses behaved *in vitro* in a manner that reflects their ability to spread *in vivo* after direct inoculation into the brain of the mouse (Dietzschold *et al.*, 1985). *In vivo*, the pathogenic virus spreads more rapidly in the CNS and infects more neurons than the avirulent virus. Could it be that the fusion function of the G was altered due to the amino acid substitution at position 333? Others have suggested, based on observations in NA and BHK cells, both of which constitutively expressed the G of rabies virus, that only the pathogenic type G (with arginine in position 333) demonstrated an ability to induce syncytium formation (cell–cell fusion) at neutral pH (pH-independent fusion) in the NA cell culture. Thus the G with arginine in position 333 without other viral proteins, as in the pathogenic virus, and not the G with glutamine in position 333 (as in the avirulent virus) has the ability to mediate virus spread among neuronal cells. Moreover, since some Gln-333 variants can kill adult immunocompetent mice when infected by stereotaxic inoculation (Yang and Jackson, 1992), it appears that the G Arg-333 is essential not only for the neuropathogenicity but also for the axonal/transsynaptic spread of the virus *in vivo*. It is apparent also that the pH-independent cell fusion induced by the rabies virus G may involve the interaction of one or more neuronal cell–specific host cell factors, which are expressed in the NA cells but not in BHK-21 cells. Another difference between the pathogenic and avirulent viruses is the ability of fixed rabies virus strains of the pathogenic phenotype to invade the CNS from a peripheral site (Kucera *et al.*, 1985; Etassami *et al.*, 2000). In these studies it was suggested that the selection of different neuronal pathways to the brain from a peripheral site of inoculation might account for the pathogenic virus reaching the brain faster than the avirulent phenotype. Yet another study shows that the difference is not in the rate and pathway of virus spread to the brain after peripheral inoculation but rather that the pathogenic virus infected many more neurons than did the avirulent virus (Jackson, 1991). In such cases, the pathogenic virus may use different sites for entry to the CNS, and the avirulent virus will fail to penetrate some of the same sites because they involve use of different receptors that the avirulent virus can no longer recognize. Since it is possible in the research efforts so far that all the rabies virus–specific receptors have not been identified or proven biologically, one can only speculate on the reasons why virus of the avirulent phenotype is sometimes unsuccessful or inefficient in spreading to the CNS.

The G of rabies virus is also of major importance immunologically for the induction of the host immune response against virus infection, and because of this, it is probably the most extensively studied rabies virus antigen (Dietzschold et al., 1988; Benmansour et al., 1991). The G induces conformational and linear epitope-specific VNA and stimulates helper as well as cytotoxic T-cell activity. Consequently, studies to functionally map and then physically locate specific epitopes within antigenic domains for binding antibody and for binding T cells to the rabies virus G have been an ongoing and extensive process. At least eight antigenic sites (I–VI, "a", and Gl) have been located on the ectodomain (amino acid residues 1–439) of the G of different virus strains (Lafon et al., 1984; Prehaud et al., 1988; Dietzschold et al., 1988, 1990; Benmansour et al., 1991). Sites I, III, VI, and "a" involve the amino acids located at positions 231, 330–338, 264, and 342, respectively. Site II is a discontinuous antigenic site that involves two separate stretches of amino acids in position 34–42 and 198–200 that presumably are linked by a disulfide bridge (Prehaud et al., 1988). Sites VI and G1 are defined as linear or nonconformational, whereas the others are conformational and readily destroyed on denaturation. Epitopes recognized by T cells have been mapped on the G using chemically cleaved and synthetic peptides or T-cell lines and clones derived from individuals immunized with rabies virus vaccine (Macfarlan et al., 1984, 1986; Celis et al., 1988a,b). These fine mapping studies have given some limited insight into the structue of the various functional domains on the G of rabies virus. To gain a fuller understanding of the function of the rabies virus G, it is necessary to determine its overall conformation and, ultimately its three-dimensional structure. However, crystallization of viral membrane glycoproteins is difficult, due to the TM domain and to oligosaccharide microheterogeneity, and attempts at crystallization of the rabies virus G have so far not been successful.

REFERENCES

Abraham, G., and Banerjee, A. K. (1976). Sequential transcription of the genes of vesicular stomatitis virus. *Proc. Natl. Acad. Sci. USA* **73**, 1504–1508.

Ackerman, H.-W., and Berthiaume, L. (1995). Rhabdoviridae. In *Atlas of Virus Diagrams*, pp. 54–56. CRC Press, Boca Raton, FL.

Ahmed, M., and Lyles, D. S. (1998). Effect of vesicular stomatitis virus matrix protein on transcription directed by host RNA polymerases I, II, and III. *J. Virol.* **72**, 8413–8419.

Anilionis, A., Wunner, W. H., and Curtis, P. J. (1981). Structure of the glycoprotein gene in rabies virus. *Nature* **294**, 275–278.

Ball, L. A., and Wertz, G. W. (1981). VSV RNA synthesis: How can you be positive? *Cell* **26**, 143–144.

Ball, L. A., and White, C. N. (1976). Order of transcription of genes of vesicular stomatitis virus. *Proc. Natl. Acad. Sci. USA* **73**, 442–446.

Banerjee, A. K. (1987). Transcription and replication of rhabdoviruses. *Microbiol. Rev.* **51**, 68–87.

Banerjee, A. K., Abraham, G., and Colonno, R. J. (1977). Vesicular stomatitis virus: Mode of transcription *J. Gen. Virol.* **34**, 1–8.

Banerjee, A. K., and Barik, S. (1992). Gene expression of vesicular stomatitis virus genome RNA. *Virology* **188**, 417–428.

Banerjee, A. K., and Chattopadhyay, D. (1990). Structure and function of the RNA polymerase of vesicular stomatitis virus. *Adv. Virus Res.* **38**, 99–124.

Barge, A., Gaudin, Y., Coulon, P., and Ruigrok, R. W. H. (1993). Vesicular stomatitis virus M protein may be inside the ribonucleoprotein coil. *J. Virol.* **67**, 7246–7253.

Barik, S., Rud, E. W., Luk, D., Banerjee, A. K., and Kang, C. Y. (1990). Nucleotide sequence analysis of the L gene of vesicular stomatitis virus (New Jersey serotype): Identification of conserved domains in L proteins of nonsegmented negative-strand RNA viruses. *Virology* **175**, 332–337.

Barr, J. N., Whelan, S. P., and Wertz, G. W. (1997a). *cis*-Acting signals involved in termination of vesicular stomatitis virus mRNA synthesis include the conserved AUAC and the U7 signal for polyadenylation. *J. Virol.* **71**, 8718–8725.

Barr, J. N., Whelan, S. P., and Wertz, G. W. (1997b). Role of intergenic dinucleotide in vesicular stomatitis virus RNA transcription. *J. Virol.* **71**, 1794–1801.

Bell, J. C., and Prevec, L. (1985). Phosphorylation sites on phosphoprotein NS of vesicular stomatitis virus. *J. Virol.* **54**, 697–702.

Benmansour, A., Brahimi, M., Tuffereau, C., Coulon, P., Lafay, F., and Flamand, A. (1992). Rapid sequence evolution of street rabies glycoprotein is related to the highly heterogeneous nature of the viral population. *Virology* **187**, 33–45.

Benmansour, A., Leblois, H., Coulon, P., Tuffereau, C., Gaudin, Y., and Flamand, A. (1991). Antigenicity of rabies virus glycoprotein. *J. Virol.* **65**, 4198–4203.

Blondel, D., Harmison, G. G., and Schubert, M. (1990). Role of matrix protein in cytopathogenesis of vesicular stomatitis virus. *J. Virol.* **64**, 1716–1725.

Blough, H. A., Tiffany, J. M., and Aaslestad, H. G. (1977). Lipids of rabies virus in BHK-21 cell membranes. *J. Virol.* **21**, 950–955.

Blumberg, B. M., Giorgi, C., and Kolakofsky, D. (1983). N protein of vesicular stomatitis virus selectively encapsidates leader RNA *in vitro*. *Cell* **32**, 559–567.

Boulger, L. R., and Porterfield, J. S. (1958). Isolation of a virus from Nigerian fruit bats. *Trans. R. Soc. Trop. Med. Hyg.* **52**, 421–424.

Bourhy, H., Kissi, B., Lafon, M., Sacramento, D., and Tordo, N. (1992). Antigenic and molecular characterization of bat rabies virus in Europe. *J. Clin. Microbiol.* **30**, 2419–2426.

Bourhy, H., Kissi, B., and Tordo, N. (1993a). Molecular diversity of the *Lyssavirus* genus. *Virology* **194**, 70–81.

Bourhy, H., Kissi, B., and Tordo, N. (1993b). Taxonomy and evolutionary studies on lyssaviruses with special reference to Africa. *Onderstepoort J. Vet. Res.* **60**, 277–282.

Bourhy, H., Tordo, N., Lafon, M., and Sureau, P. (1989). Complete cloning and molecular organization of a rabies-related virus, Mokola virus. *J. Gen. Virol.* **70**, 2063–2074.

Bracci, L., Antoni, G., Cusi, M. G., Lozzi, L., Niccolai, N., Petreni, S., Rustici, M., Santucci, A., Soldani, P., Valensin, P. E., and Neri, P. (1988). Antipeptide monoclonal antibodies inhibit the binding of rabies virus glycoprotein and alpha-bungerotoxin to the nicotinic acetylcholine receptor. *Mol. Immunol.* **25**, 881–888.

Bracho, M. A., Moya, A., and Barrio, E. (1998). Contribution of the polymerase-induced errors to the estimation of RNA virus diversity. *J. Gen. Virol.* **79**, 2921–2928.

Broughan, J. H., and Wunner, W. H. (1995). Characterization of protein involvement in rabies virus binding to BHK-21 cells. *Arch. Virol.* **140**, 75–93.

Buchholz, C. J., Retzler, C., Homann, H. E., and Neubert, W. J. (1994). The carboxy-terminal domain of Sendai virus nucleocapsid protein is involved in complex formation between phosphoprotein and nucleocapsid-like particles. *Virology* **204**, 770–776.

Burger, S. R., Remaley, A. T., Danley, J. M., Moore, J., Muschel, R. J., Wunner, W. H., and Spitalnik, S. L. (1991). Stable expression of rabies virus glycoprotein in Chinese hamster ovary cells. *J. Gen. Virol.* **72**, 359–367.

Burrage, T. G., Tignor, G. H., Hawrot, E., Smith, A. L., and Lentz, T. L. (1982). Co-localization of rabies virus and regions of high density acetylcholine receptors. *J. Cell. Biol.* **95**, 620–630.

Burrage, T. G., Tignor, G. H., and Smith, A. L. (1985). Rabies virus binding at neuromuscular junctions. *Virus Res.* **2**, 273–289.

Calain, P., and Roux, L. (1995). Functional characterization of the genome and antigenome promoters of Sendai virus. *Virology* **212**, 163–173.

Canter, D. M., Jackson, R. L., and Perrault, J. (1993). Faithful and efficient *in vitro* reconstitution of vesicular stomatitis virus transcription using plasmid-encoded L and P proteins. *Virology* **194**, 518–529.

Capone, J., and Ghosh, H. P. (1984). Association of the nucleocapsid protein N of vesicular stomatitis virus with phospholipid vesicles containing the matrix protein M. *Can. J. Biochem. Cell. Biol.* **62**, 153–158.

Carroll, A. R., and Wagner, R. R. (1979). Role of the membrane (M) protein in endogenous inhibition of *in vitro* transcription by vesicular stomatitis virus. *J. Virol.* **29**, 134–142.

Ceccaldi, P. E., Gillet, J. P., and Tsiang, H. (1989). Inhibition of the transport of rabies virus in the central nervous system. *J. Neuropathol. Exp. Neurol.* **48**, 620–630.

Celis, E., Karr, R. W., Dietzschold, B., Wunner, W. H., and Koprowski, H. (1988a). Genetic restriction and fine specificity of human T cell clones reactive with rabies virus. *J. Immunol.* **141**, 2721–2728.

Celis, E., Ou, D., Dietzschold, B., and Koprowski, H. (1988b). Recognition of rabies and rabies-related viruses by T cells derived from human vaccine recipients. *J. Virol.* **62**, 3128–3134.

Chambers, P., Millar, N. S., Platt, S. G., and Emmerson, P. T. (1986). Nucleotide sequence of the gene encoding the matrix protein of Newcastle disease virus. *Nucl. Acids Res.* **14**, 9051–9061.

Charlton, K. M., and Casey, G. A. (1979). Experimental rabies in skunks: Immunofluorescence, light and electron microscopic studies. *Lab. Invest.* **41**, 36–41.

Chenik, M., Chebli, K., and Blondel, D. (1995). Translation initiation at alternate in-frame AUG codons in the rabies virus phosphoprotein mRNA is mediated by a ribosomal leaky scanning mechanism. *J. Virol.* **69**, 707–712.

Chenik, M., Chebli, K., Gaudin, Y., and Blondel, D. (1994). *In vivo* interaction of rabies virus phosphoprotein (P) and nucleoprotein (N), existence of two N binding sites on P protein. *J. Gen. Virol.* **75**, 2889–2896.

Chenik, M., Schnell, M., Conzelmann, K. K., and Blondel, D. (1998). Mapping the interacting domain between rabies virus polymerase and phosphoprotein. *J. Virol.* **72**, 1925–1930.

Clark, H. F., Parks, N. F., and Wunner, W. H. (1981). Defective interfering particles of fixed rabies viruses: Lack of correlation with attenuation or auto-interference in mice. *J. Gen. Virol.* **52**, 245–248.

Clinton, G. M., and Huang, A. S. (1981). Distribution of phosphorserine, phosphothreonine and phosphotyrosine in proteins of vesicular stomatitis virus. *Virology* **108**, 510–514.

Clinton, G. M., Little, S. P., Hagen, F. S., and Huang, A. S. (1978). The matrix (M) protein of vesicular stomatitis virus regulates transcription. *Cell* **15**, 1455–1462.

Coll, J. M. (1995). The glycoprotein G of rhabdoviruses: Brief review. *Arch. Virol.* **140**, 827–851.

Colonno, R. J., and Banerjee, A. K. (1978). Complete nucleotide sequence of the leader RNA synthesized *in vitro* by vesicular stomatitis virus. *Cell* **15**, 93–101.

Conti, C., Hauttecoueur, B., Morelec, M. J., Bizzini, B., Orsi, N., and Tsiang, H. (1988). Inhibition of rabies virus infection by soluble membrane fraction from the rat central nervous system. *Arch. Virol.* **98**, 73–86.

Conti, C., Superti, F., and Tsiang, H. (1986). Membrane carbohydrate requirement for rabies virus binding to chicken embryo–related cells. *Intervirology* **26**, 164–168.

Conzelmann, K.-K., Cox, J. H., Schneider, L. G., and Thiel, H.-J.(1990). Molecular cloning and complete nucleotide sequence of the attenuated rabies virus SAD B19. *Virology* **175**, 485–499.

Conzelmann, K.-K., and Schnell, M. (1994). Rescue of synthetic genomic RNA analogs of rabies virus by plasmid-encoded proteins. *J. Virol.* **68**, 713–719.

Coulon, P., Derbin, C., Kucera, P., Lafay, F., Prehaud, C., and Flamand, A. (1989). Invasion of the peripheral nervous systems of adult mice by the CVS strain of rabies virus and its avirulent derivative AvOl. *J. Virol.* **63**, 3550–3554.

Coulon, P., Rollin, P., and Flamand, A. (1983). Molecular basis of rabies virulence: II. Identification of a site on the CVS glycoprotein associated with virulence. *J. Gen. Virol.* **64**, 693–696.

Cox, J. H., Dietzschold, B., and Schneider, L. G. (1977). Rabies virus glycoprotein: II. Biological and serological characterization. *Infect. Immun.* **16**, 754–759.

Cox, J. H., Dietzschold, B., Weiland, F., and Schneider, L. G. (1980). Preparation and characterization of rabies virus hemagglutinin. *Infect. Immun.* **30**, 572–577.

Craven, R. C., Harty, R. N., Paragas, J., Palese, P., and Wills, J. W. (1999). Late domain function identified I the vesicular stomatitis virus M protein by use of rhabdovirus-retrovirus chimeras. *J. Virol.* **73**, 3359–3365.

Curran, J., Boeck, R., Lin-Marq, N., Lupas, A., and Koladofsky, D. (1995). Paramyxovirus phosphoproteins form homotrimers as determined by an epitope dilution assay, via predicted coiled coils. *Virology* **214**, 139–149.

Davies, M. C., Englert, M. E., Sharpless, G. R., and Cabasso, V. J. (1963). The electron microscopy of rabies virus in cultures of chicken embryo tissues. *Virology* **21**, 642–651.

Davis, N. L., Arnheiter, H., and Wertz, G. W. (1986). Vesicular stomatitis virus N and NS proteins form multilple complexes. *J. Virol.* **59**, 751–754.

De, B. P., and Banerjee, A. K. (1985). Requirements and functions of vesicular stomatitis virus L and NS proteins in the transcription process *in vitro*. *Biochem. Biophys. Res. Commun.* **126**, 40–49.

De, B. P., Thornton, G. B., Luk, D., and Banerjee, A. K. (1982). Purified matrix protein of vesicular stomatitis virus blocks viral transcription *in vitro*. *Proc. Natl. Acad. Sci. USA* **79**, 7137–7141.

Delagneau, J.-F., Perrin, P., and Atanasiu, P. (1981). Structure of the rabies virus: Spatial relationships of the proteins G, M1, M2 and N. *Ann. Virol. (Inst Pasteur)* **132E**, 473–493.

Delarue, M., Poch, O., Tordo, N., Moras, D., and Argos, P. (1990). An attempt to unify the structure of polymerases. *Protein Eng.* **3**, 461–467.

Dietzschold, B. (1977). Oligosaccharides of the glycoprotein of rabies virus. *J. Virol.* **23**, 286–293.

Dietzschold, B., Cox, J. H., and Schneider, L. G. (1979). Rabies virus strains: A comparison study by polypeptide analysis of vaccine strains with different pathogenic patterns. *Virology* **98**, 63–75.

Dietzschold, B., Gore, M., Marchadier, D., Niu, H. S., Bunschoten, H. S., Otvos, L., Jr., Wunner, W. H., Ertl, H. C. J., Osterhous, A. D. M. E., and Koprowski, H. (1990). Structural and immunological characterization of a linear virus-neutralizing epitope of the rabies virus glycoprotein and its possible use in a synthetic vaccine. *J. Virol.* **64**, 3804–3809.

Dietzschold, B., Lafon, M., Wang, H., Otvos, L., Jr., Celis, E., Wunner, W. H., and Koprowski, H. (1987a). Localization and immunological characterization of antigenic domains of the rabies virus internal N and NS proteins. *Virus Res.* **8**, 103–125.

Dietzschold, B., Rupprecht, C. E., Tollis, M., Lafon, M., Mattei, J., Wiktor, T. J., and Koprowski, H. (1988). Antigenic diversity of the glycoprotein and nucleocapsid proteins of rabies and rabies-related viruses: Implications for epidemiology and control of rabies. *Rev. Infect. Dis.* **10**, S785–798.

Dietzschold, B., Wang, H., Rupprecht, C. E., Celis, E., Tollis, M., Ertl, H., Heber-Katz, E., and Koprowski, H. (1987b). Induction of protective immunity against rabies by immunization with rabies virus nucleoprotein. *Proc. Natl. Acad. Sci. USA* **84**, 9165–9169.

Dietzschold, B., Wiktor, T. J., Trojanowski, J. Q., Macfarlan, R. I., Wunner, W. H., Torres-Anjel, M. J., and Koprowski, H. (1985). Differences in cell-to-cell spread of pathogenic and apathogenic rabies virus *in vivo* and *in vitro*. *J. Virol.* **56**, 12–18.

Dietzschold, B., Wiktor, T. J., Wunner, W. H., and Koprowski, H. (1983a). Chemical and immunological analysis of the rabies virus glycoprotein. *Virology* **124**, 330–337.

Dietzschold, B., Wunner, W. H., Wiktor, T. J., Lopes, A. D., Lafon, M., Smith, C. L., and Koprowski, H. (1983b). Characterization of an antigenic determinant of the glycoprotein that correlates with pathogenicity of rabies virus. *Proc. Natl. Acad. Sci. USA* **80**, 70–74.

Domingo, E., Baranowski, E., Ruiz-Jarabo, C. M., Martin-Hernández, A. M., Sáiz, J. C., and Escarmis, C. (1998). Quasi-species structure and persistence of RNA viruses. *Emerg. Infect. Dis.* **4**, 521–527.

Domingo, E., and Holland, J. J. (1997). RNA virus mutations and fitness for survival. *Annu. Rev. Microbiol.* **5**, 151–178.

Egelman, E. H., Wu, S.-S., Amrien, M., Portner, A., and Murti, G. K. (1989). The Sendai virus nucleocapsid exists in at least four different helical states. *J. Virol.* **63**, 2233–2243.

Emerson, S. U. (1987). Transcription of vesicular stomatitis virus. In *The Rhabdoviruses*, R. R. Wagner (ed.), pp. 245–269. Plenum Press, New York.

Ertl, H. C. J., Dietzschold, B., Gore, M., Otvos, L., Larson, J. K., Wunner, W. H., and Koprowski, H. (1989). Induction of rabies virus-specific T-helper cells by synthetic peptides that carry dominant T-helper cell epitopes of the viral ribonucleoprotein. *J. Virol.* **63**, 2885–2892.

Ertl, H. C. J., Dietzschold, B., and Otvos, L., Jr. (1991). T-helper cell epitope of rabies virus nucleoprotein defined by tri- and tertrapeptids. *Eur. J. Immunol.* **21**, 1–10.

Etessami, R., Conzelmann, K.-K., Fadai-Ghotbi, B., Natelson, B., Tsiang, H., and Ceccaldi, P.-E. (2000). Spread and pathogenic characteristics of a G-deficeint rabies virus recombinant: An *in vitro* and *in vivo* study. *J. Gen. Virol.* **81**, 2147–2153.

Familusi, J. B., and Moore, D. L. (1972). Isolation of a rabies-related virus from the cerebrospinal fluid of a child with aseptic meningitis. *Afr. J. Med. Sci.* **3**, 93–96.

Familusi, J. B., Osunkoya, B. O., Moore, D. L., Kemp, G. E., and Fabiyi, A. (1972). A fatal human infection with Mokola virus. *Am. J. Trop. Med. Hyg.* **21**, 959–963.

Ferran, M. C., and Lucas-Lenard, J. M. (1997). The vesicular stomatitis virus matrix protein inhibits transcription form the human beta interferon promoter. *J. Virol.* **71**, 371–377.

Field, H., McCall, B., and Barrett, J. (1999). Australian bat lyssavirus infection in a captive juvenile black flying fox. *Emerg. Infect. Dis.* **5**, 438–440.

Finke, S., and Conzelmann, K.-K. (1997). Ambisense gene expression from recombinant rabies virus: Random packaging of positive- and negative-strand ribonucleoprotein complexes into rabies virions *J. Virol.* **71**, 7281–7288.

Flamand, A., Raux, H., Gaudin, Y., and Ruigrok, R. W. H. (1993). Mechanisms of rabies virus neutralization. *Virology* **194**, 302–313.

Flamand, A., Wiktor, T. J., and Koprowski, H. (1980a). Use of hybridoma monoclonal antibodies in the detection of antigenic differences between rabies and rabies-related virus proteins: I. The nucleocapsid protein. *J. Gen. Virol.* **48**, 97–104.

Flamand, A., Wiktor, T. J., Koprowski, H. (1980b). Use of hybridoma monoclonal antibodies in the detection of antigenic differences between rabies and rabies-related virus proteins: II. The glycoprotein. *J. Gen. Virol.* **48**, 105–109.

Flood, E. A., McKenzie, M. O., and Lyles, D. S (2000). Role of M protein aggregation in defective assembly of temperature-sensitive M protein mutants of vesicular stomatitis virus. *Virology* **278**, 520–533.

Fu, Z. F., Dietzschold, B., Schumacher, C. L., Wunner, W. H., Ertl, H. C. J., and Koprowski, H. (1991). Rabies virus nucleoprotein expressed in and purified from insect cells is efficacious as a vaccine. *Proc. Natl. Acad. Sci. USA* **88**, 2001–2005.

Fu, Z. F., Zheng, Y., Wunner, W. H., Koprowski, H., and Dietzschold, B. (1994). Both the N- and the C-terminal domains of the nominal phosphoprotein of rabies virus are involved in binding to the nucleoprotein. *Virology* **200**, 590–597.

Gao, Y., Greenfield, N. J., Cleverley, D. Z., and Lenard, J. (1996). The transcriptional form of the phosphoprotein of vesicular stomatitis virus is a trimer: Structure and stability. *Biochemistry* **35**, 14569–14573.

Gaudin, Y. (1997). Folding of rabies virus glycoprotein: Epitope acquisition and interaction with endoplasmic reticulum chaperones. *J. Virol.* **71**, 3742–3750.

Gaudin, Y. (2000). Rabies virus–induced membrane fusion pathway. *J. Cell Biol.* **150**, 601–611.

Gaudin, Y., Moreira, S., Benejean, J., Blondel, D., Flamand, A., and Tuffereau, C. (1999). Soluble ectodomain of rabies virus glycoprotein expressed in eukaryotic cells folds in a monomeric conformation that is antigenically distinct from the native state of the complete, membrane-anchored glycoprotein. *J. Gen. Virol.* **80**, 1647–1656.

Gaudin, Y., Raux, H., Flamand, A., and Ruigrok, R. W. H. (1996). Identification of amino acids controlling the low-pH-induced conformational change of rabies virus glycoprotein. *J. Virol.* **70**, 7371–7378.

Gaudin, Y., Ruigrok, R. W. H., and Brunner, J. (1995a). Low-pH-induced conformational changes in viral fusion proteins: Implications for the fusion mechanism. *J. Gen. Virol.* **76**, 1541–1556.

Gaudin, Y., Ruigrok, R. W. H., Knossow, M., and Flamand, A. (1993). Low-pH conformational changes of rabies virus glycoprotein and their role in membrane fusion. *J. Virol.* **67**, 1365–1372.

Gaudin, Y., Ruigrok, R. W. H., Tuffereau, C., Knossow, M., and Flamand, A. (1992). Rabies virus glycoprotein is a trimer. *Virology* **187**, 627–632.

Gaudin, Y., Tuffereau, C., Benmansour, A., and Flamand, A. (1991a). Fatty acylation of rabies virus proteins. *Virology* **184**, 441–444.

Gaudin, Y., Tuffereau, C., Durrer, P., Flamand, A., and Ruigrok, R. W. H. (1995b). Biological function of the low-pH, fusion-inactive conformation of rabies virus glycoprotein (G): G is transported in a fusion-inactive state-like conformation. *J. Virol.* **69**, 5528–5534.

Gaudin, Y., Tuffereau, C., Segretain, D., Knossow, M., and Flamand, A. (1991b). Reversible conformational changes and fusion activity of rabies virus glycoprotein. *J. Virol.* **65**, 4853–4859.

Gigant, B., Iseni, F., Gaudin, Y., Knossow, M., and Blondel, D. (2000). Neither phosphorylation nor the amino-terminal part of rabies virus phosphoprotein is required for its oligomerization. *J. Gen. Virol.* **81**, 1757–1761.

Gill, D. S., and Banerjee, A. K. (1986). Complete nucleotide sequence of the matrix protein mRNA of vesicular stomatitis virus (New Jersey serotype). *Virology* **150**, 308–312.

Gillet, J. P., Derer, P., and Tsiang, H. (1986). Axonal transport of rabies virus in the central nervous system of the rat. *J. Neuropathol. Exp. Neurol.* **45**, 619–634.

Gosztonyi, G. (1994). Reproduction of lyssaviruses: Ultrastructural composition of lyssavirus and functional aspects of pathogenesis. *Curr. Topics Microbiol. Immunol.* **187**, 43–68.

Goto, H., Minamoto, H., Ito, H., Luo, T. R., Sugiyama, M., Kinjo, T., and Kawai, A. (1995). Expression of the nucleoprotein of rabies virus in *Escherichia coli* and mapping of antigenic sites. *Arch. Virol.* **140**, 1061–1074.

Goto, H., Minamoto, N., Ito, H., Ito, N., Sugiyama, M., Kinjo, T., and Kawai, A. (2000). Mapping of epitopes and structural analysis of antigenic sites in the nucleoprotein of rabies virus. *J. Gen. Virol.* **81**, 119–127.

Gottlinger, H. G., Dorfman, T., Sodroski, J. G., and Haseltine, W. A. (1991). Effect of mutations affecting the p6 gag proteinon human immunodeficiency virus particle release. *Proc. Natl. Acad. Sci. USA* **88**, 3195–3199.

Gould, A. R., Hyatt, A. D., Lunt, R., Kattenbelt, J. A., Hengstberger, S., and Blacksell, S. D. (1998). Characterisation of a novel lyssavirus isolated from *Pteropid* bats in Australia. *Virus Res.* **54**, 165–187.

Gupta, A., Blondel, D., Choudhary, S., and Banerjee, A. (2000). Phosphoprotein (P) of rabies virus is phosphorylated by a unique cellular protein kinase and specific isomers of protein kinase C. *J. Virol.* **74**, 91–98.

György, E., Sheehan, M. C., and Sokol, F. (1971). Release of envelope glycoprotein from rabies virus by a nonionic detergent. *J. Virol.* **8**, 649–655.

Hanham, C. A., Zhao, F., and Tignor, G. H. (1993). Evidence from the anti-idiotypic network that the acetylcholine receptor is a rabies virus receptor. *J. Virol.* **67**, 530–542.

Harty, R. N., Paragas, J., Sudol, M., and Palese, P. (1999). A proline-rich motif within the matrix protein of vesicular stomatitis virus and rabies virus interacts with WW domains of cellular proteins: Implications for viral budding. *J. Virol.* **73**, 2921–2929.

Haywood, A. M. (1994). Virus receptors: Binding, adhesion strengthening, and changes in viral structure. *J. Virol.* **68**, 1–5.

Hebert, D. N., Foellmer, B., and Helenius, A. (1995). Glucose trimming and reglucosylation determine glycoprotein association with calnexin in the endoplasmic reticulum. *Cell* **81**, 425–433.

Herzog, M., Lafage, M., Montano-Hirose, J. A., Fritzell, C., Scott-Algara, D., and Lafon, M. (1992). Nucleocapsid specific T and B cell responses in humans after rabies vaccination. *Virus Res.* **24**, 77–89.

Hiramatsu, K., Mannen, K., Mifune, K., Nishizono, A., Takita-Sonoda, Y. (1993). Comparative sequence analysis of the M gene among rabies virus strains and its expression by recombinant vaccinia virus. *Virus Genes* **7**, 83–88.

Holland, J. J. (1987). Defective interfering rhabdoviruses In *The Rhabdoviruses*, R. R. Wagner (ed.), pp. 297–360. Plenum Press, New York.

Holland, J. J., De la Torre, J. C., and Steinhauer, D. A. (1992). RNA virus populations as quasispecies. *Curr. Topics Microbiol. Immunol.* **176**, 1–21.

Holloway, B. P., and Obejeski, J. F. (1980). Rabies virus–induced RNA synthesis in BHK-21 cells. *J. Gen. Virol.* **49**, 181–195.

Hsu, C.-H., and Kingsbury, D. W. (1985). Constitutively phosphorylated residues in the NS protein of vesicular stomatitis virus. *J. Biol. Chem.* **260**, 8990–8995.

Huang, A. S. (1973). Defective interfering viruses *Annu. Rev. Microbiol.* **27**, 101–117.

Huang, A. S., and Manders, E. (1972). Ribonucleic acid synthesis of vesicular stomatitis virus: IV. Transcription of standard virus in the presence of defective-interfering particles. *J. Virol.* **9**, 909–916.

Hummeler, K., Koprowski, H., and Wiktor, T. J. (1967). Structure and development of rabies virus in tissue culture. *J. Virol.* **1**, 152–170.

Hummeler, K., Tomassini, N., Sokol, F., Kuwert, E., and Koprowski, H. (1968). Morphology of the nucleoprotein component of rabies virus. *J. Virol.* **2**, 1191–1199.

Iseni, F., Barge, A., Baudin, F., Blondel, D., and Ruigrok, R. W. H. (1998). Characterization of rabies virus nucleocapsids and recombinant nulceocapsid-like structures. *J. Gen. Virol.* **79**, 2909–2919.

Iseni, F., Baudin, F., Blondel, Danielle, and Ruigrok, R. W. H. (2000). Structure of the RNA inside the vesicular stomatitis virus nucleocapsid. *RNA* **6**, 270–281.

Ito, Y., Nishizono, A., Mannen, K., Hiramatsu, K., and Mifune, K. (1996). Rabies virus M protein expressed in *Escherichia coli* and its regulatory role in virion-associated transcriptase activity. *Arch. Virol.* **141**, 671–683.

Iverson, L. E., and Rose, J. K. (1981). Localized attenuation and discontinuous synthesis during vesicular stomatitis virus transcription. *Cell* **23**, 477–484.

Iwasaki, Y., and Clark, H. F. (1975). Cell-to-cell transmission of virus in the central nervous system: II. Experimental rabies in the mouse. *Lab. Invest.* **33**, 391–399.

Iwasaki, Y., Ohtani, S., and Clark, H. F. (1975). Maturation of rabies virus by budding from neuronal cell membrane in suckling mouse brain. *J. Virol.* **15**, 1020–1023.

Iwasaki, Y., Wiktor, T. J., and Koprowski, H. (1973). Early events of rabies virus replication in tissue cultures: An electron microscopic study. *Lab. Invest.* **28**, 142–148.

Jackson, A. C. (1991). Biological basis of rabies virus neurovirulence in mice: Comparative pathogenesis study using the immunoperoxidase technique. *J. Virol.* **65**, 537–540.

Jackson, A. C., and Park, H. (1999). Experimental rabies virus infection of p75 neurotrophin receptor-deficient mice. *Acta Neuropathol.* **98**, 641–644.

Jacob, Y., Badrane, H., Ceccaldi, P.-E., and Tordo, N. (2000). Cytoplasmic dynein LC8 interacts with lyssavirus phosphoprotein. *J. Virol.* **74**, 10217–10222.

Jayakar, H. R., Murti, K. G., and Whitt, M. A. (2000). Mutations in the PPPY motif of vesicular stomatitis virus matrix protein reduce virus budding by inhibiting a late step in virion release. *J. Virol.* **74**, 9818–9827.

Kang, C. Y., and Prevec, L. (1971). Proteins of vesicular stomatitis virus: III. Intracellular synthesis and extracellular appearance of virus-specific proteins. *Virology* **46**, 678–690.

Kaplan, H. A., Welply, J. K., and Lennarz, W. J. (1987). Oligoshaccharyl transferase: The central enzyme in the pathway of glycoprotein assembly. *Biochim. Biophys. Acta.* **906**, 161–173.

Kasturi, L., Eshleman, J. R., Wunner, W. H., and Shakin-Eshleman, S. H. (1995). The hydroxy amino acid in an Asn-X-Ser/Thr sequon can influence the efficiency of N-linked core-glycosylation and the level of expression of a cell surface glycoprotein. *J. Biol. Chem.* **270**, 14756–14761.

Kawai, A., Toriumi, H., Tochikura, T. S., Takahashi, T., Honda, Y., and Morimoto, K. (1999). Nucleocapsid formation and/or subsequent conformational change of rabies virus nucleoprotein (N) is a prerequisite step for acquiring the phosphatase-sensitive epitope of monoclonal antibody 5-2-26. *Virology* **263**, 395–407.

Kemp, G. E., Causey, O. R., Moore, D. L., Odelola, A., and Fabiyi, A. (1972). Further studies on IbAn 27377, a new rabies-related etiologic agent of zoonosis in Nigeria. *Am. J. Trop. Med. Hyg.* **21**, 356–359.

Kiley, M. P., and Wagner, R. R. (1972). Ribonucleic acid species of intracellular nucleocapsids and released virions of vesicular stomatitis virus. *J. Virol.* **10**, 244–255.

King, A. A., and Crick, J. (1988). Rabies-related viruses. In *Rabies*, J. B. Campbell and K. M. Charlton (eds.), pp. 177–199. Kluwer Academic Publishers, Boston.

King, A. A., Meredith, C. D., and Thomson, G. R. (1994). The biology of Southern African lyssavirus variants. *Curr. Topics Microbiol. Immunol.* **187**, 267–295.

Kissi, B., Badrane, H., Audry, L., Lavenu, A., Tordo, N., Brahimi, M., and Bourhy, H. (1999). Dynamics of rabies virus quasi-species during serial passages in heterologous hosts. *J. Gen. Virol.* **80**, 2041–2050.

Kissi, B., Tordo, N., and Bourhy, H. (1995). Genetic polymorphism in the rabies virus nucleoprotein gene. *Virology* **209**, 526–537.

Koprowski, H., Wiktor, T. J., and Abelseth, M. K. (1985). Cross-reactivity and cross-protection: Rabies variants and rabies-related viruses. In *Rabies in the Tropics*, E. Kuwert, C. Merieux, H. Koprowski, and K. Bögel (eds.), pp. 30–39. Springer-Verlag, Berlin.

Kornfeld, R., and Kornfeld, S. (1985). Assembly of asparagine-linked oligosaccharides. *Annu. Rev. Biochem.* **54**, 631–664.

Kouznetzoff, A., Buckle, M., and Tordo, N. (1998). Identification of a region of the rabies virus N protein involved in direct binding to the Viral RNA. *J. Gen. Virol.* **79**, 1005–1013.

Kucera, P., Dolivo, M., Coulon, P., and Flamand, A. (1985). Pathways of the early propagation of virulent and avirulent rabies strains from the eye to the brain. *J. Virol.* **55**, 159–162.

Kurilla, M. G., Cabradilla, C. D., Holloway, B. P., and Keene, J. D. (1984). Nucleotide sequence and host La protein interactions of rabies virus leader RNA. *J. Virol.* **50**, 773–778.

Lafay, F., Coulon, P., Astic, L., Sauciei, D., Riche, D., Holley, A., and Flamand, A. (1991). Spread of the CVS strain of rabies virus and of the avirulent mutant AvO1 along the olfactory pathways of the mouse after intranasal inoculation. *Virology* **183**, 320–333.

Lafon, M. (1997). Rabies virus superantigen. In *Viral Superantigens*, K. Tomonari (ed.), pp. 151–170. CRC Press, Boca Raton, FL.

Lafon, M., Ideler, J., and Wunner, W. H. (1984). Investigation of antigenic structure of rabies virus glycoprotein by monoclonal antibodies. *Dev. Biol. Stand.* **57**, 219–225.

Lafon, M., Lafage, M., Martinez-Arends, A., Ramirez, R., Vuillier, F., Charron, D., Lotteau, V., and Scott-Algara, D. (1992). Evidence for a viral superantigen in humans. *Nature* **358**, 507–510.

Lafon, M., and Wiktor, T. J. (1985). Antigenic sites on the ERA rabies virus nucleoprotein and nonstructural protein. *J. Gen. Virol.* **66**, 2125–2133.

Le Gonidec, G., Rickenbach, A., Robin, Y., and Heme, G. (1978). Isolement d'une souche de virus Mokola au Cameroun. *Ann. Microbiol. (Inst. Pasteur)* **129A**, 245–249.

Le Mercier, P., Jacob, Y., and Tordo, N. (1997). The complete Mokola virus genome sequence: Structure of the RNA-dependent RNA polymerase. *J. Gen. Virol.* **78**, 1571–1576.

Lentz, T. L. (1990). The recognition event between virus and host cell receptor: A target for antiviral agents. *J. Gen. Virol.* **71**, 751–766.

Lentz, T. L., Burrage, T. G., Smith, A. L., Crick, J., and Tignor, G. H. (1982). Is the acetylcholine receptor a rabies virus receptor? *Science* **215**, 182–184.

Lentz, T. L., Hawrot, E., and Wilson, P. T. (1987). Synthetic peptides corresponding to sequences of snake venom neurotoxins and rabies virus glycoprotein bind to the nicotinic acetylcholine receptor. *Proteins* **2**, 298–307.

Leppert, M., Rittenhouse, L., Perrault, J., Summrs, D. F., and Kolakofsky, D. (1979). Plus and minus strand leader RNAs in negative strand virus-infected cells. *Cell* **18**, 735–747.

Lodmell, D. L., Sumner, J. W., Esposito, J. J., Bellini, W. J., and Ewalt, L. (1991). Raccoon poxvirus recombinant expressing the rabies virus nucleoprotein protects mice against lethal rabies virus infection. *J. Virol.* **65**, 3400–3405.

Lonberg-Holm, K. (1981). Attachment of animal virus to cells: an introduction. In *Virus Receptor*, K. Lonberg-Holm and L. Philipson (eds), pp. l–20. Chapman and Hall, New York.

Lycke, E., and Tsiang, H. (1987). Rabies virus infection of cultured rat sensory neurons. *J. Virol.* **61**, 2733–2741.

Lyles, D. S., and McKenzie, M. (1997). Activity of vesicular stomatitis virus M protein mutants in cell rounding is correlated with the ability to inhibit host gene expression and is not correlated with virus assembly function. *Virology* **229**, 77–89.

Lyles, D. S., and McKenzie, M. (1998). Reversible and irreversible steps in assembly and disassembly of vesicular stomatitis virus: Equilibria and kinetics of dissociation of nucleocapsids–M protein complexes assembled *in vivo. Biochemistry* **37**, 439–450.

Lyles D. S., McKenzie, M., Kaptur, P. E., Grant, K. W., and Jerome, W. G. (1996). Complementation of M gene mutants of vesicular stomatitis virus by plasmid-derived M protein converts spherical extracellular particles into native bullet shapes. *Virology* **217**, 76–87.

Lyles D. S., McKenzie, M., and Parce, J. W. (1992). Subunit interactions of vesicular stomatitis virus envelope glycoprotein stabilized by binding to viral matrix protein. *J. Virol.* **66**, 349–358.

Macfarlan, R. I., Dietzschold, B., and Koprowski, H. (1986). Stimulation of cytotoxic T-lymphocyte responses by rabies virus glycoprotein and identification of an immunodominant domain *Mol. Immunol.* **23**, 733–741.

Macfarlan, R. I., Dietzschold, B., Wiktor, T. J., Kiel, M., Boughten, R., Lerner, R. A., Sutcliffe, J. G., Koprowski, H. (1984). T cell responses to cleaved rabies virus glycoprotein and to synthetic peptides. *J. Immunol.* **133**, 2748–2752.

Madore, H. P., and England, J. M. (1977). Rabies virus protein synthesis in infected BHK-21 cells. *J. Virol.* **22**, 102–112.

Marsh, M., and Helenius, A. (1989). Virus entry into animal cells. *Adv. Virus Res.* **36**, 107–151.

Martinez-Arends, A., Astoul, E., Lafage, M., and Lafon, M. (1995). Activation of human tonsil lymphocytes by rabies virus nucleocapsid superantigen *Clin. Immunol. Immunopathol.* **77**, 177–184.

Masters, P., and Banerjee, A. K. (1988). Complex formation with vesicular stomatitis virus phosphoprotein NS prevents binding of nucleocapsid protein N to nonspecific RNA. *J. Virol.* **62**, 2658–2664.

Matsumoto, S. (1962). Electron microscopy of nerve cells infected with street rabies virus. *Virology* **17**, 198–202.

Matsumoto, S. (1963). Electron microscope studies of rabies virus in mouse brain. *J. Cell Biol.* **19**, 565–591.

Matsumoto, S. (1975). Electron microscopy of central nervous system infection. In *The Natural History of Rabies*, G. M Baer (ed.), pp. 217–233. Academic Press, New York.

Matsumoto, S., and Kawai, A. (1969). Comparative studies on development of rabies virus in different host cells. *Virology* **39**, 449–459.

Matsumoto, S., and Miyamoto, K. (1966). Electron-microscopic studies on rabies virus multiplication and the nature of the Negri body. *Symp. Ser. Immunobiol. Stand.* **1**, 45–54.

Matsumoto, S., Schneider, L. G., Kawai, A., and Yonezawa, T. (1974). Further studies on the replication of rabies and rabies-like viruses in organized cultures of mammalian neural tissues. *J. Virol.* **14**, 981–996.

Mayo, M. A., and Pringle, C. R. (1998). Virus taxonomy — 1997. *J. Gen. Virol.* **79**, 649–657.

Mebatsion, T., König, M., and Conselmann, K. (1996). Budding of rabies virus particles in the absence of the spike glycoprotein. *Cell* **84**, 941–951.

Mebatsion, T., Schnell, M. J., and Conzelmann, K.-K. (1995). Mokola virus glycoprotein and chimeric proteins can replace rabies virus glycoprotein in the rescue of infectious defective rabies virus particles. *J. Virol.* **69**, 1444–1451.

Mebatsion, T., Weiland, F., and Conzelmann, K.-K. (1999). Matrix protein of rabies virus is responsible for the assembly and budding of bullet-shaped particles and interacts with the transmembrane spike glycoprotein G. *J. Virol.* **73**, 242–250.

Mellon, M. G., and Emerson, S. U. (1978). Rebinding of transcriptase components (L and NS proteins) to the nucleocapsid template of vesicular stomatitis virus. *J. Virol.* **27**, 560–567.

Meredith, C. D., Rossouw, A. P., and van Praag Koch, H. (1971). An unusual case of human rabies thought to be of Chiropteran origin. *S. Afr. Med. J.* **45**, 767–769.

Minamoto, N., Tanaka, H., Hishida, M., Goto, H., Ito, H., Naruse, S., Yamamoto, K., Sugiyama, M., Kinjo, T., Mannen, K., and Mifune, K. (1994). Linear and conformation-dependent antigenic sites on the nucleoprotein of rabies virus. *Microbiol. Immunol.* **38**, 449–455.

Miyomoto, K., and Matsumoto, S. (1965). The nature of the Negri body. *J. Cell Biol.* **27**, 677–682.

Morimoto, K., Foley, H. D., McGettigan, J. P., Schnell, M. J., and Dietzschold, B. (2000). Reinvestigation of the role of the rabies virus glycoprotein in viral pathogenesis using a reverse genetics approach. *J. Neurovirol.* **6**, 373–381.

Morimoto, K., Hooper, D. C., Carbaugh, H., Fu, Z. F., Koprowski, H., and Dietzschold, B. (1998). Rabies virus quasispecies: Implications for pathogenesis. *Proc. Natl. Acad. Sci. USA* **95**, 3152–3156.

Morimoto, K., Ni, Y.-J., and Kawai, A. (1992). Syncytium formation is induced in the murine neuroblastoma cell cultures which produce pathogenic type G proteins of the rabies virus. *Virology* **189**, 203–216.

Morimoto, K, Ohkubo, A., and Kawai, A. (1989). Structure and transcription of the glycoprotein gene of attenuated HEP-Flury strain of rabies virus. *Virology* **173**, 465–477.

Morzunov, S. P., Winton, J. R., and Nichol, S. T. (1995). The complete genome structure and phylogenetic relationships of infectious hematopoietic necrosis virus. *Virus Res.* **38**, 175–192.

Murphy, F. A., and Bauer, S. P. (1974). Early street rabies virus infection in striated muscle and later progression to the central nervous system. *Intervirology* **3**, 256–268.

Murphy, F. A., Bauer, S. P., Harrison, A. K., and Winn, W. C. Jr. (1973a). Comparative pathogenesis of rabies and rabies-like viruses: Viral infection and transit from inoculation site to the central nervous system. *Lab. Invest.* **28**, 361–376.

Murphy, F. A., Bell, J. F., Bauer, S. P., Gardner, J. J., Moore, G. J., Harrison, A. K., and Coe, J. E. (1980). Experimental chronic rabies in the cat. *Lab. Invest.* **43**, 231–241.

Murphy, F. A., Fauquet, C. M., Bishop, D. H. L., Ghabrial, S. A., Jarvis, A. W., Martelli, G. P., Mayo, M. A., Summers, M. D. (eds.) (1995). *Virus Taxonomy: Sixth Report of the International Committee on Taxonomy of Viruses*, pp. 275–288. Springer-Verlag, New York.

Murphy, F. A., Harrison, A. K. (1979). Electron microscopy of the rhabdoviruses of animals. In *Rhabdoviruses*, D. H. L. Bishop (ed.), Vol. 1, pp. 65–106. CRC Press, Boca Raton, FL.

Murphy, F. A., Harrison, A. K., Washington, W. C., and Bauer, S. P. (1973b). Comparative pathogenesis of rabies and rabies-like viruses: Infection of the central nervous system and centrifugal spread of virus to peripheral tissues. *Lab. Invest.* **29**, 1–16.

Murphy, F. A., and Nathanson, N. (1994). The emergence of new virus diseases: An overview. *Semin. Virol.* **5**, 87–102.

Nadin-Davis, S. A., Casey, G. A., and Wandeler, A. (1994). A molecular epidemiological study of rabies virus in central Onatario and western Quebec. *J. Gen. Virol.* **75**, 2575–2583.

Naito, S., and Matsumoto, S. (1978). Identification of cellular actin within the rabies virus. *Virology* **91**, 151–163.

Neurath, A. R., Vernon, S. K., Dobkin, M. B., and Rubin, B. A. (1972). Characterization of subviral components resulting from treatment of rabies virus with tri(*n*-butyl)phosphate. *J. Gen. Virol.* **14**, 33–48.

Okazaki, Y., Ohno, H., Takase, K., Ochiai, T., and Saito, T. (2000). Cell surface expression of calnexin, a molecular chaperone in the endoplasmic reticulum. *J. Biol. Chem.* **275**, 35751–35759.

Patton, J., Davies, N. L., and Wertz, G. W. (1984). N protein alone satisfies the requirement for protein synthesis during RNA replication of vesicular stomatitis virus. *J. Virol.* **49**, 303–309.

Patzer, E. J., Moore, N. F., Barenholz, Y., Shaw, J. M., and Wagner, R. R. (1978). Lipid organization of the membrane of vesicular stomatitis virus. *J. Biol. Chem.* **253**, 4544–4550.

Perrin, P., Portnoi, D., and Sureau, P. (1982). Etude de l'adsorption et de la penetration du virus rabique: Interactions avec les cellules BHK21 et des membranes artificielles. *Ann. Virol. (Inst. Pasteur).* **133E**, 403–422.

Poch, O., Blumberg, B. M., Bougueleret, L., and Tordo, N. (1990). Sequence comparison of five polymerases (L proteins) of unsegmented negative-strand RNA viruses: Theoretical assignment of functional domains. *J. Gen. Virol.* **71**, 1153–1162.

Poch, O., Sauvaget, I., Delarue, M., and Tordo, N. (1989). Identification of four conserved motifs among the RNA-dependent polymerase encoding elements. *EMBO J.* **8**, 3867–3874.

Poch, O., Tordo, N., and Keith, G. (1988). Sequence of the 3386 3' nucleotides of the genome of the AVO1 strain rabies virus: structural similarities in the protein regions involved in transcription. *Biochimie* **70**, 1019–1029.

Prehaud, C., Coulon, P., Lafay, F., Thiers, C., and Flamand, A. (1988). Antigenic site II of the rabies virus glycoprotein: Structure and role in viral virulence. *J. Virol.* **62**, 1–7.

Prehaud, C., Harris, R. D., Fulop, V., Koh, C.-L., Wong, J., Flamand, A., and Bishop, D. H. L. (1990). Expression, characterization and purification of a phosphorylated rabies nucleoprotein synthesized in insect cells by baculovirus vectors. *Virology* **178**, 486–497.

Prehaud, C., Nel, K., and Bishop, D. H. L. (1992). Baculovirus-expressed rabies virus Ml protein is not phosphorylated: It forms multiple complexes with expressed rabies N protein. *Virology* **189**, 766–770.

Raux, H., Flamand, A., and Blondel, D. (2000). Interaction of the rabies virus P protein with the LC8 dynein light chain. *J. Virol.* **74**, 10212–10216.

Rayssiguier, C., Cioe, L., Withers, E., Wunner, W. H., and Curtis, P. J. (1986). Cloning of the rabies virus matrix protein mRNA and determination of its amino acid sequence. *Virus Res.* **5**, 177–190.

Reading, C. L., Penhoet, E. E., and Ballou, C. E. (1978). Carbohydrate structure of vesicular stomatitis virus glycoprotein. *J. Biol. Chem.* **253**, 5600–5612.

Reagan, K. J., and Wunner, W. H. (1985). Rabies virus interaction with various cell lines is independent of the acetylcholine receptor. *Arch. Virol.* **84**, 277–282.

Robison, C. S., and Whitt, M. A. (2000). The membrane-proximal stem region of vesicular stomatitis G protein confers efficient virus assembly. *J. Virol.* **74**, 2239–2246.

Rose, J. K., and Gallione, C. J. (1981). Nucleotide sequence of the mRNA's encoding the vesicular stomatitis virus G and M proteins determined from cDNA clones containing the complete coding regions. *J. Virol.* **39**, 519–528.

Rupprecht, C. E., Dietzschold, B., Wunner, W. H., and Koprowski, H. (1991). Antigenic relationships of lyssaviruses. In *The Natural History of Rabies*, G. M. Baer (ed.), 2nd ed., pp. 69–100. CRC Press, Boca Raton, FL.

Sacramento, D., Badrane, H., Bourhy, H., and Tordo, N. (1992). Molecular epidemiology of rabies in France: Comparison with vaccinal strains. *J. Gen. Virol.* **73**, 1149–1158.

Sacramento, D., Bourhy, H., and Tordo, N. (1991). PCR techniques as an alternative method for diagnosis and molecular epidemiology of rabies virus. *Mol. Cell. Probes* **6**, 229–240.

Sagara, J., and Kawai, A. (1992). Identification of heat shock protein 70 in the rabies virion. *Virology* **190**, 845–848.

Sagara, J., Tochikura, T. S., Tanaka, H., Baba, Y., Tsukita, S., Tsukita, S., and Kawai, A. (1998). The 21 -kDa polypeptide (VAP21) in the rabies virion is a C99-related host cell protein. *Microbiol. Immunol.* **42**, 289–297.

Sagara, J., Tsukita, S., Shigenobu, Y., Tsukita, S., and Kawai, A. (1995). Cellular actin-binding exrin-radixin-moesin (ERM) family proteins are incorporated into the rabies virion and closely associated with viral envelope proteins in the cell. *Virology* **206**, 485–494.

Sakamoto, S.-I., Ide, T., Nakatake, H., Tokiyoshi, S., Yamamotos, M, Kawai, A., and Smith, J. (1994). Studies on the antigenicity and nucleotide sequence of the rabies virus Nishigahara strain, a current seed strain used for dog vaccine production in Japan. *Virus Genes* **8**, 35–46.

Sanchez, A., De, B. P., and Banerjee, A. K. (1985). *In vitro* phosphorylation of NS protein by the L protein of vesicular stomatitis virus. *J. Gen. Virol.* **66**, 1025–1036.

Sanchez, A., Kiley, M. P., Holloway, B. P., and Auperin, D. D. (1993). Sequence analysis of the Ebola virus genome: Organization, genetic elements, and comparison with the genome of Marburg virus. *Virus Res.* **29**, 215–240.

Schlesinger, H. R., Wells, H. J., and Hummeler, K. (1973). Comparison of the lipids of intracellular and extracellular rabies viruses. *J. Virol.* **12**, 1028–1030.

Schneider, L. G. (1982). Antigenic variants of rabies virus. *Comp. Immunol. Microbiol. Infect. Dis.* **5**, 101–107.

Schneider, L. G., and Diringer, H. (1976). Structure and molecular biology of rabies virus. *Curr. Topics Microbiol. Immunol.* **75**, 153–180.

Schneider, L. G., Dietzschold, B., Dierks, R. E., Matthaeus, W., Enzmann, P. J., and Strohmaier, K. (1973). Rabies group-specific ribonucleoprotein antigen and a test system for grouping and typing rhabdoviruses. *J. Virol.* **11**, 748–755.

Schnell, M. J., Buonocore, L., Whitt, M. A., and Rose, J. A. (1996). The minimal conserved transcription stop-start signal promotes stable expression of a foreign gene in vesicular stomatitis virus. *J. Virol.* **70**, 2318–2323.

Schnell, M. J., and Conzelmann, K.-K. (1995). Polymerase activity of in vitro mutated rabies virus L protein. *Virology* **214**, 522–530.

Schnell, M. J., Mebatsion, T., and Conzelmann, K.-K. (1994). Infectious rabies viruses from cloned cDNA. *EMBO J.* **13**, 4195–4203.

Schoehn, G., Iseni, F., Mavrakis, M., Blondel, D., and Ruigrok, R. W. H. (2001). Structure of recombinant rabies virus nucleoprotein-RNA complex and identification of the phosphate binding site. *J. Virol.* **75**, 490–498.

Schütze, H., Enzmann, P.-J, Kuchling, R., Mundt, E., Niemann, H., and Mettenleiter, T. C. (1995). Complete genomic sequence of the fish rhabdovirus infectious haematopoietic necrosis virus. *J. Gen. Virol.* **76**, 2519–2527.

Seganti, L., Superti, F., Bianchi, S., Orsi, N., Divizia, M., and Pana, A. (1990). Susceptibility of mammalian, avian, fish and mosquito cell lines to rabies virus infection. *Arch. Virol.* **34**, 155–163.

Seif, I., Coulon, P., Rollin, P. E., and Flamand, A. (1985). Rabies virus virulence: Effect on pathogenicity and sequence characterization of mutations affecting antigenic site III of the glycoprotein. *J. Virol.* **53**, 926–935.

Shakin-Eshleman, S. H., Remaley, A. T., Eshleman, J. R., Wunner, W. H., and Spitalnik, S. L. (1992). N-linked glycosylation of rabies virus glycoprotein: Individual sequons differ in their efficiencies and influence on cell surface expression. *J. Biol. Chem.* **267**, 10690–10698.

Shakin-Eshleman, S. H., Wunner, W. H., and Spitalnik, S. L. (1993). Efficiency of N-linked core glycosylation at asparagine-319 of rabies virus glycoprotein is altered by deletions C-terminal to the glycosylation sequon. *Biochemistry* **32**, 9465–9472.

Shope, R. E., Murphy, F. A., Harrison, A. K., Causey, O. R., Kemp, G. E., Simpson, D. I. H., and Moore, D. L. (1970). Two African viruses serologically and morphologically related to rabies virus. *J. Virol.* **6**, 690–692.

Simon, K. O., Whitaker-Dowling, P. A., Younger, J. S., and Windell, C. C. (1990). Sequential disassembly of the cytoskeleton in BHK21 cells infected with vesicular stomatitis virus. *Virology* **177**, 289–297.

Simons, K., and Garoff, H. (1980). The budding mechanisms of enveloped animal viruses. *J. Gen. Virol.* **50**, 1–21.

Smith, J. S. (1989). Rabies virus epitopic variation: Use in ecological studies. *Adv. Virus Res.* **36**, 215–253.

Smith, J. S., Fishbein, D. B., Rupprecht, C. E., and Clark, K. (1991). Unexplained rabies in three immigrants in the United States: A virologic investigation. *New Engl. J. Med.* **324**, 205–211.

Smith, D. B., McAllister, J., Casino, C., and Simmonds, P. (1997). Virus "quasi-species': Making a mountain out of a molehill? *J. Gen. Virol.* **78**, 1511–1519.

Smith, J. S., Orciari, L. A., and Yager, P. A. (1995). Molecular epidemiology of rabies in the United States. *Semi. Virol.* **6**, 387–400.

Smith, J. S., Orciari, L. A., Yager, P. A., Seidel, H. D., and Warner, C. K. (1992). Epidemiologic and historical relationships among 87 rabies virus isolates as determined by limited sequence analysis. *J. Infect. Dis.* **166**, 296–307.

Sokol, F. (1975). Chemical composition and structure of rabies virus. In *The Natural History of Rabies*, G. M. Baer (ed.), Vol. I, pp. 79–102. Academic Press, New York.

Sokol, F., and Clark, F. (1973). Phosphoproteins, structural components of rhabdoviruses. *Virology* **52**, 246–263.

Sokol, F., Clark, H. F., Wiktor, T. J., McFalls, M. L., Bishop, D. H. L., and Obijeski, J. F. (1974). Structural phosphoproteins associated with ten rhabdoviruses. *J. Gen. Virol.* **24**, 433–445.

Sokol, F., and Koprowski, H. (1975). Structure-function relationships and mode of replication of animal rhabdoviruses. *Proc. Natl. Acad. Sci. USA* **72**, 933–936.

Sokol, F., Schlumberger, H. D., Wiktor, T. J., Koprowski, H., and Hummeler, K. (1969). Biochemical and biophysical studies on the nucleocapsid and on the RNA of rabies virus. *Virology* **38**, 651–665.

Sokol, F., Stancek, D., and Koprowski, H. (1971). Structural proteins of rabies virus. *J. Virol.* **7**, 241–249.

Spadafora; D., Canter, D. M., Jackson, R. L., and Perrault, J. (1996). Constitutive phosphorylation of the vesicular stomatitis virus P protein modulates polymerase complex formation but is not essential for transcription or replication. *J. Virol.* **70**, 4538–4548.

Stillman, E. A., and Whitt, M. A. (1997). Mutational analyses of the intergenic dinucleotide and the transcriptional start sequence of vesicular stomatitis virus (VSV) define sequences required for efficient termination and initiation of VSV transcripts. *J. Virol.* **71**, 2127–2137.

Sudol, M. (1996). Structure and function of the WW domain. *Prog. Biophys. Mol. Biol.* **65**, 113–132.

Sumner, J. W., Fakadu, M., Shaddock, J. H., Sanderlin, D. W., Esposito, J. J., and Bellini, W. J. (1991). Construction of vaccinia virus recombinants that express the rabies nucleoprotein and protective immunization of mice. *J. Virol.* **183**, 703–710.

Superti, F., Derer, M., and Tsiang, H. (1984a). Mechanism of rabies virus entry into CER cells. *J. Gen. Virol.* **65**, 781–789.

Superti, F., Hauttecoueur, B., Morelec, M. J., Goldoni, P., Bizzini, B., and Tsiang, H. (1986). Involvement of gangiosides in rabies virus infection. *J. Gen. Virol.* **67**, 47–56.

Superti, F., Seganti, L., Tsiang, H., and Orsi, N. (1984b). Role of phospholipid in rhabdovirus attachment to CER cells. *Arch. Virol.* **81**, 321–328.

Sureau, P., Rollin, P., and Wiktor, T. J. (1983). Epidemiologic analysis of antigenic variations of street rabies virus: Detection by monoclonal antibodies. *Am. J. Epidemiol.* **117**, 605–609.

Takacs, A., and Banerjee, A. (1995). Efficient interaction of vesicular stomatitis virus P protein with the L protein or the N protein in cells expressing the recombinant proteins. *Virology* **208**, 821–826.

Tanabe, K., and Matsumoto, S. (1979). Characterization of multi-layered membrane generated by rabies virus. *Microbiol. Immunol.* **23**, 763–777.

Tarbouriech, N., Curran, J., Ebel, C., Ruigrok, R. W., and Burmeister, W. P. (2000). On the domain structure and the polymerization state of the Sendai virus P protein. *Virology* **266**, 99–109.

Testa, D., Chanda, P. K., and Banerjee, A. K. (1980). Unique mode of transcription *in vitro* by vesicular stomatitis virus. *Cell* **21**, 267–275.

Thoulouze, M.-I., Lafage, M., Schachner, M., Hartmann, U., Cremer, H., and Lafon, M. (1998). The neural cell adhesion molecule is a receptor for rabies virus. *J. Virol.* **72**, 7181–7190.

Tignor, G. H., Murphy, F. A., Clark, H. F., Shope, R. E., Madore, P., Bauer, S. P., Buckley, S. M., and Meredith, C. D. (1977). Duvenhage virus: Morphological, biochemical, histopathological and antigenic relationships to the rabies serogroup. *J. Gen. Virol.* **37**, 595–611.

Tollis, M., Dietzshold, B., Volia, C. B., and Koprowski, H. (1991). Immunization of monkeys with rabies ribonucleoprotein (RNP) confers protective immunity against rabies. *Vaccine* **9**, 134–136.

Tordo, N., and Poch, O. (1988). Structure of rabies virus. In *Rabies*, J. B. Campbell and K. M. Charlton, (eds.), pp. 25–45. Kluwer Academic Publishers, Boston.

Tordo, N., Poch, O., Ermine, A., and Keith, G. (1986a). Primary structure of leader RNA and nucleoprotein genes of the rabies genome: Segmented homology with VSV. *Nucleic Acid Res.* **14**, 2671–2683.

Tordo, N., Poch, O., Ermine, A., Keith, G., and Rougeon, F. (1986b). Walking along the rabies genome: Is the large G-L intergenic region a remnant gene? *Proc. Natl. Acad. Sci. USA* **83**, 3914–3918.

Tordo, N., Poch, O., Ermine, A., Keith, G., and Rougeon, F. (1988). Completion of the rabies virus genome sequence determination: Highly conserved domains among the L (polymerase) proteins of unsegmented negative-strand RNA viruses. *Virology* **165**, 565–576.

Tordo, N., Bourhy, H., Sather, S., and Ollo, R. (1993). Structure and expression in baculovirus of the Mokola virus glycoprotein: An efficient recombinant vaccine. *Virology* **193**, 59–69.

Tordo, N., De Haan, P., Goldbach, R., and Poch, O. (1992). Evolution of negative-stranded RNA genomes. *Semin. Virol.* **3**, 341–357.

Tsiang, H. (1979). Evidence for an intraaxonal transport of fixed and street rabies virus. *J. Neuropathol. Exp. Neurol.* **38**, 286–296.

Tsiang, H. (1988). Rabies virus infection of myotubes and neurons as elements of the neuromuscular junction. *Rev. Infect. Dis.* **10** (Suppl. 4), S733–738.

Tsiang, H. (1993). Pathophysiology of rabies virus infection of the nervous system. *Adv. Virus Res.* **42**, 375–412.

Tsiang, H., Derer; M., and Taxi, J. (1983a). An *in vivo* and *in vitro* study of rabies virus infection of the rat superior cervical ganglia. *Arch. Virol.* **76**, 231–243.

Tsiang, H., De la Porte, S., Ambroise, D. J., Derer, M, and Koenig, J. (1986). Infection of cultured rat myotubes and neurons from the spinal cord by rabies virus. *J. Neuropathol. Exp. Neurol.* **45**, 28–42.

Tsiang, H., Koulakoff, A., Bizzini, B., and Berwald-Nette, Y. (1983b). Neurotropism of rabies virus: An *in vitro* study. *J. Neuropathol. Exp. Neurol.* **42**, 439–452.

Tuffereau, C., Benegean, J., Blondel, D., Kieffer, G., and Flamand, A. (1998). Low-affinity nerve-growth factor receptor (P75NTR) can serve as a receptor for rabies virus. *EMBO J.* **17**, 7250–7259.

Tuffereau, C., Fischer, S., and Flamand, A. (1985). Phosphorylation of the N and M 1 proteins of rabies virus. *Virology* **165**, 565–576.

Tuffereau, C., Leblois, H., Benejean, J., Coulon, P., Lafay, F., and Flamand, A. (1989). Arginine or lysine in position 333 of ERA and CVS glycoprotein is necessary for rabies virulence in adult mice. *Virology* **172**, 206–212.

Wertz, G. W. (1978). Isolation of possible replicative intermediate structures from vesicular stomatitis virus-infected cells. *Virology* **85**, 271–285.

Wertz, G. W., Whelan, S., LeGrone, A., and Ball, L. A. (1994). Extent of terminal complementarity modulates the balance between transcription and replication of vesicular stomatitis virus RNA. *Proc. Natl. Acad. Sci. USA* **91**, 8587–8591.

Whelan, S. P. J., and Wertz, G. W. (1999a). Regulation of RNA synthesis by the genomic termini of vesicular stomatitis virus: Identification of distinct sequences essential for transcription but not replication. *J. Virol.* **73**, 297–306.

Whelan, S. P. J., and Wertz, G. W. (1999b). The 5' terminal trailer region of vesicular stomatitis virus contains a position-dependent *cis*-acting signal for assembly of RNA into infectious particles. *J. Virol.* **73**, 307–315.

Whitt, M. A., Buonocore, L., Prehaud, C., and Rose, J. K. (1991). Membrane fusion activity, oligomerization, and assembly of the rabies virus glycoprotein. *Virology* **185**, 681–688.

WHO (1984). *WHO Expert Committee on Rabies, Seventh Report.* WHO, Geneva.

Wiktor, T. J., Dietzschold, B., Leamnson, R. N., and Koprowski, H. (1977). Induction and biological properties of defective interfering particles of rabies virus. *J. Virol.* **21**, 626–635.

Wiktor, T. J., Flamand, A., Koprowski, H. (1980). Use of monoclonal antibodies in diagnosis of rabies virus infection and differentiation of rabies and rabies-related viruses. *J. Virol. Methods* **1**, 33–46.

Wiktor, T. J., Gyorgy, E., Schlunberger, H. D., Sokol, F., and Koprowski, H. (1973). Antigenic properties of rabies virus components. *J. Immunol.* **110**, 269–276.

Wiktor, T. J., and Koprowski, H. (1978). Monoclonal antibodies against rabies virus produced by somatic cell hybridization: Detection of antigenic variants. *Proc. Natl. Acad. Sci. USA* **75**, 3938–3942.

Wiktor, T. J., and Koprwoski, H. (1980). Antigenic variants of rabies virus. *J. Exp. Med.* **152**, 99–112.

Wiktor, T. J., Macfarlan, R. I., Foggin, C. M., Koprowski, H. (1984). Antigenic analysis of rabies and Mokola virus from Zimbabwe using monoclonal antibodies. *Dev. Biol. Stand.* **57**, 199–211.

Wills, J. W., Cameron, C. E., Wilson, C. B., Xiang, Y., Bennett, R. P., and Leis, J. (1994). An assembly domain of the Rous sarcoma virus Gag protein required late in budding. *J. Virol.* **68**, 6605–6618.

Willusz, J., Kurilla, M. G., and Keene, J. D. (1983). A host protein (La) binds to a unique species of minus-sense leader RNA during replication of vesicular stomatitis virus. *Proc. Natl. Acad. Sci. USA* **80**, 5827–5831.

Wunner, W. H. (1987). Rabies viruses: Pathogenesis and immunity. In *The Rhabdoviruses*, R. R. Wagner (ed.), pp. 361–426. Plenum Press, New York.

Wunner, W. H., and Clark, H. F. (1980). Regeneration of DI particles of virulent and attenuated rabies virus: Genome characterization and lack of correlation with virulence phenotype. *J. Gen. Virol.* **51**, 69–82.

Wunner, W. H. (1991). The chemical composition and molecular structure of rabies viruses. In *The Natural History of Rabies,* G. M. Baer (ed.), pp. 31–67. CRC Press, Boca Raton, FL.

Wunner, W. H., Dietzschold, B., Smith, C. L., and Lafon, M. (1985). Antigenic variants of CVS rabies virus with altered glycosylation sites. *Virology* **140**, 1–12.

Wunner, W. H., Larson, J. K., Dietzschold, B., and Smith, C. L. (1988). The molecular biology of rabies viruses. *Rev. Infect. Dis.* **10**, S771–S784.

Wunner, W. H., Reagan, K. J., and Koprowski, H. (1984). Characterization of saturable binding sites for rabies virus. *J. Virol.* **50**, 691–697.

Yang, C., and Jackson, A. C. (1992). Basis of neurovirulence of rabies virus variant AvO 1 with stereotaxic brain inoculation in mice. *J. Gen. Virol.* **73**, 895–900.

Yang, J., Hooper, C., Wunner, W. H., Koprowski, H., Dietzschold, B., and Fu, Z. F. (1998). The specificity of rabies virus RNA encapsidation by nucleoprotein. *Virology* **242**, 107–117.

Yang, J., Koprowski, H., Dietzschold, B., and Fu, Z. F. (1999). Phosphorylation of rabies virus nucleoprotein regulates viral RNA transcription and replication by modulating leader RNA encapsidation. *J. Virol.* **73**, 1661–1664.

3

Molecular Epidemiology

JEAN S. SMITH

Rabies Section
Centers for Disease Control and Prevention
Atlanta, Georgia 30333

I. INTRODUCTION

Molecular epidemiology of a virus-induced disease such as rabies is founded on the inability of the viral polymerase to faithfully copy genetic material. Some RNA virus polymerases are particularly error prone, allowing virus populations to exist in infected hosts not as multiple copies of a discrete entity but as a collection of genetic variants (Domingo and Holland, 1994). The variation is unnoticeable by most observation methods because mutations are distributed about a relatively constant consensus sequence. Genetic drift of the consensus sequence occurs when transmission is constrained (a bottleneck) and limits passage to a subset of the virus population (a founder lineage). A founder lineage with beneficial mutations could spread quickly through a susceptible population (e.g., the

79

ability to escape immune detection would confer a higher relative fitness to a new virus lineage through the process of positive selection). More frequently, however, the founder lineage contains only neutral mutations randomly selected from the virus population through the serial bottlenecks of transmission from host to host. If molecular typing methods are sufficiently discriminating, however, a founder lineage can be distinguished from other preexisting lineages, and the information can be used to study patterns of disease transmission.

In applying the principles of molecular epidemiology to rabies, we make certain assumptions about virus transmission. The first and most important assumption is that a given virus lineage is transmitted more efficiently by a single animal species, the *reservoir* host (reviewed in Blancou,1988; Smith,1989). This species is responsible for maintaining the virus in a particular geographic area, presumably because of adaptation between virus and host (virus adaptation) but also probably because the contact that facilitates virus transmission is more common among conspecifics. Over time, a virus population that is partitioned or compartmentalized by such selective transmission accumulates numerous independently acquired mutations that provide useful markers to identify it. The molecular mechanism of virus–host adaptation is unknown, however, and we can only associate a virus variant with an animal reservoir by coupling virus typing with evidence garnered from epidemiology, surveillance, and pathogenesis studies.

If we assume that virus variants adapt to their hosts, then we would expect that the spillover cases that occur when reservoir hosts transmit rabies to other species would not ordinarily result in sustained transmission of the variant. A corollary to this assumption is that a new lineage and virus variant should evolve if sustained independent cycles of transmission in a new host species arise from the spillover event.

Methods of virus typing for rabies differ in the precision with which virus populations can be dissected. Some members of the *Lyssavirus* genus differ so significantly that serology and vaccine cross-protection tests alone are sufficient to differentiate between them (Table I). Distinctive reaction patterns between viruses and monoclonal antibodies (MAbs) have been used quite effectively to identify many of the terrestrial animal reservoirs for rabies in the United States (Table II). On the other hand, genetic typing, especially nucleotide sequence analysis, permits the most precise definition of virus type and currently has the greatest utility in epidemiologic investigations (Fig. 1).

All virus typing methods offer insight into modes of virus transmission. This chapter represents a review of progress made in the molecular epidemiology of rabies as practiced in a growing number of reference and public health laboratories worldwide. Particular emphasis is given to a discussion of the fundamentals of the molecular epidemiology of rabies and how these assumptions have been used in investigations of human cases, as a means of enhanced surveillance of animal rabies, and to monitor vaccine coverage.

II. METHODS AND DEFINITION OF TERMS

Typing of lyssavirus samples can be conducted by both antigenic and genetic methods. Although some lyssavirus species can be differentiated with hyperimmune serum, antigenic typing methods commonly rely on MAbs to identify distinctive epitopes or recognition sites that emerge or are lost when amino acid substitutions occur in viral proteins. The resolving power of an antigenic analysis is determined by, and often is proportional to, the number of MAbs used to characterize a virus and, theoretically, by the accessibility and number of nonoverlapping epitopes on viral proteins.

Genetic typing methods detect mutations in viral RNA at the nucleotide level, and different methods of genetic typing vary in their discriminatory power. The method with the highest resolution is that which determines nucleotide sequence (capable of resolving the entire genome of approximately 12,000 nucleotides). The method with the next highest resolution power is digestion with restriction enzymes, and finally, this is followed by differentiation of virus populations with specific oligonucleotide probes. Compared with antigenic typing methods, the results of genetic typing are more reproducible and readily quantified. On the other hand, genetic typing is more expensive, technically more demanding, and produces test results with increased interpretative complexity.

A. Antigenic Typing

Several laboratories have developed panels of MAbs and published the reaction patterns expected for virus variants associated with different animal reservoirs (Bourhy *et al.*, 1992; Diaz *et al.*, 1994; Mebatsion *et al.*, 1992; Nadin-Davis *et al.*, 2000; Smith, 1989). Most epidemiologic studies have used MAbs that react with the nucleocapsid (or N) protein. The N protein is produced in abundance in the brains of infected animals, and antibody recognition can be assayed using immunofluorescence methods available to almost all public health laboratories (Smith, 1989). Variation in the phosphoprotein (P) is also detectable by immunofluorescent methods (Nadin-Davis *et al.*, 2000), and Warner *et al.* (1999) demonstrated a simple histochemical method for detecting differences in the glycoprotein (G) antigens presented in formalin-fixed tissues, but antibodies to P and G proteins have not as yet gained wide use.

Although antigenic typing methods largely have been supplanted by more precise genetic methods, virus typing with MAbs provides a rapid and inexpensive method for large-scale surveillance of both new lyssavirus species (Bourhy *et al.*, 1992; Gould *et al.*, 1998) and common variants of rabies virus (Crawford-Miksza *et al.*, 1999; DeMattos *et al.*, 1996, 1999; Favi *et al.*, 1999; Kissi *et al.*, 1995; Nadin-Davis *et al.*, 2000). Antigenic typing surveys identified Mokola and Lagos

TABLE I

Currently Recognized Species in the Genus *Lyssavirus*[a]

	Rabies virus (RABV)	*Australian bat lyssavirus (ABLV)*	*Duvenhage virus (DUVV)*	*European bat lyssavirus 1 (EBLV-1)*	*European bat lyssavirus 2 (EBLV-2)*	*Mokola virus (MOKV)*	*Lagos bat virus (LBV)*
Distribution	Worldwide with the exception of Antarctica and some insular regions	Australia	South Africa, Zimbabwe, Guinea	Germany, Denmark, Holland, Poland, Russia, Ukraine, France, Spain	Holland, United Kingdom, Finland, Switzerland	Nigeria, South Africa, Cameroon, Zimbabwe, Central African Republic, Ethiopia	Nigeria, South Africa, Zimbabwe, Central African Republic, Senegal, Ethiopia
Reservoir	*Carnivora*: Wild and domestic canid species, raccoons, skunks, mongoose *Microchiroptera*: Vampire bats and almost all species of insectivorous bats that have been adequately sampled	*Megachiroptera*: Pteropid Species *Microchiroptera?*: Single cases attributed to yellow-bellied sheathtail bat (*Saccolaimus flavicentris*)	*Microchiroptera?*: Single cases attributed to *Miniopterus schreibersii*, *Nycteris gambiensis*, and *N. thebaica*	*Microchiroptera*: Almost all cases in (*Eptesicus serotinus*)	*Microchiroptera*: Almost all cases in (*Myotis dasycneme* and *M. daubentonii*)	*Insectivora?*, *Rodentia?*: Single cases in shrew (*Crocidura* sp.) and small rodent (*Lopyhromys sikapusi*), but most reported cases are from domestic cats and dogs	*Megachiroptera?*: Cases reported in *Eidolon helvum* *Micropterus pusillus*, and *Epomophorus wahlbergi*

Reported cases							
Animals	1000s per year	<100	<10	Approx. 10 per year	<10	<25	<25
Humans	1000s per year	2	1	1 confirmed, 1 suspected	1	2	0
Amino acid homology (%) with RABV N protein	—	92	86	87	85	76	79
Neutralizing titer of 2 international units of RABV immune globulin against approx. 50 infectious units of virus	1:940	1:625	1:125	1:125	1:125	1:5	1:12

[a]Data are summarized from recent review articles (Bourhy et al., 1993; Swanepoel et al., 1993; Mackenzie, 1999; Messenger et al., 2001) and unpublished data (Centers for Disease Control and Prevention).

TABLE II

Monoclonal Antibody Patterns Identifying Terrestrial Animal Reservoirs for Rabies in the United States

MAbs	Major terrestrial animal reservoirs			Minor terrestrial animal reservoirs			
	Raccoon, E US	Skunk, SC US	Skunk, NC US & CA	Dog/coyote, Texas	Fox, TX	Fox, Alaska/ New England	Fox, AZ
C4 62-15-2	Positive	Positive	Positive	Positive	Positive	Positive	Positive
CR54 6229-54	Positive	Positive	NEGATIVE	NEGATIVE	NEGATIVE	NEGATIVE	NEGATIVE
C2 62-8-1	Positive	NEGATIVE	Positive	Positive	Positive	Positive	Positive
C15 62-97-3	Positive	Positive	Positive	Positive	Positive	NEGATIVE	Positive
C10 62-52-2	Positive	Positive	Positive	Positive	Positive	Positive	NEGATIVE
C1 62-3-1	NEGATIVE	NEGATIVE	Positive	Positive	Positive	NEGATIVE	Positive
C18 62-143-2	Weak	Weak	NEGATIVE	NEGATIVE	NEGATIVE	NEGATIVE	NEGATIVE
C6/C20 62-23-4/62-164-2	Positive	Positive	Positive	Positive	Positive	Positive	Positive
C12 62-62-4	Positive	Negative	Positive	Positive	Positive	Positive	Positive

A.

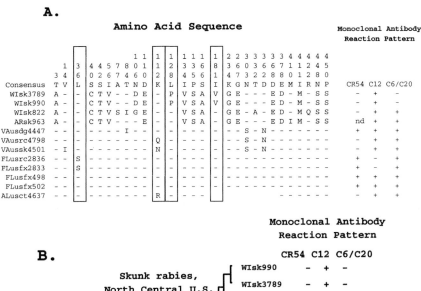

Amino Acid Sequence — Monoclonal Antibody Reaction Pattern

		1	3	4	4	5	7	8	0	1	1 1 2	1 2	1 1 1 3 3 6	1 8	2 2 3 3 3 3 3 4 4 4 4 4 3 6 0 3 6 6 7 1 1 2 4 5	CR54	C12	C6/C20
	3 4	6	0	2	6	7	4	6	0	2	8	4 5 6	1	4 7 3 2 2 8 8 0 1 2 8 0			
Consensus	T V	L	S	S	I	A	T	N	D	K	L	I P S	I	K G N T D D E M I R N P	CR54	C12	C6/C20
WIsk3789	A -	-	C	T	V	-	-	D	E	-	P	V S A	V	G E - - - E D - M - S S	-	+	-
WIsk990	A -	-	C	T	V	-	-	D	E	-	P	V S A	V	G E - - - E D - M - S S	-	+	-
WIsk822	A -	-	C	T	V	S	I	G	E	-	-	V S A	-	G E - A - E D - M Q S S	-	+	+
ARsk963	A -	-	C	T	V	-	-	-	E	-	-	V S A	-	G E - - - E D I M - S S	nd	+	+
VAusdg4447	- -	-	-	-	-	-	I	-	-	-	-	- - -	-	- - S - N - - - - - - -	+	+	+
VAusrc4798	- -	-	-	-	-	-	-	-	-	Q	-	- - -	-	- - S - N - - - - - - -	-	+	+
VAussk4501	- I	-	-	-	-	-	-	-	-	N	-	- - -	-	- - S - N - - - - - - -	-	+	+
FLusrc2836	- -	S	-	-	-	-	-	-	-	-	-	- - -	-	- - - - - - - - - - - -	+	-	+
FLusfx2833	- -	S	-	-	-	-	-	-	-	-	-	- - -	-	- - - - - - - - - - - -	+	-	+
FLusfx498	- -	-	-	-	-	-	-	-	-	-	-	- - -	-	- - - - - - - - - - - -	+	+	+
FLusfx502	- -	-	-	-	-	-	-	-	-	-	-	- - -	-	- - - - - - - - - - - -	+	+	+
ALusct4637	- -	-	-	-	-	-	-	-	-	R	-	- - -	-	- - - - - -	-	+	+

B.

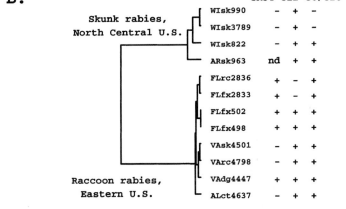

Monoclonal Antibody Reaction Pattern

	CR54	C12	C6/C20
Skunk rabies, North Central U.S. WIsk990	-	+	-
WIsk3789	-	+	-
WIsk822	-	+	+
ARsk963	nd	+	+
FLrc2836	+	-	+
FLfx2833	+	-	+
FLfx502	+	+	+
FLfx498	+	+	+
VAsk4501	-	+	+
VArc4798	-	+	+
VAdg4447	+	+	+
Raccoon rabies, Eastern U.S. ALct4637	-	+	+

Fig. 1. Identification of amino acids critical for the folding of the rabies nucleoprotein in a conformation recognized by monoclonal antibodies CR54, C12, and C6/C20. Samples very closely related by nucleotide sequence analysis may have very different reactivity with monoclonal antibodies if point mutations occur at these critical sites. Samples are identified by two-letter abbreviation for U.S. state and animal (ct, cat; dg, dog; rc, raccoon; sk, skunk; fx, fox) followed by CDC Rabies Laboratory database number. (A) The amino acid sequence predicted for the nucleoprotein gene of different antigenic variants of rabies virus associated with skunks in the north central United States and raccoons in the eastern United States. Amino acid sequence is inferred from the translation of nucleotide sequence (1350 nucleotides); only variant amino acids are shown. Spaces in the sequence for sample Alusct4637 correspond to the undetermined region of the gene. Rectangles indicate amino acid residues contributing to epitopes recognized by monoclonal antibodies CR54 (residue 112), Cl2 (residue 36), or C6/C20 (residues 128 and 181); nd = not done. (B) UPGMA tree of different antigenic variants of rabies virus associated with skunks in the north central United States and raccoons in the eastern United States shown in (A). Phylogenetic analyses were performed with DNADIST [Kimura two-parameter method and UPGMA programs of the PHYLIP package, Version 3.5] using nucleotide sequence from positions 1177–1476 (300 bp) as compared with the Pasteur rabies virus (GenBank accession no. M13215).

bat viruses in samples from dogs and cats diagnosed with rabies in Ethiopia (Mebatsion *et al.*, 1992) and South Africa (von Teichman *et al.*, 1998) and identified antigenic variants of rabies virus in animal reservoirs spanning international boundaries and diverse geographies (Diaz *et al.*, 1994; McQuiston *et al.*, 2001). Antigenic typing was used to distinguish between wild-type and vaccine virus in the massive oral vaccination campaigns against fox rabies in western Europe (Schneider *et al.*, 1988), and with very little additional effort and expense, diagnostic laboratories in the United States can provide a survey of the boundaries of raccoon-transmitted rabies needed for effective control programs for that reservoir (see Table II).

The amino acid sequence of the antigenic site recognized by a MAb is known for only a few linear epitopes that retain a reactive conformation in peptide fragments and in deletion mutants (Dietzschold *et al.*, 1983; Wunner *et al.*, 1988; Goto *et al.*, 2000). Most MAbs recognize epitopes created by the folding of a full-length protein and are mapped by functional assay (Coulon *et al.*, 1993). Functional methods do not identify the entire amino acid sequence for the epitope but may identify one or two amino acids critical for folding of the protein in the correct conformation for antibody recognition.

Figure 1, for example, details the process by which functional sites for several MAbs (see Table II) were identified. After two non reactors with MAb CR54 were found during a survey for raccoon rabies in Virginia (Sylvia Whaley, unpublished data, Virginia Department of Health), sequences of the nucleoprotein of reactive and nonreactive viruses collected from the same area revealed that a single amino acid change at position 112 had prevented recognition. The presence of lysine at position 112 was required for the reaction of antibody CR54 with the virus lineage perpetuated in raccoons in the eastern United States, but rabies viruses from skunks in North Central states did not react with CR54 despite the presence of lysine at position 112. The virus variant identified by the amino acid change could not be described as a single genetic lineage. An amino acid change affecting the binding of CR54 also was found in a sample from Alabama (Leland Wood, unpublished data, Alabama Department of Public Health), but the closest genetic relatives of the nonreactive viruses from Virginia were other virus isolates from Virginia reactive with the MAb, not the nonreactive virus from Alabama, and three different amino acid substitutions were found at position 112 in the three nonreactive viruses. Similar observations and comparisons identified the participation of leucine at position 36 in another antigenic variant in raccoons in Florida (Valerie Mock, unpublished data, Florida Department of Health) and subsequently in isolated cases in North Carolina, South Carolina, and Alabama (unpublished data, Gina Woodlief, North Carolina State Laboratory of Public Health; Marsha Tolson, South Carolina Department of Health and Environmental Control; Leland Wood, Alabama Department of Public Health). Amino acid changes at position 128 (leucine to proline) and 181 (isoleucine to valine) also produced a second antigenic variant in skunks in Wisconsin (Jim Powell, unpublished data, Wisconsin Division of Health). The variant was present in a 1983 survey but unrecognized as associated with skunks (Smith, 1989).

Clearly, MAb binding can be a complex phenomenon, and as illustrated by these findings, antigenic typing methods allow only broad conclusions about the evolutionary history or relatedness of virus groups (Bourhy *et al.*, 1992; Kissi *et al.*, 1995). No specific amino acid changes have been correlated with a host range determination despite attempts by several investigators. Comparative sequence data have revealed that some codons (triplet nucleotide sequences specific for an amino acid) in the G protein gene (Kissi *et al.*, 1999) and in the P gene (Nadin-Davis *et al.*, 1997) have higher rates of nonsynonymous change than others, which may signify localized positive selection and important structural-functional relationships. To date, such methods have failed to show a strong association between certain mutations and host species. For example, analysis of viruses from outbreaks in which spillover from foxes was suspected to have resulted in sustained transmission in skunks (Nadin-Davis *et al.*, 1993, 1997) and raccoon dogs (Bourhy *et al.*, 1999) revealed that the strongest sample associations for viruses were from the same geographic area, regardless of species source for the samples. These samples may not have been representative of sustained transmission, however, because vaccination of foxes eliminated disease from all other species in the vaccinated area (Pastoret and Brochier, 1998).

While it is likely that the molecular elements of adaptation will be revealed as more comparative studies are conducted, the genetic changes associated with adaptation may well be limited to one or a few amino acids. A striking example of this is the single amino acid at position 333 of the G protein that distinguishes pathogenic from nonpathogenic viruses arising from the ERA and CVS laboratory strains of rabies virus (Dietzschold *et al.*, 1983), and it is possible that similarly small coding changes can affect host preference as well. Without strong support from case surveillance data for host switching, the background random mutations in a virus population will obscure recognition of any functional change. In order to be reliably interpreted, antigenic variation in the virus population under survey must be understood in relation to the genetic changes that are responsible for the altered epitopes.

B. Genetic Typing

Genetic typing as a method for molecular epidemiologic investigation is increasing in use as more laboratories have the ability to amplify virus RNA by RT-PCR and nucleotide sequence analysis becomes easier to accomplish. The output of genetic typing is a phylogenetic tree, a hierarchical branching diagram that depicts relationships between samples based on models of nucleotide substitution

(Moritz and Hillis, 1996). An evolutionary root, determined by adding an out-group (i.e., a taxon that is hypothesized to be less closely related to each of the taxa under consideration than any are to each other), defines the direction of character changes on the tree. A typical outgroup for an analysis of rabies virus samples might be samples of one of the other lyssavirus species. The branches of a tree represent virus lineages, and clusters of lineages represent clades or monophyletic groups (taxa that share features that are derived from an ancestral population and set the clade apart from other samples in the analysis). The phylogenetic analysis in Fig. 1 depicts samples from rabies outbreaks in skunks and raccoons in the United States as two distinct clades.

When a nucleotide sequence is used for tree reconstruction, each position in a multiple sequence alignment is a separate character with four potential states representing the four nucleotides (A, T, G, C) possible at that position in the sequence. Since mutations continue to accumulate after lineage splitting, algorithms for tree reconstruction can be quite complex, requiring computer-based phylogeny programs. The most commonly used programs, such as PHYLIP (*http://evolution.genetics.washington.edu/phylip.html*) and PAUP (Sinauer, Sunderland, MA), provide several methods of tree reconstruction. Algorithms in distance-based methods [e.g., neighbor joining or UPGMA (unweighted pair group method using arithmetic averages)] resolve the data as a single tree based on the overall distance or difference between all pairs of sequences in an analysis. Character-based methods (e.g., maximum parsimony and maximum likelihood) analyze individual substitutions to determine the tree constructions possible for the data and then compare the trees for optimality. Maximum parsimony selects trees that minimize the total tree length (the number of evolutionary steps required to explain the sequence data); maximum likelihood defines the optimal tree as the one most likely to have occurred given the observed data and the assumed model of evolution. The choice of method used often depends on the purpose of the analysis. In many epidemiologic investigations, it is not vital that the best arrangement be found for every branch of a tree. Once an initial survey has defined the genetic variation present in an outbreak area, the important epidemiologic information is often simply the position of the sample of interest within a particular clade. For these types of analyses, which often involve very large numbers of taxa of short sequence lengths (Fig. 2, for example), distance-based methods, which are very fast, will resolve clade associations as well as maximum parsimony and maximum likelihood, which are more computationally intensive methods.

Because analysis of even a small data set produces several possible branching patterns for the phylogenetic tree, statistical methods are used to estimate the relative degree of support for a given clade. The most commonly used statistical method, the nonparametric bootstrap analysis, randomly resamples the original data with replacement to form pseudoreplicates of 100 to 1000 new data sets. When

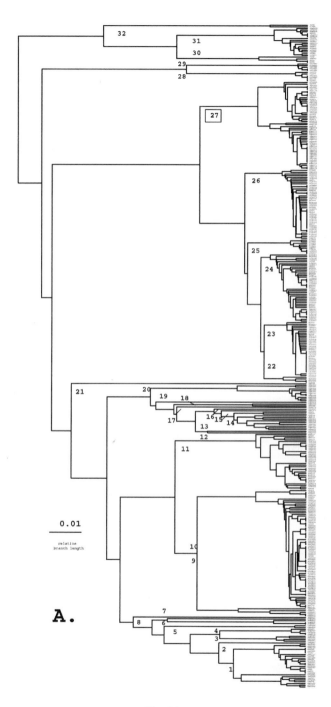

Fig. 2A.

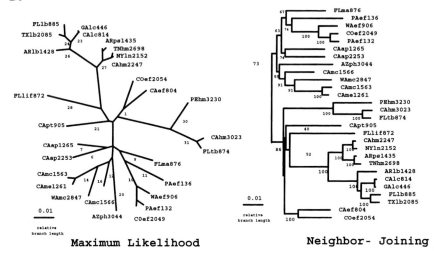

B.

Maximum Likelihood   Neighbor- Joining

Fig. 2. Genetic lineages of rabies virus in U.S. bat populations. (*A*) UPGMA tree of rabies virus found in 383 samples representing 25 U.S. bat species identified in Table III. Non U.S. bats in the UPGMA analysis include 4 samples from vampire bats *Desmodus rotundus*, from Brazil, Venezuela, and Argentina (lineage 30) and 2 samples from South American freetail bats, *Tadarida brasiliensis* (lineage 32). Phylogenetic analyses were performed using nucleotide sequence from positions 1177–1476 (300 bp). (*B*) Maximum-likelihood analysis and neighbor-joining analyses (DNAML and DNADIST programs in the PHYLIP package) using the complete N gene sequence of 1414 bp for representative rabies virus lineages found in bat populations. Samples are identified by two-letter abbreviation for U.S. state and animal origin followed by CDC Rabies Laboratory database number (hm, human; ap, *Antrozus pallidus*; ef, *Eptesicus fuscus*; ln, *Lasionycteris noctivagans*; lb, *Lasiurus borealis*; lc, *L. cinereus*; li, *L. intermedius*; ma, *Myotis austroriparius*; mc, *M. californicus*; me, *M. evotis*; ps, *Pipistrellus subflavus*; ph, *P. hesperus*; pt, *Plecotus townsendii*; tb, *Tadarida brasiliensis*). In the maximum-likelihood analysis, the numbered branches indicate the placement of the samples in the numbered sample groups in the UPGMA tree of (*A*). The numbered nodes in the neighbor-joining tree indicate the number of times each node was reproduced in 100 bootstrap resamplings of the data. Complete N gene sequences for the lineages shown are available from GenBank (accession numbers AF045166, AF394868–AF394888, and AY039224–AY039229).

the new data sets are analyzed, the proportion of times that each clade is recovered is taken as a measure of the statistical support for the grouping (see Fig. 2*B*).

    The size and location of the genomic interval for analysis and the taxa included for study are determined from the epidemiologic question under consideration. The first sequence comparisons among rabies virus samples were based on the relatively short 200 nucleotides it was possible to read from autoradiographs. When an interval of 200 nucleotides of the N protein gene was used in the analysis, the conclusions drawn from studies of genetic variation in rabies virus samples from dogs in different countries (Smith *et al.*, 1992) were similar to those of a more comprehensive study that was conducted using the entire N gene coding region of 1350 nucleotides (Kissi *et al.*, 1995). Similarly, the clades for bats are retained when the analysis is performed with 300 or 1414 nucleotides (see Fig. 2). However, short sequences often contain an insufficient number of informative characters for statistically significant support of clades and may not allow accurate reconstruction of evolutionary relationships between clades. As can be seen in Fig. 3, informative characters accumulate as longer regions of the genome are sequenced and used in the analysis.

Recombination is unknown for lyssaviruses, and phylogenetic relationships between samples have been similar regardless of the location of the genomic interval analyzed (Nel *et al.*, 1993; Nadin-Davis *et al.*, 1997; Bourhy *et al.*, 1999). Areas of the genome vary, however, in degree of evolutionary change. Protein structure and function constrain tolerable mutations in genes, whereas mutations accumulate quickly in stretches of noncoding sequence within and between genes. Although it might appear advantageous to compare samples over a rapidly evolving intergenic region, such sites can become uninformative or misleading when saturated by change. The numerous insertions, deletions, and reversions that accumulate in nontranslated regions of the lyssavirus genome produce only tentative sequence alignments for sequences from different lyssavirus species and difficult alignments even for members of the same species if samples are taken from widely differing ecologic niches. Phylogenetic reconstruction programs assume that all the nucleotides aligned at a given position represent homologous sites of the gene; thus ambiguous alignments can lead to inaccurate phylogenetic trees. For example, the extra nucleotides described for the European bat lyssavirus (EBLV-2 sample in Fig. 3) are shown adjacent to the polyadenylation signal, but in fact, the insertion could have been made as a cluster or as one or two nucleotides almost anywhere in the nontranslated region between the N and P genes. The same can be said of the deleted nucleotide in the FLUSli872 sample, although placement in this case is more constrained by the forced alignment with closely related rabies virus samples.

Perhaps the greatest drawback to interpreting rabies phylogenies correctly is not inappropriate sampling of the viral genome but inadequate sampling of the true underlying diversity of the variant in the host population. For terrestrial animal reservoirs, samples should be representative of the entire outbreak area. Physical features of the landscape can isolate virus populations (Nadin-Davis *et al.*, 1997; Bourhy *et al.*, 1999; Crawford-Miksza *et al.*, 1999), introducing unexpected genetic variability into the analysis. Because outbreaks of rabies may persist in a given area for decades at low levels, samples should represent as long a time period as possible. Localized persistence of a variant cannot be distinguished from a new introduction (Nadin-Davis *et al.*, 1994).

Rabies transmission cycles in bats are much more difficult to interpret than similar cycles in terrestrial animals and present special problems in sample

A.

```
             1371
  Consensus   GCCCTAATTC ATTTGCTGAA TTTCTAAACA AGACATATTC TAACGACCCG...
RABVVAusrc4798                                                       ...
RABVVAussk4501                                                       ...
RABVVAusdg4447                                                       ...
RABVFLusfx498                                                    t   ...
RABVFLusfx502                                                    t   ...
RABVFLusfx2833                                                   t   ...
RABVFLusrc2836                                                   t   ...
RABVALusct4637                                                  t a...


RABVFlusli872    a  c              g  t             g gt  t a...


RABVWIussk3789   t  a  c     c  c  g           g    g gt  t a...
RABVWIussk990    t  a  c     c  c  g           g    g gt  t a...
RABVWIussk822    t  a  c     c  c  g           g    g g   t a...


ABLVfruit        a  g  c        g  g     c          a gt  t   ...


ABLVinsect       g  g  c  g           c          c  g gt  tt t...


EBLV2            a     c  c     a     ct g        t  g gt  t aaga
```

B.

```
             1421
  Consensus   TAAGGAGTCG AACTTCAAGA TTGTCAACAA TAATAAATTG TTTAATTCCT CCAT..........GAAAAAAACT
RABVVAusrc4798 TAG                                                          ..........GAAAAAAACT
RABVVAussk4501 TAG                                                          ..........GAAAAAAACT
RABVVAusdg4447 TAG                                              a      c    ..........GAAAAAAACT
RABVFLusfx498  TAG                                                     c    ..........GAAAAAAACT
RABVFLusfx502  TAG                                                     c    ..........GAAAAAAACT
RABVFLusfx2833 TAG                                                     c    ..........GAAAAAAACT
RABVFLusrc2836 TAG                                           c         c    ..........GAAAAAAACT
RABVALusct4637 TAA       a                                               ..........GAAAAAAACT


RABVFlusli872  TAA.a a t      a  g      a g      c             ca  ca    t  c ..........GAAAAAAACT


RABVWIussk3789 TAA a   t    taa  t    gccgg a c ct   g c     g  ta    a t    ..........GAAAAAAACT
RABVWIussk990  TAA a   t    taa  t    gccgg a c ct   g       g  ta    a t    ..........GAAAAAAACT
RABVWIussk822  TAA a   t    taa  t    gccgg a c ct   g ca   gc ta    a t    ..........GAAAAAAACT


ABLVfruit      TAAtc  at  tgtcaggtct  gcc cta     t  tg gaa ca c cct a t t  acaa.......GAAAAAAACT


ABLVinsect     TAAct  a  .ctcaagcct gat     ta    ct  c ggaa gg tgc t   t t  ccaa.......GAAAAAAACT
EBLV2          TAAaagg g aga ctct a t at att   gt tc   cc acc tcc  a tatc aggagaaggggaaaGAAAAAAACT
```

Fig. 3. Comparison of nucleotide sequence alignments of translated (protein encoding) and nontranslated regions of the nucleoprotein gene of selected lyssavirus samples. RABV samples are identified by two-letter abbreviation for U.S. state and animal (ct, cat; dg, dog; rc, raccoon; sk, skunk; fx, fox; li, *Lasiurus intermedius*) followed by CDC Rabies Laboratory database number. Nucleotide position is determined by the sequence of the Pasteur rabies virus (GenBank accession no. M13215). GenBank accession numbers for sequences for other lyssavirus samples are as indicated in Table II in Chapter 9. (*A*) Alignment of 3′ translated sequence of the N mRNA beginning with position 1371 for selected lyssavirus samples. The open reading frame of rabies virus (RABV) and Australian bat lyssavirus (ABLV) extends through nucleotide 1420. European bat lyssavirus 2 (EBLV2) contains an additional three nucleotides of protein-encoding sequence (one codon) at the 5′ terminus of the N mRNA as compared with Pasteur rabies virus. (*B*) As compared with Pasteur rabies virus, samples of RABV and ABLV terminate translation with a stop codon (**TAA** or **TAG**) at bp 1421. The nontranslated region of ABLV contains an additional 4 nucleotides as compared with Pasteur rabies virus. EBLV2 terminates translation with a stop codon (**TAA**) at bp 1424 and contains an additional 7 to 12 nucleotides as compared with the samples of RABV and ABLV. All samples used **GAAAAAAA** as a polyadenylation signal and contained CT in the N–P intergenic region (. = insertions/deletions).

collection both because of the greater number of species that may serve as reservoir hosts and because the great vagility of some bat species permits contacts between individual animals over hundreds to thousands of miles. At least 30 different lineages are evident in the analysis of 25 U.S. bat species shown in Fig. 2. For the more reclusive species not often encountered by humans, too few samples exist to identify an associated lineage with certainty. Lineage 17, for example, is formed by a single sample from a spotted bat, *Euderma maculatum*. Despite a fairly wide range in the United States, spotted bats are one of the rarest and least known of American bats. Some lineages that are found rarely in U.S. bats may be common variants in South American bat populations. For example, the lineage 8 sample from a big free-tailed bat, *Nyctinomops macrotis*, was found more commonly in a survey of Brazilian bats (Smith, unpublished observation). Samples from hoary bats, *Lasiurus cinereus*, collected from New York to California are nearly identical (lineage 23) and share high homology with a hoary bat sample from Brazil (Smith, unpublished observation). Lineage 31 includes samples from Mexican free-tailed bats (*Tadarida barsiliensis*) collected not only from Florida to California but also from Mexico (De Mattos *et al.*, 1999). De Mattos *et al.* (2000) describe a second equally widespread lineage for virus samples collected from southern hemisphere populations of *T. brasiliensis* (lineage 32 in Fig. 2). And finally, some bat species may not support cycles of rabies transmission independent of other bat species. The 15 samples from the little brown bat, *Myotis lucifugus*, are arranged as eight different lineages (Table III), and this bat is infrequently found rabid despite its frequent submission for rabies tests (Smith *et al.*, 1995).

Because more sequence data are available for the N gene, the majority of comparative studies focus on this region of the lyssavirus genome. The database for other gene regions is increasing, however, and comparison with results from other laboratories can greatly reduce the time involved in selecting appropriate target sequences and accumulating sufficient data for the level of comparison desired for an investigation. While epidemiologic surveys rarely require more than a few hundred nucleotides for analysis, a satisfactory answer to questions of evolution and molecular mechanisms of adaptation may come only from analysis of the entire genome of every taxon under consideration. As methods of accumulating sequence data become more automated, this soon may be a reality.

C. Viral Taxonomy

The biologic and ecologic properties of an infectious agent often can be predicted from its taxonomy. Genetic differences between viruses are an easily acquired measure of evolutionary distance, and the tree structure of a phylogenetic analysis would seem an obvious way to depict the extent of relatedness

TABLE III

U.S. Bat Species Composition of Sample Groups in the Phylogenetic Analysis Depicted in Figure 2
Groups 1–14

Species	Total	1	2	3	4	5	6	7	8	9	10	11	12	13	14
Antrozous pallidus	9			1	1		3	1							
Eptesicus fuscus	117	16									65	31			
Euderma maculatum	1														
Lasionycteris noctivagans	26	1													
Lasiurus borealis	75														
Lasiurus cinereus	26														
Lasiurus ega	7	1													
Lasiurus intermedius	12														
Lasiurus seminolus	5														
Myotis austroriparius	1									1					
Myotis californicus	6												1	1	1
Myotis ciliolabrum	1														
Myotis evotis	4														4
Myotis keenii	2														1
Myotis lucifugus	15	2		1	1						1	2			2
Myotis thysanodes	2														1
Myotis velifer	5	2				2									
Myotis yumanensis	2			1	1										
Myotis sp.	11	4	1	1	1						2				1
Nycticeius humeralis	5									4					
Nyctinomops macrotis	1								1						
Pipistrellus hesperus	11														1
Pipistrellus subflavus	23														
Plecotus townsendii	2														
Tadarida brasiliensis	14														
TOTAL	383	26	1	4	4	2	3	1	1	5	68	33	1	1	11

continued

Groups 15–29 and 31[a]

Species	Total	15	16	17	18	19	20	21	22	23	24	25	26	27	28	29	31
Antrozous pallidus	9									1							2
Eptesicus fuscus	117									1	2			2			
Euderma maculatum	1			1													
Lasionycteris noctivagans	26									2				23			
Lasiurus borealis	75										35	5	34	1			
Lasiurus cinereus	26									25				1			
Lasiurus ega	7								4	2							
Lasiurus intermedius	12									1					6	5	
Lasiurus seminolus	5										1	3	1				
Myotis austroriparius	1																
Myotis californicus	6		1				1							1			
Myotis ciliolabrum	1				1												
Myotis evotis	4																
Myotis keenii	2												1				
Myotis lucifugus	15												2	4			
Myotis thysanodes	2	1															
Myotis velifer	5									1							
Myotis yumanensis	2																
Myotis sp.	11						1										
Nycticeius humeralis	5												1				
Nyctinomops macrotis	1																
Pipistrellus hesperus	11				1	1	8										
Pipistrellus subflavus	23										1	1	1	20			
Plecotus townsendii	2							1		1							
Tadarida brasiliensis	14																14
TOTAL	383	1	1	1	2	1	10	1	4	34	39	9	40	52	6	5	16

[a]The virus lineages 30 and 32 were not found in U.S. bat population.

within and among named groups of viruses. Despite these obvious attributes, few areas of virology incite as much argument and discussion as the issue of designating species names for viruses (van Regenmortel *et al.*, 2000).

   The controversy stems from the difficulty, and perhaps the impossibility in some situations, of placing viruses into different taxonomic groups based on differences in amino acid or nucleotide sequence. The abstract entity of a virus species is in fact a replicating lineage that varies continuously with time and with transmission to different host populations. We recognize one virus species as distinct from all other virus species because of genetic changes that have accumulated to a point where it is obvious that different species are present, but it is not possible to define precisely when that point is reached. "Virus species are fuzzy sets with hazy boundaries…" (van Regenmortel, 1998). Taxonomic relationships are even more difficult to develop when genetic differences between virus groups are not manifested as phenotypic differences. These same arguments apply to any organized system of nomenclature for the different viral lineages (strains, variants, subspecies) that comprise the abstract entity of a virus species.

The species and subspecies designations within the *Lyssavirus* genus are as controversial as any in virology. The need for a genus designation to encompass the viruses that cause the clinical disease rabies (see Table I) arose with the description by Shope *et al.* (1970) of two rabies-related viruses from Africa. The viruses, Lagos bat virus (LAGV) and Mokola virus (MOKV), were sufficiently similar to rabies virus that infected neurons could be detected in a fluorescent antibody test (see Chap. 9) using antisera prepared against the internal N protein of rabies virus. The two African viruses could be distinguished from rabies virus by using cross-neutralization tests with antisera prepared against their respective surface G proteins. More important from a public health perspective, human rabies immune globulin, a crucial component of rabies prophylaxis, has little or no neutralizing activity against MOKV and LAGV (see Table I). The biologic (phenotypic) change in MOKV and LAGV that eliminated cross-protective sites shared with rabies virus argues strongly for use of specific diagnostic tests to identify and distinguish MOKV and LAGV from rabies virus and specific epithets to describe these viruses and impart the public health importance of their biologic differences from rabies virus.

Although other lyssavirus species have been named, biologic distinctions among these viruses are less clear. Australian bat lyssavirus (ABLV), Duvenhage virus (DUVV), European bat lyssavirus 1 (EBLV1), and EBLV2 are readily neutralized by anti-rabies virus antibodies (see Table I). The four viruses are also difficult to distinguish from one another and from rabies virus with MAbs (Bourhy *et al.*, 1992; Gould *et al.*, 1998). Specific identification of rabies virus, ABLV, DUVV, EBLV1, and EBLV2 is based almost entirely on nucleotide sequence analyses (Fig. 4 and Table IV (Bourhy *et al.*, 1993; Gould *et al.*, 1998; Badrane *et al.*, 2001) that show these viruses as five distinct lineages. These same analyses also show that the five lineages share a common ancestry that sets them apart from MOKV and LAGV (see Fig. 4) (Badrane *et al.*, 2001). This distinctive immunologic and phylogenetic division led Badrane *et al.* (2001) to propose two subgeneric taxonomic groups for the *Lyssavirus* genus (phylogroups 1 and 2 in Fig. 4). The new grouping is intended as a guide for the development of new vaccines and public health recommendations specific for exposures to lyssaviruses resistant to traditional rabies prophylaxis.

On a finer scale, a clear and consistent system of nomenclature for the different viral lineages that comprise the abstract entity of a virus species also would

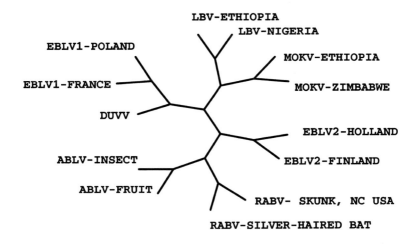

Parsimony

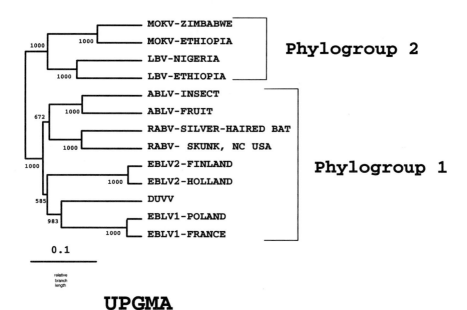

UPGMA

Fig. 4. UPGMA and parsimony analyses (DNADIST and DNAPARS programs in the PHYLIP package) using translated region of N gene (1350 bp) for representative samples of the seven lyssavirus species. The numbered nodes in the UPGMA tree indicate the number of times each node was reproduced in 1000 bootstrap resamplings of the data. GenBank accession numbers for sequence lyssavirus samples are as indicated in Table II in Chapter 9.

be of great utility in epidemiologic tracking of rabies outbreaks. When collections are small and focused on a specific geographic area, nomenclature can be personalized and uncomplicated (the skunk and raccoon rabies clades in Fig. 1, for example). This type of naming convention works well when case surveillance data have correctly identified the animal species responsible for enzootic disease maintenance in a particular geographic area, when the host species does not change over time, and when significant geographic structuring is not present in the host population. As more data accumulate, however, and the results of molecular typing are transmitted to a more general audience, an organized system of nomenclature will be needed. For example, the very complicated tree representing bat rabies in the United States does not lend itself to host-based naming of clades simply because the reservoir host is speculative for some clades and unknown for many of the other clades.

The alternative system, alphanumeric nomenclature, is more useful for rapidly evolving virus populations, such as poliovirus, in which a single variant sweeps through a host population, and patterns of transmission are reconstructed from mutations in virus samples collected for the outbreak investigation (Centers for Disease Control and Prevention, 2000a). Rabies samples for genetic analysis are almost always random submissions to public health laboratories, not study collections, and rarely is the chain of transmission known, nor can it be reconstructed from patterns of mutation. Several groups have attempted to estimate a molecular clock for the evolution of lyssavirus populations using mutational patterns (Amengual *et al.*, 1997; Sacramento *et al.*, 1992), but estimates of the date of origin of a new rabies outbreak are still most reliably demonstrated from case surveillance data.

The clades in Fig. 2 are numbered as a convenience for discussion of the samples in this chapter, but they illustrate the difficulty in presenting sequence data to any audience. Virus nomenclature should reflect both the evolutionary history of a sample and its epidemiologic significance. With increasingly large data sets and increasingly complex analyses, this goal may be difficult to attain.

III. INSIGHTS: ASPECTS OF RABIES EPIDEMIOLOGY AND PATHOGENESIS REVEALED BY MOLECULAR METHODS OF EPIDEMIOLOGIC INVESTIGATION

Rabies is unique among zoonotic diseases in that prevention of human disease is linked to the laboratory diagnosis of cases in animals. Molecular typing studies can take advantage of an abundance of animal rabies samples submitted to public health laboratories for testing. While many studies seem simply to confirm observations made from traditional case surveillance methods, virus typing often has led to unexpected disease associations and new ways of looking at traditional control programs.

A. Human Rabies Case Investigation

In what has become an increasingly familiar pattern, all four of the indigenously acquired human rabies infections in the United States during 2000 were
attributed to contact with insectivorous bats inside a home (Centers for Disease
Control and Prevention, 2000b). In no case did the contact elicit postexposure
rabies prophylaxis. Public health workers became aware of the exposures only
after a laboratory diagnosis of rabies had been made and friends and family members of the patient were questioned for incidents of bat contact reported to them
by the patient.

On the surface, these cases and 26 similar cases since 1980 (Noah *et al.*, 1998)
might not appear extraordinary. Several species of insectivorous bat use houses and
outbuildings as day roosts or hibernacula. Colonies of hundreds to thousands of
these house bats [usually big brown (*Eptesicus fuscus*), little brown (*Myotis lucifugus*), or Mexican free-tailed bats (*Tadarida brasiliensis*)] may exist seasonally in
or close to human dwellings. Rabid bats often become unable to fly, increasing the
opportunity for human contact. Because bites by bats may result in an insignificant
wound as compared with bites by terrestrial carnivores, the implications of a bat
bite often are minimized, and medical care may be thought unnecessary.

This simple explanation for human rabies exposure becomes more complicated, however, when virus samples from the cases are submitted to genetic typing. The virus variant identified in two of the four recent cases and 22 other
human case samples (Smith *et al.*, 1995) is not found commonly in house bats.
Instead, virus typing (Fig. 5) identified bats whose habits and roost preferences
do not often bring them in contact with humans, silver-haired bats (*Lasionycteris
noctivagans*) and eastern pipistrelle bats (*Pipistrellus subflavus*). Lineage 27 (see
Figs. 2 and 5) was associated with 43 of 49 samples from silver-haired and eastern pipistrelle bats but in only minority samples from other species (9 samples
representing 5 bat species; see Table III). Among the explanations compatible
with these typing results are two opposing hypotheses.

Hypothesis 1.   *Lineage 27 is present in the majority of human cases because
it is the most common variant in bat populations.*

If this hypothesis is correct, then the database used to associate lineage 27 with
silver-haired and eastern pipistrelle bats (see Fig. 2 and Table III) cannot be representative of bat populations in the United States. There is some validity to this
assumption. Only a few public health laboratories identify all submitted bats to
species, and even when identifications are made, samples from red bats and common house bats are not submitted to virus typing in numbers proportional to their
importance in human–bat interactions. A strong bias exists for the submission of
samples from less common or unusual bat species for virus typing. As more

A.　　　　　　　　　　　　　**B.**

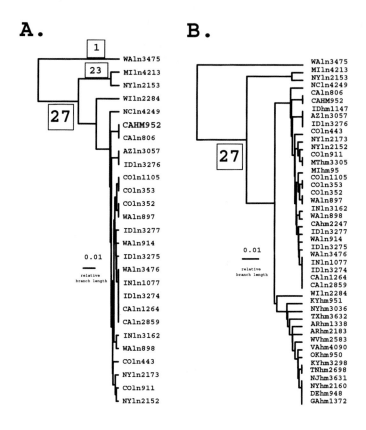

Fig. 5(A, B). Identification of silver-haired and eastern pipistrelle bats as reservoirs for the variant of rabies virus associated with most human rabies infections in the United States. (*A*) In 1958, a California woman died of rabies after a bite by a silver-haired bat, *Lasionycteris noctivagans* (ln). Nucleotide sequences for virus isolates from the woman (CAHM952) and from the bat (CAln806) were identical [positions 1177–1476 (300 bp) of the nucleocapsid gene]. The virus variant in the two samples was common in silver-haired bats throughout the United States, as indicated by the presence of the virus in 23 of 26 samples from this species (lineage 27 in Fig. 2 and Table III). This finding suggested that silver-haired bats were the reservoir for this variant of rabies virus. A virus common in hoary bats, *Lasiurus cinereus*, was found in 2 of 26 silver-haired bats (lineage 23 in Fig. 2 and Table III). The remaining sample (WAln3475) contained a virus common in big brown bats, *Eptesicus fuscus* (indicated as lineage 1 in Fig. 2 and Table III). (*B*) As more human rabies infections with this virus were identified, the topology of the phylogenetic tree changed. Virus isolates from human cases in the eastern United States clustered together separate from isolates from human cases in the western United States and separate from the silver-haired bat isolates, even from silver-haired bat samples collected in the eastern United States (see samples NcIn4249, NYln2152 and NYln2173). This finding suggested that different bat species might be involved in transmission of the virus in different areas of the United States.

continued

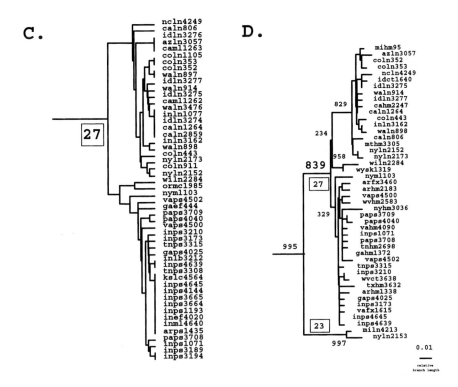

Fig. 5(C, D). Identification of silver-haired and eastern pipistrelle bats as reservoirs for the variant of rabies virus associated with most human rabies infections in the United States. (*C*) Sequence analysis identified eastern pipistrelle bats as a second reservoir for the virus found in human rabies infections. An UPGMA analysis of 383 virus samples (Fig. 2) identified a sample cluster consisting of samples from 23 of 26 silver-haired bats, 20 of 23 eastern pipistrelle bats, 4 of 16 little brown bats, 2 of 117 big brown bats, and 1 each from red, hoary, and California myotis bats (lineage 27 in Fig. 2 and Table III). Bootstrap resampling and maximum-likelihood analysis of the complete nucleocapsid gene sequence (1414 bp) supported the monophyly of lineage 27 (Fig. 2*B*). (*D*) The reservoir status of eastern pipistrelle bats may be of recent derivation. Monophyly of lineage 27 had strong statistical support by bootstrap resampling of 300 bp of nucleocapsid gene sequence for nonidentical samples (neighbor-joining analysis using ABLV as an outgroup). Samples from bats and from spillover infections in humans and terrestrial animals formed a distinct lineage separate from the lineage common in hoary bats in 839 of 1000 iterations. No support was found, however, for secondary clustering by species within lineage 27. More genetic diversity was found among samples from silver-haired bats, and a clade comprised solely of eastern pipistrelle bats was found in only 329 of 1000 iterations of the data. Samples from spillover infections are abbreviated as hm, human; ct, cat; fx, fox; sk, skunk.

surveys include all bats, it is possible that lineage 27 will be found in a larger proportion of samples from all bat species and/or eastern pipistrelle and silver-haired bats will be found to comprise a larger proportion of bats submitted for rabies testing because of human contact.

Hypothesis 1 is not supported by data gathered to date. For example, almost all bats submitted to the Indiana Department of Health from 1965 to the present have been identified to species at Indiana State University (Whitaker and Douglas, 1987). Samples from 116 bats collected during the years 1982–1999 were submitted for genetic typing (Messenger et al., in preparation). Eastern pipistrelle and silver-haired bats comprised, respectively, 2.5% and 1.6% of 6861 submissions and 7.3% and 1.5% of 342 rabies-positive bats. Samples from big brown and red bats were the most commonly submitted species (84% of all samples) and the bats more frequently found rabid (77% of all positive samples). Lineage 27 was associated with 11 of 12 eastern pipistrelle bats and 2 of 2 silver-haired bats but only 1 of 45 big brown bats, 1 of 44 red bats, and one of two little brown bats. Big brown bats in Indiana were infected most commonly with viruses of lineages 10 and 11; lineages 24, 25, and 26 were the most common lineages found in Indiana red bats, and lineage 26 was found in one little brown bat in Indiana.

There is evidence neither for frequent infection of terrestrial animals after contact with bats nor for widely disproportionate infection of terrestrial animals with the lineage 27 virus. Virus typing was conducted on 231 samples from cats and 77 samples from dogs diagnosed with rabies in public health laboratories in the United States in 1999 (McQuiston et al., 2001). Only one lineage associated with bats (lineage 10) was found in one cat sample, whereas the remaining cats and dogs were infected with the predominant terrestrial animal rabies variant in that geographic area.

Hypothesis 2.   *Incidence of contact with humans may be no greater for silver-haired and eastern pipistrelle bats than for other bats, but increased virulence of the lineage 27 virus allows for more successful transmission events to occur after superficial contact with a bat infected with a lineage 27 virus.*

Both experimental data and epidemiologic data support hypothesis 2. The lineage 27 virus replicates well at 34°C in fibroblast and epithelial cells, characteristics that could facilitate infection after superficial contact (Morimoto et al., 1996), although more experimental data are needed to confirm this observation. Certain variants associated with common bat species (e.g., lineages 24, 25, and 26 common in red bats) are underrepresented in cross-species transmission events both between bat species (see Table III) and from bats to humans (Smith et al., 1995), suggesting that virulence is not equal among all variants.

If hypothesis 2 is correct, then human rabies will remain rare in the United States because an unnoticed or unrecognized contact with silver-haired and eastern pipistrelle bats or with any animal infected with the variant of rabies virus they transmit also should be a rare event. Unfortunately, prevention of those few human deaths will be almost impossible because unnoticed or unrecognized animal contact will not elicit antirabies treatment.

The increased-virulence hypothesis carries with it an additional risk factor, however. Other bat species also have been found infected with lineage 27 (see Table III), raising the possibility of further host range expansion. Significantly, the occurrence of lineage 27 among 4 of 15 little brown bats tested, coupled with this bat's small size, broad distribution, and habit of colonizing houses, could make it an important vector species. Clearly, further study is needed to assess the potential for cross-species transmission to this and other bat species.

B. Incubation Periods

Perhaps the most dramatic findings from virus typing have confirmed the existence of extremely long incubation periods in rabies (Smith *et al.*, 1991; McColl *et al.*, 1993). Although incubation periods of 16 months to 19 years had been, reported for human rabies cases, the validity of these reports was questioned. Almost all of the cases had occurred in areas where rabies is endemic, making it impossible to rule out a second unnoticed or unrecorded exposure in the intervening period. It was not until the advent of genetic typing methods and the investigation of four rabies deaths in immigrants to the United States and Australia that the existence of this very unusual aspect of rabies pathogenesis was confirmed (Smith *et al.*, 1991; McColl *et al.*, 1993). In all four cases, the victims were young (10, 12, 13, and 18 years of age at the time of disease onset) and had emigrated from areas where dog rabies was common (Laos, Mexico, the Philippines, and Vietnam). Extensive questioning of the patients, family members, and acquaintances failed to reveal a source of exposure in the United States or Australia, virus isolates from the patients did not resemble any virus common in the United States or Australia, and the best match for the patient's virus was virus originating in and around the country of residence before emigration.

These observations are of more than epidemiologic interest because they influence the design and use of antirabies biologics. As yet, no experimental model explains virus persistence, nor at what point and for how long after entry into a wound the virus remains vulnerable to antirabies prophylaxis (Baer and Yager, 1977; Dietzschold *et al.*, 1992).

Long incubation periods are also known for naturally infected animals (Bingham *et al.*, 1994) and provide a mechanism for global spread of rabies variants along migratory routes and through human transport (Smith *et al.*, 1992).

C. Enhanced Surveillance

A description of the genetic diversity in indigenous rabies virus populations and the geographic distribution of different-genetic groups when disease-control programs are first implemented provides a mechanism for tracing transmission cycles and focusing resources in regions where rabies is persistent. Because sequence diversity in a virus population declines as intensive immunization of animals eliminates virus lineages, virus typing provides a means of evaluating control strategies. For example, recent typing of samples representative of dog rabies in Mexico and Thailand (DeMattos *et al.*, 1999; Ito *et al.*, 1999) found distinctive markers for cases originating in different regions of the country and evidence of greatest genetic diversity in national capitals where economic opportunities attract intraregional migrants with their domestic animals. For these countries, genetic heterogeneity will decline in virus samples found in capital regions only as successful rabies control programs are implemented in outlying areas. Similarly, rabies samples from the Llanos and Andean regions of Venezuela shared 99% homology with samples from Colombia (DeMattos *et al.*, 1996), suggesting that successful control programs in this region must address the wide expanse of common border and active traffic of people and their animals between the two countries.

The outcome of the surveillance analysis also can dictate the extent to which control measures must be reimplemented to eliminate residual cases. For example, virus typing of residual domestic animal rabies cases in Chile indicated that no new vaccination campaigns were necessary (Favi *et al.*, 1999). Domestic animal cases were sporadic, and antigenic and genetic typing identified insectivorous bats as the source for all 15 domestic animal rabies cases since 1980 (DeMattos *et al.*, 2000).

The phylogenetic relationships that are apparent in epidemiologic studies of rabies often lead to questions about evolutionary patterns. Certain lineages are distributed globally, whereas others are much more restricted in distribution. The *Lyssavirus* species rabies virus is found in North and South America, Europe, Asia, and Africa and a wide range of carnivore and chiropteran species serve as reservoir hosts. In contrast, almost all samples of EBLV1 are from European locations and from a single bat species, *Eptesicus serotinus* (see Table I). This adaptability is reflected in the relative complexity of a phylogenetic tree for the two lyssaviruses (see Fig. 4 and Table IV). The relatively small amount of genetic variation in samples of EBLV1 suggests a recent genetic bottleneck. Genetic analysis and geographic clustering were used to suggest a recent introduction of the virus to Europe from Africa via the south of Spain (Amengual *et al.*, 1997). Samples of EBLVI are more closely related to the African lyssavirus species DUVV than to any other lyssaviruses, raising speculation that as more DUVV samples are identified, a single lineage encompassing samples from both Africa and Europe will become evident.

Another explanation is also possible for the low genetic heterogeneity in EBLV1 and a similar lack of diversity in samples of the other European *Lyssavirus* species, EBLV2. Loss of faunal diversity in Europe concomitant with human

TABLE IV

Distance matrix of the Nucleocapsid Protein Encoding Region (1350 bp) of Representative Samples of the Seven Lyssavirus Species Described in Table I[a]

	MOKV	MOKV	LBV	LBV	ABlV	ABlV	RABV	RABV	EBLV2	EBLV2	EBLV1	EBLV1	DUVV
MOKV	—	13.4	28.7	26.4	36.8	34.5	36.2	36.1	37.9	38.3	35.9	36.5	33.8
MOKV		—	28.3	27.5	34.9	34.3	35.3	33.5	34.9	34.6	33.4	33.4	34.9
LBV			—	19.4	33.5	34.1	32.6	31.4	34.2	32.6	31.0	31.2	32.8
LBV				—	33.1	30.2	34.1	32.5	34.2	35.2	31.1	31.9	30.0
ABLV					—	18.1	28.0	27.8	29.7	30.5	27.2	27.8	28.5
ABLV						—	27.1	25.7	27.2	28.5	26.8	27.7	27.4
RABV							—	18.3	30.9	29.7	29.8	29.6	31.5
RABV								—	29.8	29.0	29.1	29.5	29.9
EBLV2									—	4.1	27.3	26.0	29.0
EBLV2										—	28.9	27.6	29.3
EBLV1											—	4.4	24.3
EBLV1												—	23.6
DUVV													—

[a]Nucleotide sequence differences between samples are given as percentages determined by Kimura two-parameter method in the program DNADIST. Figure 4 depicts a phylogenetic tree generated from the distance matrix using UPGMA.

population increases also would eliminate viral lineages. All but three of the 30 bat species recorded for Europe are listed as endangered, vulnerable, or rare (R. E. Stebbings, as cited in Brass, 1994). Two of the three nonthreatened bat species (*Eptesicus serotinus* and *Myotis daubentonii*) are the presumed reservoirs for the European lyssaviruses.

Despite relatively few samples for analysis, a surprising amount of phylogenetic diversity exists in samples of the lyssavirus species ABLV, MOKV, and LAGV (see Table IV). Evidence is accumulating for separate lyssavirus reservoirs in insectivorous and frugivorous bat species in Australia and likely multiple lineages of Australian bat lyssaviruses (Mackenzie, 1999), and although the reservoirs for the African *Lyssavirus* species are unknown, the genetic diversity in MOKV and LAGV samples (Mebatsion *et al.*, 1993; Nel *et al.*, 2000) suggests a more complicated natural history than first thought, perhaps involving several host species and certainly including a wide geographic distribution.

Some lineages within a lyssavirus species appear to be more successful than others. Phylogenetic relationships between rabies virus samples from foxes in southern Ontario and foxes in Asia suggest that transcontinental animal migration contributed to the spread of this lineage in susceptible animal populations (Kissi *et al.*, 1995). A lineage common in dog rabies samples in Africa is also represented in dog rabies samples from North and South America (Smith *et al.*, 1992; Kissi *et al.*, 1995), suggesting that human transport of domestic animals during European colonization in the nineteenth century may have contributed to the global spread of rabies.

The lineage that affects dogs is among the most adaptable of rabies viruses and contains virus samples from outbreaks maintained in skunks, foxes, coyotes, and mongooses (Smith *et al.*, 1995). One only has to examine case surveillance data for an outbreak of coyote rabies in the United States (Clark *et al.*, 1994) to appreciate how efficiently viruses of this lineage can move through an animal population. In the 27-year interval between 1961 and 1988, no more than three coyotes per year were diagnosed with rabies in Texas. In 1988, however, the identification of six rabid coyotes in a Texas county along the U.S.–Mexico border marked the beginning of an explosive epizootic. The virus transmitted in the outbreak was well adapted to dogs, and as coyotes spread the disease northward, dog-to-dog transmission of a magnitude not seen in the United States since the mass vaccination programs of the 1950s occurred in Texas. Two human deaths were attributed to the variant (Smith *et al.*, 1995), probably transmitted from rabid dogs infected through contact with rabid coyotes, and translocation of coyotes from Texas to hunting compounds was blamed for six dog rabies cases in Florida and Alabama (Centers for Disease Control and Prevention, 1995; Krebs *et al.*, 1995). The outbreak spread quickly to include 21 contiguous counties in Texas and prompted a multimillion dollar vaccination campaign for coyotes (Farry *et al.*, 1998).

It is still unknown why this variant increased in prevalence in coyotes in Texas. The variant infecting the coyotes was the most common variant in dog rabies cases in the Texas–Mexico border area for several years before the outbreak and was responsible for several human rabies deaths in the 1970s (Smith *et al.*, 1995). Although coyotes are common in this area of Texas, coyote populations have increased throughout the United States and occasionally are infected with rabies variants common in dog populations in U.S.–Mexico border areas of other states (DeMattos *et al.*, 1999). No sustained transmission was noted in these cases, however.

Some lineages of rabies virus appear to have only a limited spread. Although the lineage 31 virus associated with Mexican free-tailed bats in the United States and Mexico shares common ancestry with lineage 30 viruses associated with populations of vampire bats and lineage 32 viruses associated with South American free-tailed bats (DeMattos *et al.*, 1999), this group of viruses has a much more distant relationship with the rabies viruses found in other North American bat species (see Fig. 2 and Table II). The phylogenetic distinction between viruses affecting bats that are primarily tropical in distribution and viruses affecting bats of temperate areas of the United States becomes more interesting in the context of some explanations made for the first appearance of rabies in insectivorous bats in the United States in 1953. At that time, bat rabies was known to be common only in vampire bats. Because the initial case occurred near a Florida seaport, the origin was first hypothesized to be from the accidental introduction of rabid vampire bats into Florida with imported material from South America (Scatterday and Galton, 1954). After bat rabies cases were diagnosed throughout the United States, a more widespread dissemination from the tropics was hypothesized with free-tailed bats infected during winter while sharing caves with vampire bats in Mexico (Constantine, 1966). On their return to U.S. caves in the spring, free-tailed bats would have transmitted virus to other nonmigratory species. The nucleotide sequence analysis does suggest a fairly recent common ancestry for the rabies virus in vampire bats and free-tailed bats, lending support for a tropical origin for at least some bat rabies in the United States; however, the phylogenies offer little support for further spread in bat populations from this source.

D. Vaccine Coverage

Rabies vaccine failures are rare. Most failures are single, isolated events and involve immunocompromised animals or young animals with only a single vaccination (Eng and Fishbein, 1990; McQuiston *et al.*, 2001). No evidence exists for naturally occurring escape mutants even in areas where millions of vaccine doses were distributed in oral baiting campaigns to control wildlife rabies and despite decades of mandatory domestic animal vaccination in the United States and elsewhere.

The only true vaccination failures occur when animals vaccinated with rabies vaccines are exposed to Mokola and Lagos bat viruses. Neither laboratory animals (Shope *et al.*, 1970) nor domestic dogs and cats (van Teichman *et al.*, 1998) are protected from infection with Mokola and Lagos bat viruses by administration of vaccines prepared from rabies virus stocks. Much more information is needed about potential reservoir hosts for Mokola and Lagos bat viruses. At present, the number of cases is small, but this is almost certainly due to a lack of laboratory methods for their detection. Surveys in Ethiopia (1989–1990) and South Africa (1995–1998) identified eight new isolates in animals submitted for rabies diagnosis (Mebatsion *et al.*, 1992; von Teichman *et al.*, 1998), indicating that these lyssaviruses are a not uncommon source of rabies in some parts of Africa.

IV. CONCLUSIONS

Despite astounding progress in our ability to use molecular methods to study the epidemiology of rabies, we seem to be left with the same unanswered questions faced by biologists 50 years ago. We have no description of the forces that guide evolutionary change in lyssavirus populations. We cannot with certainty identify the genetic characteristics necessary for efficient serial transmission of a virus in a particular host animal population. We can use genetic analysis of virus populations to identify topographic features that partition animal populations and serve as barriers or deterrents to rabies transmission, but we have yet to use this information to predict epidemic spread or to guide our rabies elimination campaigns.

We often assume that the answers will come if we simply gather more data, but as the amount of genomic information increases, so does the need for professionals with a working knowledge of both biologic sciences and computational methods. If virus typing becomes a routine component of diagnosis, we can expect an explosive increase in information that must be curated in a way that it becomes useful both to scientists with a background in bioinformatics and to traditional epidemiologists and biologists as well.

The application of molecular methods has added a new dimension to the surveillance of rabies. With diligence, luck, and a few insightful scientists, we may soon arrive at a greater understanding of this ancient disease.

REFERENCES

Amengual, B., Whitby, J. E., King, A., Serra, C., and Bourhy, H. (1997). Evolution of European bat lyssaviruses. *J. Gen. Virol.* **78**, 2319–2328.
Badrane, H., Bahloul, C., Perrin, P., and Tordo, N. (2001). Evidence of two lyssavirus phylogroups with distinct pathogenicity and immunogenicity. *J. Virol.* **75**, 3268–3276.

Baer, G. M., and Yager, P. A. (1977). A mouse model for post-exposure rabies prophylaxis:.The comparative efficacy of two vaccines and of antiserum administration. *J. Gen. Virol.* **36**, 51–58.

Bingham J., Hill, F. W., and Matema, R. (1994). Rabies incubation in an African civet (*Civettictis civetta*). *Vet. Rec.* **134**, 528.

Blancou, J. (1988). Ecology and epidemiology of fox rabies. *Rev. Infect. Dis.* **10** (Suppl. 4), S606–S609.

Bourhy, H., Kissi, B., Lafon, M., Sacramento, D., and Tordo, N. (1992). Antigenic and molecular characterization of bat rabies virus in Europe. *J. Clin. Microbiol.* **30**, 2419–2426.

Bourhy, H., Kissi, B., and Tordo, N. (1993). Molecular diversity of the lyssavirus genus. *Virology* **194**, 70–81.

Bourhy, H., Kissi, B., Audry, L., Smreczak, M., Sadkowska-Todys, M., Kulonen, K., Tordo, N., Zmudzinski, J. F., and Holmes, E. C. (1999). Ecology and evolution of rabies virus in Europe. *J. Gen. Virol.* **80**, 2545–2557.

Brass, D. A. (1994). *Rabies in Bats*, p. 281. Livia Press, Ridgefield, CT.

Centers for Disease Control and Prevention (1995). Translocation of coyote rabies — Florida, 1994. *Morbid. Mortal. Weekly Rep.* **44**, 580–587.

Centers for Disease Control and Prevention (2000a). Outbreak of poliomyelitis: Dominican Republic and Haiti, 2000. *Morbid. Mortal. Weekly Rep.* **49**, 1094, 1103.

Centers for Disease Control and Prevention (2000b). Human rabies: California, Georgia, Minnesota, New York, and Wisconsin, 2000. *Morbid. Mortal. Weekly Rep.* **49**, 1111–1115.

Clark, K. A., Neill, S. U., Smith, J. S., Wilson, P. J., Whadford, V. W., and McKirahan, G. W. (1994). Epizootic canine rabies transmitted by coyotes in south Texas. *J. Am. Vet. Med. Assoc.* **204**, 536–540.

Constantine, D. G. (1966). Recent advances in our knowledge of bat rabies. *Symp. Ser. Immunobiol. Stand.* **1**, 251–254.

Coulon, P., Lafay, F., and Flamand, A. (1993). Rabies virus antigenicity: An overview. *Onderstepoort J. Vet. Res.* **60**, 271–275.

Crawford-Miksza, L. K., Wadford, D. A., and Schnurr, D. P. (1999). Molecular epidemiology of enzootic rabies in California. *J. Clin. Virol.* **14**, 207–219.

De Mattos, C. A., De Mattos, C. C., Smith, J. S., Miller, E. T., Papo, S., Utrera, A., and Osburn, B. I. (1996). Genetic characterization of rabies field isolates from Venezuela. *J. Clin. Microbiol.* **34**, 1553–1558.

De Mattos, C. A., Favi, M., Yung, V., Pavletic, C., and De Mattos, C. C. (2000). Bat rabies in urban centers in Chile. *J. Wildlife Dis.* **36**, 231–240.

de Mattos, C., de Mattos, C., Loza-Rubio, E., Aguilar-Setien, A., Orciari, L. A., and Smith, J. S. (1999). Molecular characterization of rabies virus isolates from Mexico: Implications for transmission dynamics and human risk. *Am. J. Trop. Med. Hyg.* **61**, 587–597.

Diaz, A. M., Papo, S., Rodriguez, A., and Smith, J. S. (1994). Antigenic analysis of rabies-virus isolates from Latin America and the Caribbean. *J. Vet. Med. Series B* **41**, 153–160.

Dietzschold, B., Wunner, W. H., Wiktor, T. J., Lopes, A. D., Lafon, M., Smith, C. L., and Koprowski, H. (1983). Characterization of an antigenic determinant of the glycoprotein that correlates with pathogenicity of rabies virus. *Proc. Natl. Acad. Sci. USA* **80**, 70–74.

Dietzschold, B., Kao, M., Zheng, Y. M., Chen, Z. Y., Maul, G., Fu, Z. F , Rupprecht, C. E., and Koprowski, H. (1992). Delineation of putative mechanisms involved in antibody-mediated clearance of rabies virus from the central nervous system. *Proc. Natl. Acad. Sci. USA* **89**, 7252–7256.

Domingo, E., and Holland, J. J. (1994). Mutation rates and rapid evolution of RNA viruses. In *The Evolutionary Biology of Viruses*, S. Morse (ed.), pp. 161–184. Raven Press, New York.

Eng, T. R., and Fishbein, D. B. (1990). Epidemiologic factors, clinical findings, and vaccination status of rabies in cats and dogs in the United States in 1988. *J. Am. Vet. Med. Assoc.* **197**, 201–209.

Farry, S. C., Henke, S. E., Beasom, S. L., and Fearneyhough, M. G. (1998). Efficacy of bait distributional strategies to deliver canine rabies vaccines to coyotes in southern Texas. *J. Wildlife Dis.* **34**, 23–32.

Favi, M., Yung, V., Pavletic, C., Ramirez, E., De Mattos, C. C., and De Mattos, C. A. (1999). Role of insectivorous bats in the transmission of Rabies in Chile [Spanish]. *Arch. Med. Vet.* **31**, 157–165.

Goto, H., Minamoto, N., Ito, H., Ito, N., Sugiyama, M., Kinjo, T., and Kawai, A. (2000). Mapping of epitopes and structural analysis of antigenic sites in the nucleoprotein of rabies virus. *J. Gen. Virol.* **81**, 119–127.

Gould, A. R., Hyatt, A. D., Lunt, R., Kattenbelt, J. A., Hengstberger, S., and Blacksell, S. D. (1998). Characterisation of a novel lyssavirus isolated from Pteropid bats in Australia. *Virus Res.* **54**, 165–187.

Ito, N., Sugiyama, M., Oraveerakul, K., Piyaviriyakul, P., Lumlertdacha, B., Arai, Y. T., Tamura, Y., Mori, Y., and Minamoto, N. (1999). Molecular epidemiology of rabies in Thailand. *Microbiol. Immunol.* **43**, 551–559.

Kissi, B., Tordo, N., and Bourhy, H. (1995). Genetic polymorphism in the rabies virus nucleoprotein gene. *Virology* **209**, 526–537.

Krebs, J. W., Strine, T. W., Smith, J. S., Rupprecht, C. E., and Childs, J. E. (1995). Rabies surveillance in the United States during 1994. *J. Am. Vet. Med. Assoc.* **207**, 1562–1575.

Mackenzie, J. S. (1999). Emerging viral diseases: An Australian perspective. *Emerg. Infect. Dis.* **5**, 1–8.

Mccoll, K. A., Gould, A. R., Selleck, P. W., Hooper, P. T., Westbury, H. A., and Smith, J. S. (1993). Polymerase chain reaction and other laboratory techniques in the diagnosis of long incubation rabies in Australia. *Aust. Vet. J.* **70**, 84–89.

McQuiston, J. H., Yager P. A., Smith, J. S., and Rupprecht, C. E. (2001). Epidemiology of rabies in dogs and cats in the United States during 1999. *J. Am. Vet. Med. Assoc.* **218**, 1939–1942.

Mebatsion, T., Cox, J. H., and Frost, J. W. (1992). Isolation and characterization of 115 street rabies virus isolates from Ethiopia by using monoclonal antibodies: Identification of 2 isolates as Mokola and Lagos bat viruses. *J. Infect. Dis.* **166**, 972–977.

Mebatsion, T., Cox, J. H., and Conzelmann, K. K. (1993). Molecular analysis of rabies-related viruses from Ethiopia. *Onderstepoort J. Vet. Res.* **60**, 289–294.

Morimoto, K., Patel, M., Corisdeo, S., Hooper, D. C., Fu, Z. F., Rupprecht, C. E., Koprowski, H., and Dietzschold, B. (1996). Characterization of a unique variant of bat rabies virus responsible for newly emerging human cases in North America. *Proc. Natl. Acad. Sci. USA* **93**, 5653–5658.

Moritz, C., and Hillis, D. M. (1996) Molecular systematics: Context and controversies. In *Molecular Systematics,* D. M. Hillis, C. Moritz, and B. K. Mable (eds.), pp. 1–16. Sinauer Associates, Sunderland, MA.

Nadin-Davis, S. A., Casey, G. A., and Wandeler, A. (1993). Identification of regional variants of the rabies virus within the Canadian province of Ontario. *J. Gen. Virol.* **74**, 829–837.

Nadin-Davis, S. A., Casey, G. A., and Wandeler, A. I. (1994). A molecular epidemiological study of rabies virus in central Ontario and western Quebec. *J. Gen. Virol.* **75**, 2575–2583.

Nadin-Davis, S. A., Huang, W., and Wandeler, A. I. (1997). Polymorphism of rabies viruses within the phosphoprotein and matrix protein genes. *Arch. Virol.* **142**, 979–992.

Nadin-Davis, S. A., Sampath, M. I., Casey, G. A., Tinline, R. R., and Wandeler, A. I. (1999). Phylogeographic patterns exhibited by Ontario rabies virus variants. *Epidemiol. Infect.* **123**, 325–336.

Nadin-Davis, S. A., Sheen, M., Abdel-Malik, M., Elmgren, L., Armstrong, J., and Wandeler, A. I. (2000). A panel of monoclonal antibodies targeting the rabies virus phosphoprotein identifies a highly variable epitope of value for sensitive strain discrimination. *J. Clin. Microbial.* **38**, 1397–1403.

Nel, L., Jacobs, J., Jaftha, J., von Teichman, B., and Bingham, J. (2000). New cases of Mokola virus infection in South Africa: A genotypic comparison of southern African virus isolates. *Virus Genes* **20**, 103–106.

Nel, L. H., Thomson, G. R., and Von Teichman, B. F. (1993). Molecular epidemiology of rabies virus in South Africa. *Onderstepoort J. Vet. Res.* **60**, 301–306.

Noah, D. L., Drenzek, C. L., Smith, J. S., Krebs, J. W., Orciari, L., Shaddock, J., Sanderlin, D., Whitfield, S., Fekadu, M., Olson, J. G., Rupprecht, C. E., and Childs, J. E. (1998). Epidemiology of human rabies in the United States, 1980 to 1996. *Ann. Intern. Med.* **128**, 922–930.

Pastoret, P. P., and Brochier, B. (1998). Epidemiology and elimination of rabies in western Europe. *Vet. J.* **156**, 83–90.

Sacramento, D., Badrane, H., Bourhy, H., and Tordo, N. (1992). Molecular epidemiology of rabies virus in France: Comparison with vaccine strains. *J. Gen. Virol.* **73**, 1149–1158.

Scatterday, J. E., and Galton, M. M. (1954). Bat rabies in Florida. *Vet. Med.* **49**, 133–135.

Schneider, L. G., Cox, J. H., Muller, W. W., and Hohnsbeen, K. P. (1988). Current oral rabies vaccination in Europe: An interim balance. *Rev. Infect. Dis.* **10** (Suppl. 4), S654–S659.

Shope, R. E., Murphy, F. A., Harrison, A. K., Causey, O. R., Kemp, G. E., Simpson, D. I., and Moore, D. L. (1970). Two African viruses serologically and morphologically related to rabies virus. *J. Virol.* **6**, 690–692.

Smith, J. S. (1989). Rabies virus epitopic variation: Use in ecologic studies. *Adv. Virus Res.* **36**, 215–253.

Smith,. J. S., Fishbein, D. B., Rupprecht, C. E., and Clark, K. (1991). Unexplained rabies in three immigrants in the United States: A virologic investigation. *New Engl. J. Med.* **324**, 205–211.

Smith, J. S., Orciari, L. A., Yager, P. A., Seidel, H. D., and Warner, C. K. (1992). Epidemiologic and historical relationships among 87 rabies virus isolates as determined by limited sequence analysis. *J. Infect. Dis.* **166**, 296–307.

Smith, J. S., Orciari, L. A., and Yager, P. A. (1995). Molecular epidemiology of rabies in the United States. *Semin. Virol.* **6**, 387–400.

Van Regenmortel, M. H. (1998). From absolute to exquisite specificity: Reflections on the fuzzy nature of species, specificity and antigenic sites. *J. Immunol. Methods* **216**, 37–488.

Van Regenmortel, M. H. V., Mayo, M. A., Fauquet, C. M., and Maniloff, J. (2000). Virus nomenclature: Consensus versus chaos. *Arch. Virol.* **145**, 2227–2232.

Von Teichman, B. F., De Koker, W. C., Bosch, S. J., Bishop, G. C., Meredith, C. D., and Bingham, J. (1998). Mokola virus infection: Description of recent South African cases and a review of the virus epidemiology. *J. S. Afr. Vet. Assoc.* **69**, 169–711.

Warner, C., Fekadu, M., Whitfield, S., and Shaddock, J. (1999). Use of anti-glycoprotein monoclonal antibodies to characterize rabies virus in tissues. *J. Virol. Methods* **77**, 69–74.

Whitaker, J. O., and Douglas, R. G., Jr. (1987). Bat rabies in Indiana: 1965–1984: *Proc. Ind. Acad. Sci.* **95**, 571–584.

Wunner, W. H., Larson, J. K., Dietzschold, B., and Smith, C. L. (1988). The molecular biology of rabies viruses. *Rev. Infect. Dis.* **10** (Suppl. 4), 771–784.

4

Epidemiology

JAMES E. CHILDS

Viral and Rickettsial Zoonoses Branch
Centers for Disease Control and Prevention
Atlanta, Georgia 30333

I. INTRODUCTORY CONCEPTS

Rabies is a zoonotic disease. Human infections and deaths are an unfortunate consequence of biologic processes of virus maintenance in which humans play no significant role (Fig. 1). Rabies virus and the other six recognized members of the *Lyssavirus* genus, some of which cause diseases indistinguishable from rabies in humans (Table I), are adapted to various animal species on which they depend for their existence. Details of the maintenance cycles for lyssaviruses other than rabies virus are unclear. However, rabies virus perpetuation involves introduction into a susceptible host, most typically by transmission via an animal of the same species, and then infection, dissemination, and multiplication of the virus within the host prior to reintroduction of viral progeny into a new susceptible animal. Almost without exception, the route by which rabies virus is introduced into a new host is direct, and the most important mode of transmission is by inoculation by bite of infectious virus present in saliva (McKendrick, 1941). The process by which rabies virus circulates within diverse species of mammals causing serial infections is referred to as the *maintenance* or *transmission cycle* of the virus (see Fig. 1). Since humans are rarely the source of virus for subsequent human infection, humans do not contribute to the maintenance of rabies virus or any other *Lyssavirus*. The reservoir for rabies is the animal pool that circulates rabies virus, with only occasional spillover of infection into humans.

The epidemiology of human rabies reflects the regional animal reservoir for rabies virus and the opportunity for human–animal interaction. An understanding of patterns of rabies virus maintenance within animal host populations and the degree to which rabies virus has cospeciated with particular animal hosts has been appreciated only for the last few decades. Rabies virus, serotype 1, genotype 1, of the genus *Lyssavirus*, is an assembly of virus variants or genetic lineages each closely allied to a single species of mammal. These rabies virus variants can be differentiated by their antigenic makeup (Rupprecht *et al.*, 1987; Smith, 1988), as well as by characteristic patterns of nucleotide substitutions in their RNA genome (Nadin-Davis and Casey, 1994; Sacramento *et al.*, 1991; Smith *et al.*, 1995). This molecular variation has permitted identification of primary reservoir hosts for virus variants, detailed descriptions of the geographic distribution of variants, and identification of virus spillover into animals and humans (Smith *et al.*, 1995). As an example, the distribution of genetically distinguishable variants of rabies virus in the United States can be mapped with reasonable precision (Fig. 2). These topics will be covered in detail in other chapters in this volume. An essential feature for public health programs is that regardless of this genetic and antigenic diversity, prevention of all serotype 1, genotype 1 lyssaviral infections has proved possible through pre- or postexposure treatment regimens by using the available tissue-culture-derived rabies virus vaccines and immunoglobulin products (Centers for Disease Control and Prevention, 1999a).

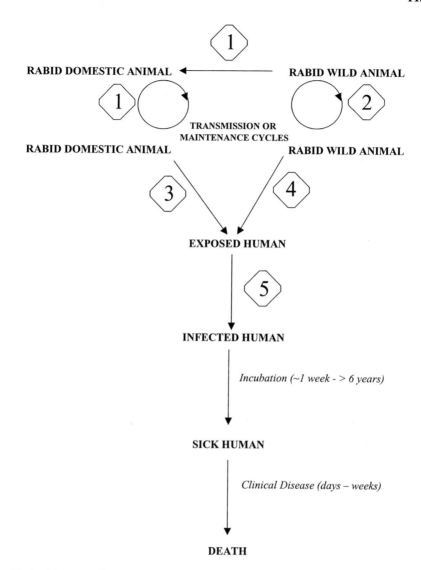

Fig. 1. The natural history of rabies, with points for the opportunity for prevention, treatment, and control indicated by numbers. The circular symbols indicate natural maintenance of rabies virus transmission among domestic dogs and wild animals. (1) Prevention and control of wildlife transmission of rabies virus or dog-to-dog maintenance of transmission by vaccination and control of domestic animals. (2) Prevention and control of wildlife transmission of rabies virus through vaccination of natural reservoir species. (3) Prevention of human exposure through avoidance and population control of rabid domestic animals. (4) Prevention of human exposure through avoidance of rabid wild animals. (5) Human infection by rabies virus can be prevented by either preexposure immunization (and appropriate postexposure treatment) or by postexposure treatment with vaccine and rabies immunoglobulin. Once a person develops clinical signs of disease, rabies is nearly always fatal. [*Modified from Hattwick (1974) and Fishbein (1991).*]

TABLE I

Current Classification of Lyssaviruses

Serotype, genotype	Major mammalian reservoirs	Distribution	Annual human deaths
Rabies (serotype 1, genotype 1)	Dogs, wild carnivores, bats	Worldwide (with exception of Australia, Antartica, and designated rabies-free countries)	~50,000
Lagos bat (serotype 2, genotype 2)	Bats	Africa: Central African Republic, Ethiopia, Nigeria, Senegal, South Africa	Never reported
Mokola (serotype 3, genotype 3)	Shrews, cats?, dogs?	Africa: Cameroon, Central African Republic, Ethiopia, Nigeria, South Africa, Zimbabwe	Occasional
Duvenhage (serotype 4, genotype 4)	Bats	Africa: South Africa, Guinea, Zimbabwe	Occasional
European bat lyssavirus 1 (genotype 5)	Bats	Europe	Occasional
European bat lyssavirus 2 (genotype 6)	Bats	Europe	Occasional
Australian bat lyssavirus (genotype 7)	Bats	Australia	Occasional

Rabies virus maintenance in animal reservoirs has served as a model system for illustrating many important concepts in infectious disease epidemiology and the theoretical modeling of the population biology of a virus and its host. Examples of these efforts include the notion of threshold density for virus transmission (Anderson *et al.*, 1981; Cruickshank *et al.*, 1999), the relevance of herd immunity for control (e.g., the critical percentage of a population immunized to eliminate or prevent rabies virus transmission and outbreaks of rabies) (Coleman and Dye, 1996), and illustrative models of spatial (Moore, 1999; Murray *et al.*, 1986) and temporal spread of an infectious disease (Smith, 1985).

II. THE EPIDEMIOLOGY OF HUMAN RABIES

A. Mortality and Morbidity Estimates

In most areas of the world, accurate estimates of human rabies deaths are impossible to obtain because surveillance systems and regional laboratories are

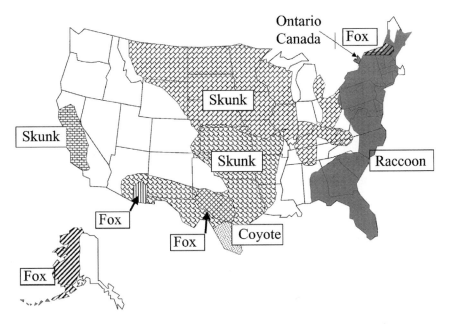

Fig. 2. The distribution of rabies virus variants in the United States by primary species or groups of terrestrial carnivore. Overlying this distribution of rabies virus variants is the reservoir present in species of bats, which includes the entire continental United States.

inadequate or nonexistent. Annual reports of 2000 human deaths in Bangladesh, 1014 in China, and 30,000 in India in the 1990s convey a rough estimate of the magnitude of mortality associated with rabies worldwide (WHO, 1993). In Latin America, 1392 deaths were recorded between 1990 and 1996 (cited in De Mattos *et al.*, 1999). As of 1997, the annual number of human deaths worldwide was estimated to be between 35,000 and 50,000 (WHO, 1999).

In 1986, the incidence of rabies per 10^6 persons per year among 30 countries with endemic disease ranged from a low of 0.1 in countries of southern Africa to 28.8 in India (Bögel and Motschwiller, 1986). Caution is warranted in accepting estimates of rabies mortality; of more than 33,000 human deaths reported in 1997, laboratory confirmation of rabies was available for less than 0.5% (WHO 1999). Sensitive, specific, and perhaps most important, widely available laboratory testing is an essential element for surveillance for any infectious disease. Worldwide, there is inadequate support for accurate, laboratory-based, rabies surveillance in humans or animals.

In addition to deaths caused by rabies, millions of persons annually receive postexposure treatment (PET) for potential exposure to rabies virus. Many of these individuals receive vaccines of nervous tissue origin (NTO), which potentially result in thousands of serious adverse reactions (Held and Adaros, 1972;

Swaddiwuthipong *et al.*, 1988). Along with the potential for adverse reactions with vaccines of NTO, there is concern over variability in antigen content. Experiences in Pakistan (Parviz *et al.*, 1998) and Nigeria (Ogunkoya and Macconi, 1986) with antirabies vaccines of little or no potency indicate that ineffective or even fake (lacking any antigenic value) biologicals may at times circulate in a number of countries.

Reviews of the incidence of neuroparalytic complications associated with vaccines of NTO indicate reaction rates of 1 in 220 to 1 in 2900 per persons vaccinated, with an average of 1.5 adverse reactions per 1000 vaccinees (Abdussalem and Bögel, 1971; Meslin *et al.*, 1994). Approximately 15% of neuroparalytic cases are fatal (Abdussalem and Bögel, 1971), and up to 25% of patients suffer permanent disability or death (Meslin *et al.*, 1994). Thus the global public health cost of rabies must be assessed in terms of human morbidity associated with disease prevention in addition to mortality.

Although vaccines of NTO are still in use in many parts of the developing world where rabies is a major public health concern, other countries have successfully adopted cell culture–derived vaccines with schedules modified from the Essen postexposure regimen (see Chap. 12). In Thailand, the number of rabies deaths has declined from more than 400 per year two decades ago to 70 in 1998 (Wilde *et al.*, 1999). This decline has been attributed largely to the adoption of modern PET regimens because dog rabies remains unchecked.

B. Rabies in Developing Nations

From the public health perspective, rabies remains a major threat only within regions of Asia, Africa, and South America where domestic dogs act as the major reservoir for the virus and the primary source for human exposures through animal bite. Within the broad category of developing countries, the geographic area of the tropics accounted for more than 99% of human deaths and approximately 90% of PETs for rabies in 1985 (Acha and Arambulo, 1985). The trend toward increasing global urbanization has meant that in 2000, approximately one-half the world's human population lives in cities compared with one-third in the 1970s (Lederberg *et al.*, 1992). Diseases such as rabies that are prone to transmission in crowded urban centers with inadequate public health infrastructures remain a constant or increasing threat in much of the world.

In general, rabies poses the greatest risk in cities where dog and human populations reach their highest population densities (Beran, 1991). Rural or sylvatic rabies (Acha and Arambulo, 1985; Turner, 1971), involving rabies virus transmission from indigenous wildlife, is a lesser threat in most regions of the world. Even in rural locations, dogs remain the most significant threat for rabies virus transmission to humans. In Mexico, where vampire bat and dog rabies co-occur, dog exposures account for approximately 81% of cases (mainly urban) and vampire bats for approximately 11% of cases (mostly rural) (De Mattos *et al.*, 1999). During an outbreak of rabies in Zimbabwe from 1980 to 1983, the majority of documented animal cases occurred in jackals (74.3% of 404 cases; *Canis mesomelus* and *C. adustus*), but dogs were the most serious threat to humans (Kennedy, 1988).

In countries where canine rabies persists, the incidence of rabies is highest among human males and among individuals less than 20 years of age (Bhatia *et al.*, 1988; Fekadu, 1982; Lakhanpal and Sharma, 1985; Wang, 1956). The age and sex distribution of human rabies deaths generally mirrors the age distribution of dog bite victims, with a large proportion of victims under the age of 15 years (Fekadu, 1982; Kale, 1977; Wang, 1956) (Fig. 3*A*).

The rate at which children are bitten by dogs and potentially exposed to rabies virus is underestimated in developed (Beck and Jones, 1985) and developing countries (Eng *et al.*, 1993). Where measured, the community impact of dog bite can be substantial, as exemplified in Hermosillo, Mexico, where approximately 2.5% of the resident population was bitten by dogs annually (Eng *et al.*, 1993). In Bangkok, 5.3% of injuries seen at an emergency room associated with a teaching hospital were due to dog bites (Bhanganada *et al.*, 1993).

An increased risk of dog bite and human rabies has been found in areas of lower socioeconomic status (SES) in developing nations, most notably in cities (Fagbami *et al.*, 1981). However, this association is not universal (Eng *et al.*, 1993). Such findings presumably reflect larger populations of free-ranging dogs in lower-SES urban areas of developing countries (WHO, 1987). The ecology of free-ranging dogs within developed countries also shows problems increasing in lower-SES neighborhoods within cities (Beck, 1973).

Human rabies deaths in developing countries occur throughout the year. Canine rabies cases show a seasonal peak during the spring and early summer in the tropics and southern hemisphere (Malaga *et al.*, 1979; Ernst and Fabrega, 1989) and in the United States (Krebs *et al.*, 1999) in association with breeding and birthing processes. In Ghana, 68% of the human rabies cases and 66% of the animal rabies cases are reported in the 6 months of July, August, September, January, February, and March, which correspond to the dry season (Addy, 1985).

The actual risk of human exposure to rabies virus in developing countries is difficult to estimate. Surveys based on the experiences of foreign citizens from developed nations travelling or working overseas provide a range of values for rabies virus exposures or postexposure treatments of 0.2–6.2 per 1000 persons per month (Table II). These values vary with location and may not accurately reflect the risk to indigenous populations. In Thailand, it is estimated that over 200,000 persons received PET using tissue culture–derived vaccines in 1997 at a cost of approximately 10 million U.S. dollars (Wilde *et al.*, 1999).

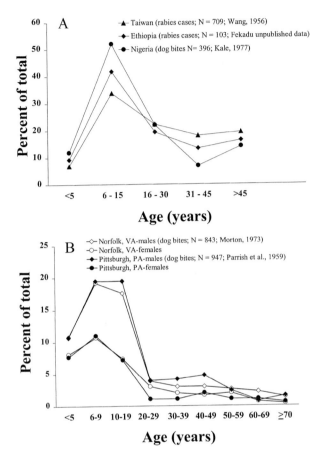

Fig. 3. (*A*) The young-age distribution of rabies cases in developing countries (illustrated by recent data from Ethiopia and past data from Taiwan) is mirrored by the age distribution of dog bite cases (illustrated with data from Nigeria). (*B*) In the developed world, dog bite is also a pediatric problem; however, the reduction of rabies in dogs and the availability of excellent biologicals for the postexposure prophylaxis for rabies have reduced human disease to a sporadic occurrence.

C. Human Rabies in Developed Nations

Historically, rabies cases among humans in developed countries showed similar patterns to the demographic profile of rabies cases occurring presently in developing countries. As an example, from 1946 (the year the Communicable Disease Center established its national rabies control program) to 1965, there were 236 cases of human rabies reported from the United States (Held *et al.*,

TABLE II

Estimated Rates of Exposure to Rabid Animals Based on the Experiences of Citizens from the United States or Other Developed Nations Who Are Stationed or Living Overseas

Continent, country or number of countries	Population	Rate of exposure to a potentially rabid animal per 1000 persons per month or rate of postexposure treatment per 1000 persons per month	Source
Africa, several	Missionaries	1.0	Arguin et al., 2000
Africa, 21	Peace Corps volunteers	2.5	Bernard and Fishbein, 1991
Asia, several	Missionaries	0.6	Arguin et al., 2000
Asia, 4	Peace Corps volunteers	2.8	Bernard and Fishbein, 1991
Asia, Nepal	Travelers	0.4	Shlim et al., 1991
Latin America, several	Missionaries	0.2	Arguin et al., 2000
Latin America, 6	Peace Corps volunteers	6.2	Bernard and Fishbein, 1991
Worldwide (several African couniries, India, Bangladesh, Ecuador, Bolivia)	Missionaries	1.3	Bjorvatn and Gundersen, 1980

1967). The vast majority of these deaths were attributable to dog exposures (81.9%), the majority of the victims were male (70%), and 51.3% of the victims were 15 years of age or younger (Held et al., 1967). The age distribution of dog bite cases in the United States is similar to that reported by developing countries (Fig. 3B) (Morton, 1973; Parrish et al., 1959).

Human rabies in developed countries where tissue culture–derived vaccines and rabies immunoglobulin are available is a very rare disease. In the United States, the number of human rabies cases has declined dramatically since the 1950s, concomitant with the decline of canine rabies (Fig. 4). There has been a median of three human cases of rabies per year since 1990 (Krebs et al., 1998a, 1999; Noah et al., 1998), and this number is higher than figures from Europe or Canada.

The history and molecular typing of rabies virus obtained from human rabies cases (Smith et al., 1995) occurring since 1980 indicate two distinctive patterns in the changing epidemiology of rabies in the United States. The indigenously acquired cases, which account for the majority of recent deaths, are now overwhelmingly attributable to variants of rabies virus maintained in wildlife reservoirs. The wildlife reservoir that has emerged as the major contributor to human deaths in the United States is found among various species of bats (see below) (Hanlon and Rupprecht, 1998; Noah et al., 1998).

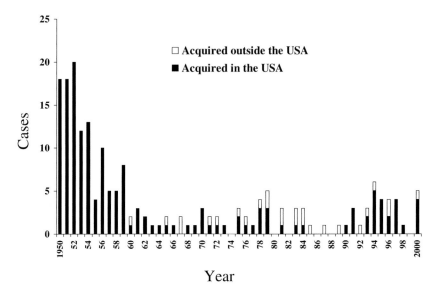

Fig. 4. Human cases of rabies in the United States, 1950–November 2000. The number has declined dramatically as a result of rabies control among dogs and because of the availability of excellent biologicals for the postexposure treatment for rabies exposures. [*Data through 1990 taken from Hattwick (1971) and Fishbein (1991); where data disagreed, numbers from Fishbein were used.*]

The other source of rabies cases diagnosed in the United States are those in which exposures to rabies virus have occurred in another country. These "imported" cases have occurred among residents of the United States (Arguin *et al.*, 2000; Centers for Disease Control and Prevention, 1982, 1983, 1997a) and among immigrants to the United States (Centers for Disease Control and Prevention, 1996a; Smith *et al.*, 1991). In every case, these individuals have been exposed to rabies through the bite of an infected dog in a country where canine rabies remains endemic. A similar situation exists in Europe, where most cases of human rabies are now imported (Delgiudice *et al.*, 1992; Muller, 1990).

Human rabies deaths in the United States occur throughout the year. Historically, the majority of human exposures occurred from spring through fall, following the peak in rabies reports among terrestrial carnivores that occurred in the winter and spring (Held *et al.*, 1967). In recent years, with the emergence of bat-associated rabies virus variants as a major contributor to human disease, a marked trend for late-summer occurrence of human cases can be observed (Fig. 5). This peak coincides with the peak reporting of rabies among bats in the fall (Childs *et al.*, 1994; Krebs *et al.*, 1999) (see below).

A disturbing trend in recent cases of human rabies in the United States has been the inability to elicit a history of animal bite from the victim or close

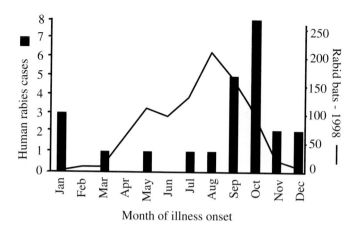

Fig. 5. Cases of human rabies (1990–November 2000) caused by variants of rabies virus associated with bats show a peak date of death in the fall. There is a marked increase in reports of rabid bats in the fall. [*Data for bats from Krebs et al. (1999).*]

family members (Noah *et al.*, 1998). Public health experts believe that a bat bite is still the most plausible explanation for these cases because documented instances of nonbite routes of infection are exceedingly rare and generally have occurred under exceptional situations (see below) that are not comparable with those described for recent cases (Gibbons and Rupprecht, 2000). The most common explanations for the lack of history of a bat bite obtained from recent rabies patients or their close personal contacts are that patients failed to report an event perceived as insignificant (Gibbons and Rupprecht, 2000) or that the bat bite went unnoticed (Feder *et al.*, 1997). The phenotype of rabies virus variants associated with bats may promote transmission via superficial wounds inflicted to peripheral body sites (Morimoto *et al.*, 1996). The indication that unnoticed or trivial contact with bats may result in rabies transmission to humans has resulted in the additional recommendation to treat individuals when bat bite cannot be ruled out (Centers for Disease Control and Prevention, 1999a).

D. Risk and Prevention of Rabies Following an Exposure

The risk of developing rabies depends on the anatomic site and severity of the bite, the species inflicting the wound, and probably the rabies virus variant. Data published by Babes (1912) and others and reviewed by Hattwick (1974) indicate that the risk of developing clinical rabies in unvaccinated persons was 50–80% following multiple, severe head bites; 15–40% following multiple, severe finger, hand, or arm bites; and 3–10% following multiple, severe leg bites inflicted by large terrestrial carnivores. In general, exposure to most body fluids (except saliva) or blood from a rabid animal (Centers for Disease Control and Prevention, 1999a) or a rabid human (Helmick *et al.*, 1987) is not regarded as reason for treatment. However, in certain circumstances, laboratory technicians reporting a definite and significant exposure (e.g., a technician cut by a broken specimen container from a rabies patient) to cerebrospinal fluid (CSF) or urine from a human rabies case have been given PET (Anderson *et al.*, 1984a). Such use of PET is prudent because rabies virus has been isolated from CSF and kidney samples obtained at autopsy from proved rabies cases (Dueñas *et al.*, 1973).

In general, modern cell culture–derived vaccines, when administered properly with antirabies immunoglobulin (RIG), are virtually 100% effective in preventing rabies after an exposure has occurred (Centers for Disease Control and Prevention, 1999a). However, vaccine failures continue to be reported when RIG was not infiltrated around the bite site (Wilde *et al.*, 1996) or when RIG was omitted in treatment (Gacouin *et al.*, 1999) (see Chap. 12). The need for administration of both vaccine and RIG for the prevention of rabies following exposure has been appreciated for decades (Baltazard and Bahmanyar, 1955). There have been recent reports of postexposure failures even when World Health Organization (WHO) treatment guidelines have been followed correctly (Hemachudha *et al.*, 1999). Explanations for these failures are not certain.

It should be noted that in the United States, all potential rabies virus exposures are treated with vaccine and human rabies immune globulin (HRIG) (Centers for Disease Control and Prevention, 1999a), whereas WHO recommendations for the most minor exposures call for vaccine alone (WHO, 1992). In addition, U.S. residents exposed to rabies virus in another country sometimes may receive PET with regimens or biologicals that are not approved for use in the United States (WHO, 1992).

In developing countries, a bite from a suspiciously acting animal generally is sufficient to ensure assessment of rabies risk and initiation of PET when required. As many as 40,000 persons annually may receive PET in the United States (Krebs *et al.*, 1998b), although frequently treatment may be recommended in situations where it is unwarranted (Noah *et al.*, 1996). Increasingly, mass human exposures to rabid animals have taxed the local availability of rabies biologicals in the United States (Rotz *et al.*, 1998). Of some surprise to public health officials, it appears that when recommendations for PET are not adhered to in an emergency room setting in the United States, most often PET is withheld when it should be recommended (Moran *et al.*, 2000). These findings suggest that closer adherence to recommended policies for deciding when to recommend PET may increase rather than decrease rabies biological use in the United States.

Unfortunately, in the United States, a clear history of animal bite was not obtained from 19 of 25 human cases that occurred between 1980 and 1995, and treatment was not sought in these instances (Noah *et al.*, 1998). It appears certain that low numbers of rabies cases will continue to be identified from persons unaware that an exposure to rabies virus has occurred.

E. Routes of Rabies Virus Transmission to Humans

Animal bite is the most important route of rabies virus transmission to humans. In a review of human rabies cases seen at Pasteur Institutes distributed around the world from 1927 to 1946, animal bites accounted for 99.8% of the 3920 cases (McKendrick, 1941). However, sporadic cases of human rabies have been described following a variety of exposures. Saliva transmission by licks to mucous membranes (Leach and Johnson, 1940), transdermal scratches contaminated with infectious material, and even improperly inactivated rabies vaccines (Para, 1965) have resulted in infection.

Although rare, human-to-human transmission of rabies has been well documented for eight recipients of transplanted corneas occurring in France (Centers for Disease Control and Prevention, 1980), the United States (Houff *et al.*, 1979), Thailand (Centers for Disease Control and Prevention, 1981b), India (Gode and Bhide, 1988), and Iran (WHO, 1994a). Rabies virus can be recovered from human fluids, including CSF (Dueñas *et al.*, 1973), eye swabs, and sedimented urine (Helmick *et al.*, 1987), so appropriate precautions are required when treating humans with rabies (Helmick *et al.*, 1987). Two cases of human rabies possibly attributable to either human bite or infectious saliva exposure to mucous membranes have been described from Ethiopia (Fekadu *et al.*, 1996). Although human transplacental transmission of rabies virus has been reported in a single case (Sipahioglu and Alpaut, 1985), infants have survived delivery from mothers infected with rabies when the child received PET (Lumbiganon and Wasi, 1990).

Under exceptional circumstances, such as use of blenders to homogenize rabies virus–infected brain material (Conomy *et al.*, 1977), infections of humans with rabies virus by airborne droplets can occur. Rabies infection possibly acquired by droplets or aerosolized virus has been described in two persons visiting Frio cave in Texas (Irons *et al.*, 1957). Millions of Mexican free-tailed bats congregate in this cave, and rabies virus is present within the bat population (Humphrey *et al.*, 1960). Experimental studies with animals and with an electrostatic precipitation device suggest that airborne transmission of rabies virus can occur under exceptional circumstances (Constantine, 1962; Winkler, 1968).

There is little documentation for natural rabies transmission by simple contact with virus-infected tissue, although isolated reports suggest infection following butchering of infected carcasses (Tariq *et al.*, 1991). In the United States, ingestion of unpasteurized milk from rabid cows has been treated as a possible exposure to virus (Centers for Disease Control and Prevention, 1999b). Scratches from a rabid animal potentially could be contaminated with virus shed in saliva and in the United States are often treated as an exposure, but documented cases of this injury leading to rabies are rare (Tuncman, 1949; see various reports in Babes, 1912).

It has been noted previously that for many of the recent human rabies cases in the United States, no history of animal bite could be solicited from the patient, relatives, or close companions. Although unusual, this situation is not unique. In Yugoslavia, from 1935–1939 and from 1946–1952, 35 cases of rabies were reported among individuals who denied any injury or contact with rabid or suspected rabid animals (Nikolic, 1952).

F. Rabies in Travelers and Overseas Personnel from Developed Nations

Rabies in residents of the United States travelling or living overseas has occurred as the result of dog bites experienced in Africa (Centers for Disease Control, 1983) and Asia (Arguin et al., 2000; Centers for Disease Control and Prevention, 1997a). Similar experiences have been reported by other countries [e.g., France (Gacouin et al., 1999)]. These cases have resulted from the failure to receive appropriate PET (Centers for Disease Control and Prevention, 1997a), failure to seek PET (Arguin et al., 2000), and presumed failure to mount sufficient immunity to rabies preexposure vaccination while concurrently receiving malaria chemoprophylaxis with chloroquine (Bernard et al., 1985).

The benefits and costs of rabies preexposure prophylaxis for travelers to rabies-endemic countries has been assessed, and although not necessarily economical (Bernard and Fishbein, 1991), the practice is likely to continue for important noneconomic reasons. The current recommendations for U.S. residents are to consider preexposure immunization when traveling to high-risk locations within countries where rabies is endemic and where access to medical care could preclude the ready availability of PET (Centers for Disease Control and Prevention, 1999a). Frequently, even staff of travel medicine clinics may be unfamiliar with recommendations for rabies preexposure vaccination for travellers going to rabies-endemic countries (Krause et al., 1999).

III. EPIDEMIOLOGY OF RABIES IN DOMESTIC ANIMALS

Rabies among domesticated animals remains the major threat for transmitting rabies virus to humans. Domestic dogs serve as a major reservoir of rabies virus in many developing countries and are capable of maintaining virus transmission in a well-defined maintenance cycle (see Fig. 1). Other domestic animals typically are involved through secondary transmission of rabies virus variants maintained by dogs or wildlife.

A. Epidemiology of Rabies in the Domestic Dog

Rabies remains endemic to dog populations throughout much of the developing world. Young dogs (<1 year of age) can be especially important in epidemic transmission of rabies virus among canines and in exposures to humans (Mitmoonpitak *et al.*, 1998; Eng *et al.*, 1993; Malaga *et al.*, 1979). Not only is the greatest proportion of dogs found in this age class, but younger dogs may be more susceptible to rabies (Beran, 1982) and less likely to have received the minimum number of vaccinations likely to confer immunity (Jenkins *et al.*, 2000).

Rabies in the domestic dog is normally a rapidly progressive, fatal disease once clinical signs develop. The 10-day confinement and observation period for previously healthy dogs that bite humans, used to great success in the United States (Jenkins *et al.*, 2000), has arisen out of this observation. However, in rare instances, dogs have been shown to recover from clinical rabies, with (Baer *et al.*, 1975) or without (Fekadu and Baer, 1980) having been vaccinated previously. Rare naturally infected dogs may excrete rabies virus for months after recovery (Fekadu *et al.*, 1981) or have prolonged incubation periods in which they shed virus prior to the development of clinical disease. The term *carriers* has been used to describe animals in which prolonged excretion of rabies virus occurs (Fekadu *et al.*, 1983). These observations and the isolation of rabies virus from healthy dogs [e.g., in Nigeria (Aghomo and Rupprecht, 1990)] are potentially important in understanding the natural history of rabies virus maintenance. Although the practical relevance of these observations to the epidemiology of rabies and its control or prevention remains unclear, some rabies specialists have used these observations to recommend immediate treatment of humans with severe exposures due to dog bite without delay pending knowledge of the dog's health (Dutta and Dutta, 1994).

1. The Distribution and Origin of Rabies Virus Associated with Dogs

In contrast to rabies virus variants found in wildlife, only limited antigenic and genetic diversity is found among rabies virus isolates from dogs from many locations in the world (Smith, 1989). Not only are rabies virus isolates from dogs in Latin America, Africa, Asia, and eastern Europe very similar to each other, they also are similar to vaccine strains of rabies virus derived from isolates made in the 1930s in the United States. RNA sequence data suggest that these antigenic similarities are not due to convergence of amino acid sequence during adaptation of different rabies variants to dogs but reflect a global reservoir of rabies in dogs that arose from a common source (Smith and Seidel, 1993; Smith *et al.*, 1992). This genetic relatedness is most likely the consequence of European colonization and the introduction of dog rabies throughout these locations through the transport of infected animals.

Although Native Americans had maintained breeds of domestic dogs for centuries prior to the arrival of European explorers (Pferd, 1987), there are no precolonial references to rabies in the Americas (Smithcors, 1958). Importation of dogs from Europe to the New World was known from the time of the second voyage of Columbus (Pferd,1987; Varner and Varner, 1983), and within a few centuries, European breeds essentially had replaced native dogs. Dog rabies was first recognized in the Greater Antilles in the eighteenth century during the time of Spanish dominion in this area and in Mexico as early as 1709 (Smithcors, 1958; Steele and Fernandez 1991). The first outbreaks of dog rabies in South America were recorded in 1803 in Peru and in 1806 in LaPlata, Argentina, among sporting dogs belonging to British officers (Steele and Fernandez, 1991).

2. Rabies among Dogs in the United States

Rabies among dogs in the United States has shown a steady decline from over a 1000 cases per year during the middle of the twentieth century to just over 100 by the century's close (Fig. 6). Rabies associated with dog bites was of greatest concern in the southeastern and south central states through 1965 (Held *et al.*, 1967). In 2000, a rabies virus variant transmitted by domestic dogs

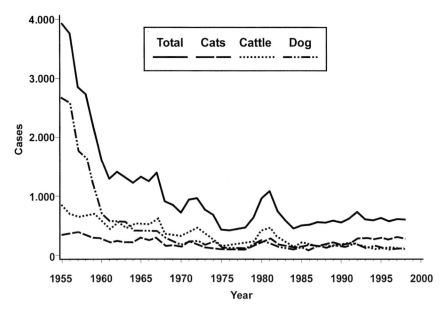

Fig. 6. Numbers of reported cases of rabies among domestic animals in the United States, 1955–1998.

remains a threat primarily in the southwestern United States along the border with Mexico (Krebs *et al.*, 1999; Clark *et al.*, 1994). In other locations, rabies infections among dogs are associated with other terrestrial carnivore reservoirs of rabies virus, such as skunks and raccoons in the continental United States and mongooses on Puerto Rico.

3. Control of Canine Rabies

Where present, canine-associated variants of rabies virus circulating among domestic dogs, particularity in urban settings, present the greatest threat to humans. However, enzootic canine rabies can be controlled or eliminated through comprehensive programs of vaccination and animal management (Bögel and Meslin, 1990) (see Chap. 13). Reservoirs of rabies in a wide variety of sylvatic species, while presenting less of a threat to human health, cannot be reached by traditional rabies control programs. As a potential source for the reintroduction of rabies to domestic animals and humans, wildlife reservoirs of rabies virus force the continuation of expensive dog rabies vaccination programs, even in areas where enzootic dog rabies has been eliminated.

The epidemiologic importance of dog vaccination and control of domestic dogs to the prevention of human rabies is illustrated clearly by the history of rabies control efforts in the United States. Programs of dog vaccination and stray animal control in the 1940s and 1950s reduced the number of dog rabies cases from thousands per year to a few hundred per year (Krebs *et al.*, 1998a; Baer and Wandeler, 1987) (see Fig. 6). A classic example of the effectiveness of mass vaccination campaigns conducted over short time intervals, coupled with stray animal control, occurred in Memphis and Shelby counties, Tennessee, in April 1948. Over a 1-week period, 23,000 dogs were vaccinated, bringing an end to an epidemic of dog rabies that had averaged more than one positive animal per day (Fig. 7A) (Tierkel *et al.*, 1950). Mass campaigns have been used effectively in Peru (Chomel *et al.*, 1988) (Fig. 7B), Malaya, Japan, Taiwan, Israel, and Zimbabwe (Bögel *et al.*, 1982). Urban dog vaccination campaigns throughout Mexico and most other Latin American countries have reduced the number of human cases dramatically since 1980 (PAHO, 1995).

Canine rabies control not only reduces the incidence of human disease but also may be a more cost-effective intervention for human rabies prevention than PET (Bögel and Meslin, 1990). In the United States, compulsory rabies vaccination laws have been credited with reducing the incidence of canine rabies (Bech-Nielsen *et al.*, 1979), and the WHO endorses national legislation in countries where such a program is affordable and enforceable (WHO, 1987).

Development of rabies vaccines for dogs and other domestic animals is a huge commercial concern, with over 28 million doses of vaccine delivered in 1997 (WHO, 1999). With new products appearing continuously, it is essential that

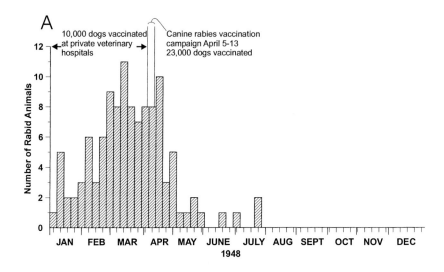

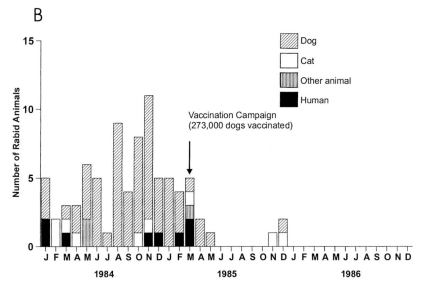

Fig. 7. Vaccination campaigns aimed at the domestic dog have been shown to be effective in (A) the United States (reproduced and modified from [Tierkel, 1959] with permission by Academic Press) and developing nations such as Peru (B) in preventing dog-to-dog transmission and dog-to-human transmission of rabies virus. [A: *Reproduced and modified from Tierkel (1959); B: Reproduced by permission from Chomel et al. (1988), from Reviews of Infectious Diseases, 10 (Supp 4), p. S699, published by The University of Chicago Press,* © *1988 by the University of Chicago.*]

coherent recommendations for animal rabies control efforts be reassessed period-
ically. Each year in the United States, a group of experts meets to review current
vaccines available for animals (predominantly dogs and cats) and to consider new
information pertinent to domestic animal and wildlife rabies control.
Recommendations from these deliberations are published annually and are
accepted widely as the national guidelines for effective rabies prevention for
domestic animals (Jenkins *et al.*, 2000).

The regulation and control of dog movement within and between countries
remain an important strategy for preventing rabies. Rabies-free locations within a
country [e.g., Hawaii in the United States (Fishbein *et al.*, 1990)] and rabies-free
nations (most notably island nations, such as the United Kingdom and Japan)
traditionally have enforced strict laws requiring 6 months of quarantine. Such
laws have kept the United Kingdom free of rabies since 1922. However, within
the last 5 years, changes in such laws have been considered or undertaken that
provide alternative measures that will shorten or do away with quarantine in many
circumstances (Cox *et al.*, 1999; Lopez, 1997; Grandien and Engvall, 1994).

4. What Level of Herd Immunity in Dog Populations is Sufficient?

Traditionally, rabies vaccination levels of 70% (critical percentage p_c) have
been reported as being essential for the elimination of dog-to-dog transmission of
rabies virus (Baer and Wandeler, 1987; Tierkel 1959). Although it is unclear how
this figure was derived, it may have originated through trial and error as the average of values suggested by veterinarians from 24 counties in New York during
rabies control programs conducted during the 1940s (Korns and Zeissig, 1948).
Undeniably, this percentage of vaccine coverage can interrupt transmission in
urban-dog rabies control programs (Beran, 1991), and the WHO has formally
adopted a minimum vaccination level of 70% for dogs at risk of entering into the
rabies transmission cycle (WHO, 1987). However, an application of epidemic
theory to rabies outbreaks in urban and rural locations estimated p_c to lie between
39% and 57%, with an upper 95% confidence interval of between 55% and 71%
(Coleman and Dye, 1996). Based on the lower estimates of p_c, the target value of
70% vaccination coverage would successfully prevent outbreaks on 96.5% of
occasions (Coleman and Dye, 1996).

5. The Ecology of the Domestic Dog: Relevance to Vaccination

The subject of what types of vaccines to use and the mechanism of their delivery to dogs is beyond the scope of this chapter. Regardless of the approach
to vaccination, it is always necessary to plan a campaign such that the maximum number of dogs are vaccinated over the shortest time interval with
the fewest dollars spent and minimum number of personnel involved. To plan

a dog-vaccination campaign adequately, information is required about the number of dogs in the targeted population (Childs *et al.*, 1998), the accessibility of these dogs (Bögel and Joshi, 1990), and the social or economic factors that might influence an owner's decision to allow his or her dog to be vaccinated (Chomel, 1993; Wandeler *et al.*, 1988). In circumstances where rabies vaccine can be distributed in oral baits, as is anticipated for dogs (Matter *et al.*, 1995; Haddad *et al.*, 1994), a measure of animal population density is required for designing optimal bait-distribution patterns through heterogeneous habitats (WHO, 1987).

B. Epidemiology of Rabies in Cats

Cats are not known to act as maintenance reservoirs for unique rabies virus variants. They are important as incidental hosts affected by spillover and can serve as important links in a chain of transmission of rabies virus to humans and other domestic animals. The last human death attributable to a cat bite in the United States occurred in 1975 in Minnesota; the rabies virus variant identified from this human case was that associated with skunks in the north central United States (Smith *et al.*, 1995) (see Fig. 2).

1. The Cat as a Source of Human Rabies Exposure

Since 1992, the cat has been the domestic animal most commonly reported rabid in the United States (see Fig. 6). In 1998, 282 cats were reported rabid, as compared with 113 dogs and 116 cattle (Krebs *et al.*, 1999). The majority of these animals were reported from the eastern United States, where the raccoon-adapted variant of rabies virus is endemic. The large and disproportionate number of rabid cats being identified in the United States presumably reflects the ongoing epidemics of wildlife rabies and the poorer vaccine coverage in this animal than is achieved for dogs (Fischman *et al.*, 1992; Nelson *et al.*, 1998). Required vaccination for cats is still not legally mandated in some states or counties. In 1996, a survey of the 50 states, the District of Columbia, and 3 of 5 territories revealed that 74% of these political units required dog vaccination compared with 52% requiring cat vaccination (Johnston and Walden, 1996). In addition, the large number of stray cats in rural environments certainly has contributed to the increase in rabies reported from this species.

The cat is the most popular pet animal in the United States, with an estimated 32.1 million households owning 64,250,000 cats during 1999–2000 [unpublished data from American Pet Products Manufacturing Association (APPMA) 1999–2000 National Pet Owners Survey; www.appma.org]. Since the late 1980s, rabid cats have been implicated more commonly than dogs as the source of potential human exposure to rabies virus in the United States (Eng and Fishbein,

1990). However, between 1996 and 1998, in emergency rooms in 11 large metropolitan areas of the United States, dog bites ($N = 1635$) were more common than cat bites ($N = 268$) (Moran *et al.*, 2000). Although a higher percentage of cat bites resulted in PET being given (7.8% versus 5.9%), dog bites resulted more often in PET being given to humans in these urban settings (Moran *et al.*, 2000). Cats have been the cause of several large-scale exposures of humans to potentially rabid animals (Rotz *et al.*, 1998), including one situation involving over 600 PETs (Noah *et al.*, 1996).

Similarly, reports from European countries from the 1950s through the 1970s indicated that cats were found rabid more frequently than dogs and were associated more frequently with human exposures (reviewed in Vaughn, 1975). Among 1104 persons receiving PET in France in 1988 following exposure to an animal proved to be rabid by laboratory testing, 88 (8%) had been bitten by a rabid dog and 285 (26%) by a rabid cat; almost half (522; 47%) were treated for contact with rabid herbivores (Sureau, 1990).

2. Characteristics of Rabid Cats and Origin of their Infection

Cats identified as rabid in the United States typically are unvaccinated animals and frequently are unowned (Fogelman *et al.*, 1993). As with dogs, the majority of rabid cats are young, and many are less than 1 year of age (Eng and Fishbein, 1990). Cats may be involved more frequently in unprovoked bites to humans and may bite women more commonly than dogs bite women (Wright, 1990).

That cats interact with terrestrial reservoirs of rabies virus and become infected with rabies virus variants maintained by these species has been well documented by molecular epidemiologic typing (Smith, 1988; Rupprecht *et al.*, 1987). In addition, cats may be more prone to interact with bats than dogs in a variety of settings (Hoff *et al.*, 1994). Bat-associated variants of rabies virus have been documented from brains of rabid cats sampled from the United States (Smith, 1988; Rupprecht *et al.*, 1987) and Latin America (Diaz *et al.*, 1994).

Spillover of rabies virus to cats occurs wherever rabies virus is endemic, and cat bites are a concern in most locations of the world. Laboratory-proved rabies in cats has been reported from Africa (Alexander *et al.*, 1993), the Middle East (Al-Qudah *et al.*, 1997), Asia (Wilde *et al.*, 1991), and Latin America (WHO, 1999), although at far lower frequency than reports of rabies among dogs. In developing countries of different regions of the world, the ratio of laboratory-confirmed rabies cases in cats to laboratory-confirmed rabies cases in dogs is of similar magnitude, varying from a low of 0.02 (106 of 5376) in Asia to a high of 0.09 in Africa (88 of 957), with the Americas (excluding Canada and the United States) at 0.06 (210 of 3643) (WHO, 1999).

Data from individual developing countries on the frequency of cat bites resulting in human PET as compared with dog bites reflect similar patterns to the data on laboratory-confirmed rabies in domestic animals. In Cambodia, animals involved in human exposures over a 1-month period included 401 dogs (98%), 6 monkeys (1.5%), and only 2 cats (0.5%) (Reynes *et al.*, 1999). In India, dogs accounted for 81% of bites received by 869 patients compared with 71 cat bites (8.2%) and 51 (5.9%) monkey bites (Bhargava *et al.*, 1996). In general, these data suggest that rabies among cats is of relatively minor importance in areas of the world where dog rabies remains endemic, a conclusion reached by Vaughn in a previous review (Vaughn, 1975).

It is important to note that cats also are involved in the transmission of other lyssaviruses to humans (see Mokola virus below). Their public health importance in the transmission of lyssaviruses cannot be assessed solely on the basis of the current situation in countries where rabies virus remains endemic in dog populations.

C. Epidemiology of Rabies in Cattle

In terms of economic impact, rabies among cattle remains a significant concern, especially in locations of Latin America from northern Argentina into Mexico within the geographic range of the vampire bat (*Desmodus rotudus*) (Acha, 1967). Much of the endemic bovine paralytic rabies is the result of vampire bat–transmitted rabies virus (Baer, 1991) (see below). In 1980, the cost of cattle rabies was estimated at $500 million (cited in Precausta and Soulebot, 1991).

In North America, cattle rabies is largely a problem where skunk-associated variants of rabies virus circulate in the central United States and raccoon-adapted rabies virus circulates in the northeastern and mid-Atlantic regions (see Fig. 2); typically over 100 cases per year are reported (see Fig. 6) (Krebs *et al.*, 1999). In southern Africa, reports of rabies in cattle is second to dog rabies among domestic animals; the jackal is also a major source of exposures (King *et al.*, 1994). Elsewhere in the world, rabies in cattle is a sporadic problem, with 3132 laboratory-confirmed cases reported in 1999, of which 57% were in the Americas (WHO, 1999).

D. Rabies in Other Domestic Animals

Rabies among horses, pigs, goats, sheep, and other domestic animals remains a sporadic occurrence wherever rabies virus is endemic. In some circumstances, such as public fairs and petting zoos in the United States, rabies in these species can result in the significant expense of large-scale human prophylaxis (Rotz *et al.*, 1998). Because of the lack of pathognomonic signs of rabies in horses, disease may not be suspected until late in the clinical course, leading to multiple human exposures (Chomel, 1999).

The ferret (*Mustelo putorius furo*) is listed as a domestic animal, and rabies vaccines suitable for use in this species are licensed (Jenkins *et al.*, 2000). Although the ferret has been involved in well-publicized reports of unprovoked attacks on infants (Hitchcock, 1994; Paisley and Lauer, 1988), it is not a significant threat to humans with regard to rabies. From 1958 through 1998, only 22 rabid ferrets were reported to the Centers for Disease Control and Prevention (CDC) (Krebs *et al.*, 1999; Krebs *et al.*, 1998a; Rupprecht *et al.*, 1996).

IV. EPIDEMIOLOGY OF RABIES IN WILDLIFE

Rabies virus transmission among wildlife, primarily involving terrestrial carnivores and bats, constitutes the reservoir for spillover infections to occur among humans and domestic animals. The major wildlife reservoirs for different variants of rabies virus vary by continent and by geographic regions within continents. Major epidemics of rabies (epizootics) occur among wildlife, and the distribution of rabies and rabies virus variants is dynamic.

Although most wildlife maintenance cycles of rabies virus appear indigenous, human translocation of wildlife has played a significant role in the distribution of wildlife rabies, as it has with dog rabies (Smith *et al.*, 1992). Examples in which variants of rabies virus have been moved inadvertently with an infected host animal include translocations of raccoons (Nettles *et al.*, 1979), coyotes (Hanlon and Rupprecht, 1998; Centers for Disease Control and Prevention, 1995a,b; Krebs *et al.*, 1994), and bats (Sasaki *et al.*, 1992).

A. Rabies in Raccoons

The epidemiology of rabies among raccoons (*Procyon lotor*) in the United States has been a public health concern since the original focus involving this species was identified in Florida in the 1940s (Kappus *et al.*, 1970). The geographic region affected by this raccoon-associated variant of rabies virus spread gradually to include Georgia by the early 1960s (Kappus *et al.*, 1970) and Alabama and South Carolina by the 1970s (Centers for Disease Control, 1981a). However, in the southeastern focus of raccoon rabies, the overall numbers of raccoons reported rabid remained relatively low in part because fewer large metropolitan and suburban centers are situated in southern than in the mid-Atlantic and northeastern regions of the United States.

In the late 1970s, a focus of rabies involving raccoons was discovered on the West Virginia–Virginia border (Jenkins *et al.*, 1988). Epidemiologic and virologic investigations suggested that this new focus was established when raccoons incubating rabies infection were translocated from southeastern states (Nettles *et al.*,

1979). Rabies viruses from the southeastern and mid-Atlantic foci were identical, as shown by antigenic and genetic typing (Rupprecht and Smith, 1994; Smith *et al.*, 1990). This rabies virus variant appeared to be highly adapted to raccoons (Smith *et al.*, 1984) and is distinguishable from variants occurring in other terrestrial carnivores serving as primary rabies virus reservoirs in other regions of the United States (Krebs *et al.*, 1998a).

This mid-Atlantic rabies epidemic has developed into one of the largest outbreaks in the history of wildlife rabies in terms of numbers of rabid animals reported and geographic extent (Jenkins and Winkler, 1987; Wilson *et al.*, 1997) (Fig. 8). More than 50,000 cases of rabies among raccoons have been reported in the United States since 1975 (Centers for Disease Control and Prevention, 2000a) (Fig. 9). Currently, the land mass affected by this epidemic is approximately 1 million km^2, in which 90×10^6 humans reside, 35% of the population of the United States (Hanlon and Rupprecht, 1998). The periodic occurrence of epidemics of rabies among raccoons has been demonstrated for an extensive area of the mid-Atlantic region of the United States, although successive epidemics are generally of smaller magnitude than the first (Childs *et al.*, 2000).

Although no human deaths have been associated with the raccoon-adapted rabies virus, the economic impact of the epidemic has been substantial. In New Jersey, two counties monitored before and during the raccoon rabies epizootic, had a more than 60-fold increase in human PETs, from 2 in 1988 to 131 in 1990 (Uhaa *et al.*, 1992). In New York, the estimated number of persons receiving PET increased from 84 in 1989, prior to the arrival of epidemic raccoon rabies, to 2905 in 1993 (Centers for Disease Control and Prevention, 1996b). Reported cases of

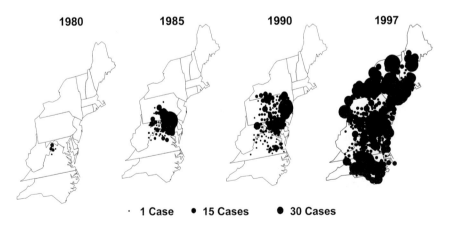

Fig. 8. The number of rabid raccoons reported by county in selected years, 1980–1997, in the mid-Atlantic region of the United States. The size of each dot is proportional to the number of cases reported by an individual county in that year.

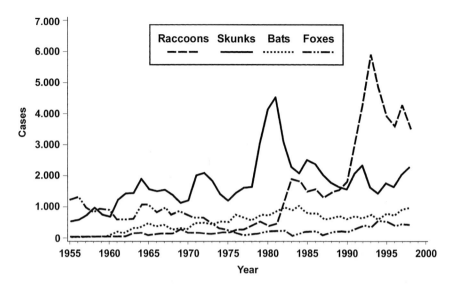

Fig. 9. Numbers of reported cases of rabies among wildlife in the United States, 1955–1998.

rabies in animals increased from 54 (bats only) to 2746 (2705 terrestrial mammals) during this period (Centers for Disease Control and Prevention, 1994). In a separate study of four upstate New York counties, the incidence of PET increased from less than 1 per 100,000 to 35 and 52 per 100,000 after the emergence of raccoon rabies (Wyatt et al., 1999). Similarly, Connecticut reported 41 persons receiving PET in 1990 (3 reported cases of rabies in bats). Following the onset of raccoon rabies, the estimated number of persons receiving PET at Connecticut hospitals increased to 260 in 1991 and to 887 during the first 9 months of 1994 (Centers for Disease Control and Prevention 1996b).

The epidemic front associated with raccoon rabies has progressed at a rate of 30 to 47 km per year (Moore, 1999; Roscoe et al., 1998; Wilson et al., 1997) through the northeastern and mid-Atlantic states. The epidemic reached into Ontario, Canada, in 1999 (Centers for Disease Control and Prevention, 2000a; Wandeler and Salsberg, 1999). In the central United States, the epidemic reached Ohio in 1996. In eastern Ohio, an oral rabies virus glycoprotein–vaccinia virus recombinant vaccine (ORV) is being distributed in an attempt to limit the further spread of epidemic rabies among raccoons (Centers for Disease Control and Prevention, 2000a; Hanlon and Rupprecht, 1998). The geographic range of the raccoon includes most of the continental United States (Kaufmann, 1982). Details of ORV campaigns against raccoons and other wildlife are given in Chap. 14.

B. Rabies in Foxes

There were no records of epizootic rabies in foxes of the United States until 1940, when an outbreak occurred in Burke County, Georgia (Johnson, 1945). Within a few years, rabies became endemic among gray foxes (*Urocyon cinereoargenteus*) in Alabama, Florida, and Tennessee. From 1940 to 1960, foxes [both gray and red (*Vulpes vulpes*)] were the wild carnivore most commonly reported rabid in the United States (see Fig. 9) (Tierkel *et al.*, 1958). Between 1946 and 1965, foxes were the most common wild animal source of human rabies reported, accounting for 4.7% of 236 cases (Held *et al.*, 1967). The last human case attributable to exposure to a rabid fox was in Kentucky in 1961 (Anderson *et al.*, 1984b). For unknown reasons, the number of rabies cases among gray foxes has declined dramatically, and endemic gray fox rabies presently is known only from relatively small areas in Texas and Arizona (Krebs *et al.*, 1999). The endemic focus in Texas is the target of an extensive ORV campaign (Krebs *et al.*, 1999).

Rabies among red foxes has been responsible for some of the most extensive epidemics of wildlife rabies ever documented in North America and Europe (Fig. 10). In North America, a major epidemic of fox rabies [involving red and arctic foxes (*Alopex lagopus*)] began in northern Canada in the 1940s (Tabel *et al.*, 1974) (see Fig. 10A). In the early 1960s, this epidemic expanded from Ontario into the northeastern states of New York, New Hampshire, Vermont, and Maine (Blancou *et al.*, 1991; Tabel *et al.*, 1974). The rabies virus variants in arctic and red foxes in Alaska and red foxes in New York are closely related (Smith *et al.*, 1995) and are reflective of a near-circumpolar distribution of fox rabies in the northern hemisphere. Arctic foxes are an occasional source of human rabies in Asia (Kuzmin, 1999).

Beginning in the 1940s, an epidemic of red fox rabies swept from eastern through western Europe, eventually affecting much of the continent (Steck and Wandeler, 1980; Wandeler *et al.*, 1974). The European epidemic of rabies among red foxes precipitated the grand-scale use of experimental oral rabies vaccination, using both modified live and recombinant vaccines, with considerable success (Brochier *et al.*, 1991; Schneider *et al.*, 1988). The topics of the ecology of red fox rabies and oral vaccination are covered in other chapters.

The origin of the European red fox variant of rabies virus is hypothesized to be the domestic dog (Bourhy *et al.*, 1999a). Physical barriers have contributed to the localized evolution of several genetic lineages of viruses found in red foxes in Europe (Bourhy *et al.*, 1999b).

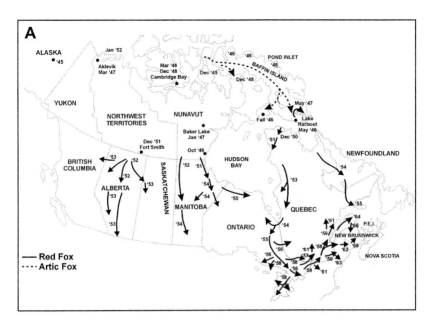

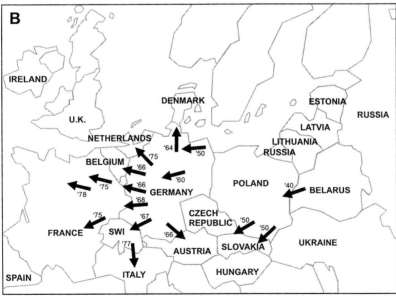

Fig. 10. Spread of fox rabies epidemics in North America (*A*) and Europe (*B*) beginning in the 1940s. [*A: Repoduced (with slight modification) from Figure 3 in Tabel (1974), with permission from Canadian Veterinary Medical Association; B: Modified from Macdonald and Voight (1985) and reproduced with permission from Academic Press.*]

C. Rabies in Skunks

Rabies among skunks has a long history in the United States. Although most of the detailed information for rabies pathogenesis and occurrence among skunks in the United States and Canada is for the striped skunk, *Mephitis mephitis* (Charlton *et al.*, 1991), the earliest reports from California in 1826 incriminate spotted skunks (genus *Spilogale*) as the source of human disease (Parker, 1975). Altogether seven species of skunks in three genera (those just mentioned and *Conepatus*, the hog-nosed skunks) exist in North America, the striped skunk is by far the most common (Parker, 1975). Since the 1950s, nine cases of human rabies associated with skunk exposures have been diagnosed in the United States and two in Canada, the last occurring in 1970 in Arizona (Anderson *et al.*, 1984b; Tabel *et al.*, 1974).

Currently, distribution of the two rabies virus variants present among skunks in the central United States (see Fig. 2) indicates distinct rabies-endemic areas that have been apparent from surveillance maps dating from the 1960s. A third variant of rabies virus circulates among skunks in California (Krebs *et al.*, 1999). In Mexico, skunks serve as reservoir hosts for unique variants of rabies virus, about which little is known concerning their public health importance (De Mattos *et al.*, 1999; Loza-Rubio *et al.*, 1999). Both *Spilogale putorius* and *Conepatus leuconotus* have been identified as rabid in Mexico (Aranda and López-de Buen, 1999). Of interest is the observation from Mexico that spotted skunks have attacked humans indoors at night as they slept (Aranda and López-de Buen, 1999) in a manner identical to that described from the United States in 1826 (Parker, 1975). Hog-nosed skunks also were involved in attacks on humans, but outside of homes (Aranda and López-de Buen, 1999).

Beginning in the 1960s and continuing until 1990, skunks were the group of terrestrial mammals most frequently reported rabid in the United States (see Fig. 9). Analyses of the temporal patterning of epidemics among skunks in North America reveal periodic major outbreaks with a period of 6 to 8 years (Gremillion Smith and Woolf, 1988), although shorter periods of 4 years have been reported from western Canada (Pybus, 1988). In general, the percentage of skunk submissions testing positive for rabies virus antigen is strongly bimodal, with peaks in the spring and fall (Gremillion Smith and Woolf, 1988). However, in Texas, Illinois, and Arkansas, the spring peak predominates (Heidt *et al.*, 1982; Pool and Hacker, 1982).

In the United States and Canada, skunk rabies is common in prairie habitat (Greenwood *et al.*, 1997; Pool and Hacker, 1982), where the disease has been postulated to be a major factor in driving the cyclic variations in skunk populations (Pybus, 1988). The possible impact of rabies on skunk populations was amply demonstrated by Greenwood *et al.* (1997), who followed a population of radio-collared animals during an epidemic in South Dakota. Estimated rates of skunk survival fell from 0.85 during April to June 1991 to 0.17 in April to July 1992 during the epidemic (Greenwood *et al.*, 1997).

D. Rabies in Bats

1. Vampire Bat–Associated Rabies

The first observation linking vampire bats (*Desmodus rotundus*) to rabies epidemics among terrestrial mammals was for cattle in Brazil in 1911 (Carini, 1911). The first human deaths attributed to bites received from vampire bats were documented on the Island of Trinidad (Pawan, 1936; Hurst and Pawan, 1931). Outbreaks of human rabies due to vampire bats continue to be reported from Brazil (Batista-da-Costa *et al.*, 1993), Peru (Lopez *et al.*, 1992), Venezuela (Caraballo, 1996), and Mexico (Martinez-Burnes *et al.*, 1997).

Vampire bats feed preferentially on livestock, and most of the economic burden they pose is through bovine paralytic rabies (Delpietro and Russo, 1996; Baer, 1991). Estimates from the 1960s place the loss of cattle at 100,000–500,000 head per year in Latin America (Acha, 1967). Because of this economic burden, vampire bats have been the target of major control efforts. Anticoagulants applied by topical treatment to the backs of captured bats subsequently released to return to roosting sites (Linhart *et al.*, 1972) or through systemic treatment of cattle (Flores-Crespo and Arellano-Sota, 1991) have been used to achieve reductions in vampire bat biting rates of 85–96% (Flores-Crespo and Arellano-Sota, 1991).

Vampire bat colonies appear to be naturally decimated by rabies virus infections, and colonies may fall to population densities incapable of maintaining transmission. Control of population density near that critical density has been recommended as a control strategy (Delpietro and Russo, 1996).

2. Insectivorous Bat–Associated Rabies

Rabies among insectivorous bats is of special interest to public health specialists in the United States because of the determination that 24 of the 32 cases of human rabies diagnosed in this country between 1990 and 2000 were caused by variants of rabies virus maintained by bat reservoirs (Centers for Disease Control and Prevention, 2000b, 1999c, 1998, 1997b; Noah *et al.*, 1998). Of these 24 bat-associated cases, 18 were caused by a variant of rabies virus found in two species of bats; the silver-haired bat (*Lasionycterus noctivagans*) and the eastern pipistrelle (*Pipistrellus subflavus*) (Noah *et al.*, 1998). In September 2000, officials in Quebec identified the first human case associated with this rabies virus variant to have occurred in Canada (Centers for Disease Control and Prevention, 2000b). In the United States, these bats typically are not submitted to laboratories for rabies testing as commonly as other species (Childs *et al.*, 1994; Baer and Smith, 1991; Baer, 1975).

Of the 39 species of bats recorded from the United States (Humphrey, 1975), at least 30 have tested positive for rabies (Constantine, 1979). Within the United

States, bats testing positive for rabies have been found from all 48 contiguous states and Alaska (Krebs *et al.*, 1999). A rabid bat also has been found in Hawaii associated with shipping containers from the mainland United States (Hanlon and Rupprecht, 1998).

The recognition of insectivorous bats as reservoirs of rabies virus dates from 1953, when rabies was first described in a bat that attacked a 7-year-old boy in Florida (Scatterday and Galton, 1954). Since that time, the number of rabid bats reported to the CDC has increased, reaching 992 in 1998 (see Fig. 9) (Krebs *et al.*, 1999). Data on rabid bats according to species have been published mostly as local accounts because most reports to the CDC do not identify the bats to species.

In North America, the species of bats exhibiting solitary lifestyles or forming small roosting colonies (the *Lasiurine* species and *Lasionycterus noctivagans*) typically have the highest prevalences of rabies when submitted for testing (Childs *et al.*, 1994; Burnett, 1989; Bigler *et al.*, 1975; Whitaker and Miller, 1974; Schneider *et al.*, 1957). In summary analyses, as many as 25% of the individuals of solitary species or species forming only small nursery colonies have tested positive for rabies, whereas typically less than 1% of the members of species that form large roosting colonies tested positive (Baer, 1975). The observation that a variant of rabies virus associated with a solitary bat species, the silver-haired bat, has been responsible for the majority of human rabies deaths in North America in the last decade increases the mystery surrounding the types of interactions that have brought about transmission of virus to humans when bites have gone unrecognized or unreported.

As expected, studies in which wild, apparently healthy bats were tested for rabies have reported a lower prevalence of infection than those recorded by rabies laboratories testing submitted specimens. In New York State, 2.9% of big brown bats (*Eptesicus fuscus*) and 0.3% of little brown bats (*Myotis lucifugus*) were found positive in colonies roosting near houses (Trimarchi and Debbie, 1977) compared with 6.3% and 0.7% among bats submitted for rabies testing (Childs *et al.*, 1994). In a similar study conducted in Massachusetts, rabies was found in 5 of 490 healthy bats (1.0%) as compared with 3 of 30 (10%) bats submitted for rabies testing (Girard *et al.*, 1965).

In North America, the peak season for bat submissions for rabies testing and the maximum prevalence of rabies are found in the late summer or early fall (Krebs *et al.*, 1999; Childs *et al.*, 1994). The submission pattern presumably reflects the interaction of increased bat activity and their presence in houses during summer months, coupled with the recruitment of juveniles born in June and July (Mills *et al.*, 1975). Juvenile bats typically are less adept at flying than are adults, and their presence in homes and lack of dexterity, which may be confused with abnormal behavior, probably result in many submissions for rabies testing.

The behavior of bats submitted for rabies testing can be correlated with the likelihood that they were rabid. In one study, bats submitted for rabies testing that had bitten a human were more than twice as likely to be rabid than those not involved in bites (Pape *et al.*, 1999). The most common types of encounters between humans and bats submitted for rabies testing include landing on a person (19% of 271 encounters), picking up a bat from the ground outside a house (18%), awaking to find a bat in a room (15%), and removing a bat from inside a structure (10%) (Pape *et al.*, 1999).

E. Other Wildlife Reservoirs

1. Rabies in Coyotes

Prior to 1988, rabies was reported only sporadically in coyotes in the southwestern United States and was confined largely to one county in southern Texas. Samples from both coyotes and dogs in this outbreak contained the same variant, suggesting that transmission of rabies virus from dogs to coyotes had resulted in enzootic maintenance among coyotes (Rohde *et al.*, 1997; Clark *et al.*, 1994). By 1991, the outbreak involved 10 counties, and 42 cases of rabies in coyotes were reported. This epidemic appeared to peak in 1995, with 80 cases of rabies reported from coyotes in Texas (Krebs *et al.*, 1995). The decline to 4 cases in each of the years 1997 and 1998 (Krebs *et al.*, 1998a; 1997) has been aided by an aggressive ORV campaign targeting coyotes and gray foxes in the state (Farry *et al.*, 1998). Variants of rabies virus associated with coyotes occasionally have been translocated with interstate shipments of these animals (Centers for Disease Control and Prevention, 1995a).

2. Rabies in Mongooses in the Caribbean

Sequence data from rabies virus isolates from mongooses in the Caribbean suggest that rabies in that reservoir originated from contact with dogs (Smith *et al.*, 1992). All mongooses present today in the Caribbean are descendants of animals brought from India to Jamaica in the 1870s for rodent control on sugar cane plantations (Everard and Everard, 1985). It is possible that rabies was introduced with these animals, although official reports of rabies in mongooses in the Caribbean were not made until 1950 in Puerto Rico (Tierkel *et al.*, 1952). Within a few years, rabies was diagnosed in mongooses in Cuba, Grenada, and the Dominican Republic (Everard and Everard, 1985). RNA sequence variation suggests that a single source for rabies introduction into mongooses cannot explain the outbreak throughout the Caribbean. Different rabies virus variants have been found in mongooses in Puerto Rico and the Dominican Republic, and these vary considerably from rabies virus obtained from mongooses from Asia (Smith *et al.*, 1992). It appears that rabies became established in mongooses separately on each island as they became infected by exposure to rabid dogs already present. The multiple introductions of dog rabies recorded for the Greater Antilles could be the source of the interisland genetic diversity observed (Malága-Alba, 1957).

3. Rabies among Rodents and Lagomorphs

Rodents and lagomorphs have never been implicated as a source of a human case of rabies in the United States and are not considered natural reservoirs. However, occasionally these animals are involved in potential rabies exposures to humans and other species (Winkler, 1991). Species in these two mammalian orders are susceptible to rabies (Winkler, 1991; Winkler et al., 1972) and consequently should be evaluated when the behavior of the animal and the history of human or domestic animal contact suggest a risk of rabies infection. Thousands of these animals are tested for rabies each year in the United States (Krebs et al., 1999), and public health officials frequently are asked to evaluate the need for PET following human exposures to these mammals (Karp et al., 1999). Although recent data are unavailable, reports from Georgia, Illinois, and Montana compiled from about 1967–1971 indicated that 11.7% of the 2516 persons treated for rabies during this interval were for exposures to rodents; none of rodents involved in these exposures were found to be rabid by laboratory testing (Winker, 1972).

Since 1980, rabies has been reported increasingly in the large native North American rodents. Most reports have involved the woodchuck (*Marmota monax*) and have occurred in the eastern United States in areas of epizootic raccoon rabies (Childs et al., 1997; Fishbein et al., 1986). The woodchuck can exhibit aggressive behavior and initiate unprovoked attacks when rabid, and human exposures have resulted (Moro et al., 1991; Winkler, 1991). Rabies also occurs sporadically in the largest rodent in North America, the beaver (*Castor canadensis*), with three cases reported from the United States in 1998 compared with 63 among woodchucks (Krebs et al., 1999).

4. Rabies among Wildlife in Africa

In South Africa, two distinct rabies virus variants have been identified from at least 30 different carnivore species belonging to four families (*Viverridae, Canidae, Mustelidae,* and *Felidae*) (King et al., 1994). There appear to be at least two distinctive maintenance cycles of rabies virus variants associated with multiple hosts, one associated with the *Canidae* [dogs, black-backed jackals (*Canis mesomelas*), and bat-eared foxes (*Otocyon megalotis*)] and a second associated with the *Viverridae* [yellow mongoose (*Cynictis penicillata*) and genets] (von Teichman et al., 1995; King et al., 1993). Crossover from each of these biotypes of rabies virus into alternative reservoir hosts has been documented, with no evidence of genetic modification in the recovered virus (Nel et al., 1997). The first irrefutable report of rabies in South Africa occurred in 1893 and could be traced to an Airedale terrier imported from England; however, it is likely that an endemic transmission cycle was already present (King *et al.*, 1994).

In East Africa, rabies virus from dogs has spilled over into other carnivore species and threatens to precipitate the extinction of the African wild dog (Macdonald, 1993; Burrows, 1992).

5. Rabies among Wildlife in Latin America

In Mexico, wildlife reservoirs for rabies virus traditionally have been regarded as the domestic dog and vampire bat. However, a unique variant of rabies virus has been described from skunks (species not specified) (De Mattos *et al.*, 1999). The identification of rabid skunks in the genera *Spilogale* and *Conepatus* and their role in human exposures were mentioned previously. Bobcats were found to be infected in Mexico with the same rabies virus variant that circulates among gray foxes in Arizona, suggesting a far wider range for this genetic lineage (De Mattos *et al.*, 1999).

In Chile, sporadic cases of urban rabies since 1980 in domestic animals suggested the existence of an additional reservoir for rabies virus other than the domestic dog or vampire bat. The examination of more than 100 rabies virus isolates obtained between 1997 and 1998 implicated the Brazilian free-tailed bat (*Tadarida brasiliensis*) as a major source of infections in domestic animals in recent decades (De Mattos *et al.*, 2000). Analyses of additional rabies virus variants identified by genetic sequencing indicate that other reservoir and maintenance cycles occur in Chile, but their epidemiologic importance remains to be elucidated (De Mattos *et al.*, 2000; Favi *et al.*, 1999).

V. EPIDEMIOLOGY OF OTHER LYSSAVIRUSES

With the exception of the two European bat lyssaviruses and the Australian bat lyssavirus, all the rabies-related viruses are endemic to Africa. The suggestion that rabies viruses radiated from a West Africa origin has been proposed (King *et al.*, 1994; Shope, 1982). Insect viruses (*Obodhiang* and *Kotokan*) related to the rabies viruses have been suggested as the relics of an ancestral virus from which the various rabies-related viruses have evolved (Shope, 1982).

A. Lagos Bat Virus, Serotype 2, Genotype 2

Lagos bat virus was isolated originally from a brain pool obtained from six *Eidolon helvum* bats collected in Nigeria (Boulger and Porterfield, 1958). Since that time, it has been identified from several African countries as far north as Ethiopia (see Table I). Most isolates of Lagos bat virus have been obtained from bats in which it can cause a fatal disease. In Natal, a die-off of *Epomorphorus* bats was attributed to Lagos bat virus infection (King *et al.*, 1994). Although no known human infections due to Lagos bat virus have been described, Lagos bat virus has been isolated from cats (cited in King *et al.*, 1994) and dogs with rabies-like diseases (Mebatsion *et al.*, 1992).

B. Mokola Virus, Serotype 3, Genotype 3

Mokola virus also appears to be widespread on the African continent (see Table I), occurring from South Africa to Nigeria in the west and Ethiopia in the north. Little is known about the epidemiology and natural history of Mokola virus. First isolated from *Crocidura* sp. shrews (*Insectivora*) captured in Nigeria (Shope *et al.*, 1970), Mokola virus has been linked to two naturally occurring human cases, of which one was fatal (Familusi and Moore, 1972; Kemp *et al.*, 1972). An isolate of Mokola virus from a rodent (*Lophuromys sikapusi*) was obtained from the Central African Republic (Saluzzo *et al.*, 1984).

Among cats and dogs, Mokola virus can cause a fatal rabies-like disease (von Teichman *et al.*, 1998; Mebatsion *et al.*, 1992; Foggin, 1983). Of public health importance are the observations that cats (von Teichman *et al.*, 1998) and dogs (Foggin, 1982) currently vaccinated against rabies virus are susceptible to Mokola virus infection. Since molecular biologic surveillance of rabies in Africa is only cursory, it is possible that human infections with Mokola virus are being attributed to rabies virus or are going undetected. In the absence of a specific Mokola virus vaccine, humans exposed to Mokola virus should be treated with the available biologicals used for rabies virus postexposure prophylaxis (von Teichman *et al.*, 1998).

C. Duvenhage Virus, Serotype 4, Genotype 4

The first isolation of Duvenhage virus was made in 1970 from a suspected case of rabies diagnosed in a man in South Africa. The man had been bitten on the lip 5 weeks previously by a bat (Meredith *et al.*, 1971). Since the original isolate, only two isolates of Duvenhage virus have been obtained, both from bats collected in South Africa. The only definitive host identification for a bat yielding an isolate of Duvenhage virus is the slit-faced bat (*Nycteris thebaica*; cited in King *et al.*, 1994), although *Miniopterus schreibersii* is also considered a likely reservoir (Meredith *et al.*, 1971). Since the original case of Duvenhage virus infection in a human was readily identifiable as rabies, it is possible that human infections are being attributed to rabies virus or are going undetected.

D. European Bat Lyssavirus 1, Genotype 5

The first report of rabies among bats in Europe dates to 1954, although the first documented case of human rabies from a bat exposure in the Old World was in 1977 (Tübingen Federal Research Centre for Virus Diseases of Animals, 1986). The European bat lyssaviruses (EBL1 and EBL2) have been characterized only recently as separate genotypes within the *Lyssavirus* genus (Bourhy *et al.*, 1993). Until 1994 (WHO, 1994b), European bat lyssavirus 1 and European bat lyssavirus 2 were considered as belonging to serogroup 4 Duvenhage viruses (Schneider and Cox, 1994), although European bat lyssavirus 1 is more closely related to Duvenhage virus than to European bat lyssavirus 2.

Human deaths associated with European bat lyssavirus 1 are rare; however, Yuli virus, recovered from a human in Russia (Selimov *et al.*, 1989), proves the potential risk posed by these viruses. Yuli is identical to isolates of European bat lyssavirus 1 from several species of bats, most notably *Eptesicus serotinus* (Perez-Jorda *et al.*, 1995; Amengual *et al.*, 1997). Numerous isolates of viruses have been made from bats collected in Europe since 1954, but unfortunately, most have not been genotyped (Schneider and Cox, 1994). In one of the most extensive surveys, isolates of an European bat lyssavirus were made from 182 of 809 (22.5%) *E. serotinus* and 4 of 92 (4.3%) of *Myotis dasycneme* tested in the Netherlands between 1987 and 1991 (Nieuwenhuijs *et al.*, 1992). It is now believed that *M. dasycneme* is a primary reservoir of European bat lyssavirus 2 (Amengual *et al.*, 1997; King *et al.*, 1990). Specimens from 1639 individuals of 11 other species were negative.

Humans exposed to potentially rabid bats in Europe are being treated with traditional rabies biologics. Human vaccine (HDCV) introduced into mice prevented infection from an European bat lyssavirus 1 isolate from *E. serotinus*, as well as from a Duvenhage virus challenge (Fekadu *et al.*, 1988). From 1987 to 1991, 174 humans were given postexposure prophylaxis after bat contact in the Netherlands (Nieuwenhuijs *et al.*, 1992).

E. European Bat Lyssavirus 2, Genotype 6

In 1985, a professional mammalogist in Finland with a special interest in bats died of a rabies-like disease that eventually was attributable to European bat lyssavirus 2 (Lumio *et al.*, 1986). The individual had been bitten by an *M. daubentoni* 51 days previously (Roine *et al.*, 1988). Finland is a country that had long been considered rabies-free, with the last case of human rabies diagnosed in 1934 and the last rabid animal in 1959 (Roine *et al.*, 1988). A single isolate of European bat lyssavirus 2 has been obtained from an *M. daubentoni* sampled in Britain (Whitby *et al.*, 1996). The occurrence of European bat lyssavirus

2 in Britain, another country considered rabies-free, presumably is a rare event because none of 1882 bats belonging to 23 species sampled from 1986 through 1995 were antigen-positive (Whitby *et al.*, 1996). Available human rabies vaccines do not appear to offer complete protection from European bat lyssavirus 2 exposure based on mouse challenge with the human isolate from Finland (Fekadu *et al.*, 1988).

F. Australian Bat Lyssavirus, Genotype 7

In 1996, a novel lyssavirus, subsequently named Australian bat lyssavirus, was described from brain samples obtained from a black flying fox (*Pteropus alecto*) collected in New South Wales, Australia (Fraser *et al.*, 1996). Within a short period, an antigenically and genetically similar virus was isolated from postmortem tissues obtained from a bat rehabilitator who died from a disease indistinguishable from rabies. This woman had been scratched or bitten by a large bat 5 weeks previously (Hooper *et al.*, 1997; Allworth *et al.*, 1996). A second human infection due to Australian bat lyssavirus was diagnosed by RT-PCR detection of RNA of Australian bat lyssavirus obtained from the saliva and nuchal biopsy from a woman dying of encephalitis 2 years after she had received a bat bite from a flying fox (Mackenzie, 1999).

The virus causing these deaths has now been demonstrated to occur in four species of flying foxes (genus *Pteropus*), as well as in the yellow-bellied sheath-tailed bat, *Saccolaimus flaviventris* (McCall *et al.*, 2000). The Australian bat lyssavirus is genetically more similar to rabies virus (serotype 1, genotype 1) than to any other member of the *Lyssavirus* genus (Gould *et al.*, 1998). In a survey of 366 sick, injured, or orphaned bats, 6% were positive for Australian bat lyssavirus by direct fluorescent antibody testing of brain impressions (McCall *et al.*, 2000).

In the treatment of persons exposed to Australian bat lyssavirus, standard HDCV and HRIG have been used, and this regimen has been shown to protect mice in experimental challenges (McCall *et al.*, 2000). Between 1996 and 1999, 205 persons potentially exposed to Australian bat lyssavirus were treated in Queensland, of which the vast majority (84%) were volunteer or professional animal handlers and bat handlers (rehabilitators) (McCall *et al.*, 2000). The majority of exposures (74%) were reported during the spring and summer (September–February) coinciding with the birthing season of the black and gray-headed (*P. poliocephalus*) flying foxes in Queensland. During birthing, many bats are orphaned and reared by bat rehabilitators (McCall *et al.*, 2000).

REFERENCES

Abdussalem, M., and Bögel, K. (1971). The problem of antirabies vaccination. In *International Conference on the Application of Vaccines against Viral, Rickettsial, and Bacterial Diseases of Man*. PAHO, No. 226. Washington, DC.

Acha, P. N. (1967). Epidemiology of paralytic bovine rabies and bat rabies. *Bull. Off. Int. Epizoot.* **67**, 343–382.

Acha, P. N., and Arambulo, P. V., III (1985). Rabies in the tropics: History and current status. In *Rabies in the Tropics*, E. Kuwert, C. Merieux, H. Koprowski, and K. Bögel (eds.), pp. 343–359. Springer-Verlag, Berlin.

Addy, P. A. K. (1985). Epidemiology of rabies in Ghana In *Rabies in the Tropics*, E. Kuwert, C. Merieux, H. Koprowski, and K. Bögel (eds.), pp. 497–519. Springer-Verlag, Berlin.

Aghomo, H. O., and Rupprecht, C. E. (1990). Further studies on rabies virus isolated from healthy dogs in Nigeria. *Vet. Microbiol.* **22**, 17–22.

Al-Qudah, K. M., Al-Rawashdeh, O. F., Abdul-Majeed, M., and Al-Ani, F. K. (1997). An epidemiological investigation of rabies in Jordan. *Acta Vet. Belgrade* **47**, 129–134.

Alexander, K. A., Smith, J, S., Macharia, M. J., and King, A. A. (1993). Rabies in the Masai Mara, Kenya: Preliminary report. *Onderstepoort J. Vet. Res.* **60**, 411–414.

Allworth, A., Murray, K., and Morgan, J. (1996). A case of encephalitis due to a lyssavirus recently identified in fruit bats. *Commun. Dis. Intell.* **20**, 504.

Amengual, B., Whitby, J. E., King, A., Cobo, J. S., and Bourhy, H. (1997). Evolution of European bat lyssaviruses. *J. Gen. Virol.* **78**, 2319–2328.

Anderson, L. J., Williams, L. P., Jr., Layde, J. B., Dixon, F. R., and Winkler, W. G. (1984a). Nosocomial rabies: Investigation of contacts of human rabies cases associated with a corneal transplant. *Am. J. Public Health.* **74**, 370–372.

Anderson, L. J., Nicholson, K. G., Tauxe, R. V., and Winkler, W. G. (1984b). Human rabies in the United States, 1960 to 1979: Epidemiology, diagnosis, and prevention. *Ann. Intern. Med.* **100**, 728–735.

Anderson, R. M., Jackson, H. C., May, R. M., and Smith, A. M. (1981). Population dynamics of fox rabies in Europe. *Nature* **289**, 765–771.

Aranda, M., and López-de Buen, L. (1999). Rabies in skunks from Mexico. *J. Wildlife Dis.* **35**, 574–577.

Arguin, P. M., Krebs, J. W., Mandel, E., Guzi, T., and Childs, J. E. (2000). Survey of rabies preexposure and postexposure prophylaxis among missionary personnel stationed outside the United States. *J. Travel Med.* **7**, 10–14.

Babes, V. (1912). *Traité de la Rage*. Baillière, Paris.

Baer, G. M. (1975). Rabies in nonhematophagous bats. In *The Natural History of Rabies*, G. M. Baer (ed.), pp. 79–97. Academic Press, New York.

Baer, G. M. (1991). Vampire bat and bovine paralytic rabies. In *The Natural History of Rabies*, G. M. Baer (ed.), pp. 389–403. CRC Press, Boca Raton, FL.

Baer, G. M., Shaddock, J. H., and Williams, L. W. (1975). Prolonging morbidity in rabid dogs by intrathecal injection of attenuated rabies vaccine. *Infect. Immun.* **12**, 98–103.

Baer, G. M., and Smith, J. S., (1991). Rabies in nonhematophagous bats. In *The Natural History of Rabies*, G. M. Baer (ed.), pp. 341–366. CRC Press, Boca Raton, FL.

Baer, G. M., and Wandeler, A. I. (1987). Rabies virus. In *Virus Infections of Carnivores*, M. J. Appel (ed.), pp. 167–182. Elsevier, New York.

Baltazard, M., and Bahmanyar, M. (1955). Essai pratique du serum anti-rabique chez les mordus par loups enrages. *Bull. WHO* **13**, 747–772.

Batista-da-Costa, M., Bonito, R. F., and Nishioka, S. A. (1993). An outbreak of vampire bat bite in a Brazilian village. *Trop. Med. Parasitol.* **44**, 219–220.

Bech-Nielsen, S., Hagstad, H. V., and Hubbert, W. T. (1979). Vaccination against dog rabies in the United States. *J. Am. Vet. Med. Assoc.* **174**, 695–699.

Beck, A.M. (1973). *The Ecology of Stray Dogs.* York Press, Baltimore.

Beck, A. M., and Jones, A. J. (1985). Unreported dog bites in children. *Public Health Rep.* **100**, 315–321.

Beran, G. W. (1982). Ecology of dogs in the central Philippines in relation to rabies control efforts. *Comp. Immunol. Microbiol. Infect. Dis.* **5**, 265–270.

Beran, G. W. (1991). Urban rabies. In *The Natural History of Rabies,* G. M. Baer (ed.), pp. 427–443. CRC Press, Boca Raton, FL.

Bernard, K. W., and Fishbein, D. B. (1991). Pre-exposure rabies prophylaxis for travellers: Are the benefits worth the cost? *Vaccine* **9**, 833–836.

Bernard, K. W., Fishbein, D. B., Miller, K. D., Parker, R. A., Waterman, S., Sumner, J. W., Reid, F. L., Johnson, B. K., Rollins, A. J., Oster, C. N., Schonberger, L. B., Baer, G. M., and Winkler, W. G. (1985). Pre-exposure rabies immunization with human diploid cell vaccine: Decreased antibody responses in persons immunized in developing countries. *Am. J. Trop. Med. Hyg.* **34**, 633–647.

Bhanganada, K., Wilde, H., Sakolsataydom, P., and Oonsombat, P. (1993). Dog-bite injuries at a Bangkok teaching hospital. *Acta Trop. (Basel)* **55**, 249–255.

Bhargava, A., Deshmukh, R., Ghosh, T. K., Goswami, A., Prasannaraj, P., Marfatia, S. P., and Sudarshan, M. K. (1996). Profile and characteristics of animal bites in India. *J. Assoc. Physicians India* **44**, 37–38.

Bhatia, R., Bhardwaj, M., and Sehgal, S. (1988). Canine rabies in and around Delhi: A 16-year study. *J. Commun. Dis.* **20**, 104–110.

Bigler, W. J., Hoff, G. L., and Buff, E. E. (1975). Chiropteran rabies in Florida: A twenty-year analysis, 1954 to 1973. *Am. J. Trop. Med. Hyg.* **24**, 347–352.

Bjorvatn, B., and Gundersen, S. V. (1980). Rabies exposure among Norwegian missionaries working abroad. *Scand. J. Infect. Dis.* **12**, 257–264.

Blancou, J., Aubert, M. F. A., and Artois, M. (1991). Fox rabies. In *The Natural History of Rabies,* G. M. Baer (ed.), pp. 257–290. CRC Press, Boca Raton, FL.

Bögel, K., Andral, L., Beran, G., Schneider, L. G., and Wandeler, A. (1982). Dog rabies elimination. *Int. J. Zoonoses* **9**, 97–112.

Bögel, K., and Motschwiller, E. (1986). Incidence of rabies and post-exposure treatment-in developing countries. *Bull. WHO* **64**, 883–887.

Bögel, K., and Meslin, F. X. (1990). Economics of human and canine rabies elimination: Guidelines for programme orientation. *Bull. WHO* **68**, 281–291.

Bögel, K., and Joshi, D. D. (1990). Accessibility of dog populations for rabies control in Kathmandu valley, Nepal. *Bull. WHO* **68**, 611–617.

Boulger, L. R., and Porterfield, J. S. (1958). Isolation of a virus from a Nigerian fruit bat. *Trans. R. Soc. Trop. Med. Hyg.* **52**, 421–424.

Bourhy, H., Kissi, B., and Tordo, N. (1993). Molecular diversity of the *Lyssavirus* genus. *Virology* **194**, 70–81.

Bourhy, H., Kissi, B., Audry, L., Smreczak, M., Sadkowska-Todys, M., Kulonen, K., Tordo, N., Zmudzinski, J. F., and Holmes, E. C. (1999a). Ecology and evolution of rabies virus in Europe. *J. Gen. Virol.* **80**, 2545–2557.

Bourhy, H., Kissi, B., Audry, L., Smreczak, M., Sadkowska-Todys, M., Kulonen, K., Tordo, N., Zmudzinski, J. F., and Holmes, E. C. (1999b). Ecology and evolution of rabies virus in Europe. *J. Gen. Virol.* **80**, 2545–2557.

Brochier, B., Kieny, M. P., Costy, F., Coppens, P., Bauduin, B., Lecocq, J. P., Languet, B., Chappuis, G., Desmettre, P., and Afiademanyo, K. (1991). Large-scale eradication of rabies using recombinant vaccinia-rabies vaccine. *Nature* **354**, 520–522.

Burnett, C. D. (1989). Bat rabies in Illinois: 1965 to 1986. *J. Wildlife Dis.* **25**, 10–19.

Burrows, R. (1992). Rabies in wild dogs. *Nature* **359**, 277.

Caraballo, A. J. (1996). Outbreak of vampire bat biting in a Venezuelan village. *Rev. Saude Publica.* **30**, 483–484.

Carini, A. (1911). Sur une grande épizootie de rage. *Ann. Inst. Pasteur (Paris)* **25**, 843–846.

Centers for Disease Control (1980). Human-to-human transmission of rabies via a corneal transplant — France. *Morb. Mortal. Weekly Rep.* **29**, 25–26.

Centers for Disease Control (1981a). *Rabies Surveillance Annual Summary 1978.* HHS Publication No. (CDC) 82-8255, Washington, DC, pp. 1–20.

Centers for Disease Control (1981b). Human-to-human transmission of rabies via corneal transplant — Thailand. *Morb. Mortal. Weekly Rep.* **30**, 473–474.

Centers for Disease Control (1982). Human rabies — Rwanda. *Morb. Mortal. Weekly Rep.* **31**, 135.

Centers for Disease Control (1983). Human rabies — Kenya. *Morb. Mortal. Weekly Rep.* **32**, 494–495.

Centers for Disease Control and Prevention (1994). Raccoon rabies epizootic — United States, 1993. *Morb. Mortal. Weekly Rep.* **43**, 269–273.

Centers for Disease Control and Prevention (1995a). Translocation of coyote rabies — Florida, 1994. *Morb. Mortal. Weekly Rep.* **44**, 580–581, 587.

Centers for Disease Control and Prevention (1995b). Human rabies — Alabama, Tennessee, and Texas, 1994. *Morb. Mortal. Weekly Rep.* **44**, 269–272.

Centers for Disease Control and Prevention (1996a). Human rabies — Florida, 1996. *Morb. Mortal. Weekly Rep.* **45**, 719–727.

Centers for Disease Control and Prevention (1996b). Rabies postexposure prophylaxis — Connecticut, 1990–1994. *Morb. Mortal. Weekly Rep.* **45**, 232–234.

Centers for Disease Control and Prevention (1997a). Human rabies — New Hampshire, 1996. *Morb. Mortal. Weekly Rep.* **46**, 267–270.

Centers for Disease Control and Prevention (1997b). Human rabies — Montana and Washington: 1997. *Morb. Mortal. Weekly Rep.* **46**, 770–774.

Centers for Disease Control and Prevention (1998). Human rabies — Texas and New Jersey, 1997, *Morb. Mortal. Weekly Rep.* **47**, 1–5.

Centers for Disease Control and Prevention (1999a). Human rabies prevention — United States, 1999: Recommendations of the Advisory Committee on Immunization Practices (ACIP). *Morb. Mortal. Weekly Rep.* **48**, 1–21.

Centers for Disease Control and Prevention (1999b). Mass treatment of humans who drank unpasteurized milk from rabid cows — Massachusetts, 1996–1998. *Morb. Mortal. Weekly Rep.* **48**, 228–229.

Centers for Disease Control and Prevention (1999c): Human rabies — Virginia, 1998. *Morb. Mortal. Weekly Rep.* **48**, 95–97.

Centers for Disease Control and Prevention (2000a). Update: Raccoon rabies epizootic — United States and Canada, 1999. *Morb. Mortal. Weekly Rep.* **49**, 31–35.

Centers for Disease Control and Prevention (2000b). Human rabies — California, Georgia, Minnesota, New York, and North Dakota, 2000. *Morb. Mortal. Weekly Rep.* **49**, 1111–1115.

Charlton, K. M., Webster, W. A., and Casey, G. A. (1991). Skunk rabies. In *The Natural History of Rabies*, G. M. Baer (ed.), pp. 307–324. CRC Press, Boca Raton, FL.

Childs, J. E., Trimarchi, C. V., and Krebs, J. W. (1994). The epidemiology of bat rabies in New York State, 1988–1992. *Epidemiol. Infect.* **113**, 501–511.

Childs, J. E., Colby, L., Krebs, J. W., Strine, T., Feller, M., Noah, D., Drenzek, C., Smith, J. S., and Rupprecht, C. E. (1997). Surveillance and spatiotemporal associations of rabies in rodents and lagomorphs in the United States, 1985–1994. *J. Wildlife Dis.* **33**, 20–27.

Childs, J. E., Robinson, L. E., Sadek, R., Madden, A., Miranda, M. E., and Miranda, N. L. (1998). Density estimates of rural dog populations and an assessment of marking methods during a rabies vaccination campaign in the Philippines. *Prev. Vet. Med.* **33**, 207–218.

Childs, J. E., Curns, A. T., Dey, M. E., Real, L. A., Feinstein, L., Bjørnstad, O. N., and Krebs, J. W. (2000). Predicting the local dynamics of epizootic rabies among raccoons in the United States. *Proc. Natl. Acad. Sci. USA* **97**, 13666–13671.

Chomel, B. B. (1993). The modern epidemiological aspects of rabies in the world. *Comp. Immunol. Microbiol. Infect. Dis.* **16**, 11–20.

Chomel, B. B. (1999). Rabies exposure and clinical disease in animals. In *Rabies: Guidelines for Medical Professionals*, pp. 20–26. Veterinary Learning Systems, Trenton, NJ.

Chomel, B., Chappuis, G., Bullon, F., Cardenas, E., de Beublain, T. D., and Lombard, M. (1988). Mass vaccination campaign against rabies: Are dogs correctly protected? *Rev. Infect. Dis.* **10**, S697–S702.

Clark, K. A., Neill, S. U., Smith, J. S., Wilson, P. J., Whadford, V. W., and McKirahan, G. W. (1994). Epizootic canine rabies transmitted by coyotes in south Texas. *J. Am. Vet. Med. Assoc.* **204**, 536–540.

Coleman, P. G., and Dye, C. (1996). Immunization coverage required to prevent outbreaks of dog rabies. *Vaccine* **14**, 185–186.

Conomy, J. P., Leibovitz, A., McCombs, W., and Stinson, J. (1977). Airborne rabies encephalitis: Demonstration of rabies virus in the human central nervous system. *Neurology* **27**, 67–69.

Constantine, D. G. (1962). Rabies transmission by nonbite route. *Public Health Rep.* **77**, 287–289.

Constantine, D. G. (1979). An updated list of rabies-infected bats in North America. *J. Wifdlife Dis.* **15**, 347–349.

Cox, M., Barbier, E. B., White, P. C. L., Newton-Cross, G. A., Kinsella, L., and Kennedy, H. J. (1999). Public preferences regarding rabies-prevention policies in the UK. *Prev. Vet. Med.* **41**, 257–270.

Cruickshank, I., Gurney, W. S. C., and Veitch, A. R. (1999). The characteristics of epidemics and invasions with thresholds. *Theor. Popul. Biol.* **56**, 279–292.

De Mattos, C. C., De Mattos, C. A., Loza-Rubio, E., Aguilar-Setien, A., Orciari, L. A., and Smith, J. S. (1999). Molecular characterization of rabies virus isolates from Mexico: Implications for transmission dynamics and human risk. *Am. J. Trop. Med. Hyg.* **61**, 587–597.

De Mattos, C. A., Favi, M., Yung, V., Pavletic, C., and De Mattos, C. C. (2000). Bat rabies in urban centers in Chile. *J. Wildlife Dis.* **36**, 231–240.

Delgiudice, P., Bernard, E., Rollin, P., Bertrand, F., and Dellamonica, P. (1992). A French case of rabies in Europe. *Eur. J. Clin. Microbiol. Infect. Dis.* **11**, 479.

Delpietro, H. A., and Russo, R. G. (1996). Ecological and epidemiological aspects of attacks by vampire bats in relation to paralytic rabies in Argentina, and an analysis of proposals for control. *Rev. Sci. Tech. Int. Epizoot.* **15**, 971–984.

Diaz, A. M., Papo, S., Rodriguez, A., and Smith, J. S. (1994). Antigenic analysis of rabies-virus isolates from Latin America and the Caribbean. *J. Vet. Med. Series B.* **41**, 153–160.

Dueñas, A., Belsey, M. A., Escobar, J., Medina, P., and Sanmartin, C. (1973). Isolation of rabies virus outside the human central nervous system. *J. Infect. Dis.* **127**, 702–704.

Dutta, J. K., and Dutta, T. K. (1994). Rabies in endemic countries. *Br. Med. J.* **308**, 488–489.

Eng, T. R., and Fishbein, D. B. (1990). Epidemiologic factors, clinical findings, and vaccination satus of rabies in cats and dogs in the United States in 1988. National Study Group on Rabies. *J. Am. Vet. Med. Assoc.* **197**, 201–209.

Eng, T. R., Fishbein, D. B., Talmante, H. E., Hall, D. B., Chavez, G. F., Dobbins, J. G. Muro, F. J. Bustos, de los Angles, J. L., and Munguia, A. (1993). Urban epizootic of rabies in Mexico: Epidemiology and impact of animal bite injuries. *Bull. WHO* **71**, 615–624.

Ernst, S. N., and Fabrega, F. (1989). A time series analysis of the rabies control programme in Chile. *Epidemiol. Infect.* **103**, 651–657.

Everard, C. O. R., and Everard, J. D. (1985). Mongoose rabies in Grenada. In *Population Dynamics of Rabies in Wildlife*, P. J. Bacon (ed.), pp. 43–67. Academic Press, New York.

Fagbami, A.H., Anosa, V. O., and Ezebuiro, E. O. (1981). Hospital records of human rabies and antirabies prophylaxis in Nigeria 1969–1978. *Trans. R. Soc. Trop. Med. Hyg.* **75**, 872–876.

Familusi, J. B., and Moore, D. L. (1972). Isolation of a rabies related virus from the cerebrospinal fluid of a child with "aseptic meningitis." *Afr. J. Med. Sci.* **3**, 93–96.

Farry, S. C., Henke, S. E., Beasom, S. L., and Fearneyhough, M. G. (1998). Efficacy of bait distributional starategies to deliver canine rabies vaccines to coyotes in southern Texas. *J. Wildlife Dis.* **34**, 23–32.

Favi, M., Yung, V., Pavletic, C., Ramirez, E., De Mattos, C. C., and De Mattos, C. A. (1999). Role of insectivorous bats in the transmission of rabies in Chile [Spanish]. *Arch. Med. Vet.* **31**, 157–165.

Feder, H. M., Jr., Nelson, R., and Reiher, H. W. (1997). Bat bite? *Lancet* **350**, 1300.

Fekadu, M. (1982). Rabies in Ethiopia. *Am. J. Epidemiol.* **115**, 266–273.

Fekadu, M., and Baer, G. M. (1980). Recovery from clinical rabies of 2 dogs inoculated with a rabies virus strain from Ethiopia. *Am. J. Vet. Res.* **41**, 1632–1634.

Fekadu, M., Endeshaw, T., Alemu, W., Bogale, Y., Teshager, T., and Olson, J. G. (1996). Possible human-to-human transmission of rabies in Ethiopia. *Ethiop. Med. J.* **34**, 123–127.

Fekadu, M., Shaddock, J. H., and Baer, G. M. (1981). Intermittent excretion of rabies virus in the saliva of a dog two and six months after it had recovered from experimental rabies. *Am. J. Trop. Med. Hyg.* **30**, 1113–1115.

Fekadu, M., Shaddock, J. H., Chandler, F. W., and Baer, G. M. (1983). Rabies virus in the tonsils of a carrier dog. *Arch. Virol.* **78**, 37–47.

Fekadu, M., Shaddock, J. H., Sanderlin, D. W., and Smith, J. S. (1988). Efficacy of rabies vaccines against Duvenhage virus isolated from European house bats (*Eptesicus serotinus*), classic rabies and rabies-related viruses. *Vaccine* **6**, 533–539.

Fischman, H. R., Grigor, J. K., Horman, J. T., and Israel, E. (1992). Epizootic of rabies in raccoons in Maryland from 1981 to 1987. *J. Am. Vet. Med. Assoc.* **201**, 1883–1886.

Fishbein, D. B. (1991). Rabies in humans. In *The Natural History of Rabies*, G. M. Baer (ed.), pp. 519–549. CRC Press, Boca Raton, FL.

Fishbein, D. B., Belotto, A. J., Pacer, R. E., Smith, J. S., Winkler, W. G., Jenkins, S. R., and Porter, K. M. (1986). Rabies in rodents and lagomorphs in the United States, 1971–1984: Increased cases in the woodchuck (*Marmota monax*) in mid-Atlantic states. *J. Wildlife Dis.* **22**, 151–155.

Fishbein, D. B., Corboy, J. M., and Sasaki, D. M. (1990). Rabies prevention in Hawaii. *Hawaii Med. J.* **49**, 98–101.

Flores-Crespo, R., and Areeano-Sota, C. (1991). Biology and control of the vampire bat. In *The Natural History of Rabies*, G. M. Baer (ed.), pp. 461–476. CRC Press. Boca Raton, FL.

Fogelman, V., Fischman, H. R., Horman, J. T., and Grigor, J. K. (1993). Epidemiologic and clinical characteristics of rabies in cats. *J. Am. Vet. Med. Assoc.* **202**, 1829–1833.

Foggin, C. M. (1982). A typical rabies virus in cats and a dog in Zimbabwe. *Vet. Rec.* **110**, 338.

Foggin, C. M. (1983). Mokola virus infection in cats and a dog in Zimbabwe. *Vet. Rec.* **113**, 115–116.

Fraser, G. C., Hooper, P. T., Lunt, R. A., Gould, A. R., Gleeson, L. J., Hyatt, A. D., Russell, G. M., and Kattenbelt, J. A. (1996). Encephalitis caused by a lyssavirus in fruit bats in Australia. *Emerg. Infect. Dis.* **2**, 327–331.

Gacouin, A., Bourhy, H., Renaud, J. C., Camus, C., Suprin, E., and Thomas, R. (1999). Human rabies despite postexposure vaccination. *Eur. J Clin. Microbiol. Infect. Dis.* **18**, 233–235.

Gibbons, R. V., and Rupprecht, C. (2000). Twelve common questions about human rabies and its prevention. *Infect. Dis. Clin. Pract.* **9**, 202–207.

Girard, K. F., Hitchcock, H. B., Edsall, G., and MacCready, R. A. (1965). Rabies in bats in southern New England. *New Engl. J. Med.* **272**, 75–80.

Gode, G. R., and Bhide, N. K. (1988). Two rabies deaths after corneal grafts from one donor. *Lancet* **2**, 791

Gould, A. R., Hyatt, A. D., Lunt, R., Kattenbelt, J. A., Hengstberger, S., and Blacksell, S. D. (1998). Characterisation of a novel lyssavirus isolated from *Pteropid* bats in Australia. *Virus Res.* **54**, 165–187.

Grandien, M., and Engvall, A. (1994). Quarantine to be abolished for dogs and cats: New regulations for import of pets from EU/EFTA countries [Swedish]. *Lakartidningen* **91**, 373–374.

Greenwood, R. J., Newton, W. E., Pearson, G. L., and Schamber, G. J. (1997). Population and movement characteristics of radio-collared striped skunks in North Dakota during an epizootic of rabies. *J. Wildlife Dis.* **33**, 226–241.

Gremillion Smith, C., and Woolf, A. (1988). Epizootiology of skunk rabies in North America. *J. Wildlife Dis.* **24**, 620–626.

Haddad, N., Ben Khelifa, R., Matter, H., Kharmachi, H., Aubert, M. F., Wandeler, A., and Blancou, J. (1994). Assay of oral vaccination of dogs against rabies in Tunisia with the vaccinal strain SADBern *Vaccine* **12**, 307–309.

Hanlon, C. A., and Rupprecht, C. E. (1998). The reemergence of rabies. In *Emerging Infections*, W. M. Scheld, D. Armstrong, and J. M. Hughes (eds.), pp. 59–80. ASM Press, Washington, DC.

Hattwick, M. A. W. (1974). Human rabies. *Public Health Rev.* **3**, 229–274.

Heidt, G. A., Ferguson, D. V., and Lammers, J. (1982). A profile of reported skunk rabies in Arkansas: 1977–1979. *J. Wildlife Dis.* **18**, 269–277.

Held, J. R., and Adaros, H. L. (1972). Neurological disease in man following administration of suckling mouse brain antirabies vaccine. *Bull. WHO* **46**, 321–327.

Held, J. R., Tierkel, E. S., and Steele, J. H. (1967). Rabies in man and animals in the United States, 1946–1965. *Public Health Rep.* **82**, 1009–1018.

Helmick, C. G., Tauxe, R. V., and Vernon, A. A. (1987). Is there a risk to contacts of patients with rabies? *Rev. Infect. Dis.* **9**, 511–518.

Hemachudha, T., Mitrabhakdi, E., Wilde, H., Vejabhuti, A., Siripataravanit, S., and Kingnate, D. (1999). Additional reports of failure to respond to treatment after rabies exposure in Thailand. *Clin. Infect. Dis.* **28**, 143–144.

Hitchcock, J. C. (1994). The European ferret, *Mustela putorius* (family *Mustelidae*), its public health, wildlife and agricultural significance. In *Proc. 16th Vert. Pest Conf.*, pp. 207–212.

Hoff, G., Mellon, G., Thomas, M., and Giedinghagen, D. (1994). Bats, cats, and rabies in an urban community. *South. Med. J.*

Hooper, P. T., Lunt, R. A., Gould, A. R., Samaratunga, H., Hyatt, A. D., Gleeson, L. J., Rodwell, B. J., Rupprecht, C. E., Smith, J. S., and Murray, P. K. (1997). A new lyssavirus: The first endemic rabies-related virus recognized in Australia. *Bull. Inst. Past.* **95**, 209–218.

Houff, S. A., Burton, R. C., Wilson, R. W., Henson, T. E., London, W. T., Baer, G. M., Anderson, L. J., Winkler, W. G., Madden, D. L., and Sever, J. L. (1979). Human-to-human transmission of rabies virus by corneal transplant. *New Engl. J. Med.* **300**, 603–604.

Humphrey, G. L., Kemp, G. E., and Wood, E. G. (1960). A fatal case of rabies in a woman bitten by an insectivorous bat. *Public Health Rep.* **75**, 317–326.

Humpery, S. R. (1975). Nursery roosts and community diversity of *Nearctic* bats. *J. Mammal.* **56**, 321–346.

Hurst, E. W., and Pawan, J. L. (1931). An outbreak of rabies in Trinidad without history of bites and with the symptoms of acute ascending paralysis. *Lancet.* **2**, 622–625.

Irons, J. V., Eads, R. B., Grimes, J. E., and Conklin, A. (1957). The public health importance of bats. *Texas Rep. Biol. Med.* **15**, 292–298.

Jenkins, S. R., Auslander, M., Conti, L., Johnson, R. H., Leslie, M. J., Sorhage, F. E., Briggs, D. J., Childs, J. E., Currier, M., Frank, N., Watson, B., Miller, R. B., Rupprecht, C. E., and Trimarchi, C. V. (2000). Compendium of animal rabies prevention and control, 2000. *J. Am. Vet. Med. Assoc.* **216**, 338–343.

Jenkins, S. R., Perry, B. D., Winkler, W. G. (1988). Ecology and epidemiology of raccoon rabies. *Rev. Infect. Dis.* **10**, (Suppl. 4), S620–S625.

Jenkins, S. R., and Winkler, W. G. (1987). Descriptive epidemiology from an epizootic of raccoon rabies in the Middle Atlantic states, 1982–1983. *Am. J. Epidemiol.* **126**, 429–437.

Johnson, H. N. (1945), Fox rabies. *J. Med. Assoc. Ala.* **14**, 268–271.

Johnston, W.B., and Walden, M. B. (1996). Results of a national survey of rabies control procedures. *J. Am. Vet. Med. Assoc.* **208**, 1667–1672.

Kale, O. O. (1997). Epidemiology and treatment of dog bites in Ibadan: A 12-year retrospective study of cases seen at the University College Hospital Ibadan (1962–1973). *Afr. J. Med. Sci.* **6**, 133–140.

Kappus, K. D., Bigler, W. J., McLean, R. G. and Trevino, H. A. (1970). The raccoon as an emerging rabies host, *J. Wildlife Dis.* **6**, 507.

Karp, B. E., Ball, N. E., Scott, C. R., and Walcoff, J. B. (1999). Rabies in two privately owned domestic rabbits. *J. Am. Vet. Med. Assoc.* **215**, 1824–1827.

Kaufmann, J. H. (1982). Raccoon and allies (*Procyon lotor* and allies). In *Wild Mammals of North America: Biology, Management, Economics*, J. A. Chapman and G. A. Feldhamer (eds.), pp. 567–585. Johns Hopkins University Press, Baltimore.

Kemp, G. E., Causey, O. R., Moore, D. L., Odelola, A., and Fabiyi, A. (1972). Mokola virus: Further studies on IbAn 27377, a new rabies-related etiologic agent of zoonosis in Nigeria. *Am. J. Trop. Med. Hyg.* **21**, 356–359.

Kennedy, D. J. (1988). An outbreak of rabies in northwestern Zimbabwe, 1980 to 1983. *Vet. Rec.* **122**, 129–133.

King, A., Davies., and Lawrie, A. (1990). The rabies viruses of bats. *Vet. Microbiol.* **23**, 165–174.

King, A. A., Meredith, C. D., and Thomson, G. R. (1993). Canid and viverrid rabies viruses in South Africa. *Onderstepoort J. Vet. Res.* **60**, 295–299.

King, A. A., Meredith, C. D., and Thomson, G. R. (1994). The biology of southern African lyssavirus variants. *Curr. Top. Microbiol. Immunol.* **187**, 267–295.

Korns, R. F., and Zeissig, A. (1948). Dog, fox, and cattle rabies in New York State evaluation of vaccination in dogs. *Am. J. Public Health* **38**, 50–65.

Krause, E., Grundmann, H., and Hatz, C. (1999). Pretravel advice neglects rabies risk for travelers to tropical countries. *J. Travel Med.* **6**, 163–167.

Krebs, J. W., Strine, T. W., Smith, J. S., Rupprecht, C. E., and Childs, J. E. (1994). Rabies surveillance in the United States during 1993. *J. Am. Vet. Med. Assoc.* **205**, 1695–1709.

Krebs, J. W., Strine, T. W., Smith, J. S., Rupprecht, C. E., and Childs, J. E. (1995). Rabies surveillance in the United States during 1994. *J. Am. Vet. Med. Assoc.* **207**, 1562–1575.

Krebs, J. W., Smith, J. S., Rupprecht, C. E., and Childs, J. E. (1997). Rabies surveillance in the United States during 1996. *J. Am. Vet. Med. Assoc.* **211**, 1525–1539.

Krebs, J. W., Smith, J. S., Rupprecht, C. E., and Childs, J. E. (1998a). Rabies surveillance in the United States during 1997. *J. Am. Vet. Med. Assoc.* **213**, 1713–1728.

Krebs, J. W., Long-Marin, S. C., and Childs, J. E. (1998b). Causes, costs, and estimates of rabies postexposure prophylaxis treatments in the United States. *J. Pubic Health Manag. Pract.* **4**, 57–63.

Krebs, J. W., Smith, J. S., Rupprecht, C. E., and Childs, J. E. (1999). Rabies surveillance in the United States during 1998. *J. Am. Vet. Med. Assoc.* **215**, 1786–1798.

Kuzmin, I. V. (1999). An arctic fox rabies virus strain as the cause of human rabies in Russian Siberia. *Arch. Virol.* **144**, 627–629.

Lakhanpal, U., and Sharma, R. C. (1985). An epidemiological study of 177 cases of human rabies. *Int. J. Epidemiol.* **14**, 614–617.

Leach, C. N., and Johnson, H. N. (1940). Human rabies with special reference to virus distribution and titer. *Am. Soc. Trop. Med. Hyg.* **20**, 335–340.

Lederberg, J., Shope, R. E., and Oaks, S. C., Jr. (1992). *Emerging Infections.* National Academy Press, Washington, DC.

Linhart, S. B., Flores Crespo, R., and Mitchell, G. C. (1972). Control of vampire bats by means of an anticoagulant [Spanish]. *Bol. Sanit. Panama.* **73**, 100–109.

Lopez, A., Miranda, P., Tejada, E., and Fishbein, D. B. (1992). Outbreak of human rabies in the Peruvian jungle. *Lancet* **339**, 408–411.

Lopez, T. (1997). Quarantine changes take effect in Hawaii. *J. Am. Vet. Med. Assoc.* **211**, 817–819.

Loza-Rubio, E., Aguilar-Setien, A., Bahloul, C., Brochier, B., Pastoret, P. P., and Tordo, N. (1999). Discrimination between epidemiological cycles of rabies in Mexico. *Arch. Med. Res.* **30**, 144–149.

Lumbiganon, P., and Wasi, C. (1990). Survival after rabies immunisation in newborn infant of affected mother. *Lancet* **336**, 319–320.

Lumio, J., Hillbom, M., Roine, R., Ketonen, L., Haltia, M., Valle, M., Neuvonen, E., and Lahdevirta, J. (1986). Human rabies of bat origin in Europe. *Lancet* **1**, 378.

Macdonald, D. W. (1993). Rabies and wildlife: A conservation problem? *Onderstepoort J. Vet. Res.* **60**, 351–355.

Macdonald, D. W., and Voight, D. R. (1985). The biological basis of rabies models. In *Population Dynamics of Rabies in Wildlife*, P. J. Bacon (ed.), pp. 71–108. Academic Press, New York.

Mackenzie, J. S. (1999). Emerging viral diseases: An Australian perspective. *Emerg. Infect. Dis.* **5**, 1–8.

Malaga, H., Lopez Nieto, E., and Gambirazio, C. (1979). Canine rabies seasonality. *Int. J. Epidemiol.* **8**, 243–245.

Malága-Alba, A. (1957). Rabies in wildlife in middle America. *J. Am. Vet. Med. Assoc.* **130**, 386–390.

Matter, H. C., Kharmachi, H., Haddad, N., Ben Youssef, S., Sghaier, C., Ben Khelifa, R., Jemli, J., Mrabet, L., Meslin, F. X., and Wandeler, A. I. (1995). Test of three bait types for oral immunization of dogs against rabies in Tunisia. *Am. J. Trop. Med. Hyg.* **52**, 489–495.

McCall, B. J., Epstein, J. H., Neill, A. S., Heel, K., Field, H., Barrett, J., Smith, G. A., Selvey, L. A., Rodwll, B., and Lunt, R. (2000). Potential exposure to Australian bat lyssavirus, Queensland, 1996–1999. *Emerg. Infect. Dis.* **6**, 259–264.

McKendrick, A. G. (1941). A ninth analytical review of reports from Pasteur Institutes. *Bull. WHO* **9**, 31–78.

Mebatsion, T., Cox, J. H., and Frost, J. W. (1992). Isolation and characterization of 115 street rabies isolates from Ethiopia by using monoclonal antibodies. *J. Infect. Dis.* **166**, 972–977.

Meredith, C. D., Rossouw, A. P., and Van Pragg Koch, H. (1971). An unusual case of human rabies thought to be of chiropteran origin. *S. Afr. Med. J.* **45**, 767–769.

Meslin, F.-X., Fishbein, D. B., and Matter, H. C. (1994). Rationale and prospects for rabies elimination in developing countries. *Curr. Top. Microbiol. Immunol.* **187**, 1–26.

Mills, R. S., Barrett, G. W., and Farrell, M. P. (1975). Population dynamics of the big brown bat (*Eptesicus fuscus*) in southwestern Ohio. *J. Mamm.* **56**, 591–604.

Mitmoonpitak, C., Tepsumethanon, V., and Wilde, H. (1998). Rabies in Thailand. *Epidemiol. Infect.* **120**, 165–169.

Moore, D. A. (1999). Spatial diffusion of raccoon rabies in Pennsylvania, USA. *Prevent. Vet. Med.* **40**, 19–32.

Moran, G. J., Talan, D. A., Mower, W., Newdow, M., Ong, S., Nakase, J. Y., Pinner, R. W., and Childs, J. E., for the Emergency ID Net Study Group (2000). Appropriateness of emergency department rabies post-exposure prophylaxis for animal exposures in the United States. *JAMA* **284**, 1001–1007.

Morimoto, K., Patel, M., Corisdeo, S., Hooper, D. C., Fu, Z. F., Rupprecht, C. E., Koprowski, H., and Dietzschold, B. (1996). Characterization of a unique variant of bat rabies virus responsible for newly emerging human cases in North America. *Proc. Natl. Acad. Sci. USA* **93**, 5653–5658.

Moro, M. H., Horman, J. T., Fischman, H. R., Grigor, J. K., and Israel, E. (1991). The epidemiology of rodent and lagomorph rabies in Maryland, 1981 to 1986. *J. Wildlife Dis.* **27**, 452–456.

Morton, C. (1973). Dog bites in Norfolk, Va. *Health Serv. Rep.* **88**, 59–64.

Muller, W. W. (1990). Review of reported rabies cases data in Europe to the WHO from 1977 to 1990. *Rabies Bull. Eur.* **14**, 10–12.

Murray, J. D., Stanley, E. A., and Brown, D. L. (1986). On the spatial spread of rabies among foxes. *Proc. R. Soc. Lond. [Biol.]* **229**, 111–150.

Nadin-Davis, S. A., and Casey, G. A. (1994). A molecular epidemiological study of rabies virus in central Ontario and western Quebec. *J. Gen. Virol.* **75**, 2575–2583.

Nel, L., Jacobs, J., Jaftha, J., and Meredith, C. (1997). Natural spillover of a distinctly *Canidae*-associated biotype of rabies virus into an expanded wildlife host range in southern Africa. *Virus Genes* **15**, 79–82.

Nelson, R. S., Mshar, P. A., Cartter, M. L., Adams, M. L., and Hadler, J. L. (1998). Public awareness of rabies and compliance with pet vaccination laws in Connecticut, 1993. *J. Am. Vet. Med. Assoc.* **212**, 1552–1555.

Nettles, V. F., Shaddock, J. H., Sikes, R. K., and Reyes, C. R. (1979). Rabies in translocated raccoons. *Am. J. Public Health.* **69**, 601–602.

Nieuwenhuijs, J., Haagsma, J., and Lina, P. (1992). Epidemiology and control of rabies in bats in the Netherlands. *Rev. Sci. Tech.* **11**, 1155–1161.

Nikolic, M. (1952). Tollwuttodesfälle bei menschen ohne verletzungen oder kontakt mit einem tollwütigen oder an tollwut verdächtigen tiere. *Arch. Hyg. Bakteriol.* **136**, 80–84.

Noah, D. L., Smith, G. M., Gotthardt, J. C., Krebs, J. W., Green, D., and Childs, J. E. (1996). Mass human exposure to rabies in New Hampshire: Assessment of exposures and adverse reactions. *Am. J. Public Health.* **86**, 1149–1151.

Noah, D. L., Drenzek, C. L., Smith, J. S., Krebs, J. W., Orciari, L., Shaddock, J., Sanderlin, D., Whitfield, S., Fekadu, M., Olson, J. G., Rupprecht, C. E., and Childs, J. E. (1998). The epidemiology of human rabies in the United States, 1980 to 1996. *Ann. Intern. Med.* **11**, 922–930.

Ogunkoya, A. B., and Macconi, F. (1986). Emergence of antirabies vaccine of unknown origin for human treatment in Nigeria. *Vaccine* **4**, 77–78.

PAHO (1995). La situacion de la rabia en America Latina de 1990 a 1994. *Bol. Sanit. Panama* **119**, 451–456.

Paisley, J. W., and Lauer, B. A. (1988). Severe facial injuries to infants due to unprovoked attacks by pet ferrets. *JAMA* **259**, 2005–2006.

Pape, W. J., Fitzsimmons, T. D., and Hoffman, R. E. (1999). Risk for rabies transmission from encounters with bats, Colorado, 1977–1996. *Emerg. Infect. Dis.* **5**, 433–437.

Para, M. (1965). An outbreak of post-vaccinal rabies (rage de laboratoire) in Fortaleza, Brazil, in 1960. *Bull. WHO* **33**, 177–182.

Parker, R. L. (1975). Rabies in skunks. In *The Natural History of Rabies*, G. M. Baer (ed.), Vol. II, 41–51. Academic Press, New York.

Parrish, H. M., Clack, F. B., Brobst, D., and Mock, J. F. (1959). Epidemiology of dog bites. *Public Health Rep.* **74**, 891–903.

Parviz, S., Luby, S., and Wilde, H. (1998). Postexposure treatment of rabies in Pakistan. *Clin. Infect. Dis.* **27**, 751–756.

Pawan, J. L. (1936). The transmission of paralytic rabies in Trinidad by the vampire bat (*Desmodus rotundus murinus*, Wagner 1804). *Ann. Trop. Med. Parasitol.* **30**, 101–129.

Perez-Jorda, J. L., Ibanez, C., Munoz-Cervera, M., and Tellez, A. (1995). Lyssavirus in *Eptesicus serotinus* (*Chiroptera: Vespertilionidae*). *J. Wildlife Dis.* **31**, 372–377.

Pferd, W., III (1987). *Dogs of the American Indians*. Denlinger's, Fairfax, VA.

Pool, G. E., and Hacker, C. S. (1982). Geographic and seasonal distribution of rabies in skunks, foxes and bats in Texas. *J. Wildlife Dis.* **18**, 405–418.

Precausta, P., and Soulebot, J. P. (1991). Vaccines for domestic animals. In *The Natural History of Rabies*, G. M. Baer (ed.), pp. 445–459. CRC Press, Boca Raton, FL.

Pybus, M. J. (1988). Rabies and rabies control in striped skunks (*Mephitis mephitis*) in three prairie regions of western North America. *J. Wildlife Dis.* **24**, 434–449.

Reynes, J. M., Soares, J. L., Keo, C. Ong, S., Heng, N. Y., and Vanhoye, B. 1999. Characterization and observation of animals responsible for rabies post-exposure treatment in Pnom Penh, Cambodia. *Onderstepoort J. Vet. Res.* **66**, 129–133.

Rohde, R. E., Neill, S. U., Clark, K. A., and Smith, J. S. (1997). Molecular epidemiology of rabies epizootics in Texas. *Clin. Diagn. Virol.* **8**, 209–217.

Roine, R. O., Hillbom, M., Valle, M., Haltia, M., Ketonen, L., Neuvonen, E., Lumio, J., and Lahdevirta, J. (1988). Fatal encephalitis caused by a bat-borne rabies-related virus: Clinical findings. *Brain* **111**, 1505–1516.

Roscoe, D. E., Holste, W. C., Sorhage, F. E., Campbell, C., Neizgoda, M., Buchannan, R., Diehl, D., Niu, S., and Rupprecht, C. E. (1998). Efficacy of an oral vaccinia-rabies glycoprotein recombinant vaccine in controlling epidemic raccoon rabies in New Jersy. *J. Wildlife Dis.* **34**, 752–763.

Rotz, L. D., Hensley, J. A., Rupprecht, C. E., and Childs, J. E. (1998). Large-scale human exposures to rabid or presumed rapid animals in the United States: 22 cases (1990–1996). *J. Am. Vet. Med. Assoc.* **212**, 1198–1200.

Rupprecht, C. E., Glickman, L. T., Spencer, P. A., and Wiktor, T. J. (1987). Epidemiology of rabies virus variants: Differentiation using monoclonal antibodies and discriminant analysis. *Am. J. Epidemiol.* **126**, 298–309.

Rupprecht, C. E., and Smith, J. S. (1994). Raccoon rabies: The re-emergence of an epizootic in a densely populated area. *Semin. Virol.* **5**, 155–164.

Rupprecht, C. E., Smith, J. S., Krebs, J., Niezgoda, M., and Childs, J. E. (1996). Current issues in rabies prevention in the United States health dilemmas: Public coffers, private interests. *Public Health Rep.* **111**, 400–407.

Sacramento, D., Bourhy, H., and Tordo, N. (1991). PCR technique as an alternative method for diagnosis and molecular epidemiology of rabies virus. *Mol. Cell Probes* **5**, 229–240.

Saluzzo, J. F., Rollin, P. E., Dauget, C., Digoutte, J. P., Georges, A. J., and Sureau, P. (1984). Premier isolement du virus mokola a partir d'un rongeur (*Lophuromys sikapusi*). *Ann. Virol.* (*Inst. Pasteur*). **135**, 57–66.

Sasaki, D. M., Middleton, T. R., Sawa, T. R., Christensen, C. C., and Kobyashi, G. Y. (1992). Rabid bat diagnosed in Hawaii. *Hawaii Med. J.* **51**, 181–185.

Scatterday, J. E., and Galton, M. M. (1954). Bat rabies in Florida. *Vet. Med.* **49**, 133–135.

Schneider, L. G. and Cox, J. H. (1994). Bat lyssaviruses in Europe. *Curr. Top. Microbiol. Immunol.* **187**, 207–218.

Schneider, L. G., Cox, J. H., Muller, W. W., and Hohnsbeen, K. P. (1988). Current oral rabies vaccination in Europe: an interim balance. *Rev. Infect. Dis.* **10** (Suppl. 4), S654–S659.

Schneider, N. J., Scatterday, J. E., Lewis, A. L., Jennings, W. L., Venters, H. D., and Hardy, A. V. (1957). Rabies in bats in Florida. *Am. J. Public Health* **47**, 983–989.

Selimov, M. A., Tatarov, A. G., Botvinkin, A. D., Klueva, E. V., Kulikova, L. G., and Khismatullina, N. A. (1989). Rabies-related Yuli virus: Identification with a panel of monoclonal antibodies. *Acta Virol.* **33**, 542–546.

Shlim, D. R., Schwartz, E., and Houston, T. (1991). Rabies immunoprophylaxis strategy in travelers. *J. Wilderness Med.* **2**, 15–21.

Shope, R. E. (1982). Rabies-related viruses. *Yale J. Biol. Med.* **55**, 271–275.

Shope, R. E., Murphy, F. A., Harrison, A. K., Causey, O. R., Kemp, G. E., Simpson, D. I. H., and Moore, D. L. (1970). Two African viruses serologically and morphologically related to rabies virus. *J. Virol.* **6**, 690.

Sipahioglu, U., and Alpaut, S. (1985). Transplacental rabies in humans (original in Turkish). *Mikrobiyol. Bul.* **19**, 95–99.

Smith, A. D. M. (1985). A continuous time deterministic model of temporal rabies. In *Population Dynamics of Rabies in Wildlife*, P. J. Bacon (ed.), pp. 131–146. Academic Press, New York.

Smith, J. S. (1989). Rabies virus epitopic variation: Use in ecologic studies. *Adv. Virus Res.* **36**, 215–253.

Smith, J. S., Sumner, J. W., Roumillat, L. F., Baer, G. M., and Winkler, W. G. (1984). Antigenic characteristics of isolates associated with a new epizootic of raccoon rabies in the United States. *J. Infect. Dis.* **149**, 769–774.

Smith, J. S. (1988). Monoclonal antibody studies of rabies in insectivorous bats of the United States. *Rev. Infect. Dis.* **10** (Suppl. 4), S637–S643.

Smith, J. S., Yager, P. A., Bigler, W. J., and Hartwig, E. C. J. (1990). Surveillance and epidemiologic mapping of monoclonal antibody–defined rabies variants in Florida. *J. Wildlife Dis.* **26**, 473–485.

Smith, J. S., Fishbein, D. B., Rupprecht, C. E., and Clark, K. (1991). Unexplained rabies in three immigrants in the United States: A virologic investigation. *New Engl. J. Med.* **324**, 205–211.

Smith, J. S., Orciari, L. A., Yager, P. A., Seidel, H. D., and Warner, C. K. (1992). Epidemiologic and historical relationships among 87 rabies virus isolates as determined by limited sequence analysis. *J. Infect. Dis.* **166**, 296–307.

Smith, J. S., and Seidel, H. D. (1993). Rabies: A new look at an old disease. *Prog. Med. Virol.* **40**, 82–106.

Smith, J. S., Orciari, L. A., and Yager, P. A. (1995). Molecular epidemiology of rabies in the United States. *Semin. Virol.* **6**, 387–400.

Smithcors, J. F. (1958). The history of some current problems in animal diseases: VII. Rabies. *Vet. Med.* **53**, 149–154.

Steck, F., and Wandeler, A. (1980). The epidemiology of fox rabies in Europe. *Epidemiol. Rev.* **2**, 71–96.

Steele, J. H., and Fernandez, P. J. (1991). History of rabies and global aspects. In *The Natural History of Rabies*, G. M. Baer (ed.), pp. 1–24. CRC Press, Boca Raton, FL.

Sureau, P. (1990). Recent data on the epidemiology and prophylaxis of human rabies in France. *Comp. Immunol. Microbiol. Infect. Dis.* **13**, 107–110.

Swaddiwuthipong, W., Weniger, B. G., Wattanasri, S., and Warrell, M. J. (1988). A high rate of neurological complications following Semple anti-rabies vaccine. *Trans. R. Soc. Trop. Med. Hyg.* **82**, 472–475.

Swanepoel, R., and Foggin, C. M. (1978). The occurrence, diagnosis, treatment and control of rabies in Rhodesia. *Central Afr. J. Med.* **24**, 107–114.

Tabel, H., Corner, A. H., Webster, W. A., and Casey, C. A. (1974). History and epizootiology of rabies in Canada. *Can. Vet. J.* **15**, 271–281.

Tariq, W. U., Shafi, M. S., Jamal, S., and Ahmad, M. (1991). Rabies in man handling infected calf. *Lancet* **337**, 1224–1234.

Tierkel, E. S. (1959). Rabies. *Adv. Vet. Sci.* **5**, 183–226.

Tierkel, E. S., Graves, L. M., and Wadley, S. L. (1950). Effective control of an outbreak of rabies in Memphis and Shelby County, Tennessee. *Am. J. Public Health* **40**, 1084–1088.

Tierkel, E. S., Arbona, G., Rivera, A., and de Juan, A. (1952). Mongoose rabies in Puerto Rico. *Public Health Rep.* **67**, 274–278.

Tierkel, E. S., Chadwick, V. D., Cerosaletti, M. J., Cox, H. R., Dwyer, E. M., Grennan, T. J., and Mann, J. W. (1958). Report of Committee on Rabies. In *Sixty-Second Annual Proceedings of the U.S. Livestock Sanitary Association*, pp. 253–259.

Trimarchi, C. V., and Debbie, J. G. (1977). Naturally occurring rabies virus and neutralizing antibody in two species of insectivorous bats of New York State. *J. Wildlife Dis.* **13**, 366–369.

Tübingen Federal Research Centre for Virus Diseases of Animals. (1986). *Rabies Bulletin Europe.* Tübingen.

Tuncman, Z. M. (1949). A rare case of rabies without a bite. *Trop. Dis. Bull.* **46**, 139.

Turner, G. S. (1971). Rural rabies. *Rural Med.* **2**, 108–112.

Uhaa, I. J., Dato, V. M., Sorhage, F. E., Beckley, J. W., Roscoe, D. E., Gorsky, R. D., and Fishbein, D. B. (1992). Benefits and costs of using an orally absorbed vaccine to control rabies in raccoons. *J. Am. Vet. Med. Assoc.* **201**, 1873–1882.

Varner, J. G., and Varner, J. J. (1983). *Dogs of Conquest.* University of Oklahoma Press, Norman, UK.

Vaughn, J. B. (1975). Cat rabies. In *The Natural History of Rabies*, G. M. Baer (ed.), pp. 139–154. Academic Press, New York.

von Teichman, B. F., de Koker, W. C., Bosch, S. J., Bishop, G. C., Meredith, C. D., and Bingham (1998). Mokola virus infection: Description of recent South African cases and a review of the virus epidemiology. *J. S. Afr. Vet. Med. Assoc.* **69**, 169–171.

von Teichman, B. F., Thomson, G. R., Meredith, C. D., and Nel, L. H. (1995). Molecular epidemiology of rabies virus in South Africa: Evidence for two distinct virus groups. *J. Gen. Virol.* **76**, 73–82.

Wandeler, A., Wachendorfer, G., Forster, U., Krekel, H., Schale, W., Muller, J., and Steck, F. (1974). Rabies in wild carnivores in central Europe: I. Epidemiological studies. *Zentralbl. Veterinarmed. B* **21**, 735–756.

Wandeler, A. I., Budde, A., Capt, S., Kappeler, A., and Matter, H. (1988). Dog ecology and dog rabies control. *Rev. Infect. Dis.* **10** (Suppl. 4), S684–S688.

Wandeler, A. I., and Salsberg, E. B. (1999). Raccoon rabies in eastern Ontario. *Can. Vet. J.* **40**, 731.

Wang, S. P. (1956). Statistical studies of human rabies in Taiwan. *J. Formosan Med. Assoc.* **55**, 548–554.

Whitaker, J. O., and Miller, W. A. (1974). Rabies in bats of Indiana: 1968–1972. *Proc. Ind. Acad. Sci.* **83**, 469–472.

Whitby, J. E., Johnstone, P., Parsons, G., King, A. A., and Hutson, A. M. (1996). Ten-year survey of British bats for the existence of rabies. *Vet. Rec.* **139**, 491–493.

WHO (1987). *Guidelines for Dog Rabies Control.* World Health Organization, Geneva.

WHO Expert Committee on Rabies (1992). *Eighth Report.* World Health Organization, Geneva.

WHO (1993). *Report of the Symposium on Rabies Control in Asian Countries.* World Health Organization, Geneva.

WHO (1994a). Two rabies cases following corneal transplantation. *Wkly. Epidemiol. Rec.* **44**, 330.

WHO (1994b). *WHO Workshop on Genetic and Antigenic Molecular Epidemiology of Lyssaviruses.* World Health Organization, Geneva, pp. 1–14.

WHO (1999). *World Survey of Rabies No 33 for the Year 1997.* World Health Organization, Geneva, pp. 1–29.

Wilde, H., Chutivongse, S., Tepsumethanon, W., Choomkasien, P., Polsuwan, C., and Lumbertdacha, B. (1991). Rabies in Thailand: 1990. *Rev. Infect. Dis.* **13**, 644–652.

Wilde, H., Sirikawin, S., Sabcharoen, A., Kingnate, D., Tantawichien, T., Harischandra, P. A., Chaiyabutr, N., de Silva, D. G., Fernando, L., Liyanage, J. B., and Sitprija, V. (1996). Failure of postexposure treatment of rabies in children. *Clin. Infect. Dis.* **22**, 228–232.

Wilde, H., Tipkong, P., and Khawplod, P. (1999). Economic issues in postexposure rabies treatment. *J. Trav. Med.* **6**, 238–242.

Wilson, M. L., Bretsky, P. M., Cooper, G. H., Jr., Egbertson, S. H., Van Kruiningen, H. J., and Cartter, M. L. (1997). Emergence of raccoon rabies in Connecticut, 1991–1994: Spatial and temporal characteristics of animal infection and human contact. *Am. J. Trop. Med. Hyg.* **57**, 457–463.

Winkler, W. G. (1968). Airborne rabies virus isolation. *Bull. Wildlife Dis. Assoc.* **4**, 37–40.

Winkler, W. G. (1972). Rodent rabies in the United States. *J. Infect. Dis.* **126**, 565–567.

Winkler, W. G. (1991). Rodent rabies. In *The Natural History of Rabies*, G. M. Baer (ed.), pp. 405–410. CRC Press, Boca Raton, FL.

Winkler, W. G., Schneider, N. J., and Jennings, W. L. (1972). Experimental rabies infection in wild rodents. *J. Wildlife Dis.* **8**, 99–103.

Wright, J. C. (1990). Reported cat bites in Dallas: Characteristics of the cats, the victims, and the attack events. *Public Health Rep.* **105**, 420–424.

Wyatt, J. D., Barker, W. H., Bennett, N. M., and Hanlon, C. A. (1999). Human rabies postexposure prophylaxis during a raccoon rabies epizootic in New York, 1993 and 1994. *Emerg. Infect. Dis.* **5**, 415–423.

5

Animal Rabies

MICHAEL NIEZGODA, CATHLEEN A. HANLON, and
CHARLES E. RUPPRECHT

Rabies Section
Centers for Disease Control and Prevention
Atlanta, Georgia 30333

I. INTRODUCTION

Rabies is an acute viral encephalitis. As the inquisitive reader casually begins this page, literally tens of thousands of animals, if not more, are dying from rabies around the globe. These stories vary but repeat daily as the players change. In an

163

impoverished rural Chinese village, a stray rabid dog is butchered, and its organs are not wasted but become the evening meal. In Germany, an exhausted red fox in the terminal stages of disease slowly drowns in a shallow mountain stream, a major source of water for the small town below. In the United States, an Amish farmer tries in vain to extract the last few drops of milk from the udder of his oddly bellowing Holstein. A stricken Alaskan wolf strains to mark a scent post with urine, soon visited by another male. On the Serengeti Plains, an ataxic wildebeest faces evisceration by a pack of African wild dogs in hot pursuit. A multitude of arthropods in a living guano field feast on the flesh of a fallen pregnant Mexican free-tail bat, its brain laden with virus. An unfortunate paretic skunk falls into the spring compost and eventually becomes part of the green silage for foraging Iowa cattle. Fresh from its deadly encounter with an ataxic coyote, a bloodied Texas sheepdog runs into the farmhouse kitchen and straight into the arms of an expectant youngster. At the first light in Georgia, a solitary crow picks through a still warm road-killed raccoon, paralyzed from the disease the night before. Dramatic as some of the scenarios may sound, their ultimate significance in disease perpetuation is highly debatable, owing to the alleged primary importance of a bite in virus transmission.

Animals are dynamic viral vessels. They form a key part of the epidemiologic triad, and their populations are simulated in the construction of disease models of rabies. Those interested in the basic form and function of rabies must use the building blocks provided by animals. Routine rabies diagnosis occurs in animal tissues. Rabies is the most important viral zoonosis and an occupational hazard to all those exposed to particular animals, intentionally or accidentally. Preventive public health practices of leashing, confinement, observation, quarantine, and so on relate directly to animals. Pure, potent, safe, and effective rabies vaccines are developed through the use of animals. Rabies elimination is a desirable human goal, but elimination of rabies reservoir populations is neither achievable nor desirable. Thus, with rabies, it all begins and ends with animals. The objectives of this chapter are to review some of the basic principles of animal rabies related to host range, susceptibility, clinical signs, differential diagnosis, and transmission; to provide salient examples of these topics in selected domestic and wildlife species; and to provoke a discussion on certain research issues in need of further inspection.

II. HOST RANGE

Rabies is a disease of mammals caused by viral representatives in the genus *Lyssavirus*, family *Rhabdoviridae*. Rhabdoviruses as a group can replicate in vertebrates, plants, or invertebrates. Mokola is the only lyssavirus considered as a remote possible bridge among such diverse host types because it is reported to be able to replicate in insect cells, at least under laboratory conditions (Buckley,

1975; Aitken *et al.*, 1984). Similarly, rabies virus can replicate *in vitro* in certain cold-blooded vertebrate tissues (Clark and Kritchevsky, 1972; Seganti *et al.*, 1990), but no successful *in vivo* attempts have been reported. Birds are susceptible to experimental rabies infection (Yamaoka, 1962; Schneider and Burtscher, 1967; Jorgenson and Gough, 1976), but the virus appears to be largely restricted to the central nervous system (CNS) and is apparently neutralized effectively by host defenses. Perhaps due to such autosterilization, virus may not readily reach relevant exit portals, such as the saliva, and hence would be at a dead end. Although there were earlier, unconfirmed reports, there have been no recent documentations of natural cases of rabies in birds (despite more sophisticated diagnostic techniques available), and serologic surveys of birds of prey have not detected evidence of antibodies to rabies virus (Shannon *et al.*, 1988).

Viral adaptation to certain common animals having a relatively narrow range of metabolically regulated internal temperatures might be a useful way, akin to a mobile incubator, for the virus to establish itself in a new environment. Abundant homeotherms with teeth and complex social repertoires seem ideal, particularly if relatively deep intramuscular inoculation of virus is needed to reach the vicinity of neuromuscular junctions or, alternatively, copious salivary contamination of mucous membranes and neural receptors with virus prior to direct infection of the CNS. Teeth were possessed by now-extinct avian predecessors (Hou *et al.*, 1996), but their notable absence and the much more limited development of salivary glands in extant avian species, coupled with differences in the sociobiology and demography of birds versus mammals, may have been significant in support of the differential lyssavirus affinities between birds and mammals.

These proximate speculations do not begin to explain the divergence of lyssaviruses from other rhabdoviruses, the origins of neurotropism, or the ultimate selection of certain vertebrate groups over others. However, the paucity of recognized isolates in birds appears odd, considering rhabdovirus plasticity, adaptability, and persistence otherwise, as evidenced by their widespread occurrence in plants, invertebrates, fishes, amphibians, reptiles, and mammals. Similarly, given more than 4000 mammalian species, all of which are susceptible to rabies in theory, relatively few qualify as major reservoir hosts. All rabies reservoirs are also known vectors, capable of disease transmission, but not all mammalian vectors are also reservoirs.

III. SUSCEPTIBILITY AND TRANSMISSION

Successful lyssavirus infection depends on three main events: initial direct contact with the surface of a receptive host cell; viral uncoating, nucleic acid replication, gene transcription, and protein translation in the intracytoplasmic environment, culminating in viral assembly at the cell membrane; and egress from the cells of the old host to renew the process (see Chap. 2). The viral strategy of entrance, self-production, and exit of progeny, extrapolated from the biochemical, cellular, and tissue levels of organization to an entire organism, forms the basis of susceptibility, or the innate capability of an animal to become rabid and infectious to other hosts. In theory, a single virion can initiate the process, but in actuality, multiple infectious units are needed for a productive encounter. A very susceptible species would be one in which few infectious particles would be required to induce a productive infection.

Trends in species susceptibility are greatly influenced by host species attributes and, perhaps to a lesser extent, by individual host factors, such as immunologic status and age. Generalities about species susceptibility may be inferred from selected sets of experimental data and within the limitations of epidemiologic observations. However, specific species attributes have not been characterized exhaustively due in part to confounding variables such as virus variant, ecologic characteristics of the hosts that affect exposure risk and outcome, and surveillance bias, which limits the source and number of specimens examined. From a practical standpoint, so-called high-risk species include certain canids (i.e., dogs, foxes, and coyotes), viverrids (i.e., the mongoose and its allies), procyonids (i.e., the common raccoon and its relatives), skunks, and bats. Moderate-risk species consist of felids, mustelids (i.e., badgers, ferrets, and minks), ungulates, and primates. Low-risk species comprise monotremes, marsupials, insectivores, rodents, and lagomorphs, among others. The only North American marsupial, the opossum (*Didelphis virginianus*), appears relatively resistant to experimental infection (Beamer *et al.*, 1960), also reflected by consistently low numbers of naturally occurring cases. One of the greatest sources of infection for the opossum is the raccoon, most likely due to ecologic overlap of the two species in the suburban environment. The virtual absence of substantial reports despite the diversity of marsupials widely and abundantly distributed throughout Australia and South America argues in part for fundamental taxonomic differences in virus–host response. Nonetheless, any individual mammalian species is still considered susceptible to rabies, even marine representatives, as demonstrated by a case report in a ringed seal from Norway (Odegaard and Krogsrud, 1981). This animal was wounded and appeared confused. It deteriorated over the course of 5 days and later became aggressive. Rabies was confirmed by immunofluorescent testing (Dean *et al.*, 1996) of the brain, and the case was presumed to be due to an epizootic of rabies among arctic foxes in the area.

It is unclear how mammalian reservoirs and associated viral variants may have coevolved. The greatest genetic differences exist between virus variants of terrestrial species and those found in bats. The capacity to distinguish among variants has become more precise in the past 25 years due to the advent of monoclonal antibodies for antigenic characterization (Wiktor and Koprowski, 1978) and, later, the development of the reverse-transcriptase polymerase chain reaction

(RT–PCR) assay and genetic sequencing to elucidate differences (Smith, 1996; Tordo, 1996). This level of distinction has led to a clearer understanding of the likely sources of rabies in different animals. Reservoirs are those mammals capable of sustained intraspecies maintenance of a virus variant within a geographic area. Critical components of the reservoir in the virus–host interaction would necessarily include distribution, abundance, population density, and contact rate. In addition, virus maintenance also may take advantage of potentially competent coexisting vector species (Bell, 1980; Childs et al., 1994). Vector species may overlap closely with the primary reservoir in ecologic and behavioral characteristics, as well as in temporal and spatial patterns in a rabies-enzootic area. A recent example is the description of a canid viral variant maintained and perpetuated in domestic dogs at the Texas–Mexico border. In the 1980s, the variant demonstrated emergent properties through its dramatic spread through a newly recognized reservoir — the coyote (Clark et al., 1994; Krebs et al., 2000). Equally interesting was the apparent retention of its capacity for dog-to-dog transmission, evident in border communities where rabies vaccination of domestic dogs was low.

In addition to the host species, equally important facets in basic measurement of susceptibility include specific attributes of the rabies virus variant, its origin and passage history, the concentration of virus, the type of inoculum, and the route of exposure. Transmission does not occur through intact skin. Such trivial contact is not considered an exposure to rabies. Are other activities, such as predation, scavenging, or repeated exposure to fomites, important to viral maintenance? As to specific niche, lyssaviruses replicate predominantly in mammalian neural tissue and do not persist outside animals. The synergy of ultraviolet radiation, pH extremes, organic solvents, desiccation, excessive heat, and putrefaction lead to a relatively rapid diminution of viral load, usually on the order of days (Lewis and Thacker, 1974). Thus it is unlikely that the abiotic environment is important in transmission.

A bite seems the most reliable route of exposure leading to infection (CDC, 1999). Oral exposure may result in infection, albeit with relatively low efficiency. Consumption of infected carcasses by carnivores may be the most relevant example of this scenario. For example, transmission could be enhanced through penetration of the oral or esophageal mucosa by bone fragments contaminated with highly infectious material, such as brain and salivary gland tissue. This mechanism has been hypothesized to contribute to the maintenance of arctic fox rabies, where contact between potential hosts is minimal but where transmission may be facilitated due to the preservation of virus in carcasses under polar conditions (Crandell, 1991). Infectious virus may be recovered months later in a frozen fox carcass during winter but could be inactivated within hours during the summer within the decomposing tissues of a road-killed raccoon in the Florida sun. Similarly, contamination of other mucous membranes, such as the eyes and nose, is considered a potential exposure to rabies. However, this is largely based on human infection following corneal transplantation (Anderson *et al.*, 1984; CDC, 1999) and a few case histories in which mucous membranes may have been contaminated, but the possibility of a bite could not be excluded completely. In context, during limited experimental studies in Syrian hamsters (generally believed to be highly susceptible to rabies), ocular instillation by drop of a virulent canine isolate of virus did not result in rabies, despite months of observation (C. Hanlon, unpublished data). Perhaps multiple direct applications to the surfaces of the cornea, to mimic minor abrasions from a rasping tongue, would have resulted in a different outcome. Depending on dose, oral exposure to rabies virus may not elicit a fatal infection. A proportion of animals may develop clinical rabies, whereas others may become immune. Intranasal exposure may result in infection more readily than by the oral route (Charlton and Casey, 1979) but is less efficient than intramuscular inoculation. Aerosol transmission of rabies can occur under some field conditions, but these involve unusual circumstances (CDC, 1999). Aerosol infection has been suggested as a result of laboratory accidents (CDC, 1972, 1977), in an unusual cave setting involving millions of Mexican free-tailed bats (Constantine, 1962), and in experimental studies with a unique bat rabies virus variant (Winkler *et al.*, 1972). Direct contamination of an open wound with infectious material (i.e., saliva and CNS tissue) is considered an exposure to rabies and may cause the disease.

The virus variant profoundly affects host susceptibility to infection and seems uniquely adapted to each reservoir species. Virus variants may possess characteristics that can directly influence tropism, host behavior, or clinical outcome (Baer *et al.*, 1977; Flamand *et al.*, 1993; Wilbur and Aubert, 1996). Thus susceptibility of a species to a virus, for which the species is not a natural reservoir, will vary. Moreover, viral pathogenesis within a "spillover" or "victim" species may differ substantially from that found in the reservoir species. For example, a "canine" virus variant in a raccoon may produce a hyperacute encephalitis, sometimes resulting in rather sudden death prior to substantial viral shedding in the saliva (Wandeler *et al.*, 1994; Hamir *et al.*, 1996). In contrast, a "raccoon" variant in a dog may behave differently, with selection eventually enhancing mechanisms that could favor survival and transmission in a new environment.

IV. CLINICAL COURSE

There are no known definitive or species-specific clinical signs of rabies beyond acute behavioral alterations (Blancou *et al.*, 1991; Charlton *et al.*, 1991; Winkler and Jenkins, 1991; Brass, 1994). To paraphrase, in rabies, "... the abnormal becomes typical ...." Severity and variation of signs may be related to the specific site(s) of the primary CNS lesion(s) or to viral strain, dose, and route of infection (Smart and Charlton, 1992; Hamir *et al.*, 1996). The prodromal period usually follows a bite by several weeks. However, periods of less than 10 days to several months are well documented (Charlton, 1994). Severe and multiple bites to the head and neck and bites to highly innervated areas may result in shorter incubation periods. At the end of the incubation period, the disease progresses through a short prodromal stage to encephalopathy and death, usually within days.

Initial signs of rabies are nonspecific and may include anorexia, lethargy, fever, dysphagia, vomiting, stranguria, straining to defecate, and diarrhea. A gradual and subtle alteration in behavior, such as increased aggressiveness in a normally even-tempered animal or vice versa, and a qualitative change in phonation, as well as increased vocalization, may be noted fairly early in the clinical course. In addition to behavioral abnormalities, cranial nerve manifestations may include facial asymmetry, trismus, choking, a lolling tongue, drooling, drooping of the lower jaw, prolapse of the third eyelid, and anisocoria.

An acute neurologic period usually follows the brief prodromal period by 1 to 2 days. A generalized excitative increase in neurologic activity is observed, associated with hyperesthesia to auditory, visual, or tactile stimuli and sudden and seemingly unprovoked agitation and extreme aggressive behavior (furious rabies) toward animate or inanimate objects. Wild animals may lose their apparent wariness of humans. Domestic species and other animals alter their activity cycles, seek solitude, or become more gregarious. Head tilt, head pressing or butting, and "star gazing" may be observed.

Similar to the paraesthesia reported by infected humans, animals may be observed grooming or scratching at the known or presumed site of virus exposure most likely in response to altered sensation, probably due to viral excitation of sensory ganglia. This abnormal behavior may progress to self-mutilation and even self-consumption of body parts, particularly appendages. In males, aberrant grooming of the penis may lead to gross trauma. During the clinical period, animals may attack inanimate objects (cages, sticks, moving vehicles) or other animals with no apparent response to pain, such as cessation of the activity, following tooth or bone fracture or extensive tissue trauma, particularly to the tongue and facial structures (Fig. 1).

The clinical presentation of rabies often is generalized as being either *furious* or *dumb*. Furious rabies is a clinical presentation that consists predominantly of profound agitation and aggression. With dumb rabies, aggression may be completely lacking, but paralysis may be paramount. Clinical manifestations may include progressively anorexia, depression, cranial nerve signs, and increased salivation, sometimes profuse with a stringy or ropey characteristic. Paresis may occur and progress to paralysis and death. These two extreme clinical presentations likely may reflect differences in viral infection within specific areas of the CNS. An individual animal alternatively may manifest both these generalized forms, with the furious signs first and then the dumb signs, or vice versa, as the clinical course progresses. Profound characteristic neurologic manifestations of

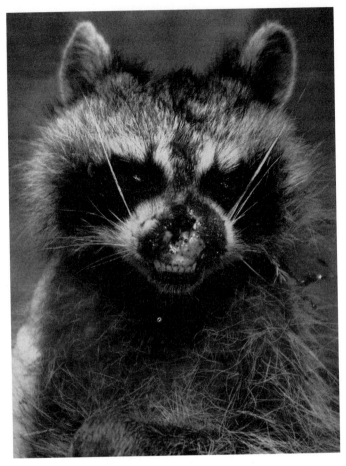

Fig. 1.   A confirmed rabid raccoon with self-mutilation from New York State. (Photograph courtesy of Ward Stone, New York State Department of Environmental Conservation, Wildlife Pathology Unit.)

human rabies (Hemachuda, 1994), namely, true hydrophobia and aerophobia, have not been documented in other animals.

The disease has a rapidly declining clinical course, worsening progressively within each time period. Most clinical periods are less than 1 week to 10 days, although exceptions have been reported, particularly in reservoir species, such as illness as long as 17 days in a fox and shedding of virus 30 days prior to death (Blancou *et al.*, 1991) or 18 days prior to death in a skunk (Parker and Wilsnack, 1966). While recovery from rabies may occur, it is quite rare (Baer and Olson, 1972). Recovery may be complete, or it may involve neurologic sequelae.

As the CNS infection progresses, signs may include extreme tremors, paresis, ataxia, and paralysis. There may be additional CNS excitation with pronounced hyperactivity, disorientation, confusion, photophobia, pica, incoordination, and convulsive seizures. Autonomic systemic excitation also may result in labile hypertension, hyperventilation, muscle tremors, priapism, altered libido, hypothermia, or hyperthermia. Ascending, flaccid, symmetric, or asymmetric paralysis eventually leads to respiratory and cardiac failure. Ultimately, rabies most often culminates in coma and generalized multiorgan failure with death in 1–10 days (or rarely more) after primary signs, or it may result in acute death with no premonitory suspicion.

Curiously, reported signs in rabies from different species range the gamut from subtle neurologic illness to maniacal frenzy, the stuff of literature and legend. In contrast to these dramatic scenarios, common mammalian behaviors also may contribute to transmission of virus. For example, many mammalian males mount and stabilize the female during copulation by holding at the nape of the neck with their teeth, combining the potential excretion of virus in the saliva prior to overt clinical signs with an obvious need for mechanical manipulation during procreation, even among less social species. Teeth and the oral cavity (with its associated secretions) are used daily for multiple and critical mammalian behaviors. Beyond obvious foraging activities such as predation and aggressive encounters during resource defense, these can include stimulation of the urogenital reflex of the neonate by the mother, carrying of infants, food begging, food sharing, play, and grooming. Viral excretion during the prodromal phase, when the individual may appear normal but is gradually lapsing into nonspecific episodes of illness, may be a more important opportunity for transmission than later mania. Exhibition of more extreme forms of behavior does occur but may not be needed to the extent believed, particularly if the encounters are initiated by the unaffected animal rather than by the obviously diseased conspecific. No doubt, rabies changes host behavior and virtually ensures its own transmission in the process, but exploitation of routine social activities could be the norm.

V. DIFFERENTIAL DIAGNOSIS

Rabies should be considered strongly in the differential diagnosis of any mammal presenting with signs compatible with an acute encephalitis, particularly in high-risk taxa such as the *Carnivora* and *Chiroptera*. Depending on the species in question, signs of rabies may appear clinically similar to a number of viral, bacterial, mycotic, protozoal, helminth, or other acquired conditions (Table I). Moreover, rabies may be mimicked by a multitude of noninfectious diseases.

TABLE I

Major Differential Diagnoses for an Acute Encephalitis Compatible with Rabies

Viral
  Canine distemper
  Pseudorabies (Aujeszky's disease)
  Feline infectious peritonitis
  Herpes myelitis
  Eastern equine encephalitis/western
    EE/Venezuelan EE
  Equine herpesvirus 1
    encephalomyelopathy
  Porcine enteroviral encephalomyelitis
  Malignant catarrhal fever
  Infectious canine hepatitis
  Borna disease

Bacterial
  Botulism
  Tetanus
  Listeriosis
  Sporadic bovine encephalomyelitis
  Parahypophyseal abscess
  Rocky Mountain spotted fever

Fungal
  Cryptococcosis
  Blastomycosis

Protozoal
  Toxoplasmosis
  Equine protozoal myelitis
  Neosporosis

Parasitic
  Baylisascariasis
  Parelaphostrongylosis
  Strongylosis

Neoplastic
  Lymphosarcoma
  Osteosarcoma
  Fibrosarcoma
  Meningioma
  Metastatic neoplasia

Traumatic
  Intervertebral disk disease
  Hit by car
  Gunshot
  Esophageal foreign body

Toxic
  Heavy metals
  Chlorinated hydrocarbons
  Organophosphates

Metabolic
  Ketosis (acetonemia, ketonemia)
  Puerperal hypocalcaemia (milk fever)
  Hypomagnesaemia

Developmental/inherited
  Hydrocephalus
  Cerebellar hypoplasia

Other/idiopathic
  Transmissible spongiform encephalopathies
  Tick paralysis
  Acute idiopathic polyradiculoneuritis
    (coonhound paralysis)
  Idiopathic trigeminal neuropathy
  Polioencephalomalacia
  Thromboembolic encephalopathy

VI. A QUESTION OF IMMUNITY?

Immunity to rabies can involve both anatomic defenses, such as intact, heavily furred, or cornified skin that aids in protection against bites (or licks), and nonspecific inflammatory responses to foreign substances, as well as specifically induced responses to viral antigens (Lodmell, 1983; Xiang *et al.*, 1995). Intact virus can induce high lymphokine secretion, but induction of protective antiviral immunity is based primarily on response to the glycoprotein (G protein). It is the only *Lyssavirus* antigen known to induce virus-neutralizing antibody (VNA) and plays a critical role in eliciting immunity (Foley *et al.*, 2000). Nevertheless, there is not always a clear relationship between level of VNA and resistance to rabies, suggesting that other antigens and immune effector mechanisms likely are involved in protection against lethal infection. Besides the G protein, internal *Lyssavirus* antigens may possess the capacity to enhance immune responsiveness, characterized either as superantigens (Lafon, 1994) or as powerful adjuvants.

Viral exposure may or may not lead to a productive viral infection, which may or may not result in detectable immune responses (Niezgoda *et al.*, 1997). Demonstration of rabies antibody in serum only indicates exposure to viral antigen. The outcome following exposure depends in part on a complex interplay of viral and host factors (Nathanson and Gonzalez-Scarano, 1991). During the centripetal transport of limited numbers of virions to the brain, especially during long incubation periods, insufficient antigenic mass may be present for detection, which may fail to induce an appropriate response. In contrast, highly neural invasive strains might be quite immunogenic, but the host response could be slow or inadequate to prevent or clear CNS replication in time, given the rather immunologically privileged location of replication. If detected at all, rabies-specific antibodies can be found at the onset of illness but may appear more commonly concomitant with terminal stages of disease. Rabies VNA may interfere with salivary excretion of infectious virus (Charlton *et al.*, 1987). Antibody detection in the cerebrospinal fluid (CSF) of rabies suspects is considered a reliable indication of present or past CNS infection and possible recovery (Fekadu, 1991a, 1991b). The finding of lymphocytic pleocytosis in the CSF of some survivors to infection, without antibody, has not been explained adequately (Hanlon *et al.*, 1989).

Rates of specific acquired immunity to rabies in naturally exposed animals vary. European red foxes appear to seldom have significant VNA, usually less than a fraction of surveyed populations (Blancou *et al.*, 1991). A seroprevalence of 2–10% has been reported in some insectivorous bats (Trimarchi and Debbie, 1977) but could be considerably higher in some highly colonial species. Among raccoons, the presence of VNA varied from 1–3% in epizootic areas of the mid-Atlantic states (Winkler and Jenkins, 1991) to more than 20% of those sampled in Florida (Bigler *et al.*, 1983). In mongoose from Grenada, where the presence of rabies VNA ranged from 9% to upwards of 55%, seroprevalence was inversely proportional to the number of reported rabies cases, and animals with preexisting VNA responded with higher titers on rabies vaccination (Everard and Everard, 1988). These observations suggest that natural immunity to rabies varies based on circumstances (Rosatte and Gunson, 1984; Black and Wiktor, 1986; Orr *et al.*, 1988; Follman *et al.*, 1994), depending in part on the species and the virus variant (Niezgoda *et al.*, 1998).

On average, productive infection in a single animal is adequate to maintain a chain of transmission. With regard to dose, inoculation of a high viral load may result in a relatively short incubation period with less opportunity for shedding of virus in the saliva. Conversely, infection with lower amounts of virus may result in longer incubation and clinical periods and greater viral shedding over time. A balance may exist between the minimum amount of virus produced per unit infection and the basic susceptibility of an individual host, while evading immune defenses.

VII. RESERVOIRS AND OTHER LYSSAVIRUSES

Rabies virus is the representative type species and most significant member of the *Lyssavirus* genus as concerns relative distribution, abundance, and public health and veterinary impact. Not surprisingly, most scientific focus has concentrated on this classic agent, and the principal applied attributes of rabies virus are felt to be largely interchangeable with the rabies-related lyssaviruses with regard to features such as incubation period and clinical signs.

Although not currently recognized as major zoonotic threats, the nonrabies lyssaviruses (Lagos bat, Mokola, Duvenhage, European bat, and Australian bat viruses) may pose future public health problems because of the opportunity for international translocation and local establishment. This latter concern could be compounded because traditional rabies virus vaccines do not always provide adequate protection (Dietzschold *et al.*, 1988). Two rhabdoviruses, Obodhiang and Kotonkan, isolated from invertebrates in Africa by intracerebral inoculation of mice, were seemingly aligned with the rabies-like viruses on the basis of initial serology at one time but do not produce rabies in the traditional sense and await further genetic characterization (Shope, 1975).

When the prototypic rabies-related candidate, Lagos bat virus, was isolated during 1956 from one of seven pooled brain samples of 42 straw-colored fruit bats, *Eidolon helvum*, shot while roosting in a tree on Lagos island, Nigeria, no suggestion of abnormal behavior was noted in this presumed host (Boulger and Porterfield, 1958) nor in a mist-netted dwarf epauletted bat, *Micropteropus pusillus*, during 1974 from the Central African Republic (Sureau *et al.*, 1977). However, widespread morbidity and mortality were associated with later isolations of Lagos bat virus among Wahlberg's epauletted fruit bat, *Epomophorus wahlbergi*, in Natal, with the reproduction of a typical rabies-like syndrome and Negri bodies following experimental infection of animals (Meredith and Standing, 1981; Crick *et al.*, 1982; King *et al.*, 1994). Besides further isolations in bats, a diagnosis was made from a domestic cat in Natal (King and Crick, 1988), whereas another cat showing atypical clinical signs but suspected of being rabid also was found infected with Lagos bat virus in Zimbabwe (Foggin, 1988). In Ethiopia, a dog having rabies-like signs was reported infected with Lagos bat virus (Mebatsion *et al.*, 1992a). Recently, a fruit bat, *Rousettus aegyptiucus*, imported from North Africa for the pet trade was diagnosed with Lagos bat virus after exposing its French owner (Jaussaud *et al.*, 2000). Lagos bat virus has not, as yet, been incriminated in any fatal human cases.

Somewhat similar to the accidental discovery of Lagos bat virus, a 1968 arbovirus survey in Nigeria resulted in isolation from viscera of four shrews, *Crocidura* sp. (one found dead), another new agent, Mokola, only later appreciated as a rabies-related virus (Shope *et al.*, 1970; Kemp *et al.*, 1972). Again, no description was offered of any associated illness in these animals. Mokola virus was implicated in the death of a child in Nigeria (Familusi *et al.*, 1972). It also was claimed to have been isolated during 1969 from the CSF of another patient suffering from aseptic meningitis (with no known source of exposure) who later recovered (Familusi and Moore, 1972). Elsewhere, Mokola virus was identified from the organs of a *Crocidura* shrew during 1974 in Cameroon (le Gonidec *et al.*, 1978), from a harsh-furred mouse, *Lophuromys sikapusi*, in the Central African Republic (Saluzzo *et al.*, 1984), from cats and a dog in Zimbabwe (Foggin, 1982, 1983, 1988), and retrospectively, from a cat in 1970 that had attacked residents of a seaside town near Durban (King *et al.*, 1994). Thereafter, during 1995, cats from the eastern cape were found infected with Mokola virus (Meredith *et al.*, 1996). Within a few months of this case, two further Mokola virus infections of cats were diagnosed in the same district. Similarly, in Ethiopia, the occurrence of Mokola virus infection in a single cat was recorded (Mebatsion *et al.*, 1992b). Clearly, although a determination of the ultimate reservoir for Mokola virus is only speculative, small mammals such as insectivores or rodents, among others (possibly bats), appear to be involved in its maintenance, and the domestic cat serves as an important predatory sentinel for future introspection.

During 1970, a case of classic rabies was reported in a man from north of Pretoria, who while asleep had been bitten on the lip by a bat, possibly the long-fingered bat, *Miniopterus schreibersii* (Meredith *et al.*, 1971). Brain specimens from the patient were negative when examined by the fluorescent antibody test, but Negri bodies were observed in Purkinje cells, and eventual characterization allowed discovery of a new rabies-related agent, Duvenhage virus (Tignor *et al.*, 1977). Confirmation of the relationship between Duvenhage virus and certain *Chiroptera* occurred when isolation was made from the brain of a sick bat, suggestive of *Miniopterus* (Schneider *et al.*, 1985), as well as from a common slit-faced bat, *Nycteris thebaica*, during a survey in Zimbabwe (Foggin, 1988). As with Lagos bat and Mokola viruses, the natural history of Duvenhage virus is not well understood.

Existence of rabies among European bats was suspected as early as the 1950s, but distinct confirmation and characterization of this phenomenon required several more decades (Schneider and Cox, 1994). Two unique lyssaviruses have been described, the European bat virus variants, subtypes I and II (Muller, 1988; Bourhy *et al.*, 1992; Perez-Jorda *et al.*, 1995). Reservoirs seem to be insectivorous bats (both *Eptesicus* and *Myotis* spp.), responsible for limited human fatalities. With the exception of a rabid sheep, additional domestic or wildlife cases have not been confirmed after active disease surveillance. Hundreds of rabid bats have been identified throughout Europe over the past 20 years, including a report from Great Britain (Whitby *et al.*, 2000).

Without definitive evidence of prior rabies establishment in Australia, during the spring of 1996, a novel virus infection was uncovered in a single black flying fox, *Pteropus alecto* (Fraser *et al.*, 1996). As is often the case for other rabies-like agents, it was only submitted to a veterinary laboratory during routine examination for another purpose: surveillance for a recently discovered paramyxovirus (Murray *et al.*, 1995). This new Australian bat virus possessed typical rhabdovirus morphology, was diagnosed using standard antirabies reagents, and caused a nonsuppurative meningoencephalitis consistent with lesions produced by other lyssaviruses. Thereafter, Australian bat virus was isolated from grayheaded *P. poliocephalus* and little red *P. scapulatus* flying foxes and from a yellow-bellied sheath-tail bat, *Saccolaimus flaviventris* (Tidemann *et al.*, 1997). Seemingly, these bat lyssaviruses are distributed throughout New South Wales, Queensland, Victoria, and the Northern Territory (Speare *et al.*, 1997) (if not elsewhere), have been documented at least since 1995 (if not earlier), and have caused at least two human deaths to date, both related to bat exposure (Allworth *et al.*, 1996; Hanna *et al.*, 2000). The Australian bat lyssaviruses are quite similar to classic rabies viruses by antigenic and genetic characterization, confirmed by cross-protection studies with commercial human and animal rabies vaccines (Rupprecht *et al.*, 1996), while representing a distinct subtype (Gleeson, 1997). In all practical respects, the clinical syndrome is not different from that described previously for rabid bats (Field *et al.*, 1999). Although undetected in prior surveys of bats in Malaysia (Tan *et al.*, 1969) or the Philippines (Beran *et al.*, 1972), rabies was reported during 1978 from a gray-headed flying fox found dead in India (Pal *et al.*, 1980). When interpreted in light of the Australian data, it strongly suggests that lyssaviruses may be more prevalent among Asian–Pacific bat populations than previously realized.

Within each lyssavirus serotype and genotype there are numerous viral variants that exist as quasi-species, heterogeneous mutant viral populations subject to Darwinian evolution and punctuated equilibrium (Eigen and Biebricher, 1988;

Nichol *et al.*, 1993) that may further complicate any in-depth studies of overt susceptibility, incubation periods, associated clinical signs, and related outcome in a relevant host.

VIII. RABIES IN DOMESTIC ANIMALS

A. Dog

On a global basis, the domestic dog remains the most important reservoir of rabies in overall case numbers and with regard to transmission to humans. In regions where strict control of free-ranging dogs and mandatory parenteral rabies vaccination are enforced, canine rabies virus variants have been eliminated successfully. Examples of such areas include Great Britain, Japan, Canada, and the United States. Recently, numerous countries in Latin America have made tremendous progress in the application of stray dog control and mass vaccination with consequent control of canine rabies and markedly reduced human rabies over large geographic areas. Although canine rabies has been eliminated in most European countries, canine rabies remains largely uncontrolled throughout most of Asia and Africa.

An additional aspect of canine rabies is its impact on other animals. True wild dogs, *Lycaon pictus*, are among the most endangered carnivores in Africa (Gascoyne *et al.*, 1993). In 1990, an adult *Lycaon* was found dead due to rabies in the Serengeti Region of Tanzania. Rabies also was suspected but not confirmed in one adult and six pups of the same pack. In response, two *Lycaon* packs in the Serengeti National Park were given inactivated rabies vaccine either by dart or by parenteral inoculation following sedation, demonstrating the need for veterinary intervention in wildlife conservation directly related to dog rabies.

The incubation period of rabies in dogs may be as short as 10 days or as long as several months. A commonly imposed quarantine period for an exposed dog (and often cat, ferret, horse, cow, and other animals) is 6 months. This period is based on epizootiologic and experimental evidence that if an exposed dog will develop rabies from an exposure, there is a strong likelihood that it will occur within 6 months of the exposure. At the beginning of the clinical course, nonspecific signs may include anorexia, fever, dysphagia, and a change in behavior, such as being more reclusive than normal or showing signs of restlessness. The animal may be startled more easily by noise, light, or touch. As each day passes, other clinical abnormalities may appear, and the initial signs may become more pronounced. Substantial injury may occur due to aggression toward objects or other animals. Self-mutilation may occur. Salivation may appear profuse due to the inability to swallow (Fig. 2). Dehydration and anorexia secondary to dysphagia may result in acute weight loss. Tremors, ataxia, paresis, paralysis, and generalized seizures may

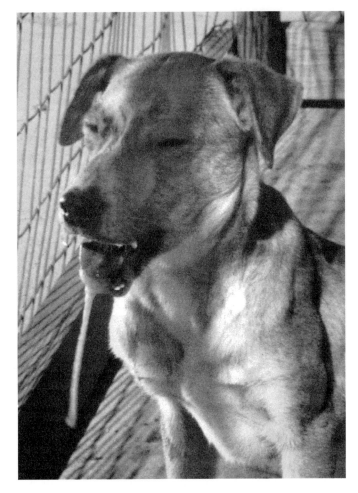

Fig. 2.   A rabies-infected domestic dog with thick, ropey saliva.

develop. The actual physiologic mechanism resulting in death can vary but may result from profound autonomic dysfunction producing alternations in respiration, body temperature, blood pressure, and cardiac rhythm.

When a dog potentially has exposed a person to rabies through a bite or other exposure route, the dog commonly is subjected to a 10-day confinement and observation period. The 10-day time period is derived from experimental observations of clinical shedding of rabies virus (Vaughn *et al.*, 1965), as well as supportive field data. If a dog is capable of shedding virus in its saliva (which necessarily has developed after CNS infection) at the time it bit someone, the dog reliably may be expected to develop clinical signs of rabies within the 10-day confinement and observation period. If the dog remains alive and well, there are no substantive epizootiologic data to contradict the presumption that there was no virus in the dog's saliva at the time of the bite.

There are occasional reports in the literature of apparent exceptions to the widely practiced public health rabies management protocol in North America of a 10-day confinement and observation period for a biting dog. In one report, four beagles were inoculated with mouse brain–passaged saliva from an apparently healthy dog from Ethiopia that had been reported to excrete virus intermittently (Fekadu, 1972; Fekadu et al., 1981, 1983). Two inoculated dogs remained clinically normal. Two dogs developed signs of rabies but apparently recovered. One later died of a bacterial pneumonia. Salivary swabs from the surviving dog were collected routinely and inoculated into mice. Virus was reported to have been present in samples taken on days 42, 169, and 305 after inoculation. The amount of virus was extremely low, less than 10 infectious particles. In a related study, 39 dogs were injected intramuscularly with either an Ethiopian strain or a Mexican strain of rabies virus. Virus was recovered from the submaxillary salivary glands of 9 of 17 dogs that died following inoculation with the Ethiopian virus variant. Four of these dogs were reported to have virus in the saliva up to 13 days before overt signs of rabies were observed. Virus was recovered from the submaxillary salivary glands of 16 of 22 dogs that died following inoculation with the Mexican virus variant. Eight of these dogs also excreted virus in the saliva up to 7 days before definitive signs of rabies were observed (Fekadu et al., 1982, 1983). Observations in Asia suggest that, on rare occasions, a dog under a 10-day observation period can still be alive and apparently healthy, whereas the bitten human may develop signs and symptoms of rabies during that period (Somayajulu and Reddy, 1989) The veracity of these reports is unknown. It is possible that a different dog may have bitten a patient several weeks to several months prior to the temporally associated situation. However, if these observations have merit, two potential interpretations may be possible. The dogs may be remaining healthy and shedding rabies virus for longer than the expected 10-day period prior to clinical development of rabies. Alternatively, these dogs may reflect the possibility of recovery from rabies with the potential for intermittent shedding. In the past 20 years, virus detection and identification techniques have advanced greatly in sophistication and sensitivity, yet there has been a conspicuous lack of additional reports of similar findings. No such field observations have come from North or South America. It is unknown if these occasional observations simply reflect rare events or if they have more profound implications as to the difficulty of canine rabies control in Asia, Africa, and possibly elsewhere.

Recently, a purported antemortem latex agglutination (LA) test for rabies virus antigen has been developed for evaluation of dog saliva (Kasempimolporn et al., 2000). Rabies virus antigen is detected by agglutination on a glass slide using latex particles coated with gamma-globulin. In the study of paired saliva and brain specimens from 238 dogs, the LA test using saliva was 99% specific and 95% sensitive compared with the direct fluorescent antibody test on brain impressions. It is still unfortunate that for most species, besides dogs, cats, and ferrets (CDC, 1999), an animal must be euthanized to rule out rabies definitively. The obvious disadvantage of a potential antemortem test is the biologic potential for intermittent shedding of rabies virus in the saliva of an infected animal, even during a typically short clinical course (Vaughn *et al.*, 1965). Moreover, the test itself would require rigorous controlled evaluation with acceptable levels at no less than a virtually 100% sensitivity if it were ever to be considered as a primary diagnostic tool to facilitate human exposure determinations. A false-negative test would have severe implications if human rabies postexposure prophylaxis decisions were to be based on such a test. Certainly it would seem prudent to conduct further research on the pathogenesis of prominent canine rabies virus variants employing traditional and novel viral detection methods. The findings of such studies either would support the current practices of dog (as well as cat and ferret) management in the face of human exposure or would provide enhanced experimental data on which to frame optimal human rabies prevention.

B. Cat

In developed countries where canine rabies has been controlled but where wildlife rabies predominates, the cat is one of the most important domestic animals. In the United States, the leading domestic animal diagnosed with rabies is the cat, with a total of 2173 positive animals and an average of 272 annual cases (range 189–300) from 1991–1998 (Krebs *et al.*, 1999). The impact of rabies in cats is reflected in the relatively large numbers of humans exposed, typically involving caregivers of the cat and veterinary hospital staff. One of the most dramatic cases occurred when a kitten was offered for sale in a pet store where customers could freely pet the animals, after which at least 665 persons received postexposure prophylaxis (Noah *et al.*, 1996). Although most states and localities require registration of dogs coupled with proof of rabies vaccination, few have extended similar regulations to cats. Thus cats are less commonly vaccinated against rabies. Also, when cats are allowed outdoors by owners, cats are more commonly unrestricted and unsupervised in comparison with dogs and roam frequently at night. In many communities, free-ranging cats are more likely to be tolerated than free-ranging dogs. Recent controversy has erupted regarding the maintenance of feral cat colonies by humans through provision of shelter, food, and limited veterinary care that may include surgical neutering to limit colony size.

In the United States, cats along the East Coast from Florida to Maine are infected most commonly with the raccoon rabies virus variant. In the Midwest and

California, cats are likely to be infected with the predominant skunk rabies virus variant. In suburban and urban settings, raccoons and skunks often are tolerant of human presence and, along with dogs and cats, forage on food offered intentionally for domestic animals and sometimes offered for wild animals, as well as from unintended garbage sources. This may enhance opportunities for conflict that may contribute directly to rabid raccoons and skunks infecting cats and dogs.

Another source of rabies in cats is from bats. Since insectivorous bats and their associated rabies virus variants are distributed widely throughout North America, this provides a constant potential source of infection for cats. Encounters between rabid bats and cats are not surprising given the nocturnal activity patterns of bats and cats, as well as a cat's propensity to investigate and capture small animals, such as bats. Cats are susceptible to rabies virus of bat origin and can shed the virus in their saliva (Trimarchi *et al.*, 1986). In light of these findings, it is not surprising that rabid cats have outnumbered dogs by a margin of two to one in the United States for the past 8-year period. Moreover, among 209 rabies-positive cat samples provided to the Centers for Disease Control and Prevention (CDC) from various state health departments within the United States, 11% (4 of 47) were bat-associated variants (J. S. Smith, personal communication), a statistically significant higher rate than that of bat-associated variants found in dogs (3 of 157, 2%; $p < 0.0001$).

Based on a seminal study published nearly 30 years ago (Vaughn *et al.*, 1963), a 10-day confinement and observation period is considered an option to euthanasia and testing of a cat to rule out rabies exposure when a cat has bitten a human (CDC, 1999). Two subsequent studies raised interesting questions about potential chronic and recrudescent rabies in the cat (Perl *et al.*, 1977; Murphy *et al.*, 1980). Since these original studies were conducted, virus detection and identification techniques have advanced greatly in sophistication and sensitivity. Similar to the need for rabies pathogenesis studies in dogs, it would seem prudent to conduct further research on the pathogenesis of important rabies variants employing traditional and novel viral detection methods. Again, the findings of such studies either would support the current practices of cat management in the face of human exposure or would provide enhanced experimental data on which to frame optimal human rabies prevention.

C. Livestock

Most reports of rabies in livestock involve cattle and, occasionally, horses, but other domestic species have been reported (Baer and Olson, 1972; Bergeron *et al.*, 1981). The greatest economic and public health impact of rabies in cattle occurs in Latin America (Martinez-Burnes *et al.*, 1997; Delpietro and Russo, 1996; Lord, 1992). The major source of infection is from vampire bats, predominantly the common vampire bat (*Desmodus rotundus*). Cattle also may be infected from dogs, foxes, or jackals in areas where such rabies is endemic. In North America, predominant sources of infection are from wild carnivore species such as from skunks in the Midwest and raccoons in the East. In addition, cattle infrequently may become infected with insectivorous bat rabies virus variants. Among 47 rabies-positive bovine samples provided to the CDC from various state health departments within the United States, 8% (4 of 47) were bat-associated variants (J. S. Smith, personal communication).

Hudson (1996a) provided a description of clinical signs of rabies in cattle and sheep. In the diseased cattle ($n = 20$), the average incubation period was 15 days, and the average morbidity period was nearly 4 days. Major clinical signs included excessive salivation (100%), behavioral change (100%), muzzle tremors (80%), vocalization (bellowing, 70%), aggression, hyperesthesia and/or hyperexcitability (70%), and pharyngeal paresis/paralysis (60%). The furious form of rabies was seen in 70% of the cattle and in 80% of sheep ($n = 5$). In many cases, rabies may be considered only in retrospection (Stoltenow *et al.*, 1999). Often the animal exhibits signs of choking, and well-intentioned individuals may insert a hand in the mouth to search for a foreign body.

In a similar study among 21 experimentally infected horses, the average incubation period was 12 days, and average morbidity was nearly 6 days (Hudson *et al.*, 1996b). Naive animals had significantly shorter incubation and morbidity periods ($p < 0.05$) than test animals vaccinated with products under development. Tremor of the muzzle was observed most frequently (81%) and the most common initial sign. Other common signs were pharyngeal spasm or pharyngeal paresis (71%), ataxia or paresis (71%), and lethargy or somnolence (71%). Although some initial presentations began as the dumb form, ultimately, 43% of horses developed furious rabies.

An animal's clinical response to supportive therapy, as well as results of specific diagnostic tests, may confirm a diagnosis other than rabies. With rabies, the clinical course will worsen intractably and invariably is fatal. Despite reports of survivorship among other animals, such as humans, dogs, cats, ferrets, and raccoons, there have been no such reports in cattle and horses, probably due in part to limitations in intensive clinical management as well as increased physiologic complications due to ponderous size (e.g., rhabdomyolysis). In equids, ataxia may be pronounced after involvement of the brainstem and cerebellum due in no small part to the substantial balancing act these animals perform on a single toe.

D. Ferrets

Ferrets are popular pets in the United States. During 1990, an inactivated rabies vaccine was licensed for use in these domestic carnivores (Rupprecht *et al.*, 1990). However, the potential rabies virus shedding period of ferrets remained uncharacterized, even though a preliminary study using a fox virus found no evidence for excretion in the saliva (Blancou et al., 1982). This situation presented a dilemma for public health officials for the management of those occasions when a person was bitten by a pet ferret. There was no scientifically defined confinement period for which a biting ferret, regardless of vaccination status, could be observed for signs of rabies. Due to the lack of experimental data on ferret response to rabies virus infection, recommendations were to euthanize the ferret and test the brain for rabies virus, even in low-risk situations, such as if the ferret was vaccinated, appeared clinically normal, and the bite was provoked. Clearly, this was unlike the management of the biting dog and cat, in which an observation and confinement period of at least 10 days was recommended. Before recommendations could be made regarding an observation period for biting ferrets, basic parameters of rabies pathogenesis in ferrets needed to be defined (Anonymous, 1990).

To answer a number of basic questions about ferret response to rabies virus infection, studies were designed to determine ferret response using rabies virus variants obtained from important reservoir species in the United States, including primary isolates from naturally infected skunks, raccoons, and coyotes, among others. Susceptibility, incubation and morbidity period, clinical signs, serologic response, and viral shedding were investigated by routine procedures (Niezgoda et al., 1997).

The pathogenesis of rabies in domestic ferrets with regard to overt susceptibility, aggressive behavior, spread of virus to the salivary glands, and excretion was found to vary significantly depending on the rabies virus variant. For example, 6 of 12 (50%) ferrets given a raccoon rabies virus variant at a viral dose of $10^{5.8}$ $MICLD_{50}$ succumbed to infection (Niezgoda et al., 1998), whereas 10 of 10 (100%) ferrets that received a North Central skunk rabies virus variant at $10^{5.5}$ $MICLD_{50}$ succumbed (Niezgoda et al., 1997). In contrast, 12 of 20 (60%) ferrets that received a North Central skunk rabies virus variant at doses that ranged $10^{3.5}$ to $10^{2.5}$ $MICLD_{50}$ succumbed to infection, whereas 12 of 12 (100%) ferrets that received a canine rabies virus variant at doses that ranged $10^{3.3}$ to $10^{2.3}$ $MICLD_{50}$ died. At a higher dose, only 2 of 10 (20%) ferrets that received a raccoon rabies virus variant at $10^{4.0}$ $MICLD_{50}$ succumbed. Overall clinical signs were consistent with an acute viral infection of the CNS and included ataxia, paresis, paraparesis, paralysis, lethargy, tremors, bladder atony, fever, and weight loss. Morbidity periods also were similar at 4 to 5 days, regardless of virus variant, but aggressive behavior in ferrets varied significantly with different viruses. For example, none of 33 rabid ferrets that received a North Central skunk rabies virus variant showed signs of aggressive behavior. Only 2 of 19 (11%) rabid ferrets that received a raccoon rabies virus isolate were aggressive. In contrast, 10 of 10 (100%) rabid ferrets that received a canine rabies virus variant were aggressive. In addition, viral excretion and salivary gland infection results varied significantly depending on the rabies virus variant. No ferrets succumbing to a North Central skunk rabies virus variant had detectable virus in their saliva, and only 1 of 33 (3%) had detectable virus in their salivary glands. In contrast, in ferrets that received a raccoon rabies virus isolate, 12 of 19 (63%) rabid ferrets had detectable virus in their salivary glands, and 9 (47%) shed virus in their saliva. Shedding of virus in saliva was largely concomitant with clinical signs of rabies. The antibody response of ferrets also varied significantly depending on the virus variant. In ferrets inoculated with the North Central skunk rabies virus variant, 14 of 33 (42%) rabid ferrets had rabies VNA, and 5 of 17 (29%) survivors seroconverted. In ferrets given the raccoon rabies virus isolate, 2 of 19 (11%) rabid ferrets had rabies VNA, and only 1 of 32 (3%) survivors seroconverted. Interestingly, surviving ferrets tended to seroconvert at about the same time that infected members of the same experimental cohort died. Obviously, in the same species, multiple parameters of pathobiology will change, even at the same relative dose and route, as the virus variant in question varies. In addition, when the identical virus variant is used in different species, the clinical response may vary significantly (Fig. 3).

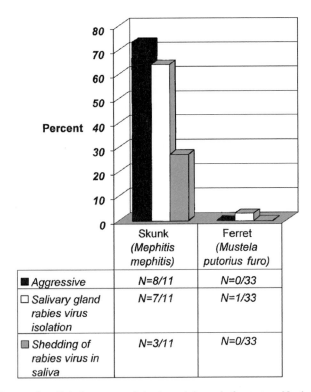

	Skunk (Mephitis mephitis)	Ferret (Mustela putorius furo)
■ Aggressive	N=8/11	N=0/33
□ Salivary gland rabies virus isolation	N=7/11	N=1/33
■ Shedding of rabies virus in saliva	N=3/11	N=0/33

Fig. 3. Comparative clinical response of skunks and domestic ferrets to a North Central skunk rabies virus variant.

Based on the data generated in these published studies and a subsequent unpublished study using a number of bat variants, the Compendium of Animal Rabies Control (CDC, 1998) supported the option of a 10-day confinement and observation period for a ferret that bites a person as an alternative to euthanasia and diagnostic testing to rule out rabies.

E. Wolf Hybrids

As with ferrets, the keeping of wolf–dog hybrids as pets has been challenging not only with regard to rabies prevention but also for many regulatory agencies responsible for public interests and protection (Jay *et al.*, 1994; Johnson, 1995; Overall, 2000). Whether or not these animals are suitable pets will continue to be debated fiercely for the foreseeable future. Nonetheless, at this time, there is no objective scientific method to determine the difference between the genetic makeup of a dog versus a wolf, nor of combinations in between. Due to this lack of capacity for distinction, it is illogical to assume that wolf hybrids would differ substantially in their immunologic capacity to respond to parenteral inoculation of rabies vaccines with demonstrated efficacy in dogs. Therefore, the U.S. Department of Agriculture, Animal and Plant Health Inspection Service, Veterinary Biologics, has deliberated on this generalization on the approval of the use of licensed vaccines for dogs in offspring of wolves and dogs (CDC, 2000a). However, there remains a complete void with regard to rabies pathogenesis and viral shedding studies in wolves. Wolves have been of historical importance in human exposures and present some of the highest case/fatalities per occurrence. Similar to the situation in 1990 with ferrets as to approved rabies vaccines, there is lack of scientific data with regard to virus shedding needed to establish safe confinement and observation periods for the times when animals, vaccinated or not, bite people.

IX. WILDLIFE RESERVOIRS

The potential role of wildlife in rabies maintenance often has been obscured by ubiquitous urban dog rabies and the higher prominence placed on domestic animals due to the human–pet bond and the economic value of livestock (Smith and Seidel, 1993). For example, despite the plethora of mammals found throughout Africa, recognition of the complexity of the disease among wildlife has been very slow to emerge. Given deficiencies in general surveillance of wildlife diseases, recognition may require notoriety related to perceived threats to endangered species and dramatic losses, such as among wild dogs, the Ethiopian wolf, and kudu (Rottcher and Sawchuk, 1978; Sawchuk and Rottcher, 1978; Gascoyne *et al.*, 1993; Sillero-Zubiri *et al.*, 1996; Creel *et al.*, 1997; Whitby *et al.*, 1997). In contrast, in southern Africa, many indigenous inhabitants long believed the bite of certain wild mammals would lead to a fatal disease, principally from viverrids (e.g., mongoose, civet, and genet). Recognized today, the yellow mongoose (*Cynictis penicillata*), is a common, widely distributed rabies host involved in maintaining endemic disease in the region (King *et al.*, 1994).

A. Fox

With its occurrence in Eurasia, North America, and northern Africa and introduction to Australia, the red fox (*Vulpes vulpes*) is one of the most widely distributed and abundant wild carnivores in the world. Perhaps more is known about rabies in this fox than in any other wild mammal, not only related to its significance as a major reservoir but also due to the influence of directed research during the past 30 years, coordinated by the World Health Organization (WHO) (Wandeler, 1980).

Descriptions of rabies among foxes (and other canids) were not uncommon in western and central Europe throughout the Middle Ages (Steck, 1968; Wilkinson, 1988; Steele and Fernandez, 1991). Possible confusion with other diseases, such as canine distemper, and the possibility of species misidentification are both dilemmas for all such historical accounts. Nevertheless, by the nineteenth century, rabies in the red fox seemed prevalent throughout Europe. Oddly, fox rabies largely disappeared during the first decades of the twentieth century but reemerged during the 1930s and spread throughout much of mainland Europe until the relatively recent advent of oral vaccination (Wandeler *et al.*, 1974; Bögel *et al.*, 1976; Toma and Andral, 1977; Steck and Wandeler, 1980; Steele and Fernandez, 1991; Blancou *et al.*, 1991). In North America during the middle to late 1700s, reports of rabid foxes and dogs were common throughout the mid-Atlantic British Colonies, probably exacerbated by a cultural predilection for fox hunting and hence European fox introductions and widespread translocation. One of the first descriptions of the disease in Canada did not occur until 1819, when the governor general was bitten by a pet fox and died (Steele and Fernandez, 1991; Jackson, 1994). The disease may have been present in the New World for centuries (Crandell, 1991). Description of a major rabies outbreak among Arctic (*Alopex lagopus*) and red foxes did not occur until well into the mid-twentieth century, spreading into southern Canada and the United States by the 1950s (Johnston and Beauregard, 1969; Tabel *et al.*, 1974).

Foxes have appeared quite susceptible to experimental infection. The amount of virus needed to productively infect half of red foxes in captivity varied from less than or equal to 1–5 $MICLD_{50}$ in the masseter, neck, or cervical muscles (and intradermally in the ear) to 16 $MICLD_{50}$ or more in the gluteal muscles (Sikes, 1962; Parker and Wilsnack, 1966; Black and Lawson, 1970; Winkler, 1975;

Wandeler, 1980; Blancou *et al.*, 1991). Foxes were more resistant to rabies when infected by isolates of canine, bat, or raccoon dog origin, among others (Blancou *et al.*, 1991). By other routes, it took approximately 5 more logs of rabies virus to infect foxes orally than parenterally (Wandeler, 1980). Minimum incubation periods ranged from as short as 4 days to longer than 15 months. Most appeared between 2 weeks and 3 months, inversely related to dose, as were the proportion of foxes that have virus in the salivary glands and the relative quantity of virus recovered (Wandeler, 1980; Blancou *et al.*, 1991). Thus, in theory, the greater the infective dose, the more foxes that can develop rabies but the fewer that may transmit to conspecifics because of the decreased probability of salivary shedding. Conversely, small inocula may result in fewer productive infections but a greater proportion of animals that could shed virus in the saliva. Considering that most foxes tend to excrete, on average, between 3 and 4 logs of virus, this appears to be more than adequate to ensure infectious chains of transmission given the extreme susceptibility of the species to selected viral variants. Short morbidity periods of 2–3 days are the usual rule regardless of dose but have ranged from less than 1 to over 14 days (Wandeler, 1980; Aubert, 1992). Signs are variable but commonly include anorexia, restlessness, hyperactivity, ataxia, and aggression (George *et al.*, 1980). Radio-tracked rabid foxes seem to experience abnormal behaviors, such as spatial-temporal alterations and frequent prostration, and may acquire wounds from normal foxes responding to territorial incursion (Artois and Aubert, 1985). Virus may be excreted in the saliva concomitant with or as long as a month before obvious clinical signs (Aubert *et al.*, 1992). Unlike the case for some other mammals, herd immunity is not believed to be important in red foxes. Insufficient explanations have appeared as to why fox rabies halted midstream in France (Blancou *et al.*, 1991) or seemingly disappeared in the United States during the 1970s (Winkler, 1975).

Approximately 20 extant "fox" species are presumed to exist throughout the world (Nowak, 1991). Although many possess solitary habits and occupy only geographic remnants of a former domain, others are widespread and seem to meet basic social criteria for a successful rabies reservoir. Nevertheless, with the exception of the Arctic and gray foxes (*Urocyon cinereoargenteus*) that have distinct associated rabies virus variants and are regionally important in the epidemiology of the polar and western American regions, related information on other foxes is scanty in this regard. Some biologic limitations appear obvious, most related to direct human depredation or encroachment and subsequent habitat loss. Such a tale holds for many representatives among the genus *Vulpes* in the Old World, such as the quite social Eurasian corsac fox of the steppe and desert zones; Blanford's fox; the Bengal fox in India, Pakistan, and Nepal; and the Tibetan sand fox. An apparent exception to these may be the common sand fox (*V. reuppelli*) reported from the desert zones of Morocco and Niger to Afghanistan and Somalia, in which recent reports to the WHO support the notion of a possible rabies reservoir on the Arabian peninsula. Alternatively, the Fennec fox *Fennecus zerda*) seems confined to the North African desert biome, and the Cape fox has been severely persecuted in its restricted occurrence in dry areas of southern Africa. Little is known of the otherwise rather gregarious pale fox, found throughout Senegal to the Sudan. The bat-eared fox (*Otocyon megalotis*) has been reported from Ethiopia to southern Africa and is considered to be important occasionally in the local epidemiology of rabies, but it too declines near human habitation and suffers destruction via domestic dogs. The New World Channel Islands fox (*Urocyon littoralis*) is restricted to offshore sites of southwestern California, and the kit and swift foxes are endangered species with extremely fragmented distributions, having disappeared over much of their former ranges. The hoary fox (Lycalopex) is confined to Brazil, where it is often killed for presumed predation on fowl. The Culpeo fox (*Pseudalopex*) and its allies extend over a fairly wide swath of South America from the equator to Argentina, but these are habitat specialists and may be limited in population density while restricted to sanctuaries among park reserves. One possible candidate deserving of further study is the crab-eating fox (*Cerdocyon thous*). Populations of this 3 to 8-kg canid occur in a variety of savanna to woodland habitats from Columbia to Argentina, are omnivorous and locally abundant, and could prove to be an important species of concern in Latin America, given adequate attention to rabies surveillance.

B. Raccoon

The common raccoon (*Procyon lotor*) is widely distributed from Canada through Central America and was introduced into Russia and western Europe (Kaufmann, 1982) as well as onto a number of islands, including Japan. Over the past 50 years, raccoons have become recognized as a significant host of wildlife rabies in North America. Persuasive explanations for the original nidus in Florida during the 1940s remain speculative. The disease in raccoons spread gradually into the southeastern United States over the next 30 years. Due to their importance in the fur trade and in hunting, it was not unusual for raccoons to be moved between regions. Rabid raccoons were discovered in some of these shipments (Nettles *et al.*, 1979). In the late 1970s, a new focus of rabid raccoons appeared in the mid-Atlantic region. By 1991, the number of reported rabid raccoons had outnumbered rabid skunks. In the year 2000, the affected area stretched east of the Appalachian Mountains from eastern Ontario to Florida and westward into Alabama and Ohio, making the raccoon the single most important rabies reservoir in the United States (CDC, 2000b). The large geographic range exploited by raccoons in North America is coupled with their adaptability and high density in some suburban and urban environments. Together with the existence of a persistent viral variant (Smith *et al.*, 1984), raccoon rabies is a particularly salient testament to reemerging disease (Hanlon and Rupprecht, 1998).

Despite its relevance as a reservoir, rabies pathogenesis in raccoons is neither well understood nor well described experimentally. Most published responses of raccoons to rabies virus infection have been conducted using a number of other isolates, including a fox (Sikes and Tierkel, 1961), a bat (Constantine, 1966a), a skunk (Hill and Beran, 1992a; Hill *et al.*, 1993), and a dog (Rupprecht *et al.*, 1988). Experimental studies investigating the pathogenesis of raccoon rabies virus in raccoons are limited (Winkler *et al.*, 1985; McLean, 1975; Winkler and Jenkins, 1991), hampered in no small way by the lack of a means to definitively characterize such variants prior to the advent of monoclonal antibodies in 1978 (Wiktor and Koprowski, 1978).

In a recent study of rabies in raccoons, animals were inoculated with rabies virus several times over one year, and their responses were monitored (Niezgoda *et al.*, 1991). The incubation period was independent of viral dose and was approximately 50 days (range 23–92 days), and the morbidity period was approximately 4–5 days (range 2–10 days) (Table II). Not all raccoons succumbed nor seroconverted. All raccoons euthanized with clinical signs of rabies contained rabies virus antigen in their CNS, whereas all survivors were free of antigen at final necropsy.

Not unexpectedly, raccoons may lack discernible clinical signs following exposure to a rabid animal (McLean, 1975) for a variety of reasons. Rabies virus may not be shed from the infected animal during the exposure event, or the concentration of excreted virus may be minimal, or the severity of the exposure could be limiting. Likely, raccoons may be exposed, develop a detectable response, and then develop apparent immunity. In contrast, no antibodies may be detected following multiple rabies exposures but with protective immunity ensuing nonetheless.

Based on both laboratory and field observations, several theoretical groups may exist in free-ranging raccoons depending on local rabies epidemiology (Fig. 4). For example, in a study conducted in four different areas of Pennsylvania, the lowest geometric mean titer (GMT) of rabies VNA was found in a "rabies-free" area. A higher GMT was found at the perceived front to two areas, and the highest was found within a rabies epizootic area (Winkler and Jenkins, 1991). All these antibody-positive raccoons were normal clinically when originally live-trapped. Additionally, in raccoons we live-trapped during a raccoon rabies epizootic in Philadelphia's Fairmount Park during 1990, only 1 of 14 clinically rabid animals had detectable rabies antibody, and all were later confirmed rabid by laboratory diagnosis. Hence detection of rabies antibody in a free-ranging raccoon only shows that exposure to rabies virus antigen has occurred, and detectable responses may be reflective of immunity rather than indicative of a viral incubation phase or ensuing illness per se.

Similarly, rabid raccoons that succumb to a productive infection can present either as antibody-positive or antibody-negative (see Table II). Experimental data

TABLE II

Susceptibility and Virus Neutralizing Antibody Induction in Raccoons Following Four Serial Rabies Virus Inoculations

Inoculum MICLD	Raccoon no.	Rabies VNA titers Day (rabies inoculation 1–4)[a]								Survivorship[b] (VNA titer)	Morbidity period (d)
		0 (1)	36	163 (2)	170	248 (3)	254	370 (4)	386		
$10^{4.5}$	77	<5	15	<5	<5	15	<5	<5	<5	S	
	75	<5	<5	<5	<5	<5	<5	<5	<5	S	
	79	<5	<5	—	—	—	—	—	—	D97 (32,805)	5
	89	<5	15	—	—	—	—	—	—	D89 (10,935)	2
	83	<5	—	—	—	—	—	—	—	D29 (135)	6
$10^{3.8}$	61	<5	<5	<5	<5	<5	45	45	45	S	
	63	<5	<5	15	<5	<5	234	<5	45	S	
	55	<5	15	<5	<5	<5	<5	<5	15	S	
	57	<5	<5	—	—	—	—	—	—	D43 (26)	2
	59	<5	15	—	—	—	—	—	—	D50 (2,104)	5
$10^{3.1}$	69	<5	15	<5	15	<5	15	<5	15	S	
	65	<5	15	<5	135	<5	15	<5	45	S	
	73	<5	<5	15	<5	—	—	—	—	D27[c] (ND)[d]	1
	67	<5	135	—	—	—	—	—	—	D41 (ND)	10
	49	<5	—	—	—	—	—	—	—	D35 (3,645)	4

[a]Raccoons were inoculated after initial inoculation on days 163, 248, and 370 with a raccoon salivary gland suspension obtained from naturally infected raccoons from Pennsylvania consisting of $10^{4.7}$, $10^{5.1}$, and $10^{4.1}$, $MICLD_{50}$ respectively. All raccoons received the inoculum by intramasseter inoculation.

[b]S, survived; D, day euthanatized/died. All raccoons that died contained rabies virus antigen in brain tissue by the direct fluorescent antibody test.

[c]Raccoon 73 died 27 days following the second inoculation.

[d]ND = not done.

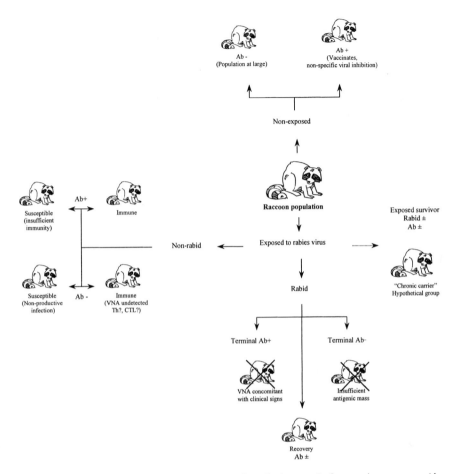

Fig. 4. Potential outcome of rabies exposure and serologic status in free-ranging raccoons. Ab, antibody-positive ($+$), -negative ($-$) for rabies virus neutralizing antibodies (VNA); Ab $\pm$: may or may not have VNA; Rabid $\pm$, may or may not develop clinical rabies; rabies virus primed helper T cells, Th; cytotoxic T-lymphocytes, CTL; X, succumbed to rabies.

suggest that raccoons in terminal stages of disease probably will be seropositive, whereas during earlier stages it would not be unusual for an animal to be antibody-negative. Also, if seroconversion does occur at all, the GMT may be higher in raccoons that succumb to infection in comparison with those which are exposed and seroconvert without detectable illness. Under common field scenarios, rabid raccoons may succumb much earlier than under laboratory situations with supportive veterinary care due to a variety of adverse environmental conditions and probably would appear as antibody-negative.

In areas believed to be free of terrestrial rabies based on surveillance (such as much of the eastern United States immediately prior to the late 1970s), a majority of raccoons are presumed to be largely naive, nonexposed, antibody-negative animals. Occurrence of minimal seroprevalence (i.e., in the range of 0–3%) in low to nonenzootic areas may be coincident to rare rabies exposures, such as a raccoon consuming an infected bat. Supposed detection of some low "titers" may be artifactual, due to nonspecific viral inhibitors within serum (Hill and Beran, 1992a; Hill *et al.*, 1992b, 1993). Alternatively, intentional human intervention through parenteral immunization with inactivated rabies vaccine via wildlife rehabilitation, purposeful trap-vaccinate-release programs, or more recently, programs evaluating the effect of oral rabies vaccination on wildlife also could account for antibody.

Categorically, to include a complete theoretical outcome following exposure, a certain small fragment of a subcompartment of raccoons could be exposed to rabies, develop organic disease, yet recover, with or without obvious sequelae. Nevertheless, documented recovery from clinical rabies is quite rare. A single report exists of an experimentally infected raccoon that showed compatible clinical signs but recovered; it had been vaccinated previously (Rupprecht *et al.*, 1988). Moreover, it is difficult to comprehend how an acute encephalomyelitis such as rabies could be cleared successfully and spontaneously without some residual neurologic damage. The probability for survival in the field for such an obviously debilitated animal assuredly would be low. To date, there is no discrete experimental evidence supporting any chronic carrier state in raccoons, i.e., infected animals that shed virus in the saliva but remain clinically normal. Rather, a scheme of exposure leading to clinical rabies and death or the induction of protective immunity seems a much better fit with current experimental and field data.

C. Skunk

Although tales of rabies in foxes were detailed in the New World as early as the eighteenth century, it took another hundred years for the same case to be made for skunks during western explorations. These small to moderate-sized carnivores with specialized anal glands are widespread in parts of North America, consisting of at least four different species and several subspecies. By the mid-1800s, rabies in skunks was reported from the American prairies, and the disease spread north into Canada by the next century. Rabid skunks were noted to be tenacious biters, and at times rabies seemed so prevalent that some proposed the name *rabies mephitica* to describe the disease in spotted skunks (Steele and Fernandez, 1991). Today in North America, reports of rabies in skunks occur mainly in four geographic regions: (1) the eastern United States, (2) the north central United States and the Canadian provinces of Manitoba, Saskatchewan, and Alberta, (3) California, and (4) the south central United States and Mexico (Aranda and

Lopez-de, 1999; Crawford-Miksza *et al.*, 1999; de Mattos *et al.*, 1999; Gremillion-Smith and Woolf, 1988). Rabies in these areas (in skunks and, to a large extent, in other terrestrial mammals) is caused mainly by four different street virus variants. In the eastern United States, cases are primarily related to spillover from infected raccoons, whereas in the other three, the viruses are adapted to skunks as the primary reservoir. Earlier work suggested that basic differences in host susceptibility would help to explain geographic patterns of maintenance, in that red foxes could succumb relatively quickly to large doses of virus inoculated by rabid skunks (Sikes, 1962). This observation was not found to be universally true and predated the discovery of antigenic variants of rabies virus. Moreover, the role of several independently maintained rabies virus variants and different skunk species is not understood precisely. Other experimental studies do suggest that species specificity of enzootic rabies is due, at least partly, to host immune response and differences in the route, dose, and pathogenicity of these variants of rabies virus (Charlton *et al.*, 1987, 1988, 1996).

Besides route of inoculation and virus dose, the rabies virus variant also may produce different outcomes in skunks. For example, groups of skunks were inoculated intramuscularly with different dilutions of virus from salivary glands of naturally infected skunks in Canada and the United States collected in areas reflective of either the red fox or raccoon rabies outbreak. While there was no significant difference in basic susceptibility, incubation period, or the spectrum of clinical signs, skunks infected with the rabies isolate from the United States exhibited a morbidity period and shed virus in the saliva over 2–3 days. However, skunks infected with the Canadian isolate were clinically rabid and shed virus in the saliva for an average of 1 week, suggestive of significant differences in the infective potential of the two different variants (Charlton *et al.*, 1988, 1991; Hill *et al.*, 1993).

Other research using skunks suggests a major role for muscle tissue during the incubation period of rabies (Charlton *et al.*, 1997). Two months after inoculation, muscle at the inoculation site contained viral RNA, even though other relevant tissues on the route of viral migration and early entrance into the CNS were negative. The location of viral antigen was striated muscle fibers and fibrocytes, confirming earlier observations that indicated that virus may replicate in local tissues prior to invasion of the nervous system.

Rabies virus strains may use different cell populations in the CNS of skunks, even by the same route of infection. For example, examination of the cerebellum of skunks infected experimentally with either a skunk isolate of street rabies virus or the fixed virus strain (CVS) revealed a differential response based on viral inoculum (Jackson *et al.*, 2000). The skunk rabies virus variant displayed prominent infection of glial cells, with a relatively small amount of antigen in the perikarya of Purkinje cells. In contrast, the highly adapted CVS strain showed many intensely labeled Purkinje cells and relatively few infected glial cells. Previously, it was suggested that the relative accumulations and effects of different rabies viruses in the CNS could account for either furious or paralytic phases of the disease (Smart and Charlton, 1992). Thus, while lyssaviruses are highly neurotropic, different viruses can show a predilection for various neural elements and locations.

Experimental studies have shed some light on the pathobiology of rabies in skunks, but fewer observations have been made from naturally infected animals. Rabies virus may be detected in a number of glands, particularly in the end stages of disease, but the submandibular salivary glands seem to be one of the sites most consistently infected, with high concentrations of virus (Charlton *et al.*, 1984; Howard, 1981a,b). Other incidental findings have been reported. During necropsy of one pregnant skunk, rabies virus was discovered in the CNS of a single fetus, but the significance of this observation is unclear (Howard, 1981c). The behavior of normal and rabid striped skunks recently was reported unexpectedly during an unrelated radiotelemetry study in North Dakota (Greenwood *et al.*, 1997). In 1991, only 1 of 23 skunks under study was found to be rabid, whereas during 1992, 35 of 50 (70%) were diagnosed as rabid. The estimated survival rate of skunks was 0.85 during the spring of 1991 but dropped to 0.17 during the same season in 1992. Nearly a third of rabid skunks were located below ground. No differences were observed between healthy and rabid skunks in estimated mean rate of travel per hour, distance traveled per night, or home range. Among rabid skunks, mean rate of travel and distance traveled per night tended to decrease with the onset of illness. Mean home ranges of male skunks were greater than for females before illness but not after the demonstration of clinical signs. Home range of females did not differ when compared before or after signs of rabies. Rabid animals were more spatially clumped than expected, but no relationship was detected between locations of rabid skunks and dates of death. This research not only provided a glimpse of how rabies may affect an animal's use of space but also provided an estimate of the relative impact of rabies on a local population. It also exemplifies how many rabies cases typically can escape routine surveillance due to the circumstances surrounding an animal's demise, such as predation or carcass loss.

As with any wild animal, clinical signs of rabies are difficult to discern, and skunks should not be kept as pets. Illustrative of this point, an apparent outbreak of rabies was reported within a colony of captive striped skunks. One of the animals had been infected in the wild and developed clinical illness approximately 7 weeks after capture. This female transmitted the virus to three of her five offspring and to one other adult. The disease spread when the infants were orphaned and adopted by lactating females. Although the animals were in close contact with each other, the infection spread quite slowly. Furious rabies was not detected. Usually, rabid skunks were found dead without obvious prior clinical signs.

In the raccoon rabies enzootic area of the United States, skunks are the most frequently reported species after raccoons (Krebs *et al.*, 1999). To date, all skunks examined have been associated with the raccoon rabies virus variant and appear to be related to infection from raccoons based on spatial and temporal submission patterns. However, on a few occasions (e.g., in Massachusetts and Rhode Island), rabid skunks have outnumbered rabid raccoons. Whether this variant will evolve toward independent rabies transmission in skunks remains to be seen. Such a phenomenon would hamper oral vaccination plans for raccoons in the region substantially due to the absence of an effective rabies vaccine for skunks.

D. Coyote

The coyote (*Canis latrans*) is a highly adaptable and behaviorally variable "carnivore" that actually is quite omnivorous, exploiting both western rangelands and eastern suburbs. It occurs widely throughout North America from Alaska to Panama. With the near extirpation of the gray wolf, the coyote appears to be in a range expansion and more numerous than in the past (Vila *et al.*, 1999). Flexibility in social organization prevails, from solitary individuals with transient home ranges in excess of 50 km^2 to monogamous pair bonds and small packs.

Given the limitations imposed by predation and competition from wolf populations, it is doubtful that the coyote doubled as an adequate reservoir for rabies in times past. Few accounts in the New World suggest any major problem prior to reports from North America in the twentieth century. For example, during 1952–1954, a large rabies outbreak in Alberta, Canada, involved foxes, wolves, and coyotes, but the primary role of the latter species is questionable. In the United States, during 1915–1917, coyotes were involved in an extensive epizootic that extended over portions of California, Oregon, Nevada, and Utah (Humphrey, 1971). From California alone in this period, records from the state public health department confirmed infection via laboratory examination in at least 94 coyotes, 64 cattle, 31 dogs, 8 sheep, 6 horses, 3 bobcats, 1 cat, 1 goat, and 1 human. These records only serve to underscore the magnitude of the outbreak, considering the hundreds of miles from the field sites to the laboratory. In the same period, at least 192 rabid coyotes were diagnosed in Nevada. Trapping and poisoning campaigns ensued, resulting in the destruction of thousands of coyotes and dogs and hundreds of other species representatives, and the epizootic eventually abated, even if the enzootic focus did not.

Were coyotes the reservoir that infected dogs and other species, or were rabid dogs the instigation that eventually spilled over to coyotes? Some believe that rabies in coyotes was present in Oregon as early as 1910, but this does not explain adequately how or why (Mallory, 1915). Others insinuate that "… the disease gradually spread, traveling northward through California and being introduced into Oregon in 1912 by a sheep dog taken across the mountains from Redding, California, to Wallowa County in that state, where this infected dog in a fight with a coyote, first introduced the disease …" (Records, 1932). As with many rabies tales, the chicken or egg origin to this outbreak (and others) cannot be resolved easily but does point out the intrinsic historical relationship between poorly supervised, unvaccinated dogs and wildlife disease. Similarly, coyotes in northern Baja were believed to act as vehicles behind the persistent infections that started during 1958 along the California–Mexico border thought related in part to long-distance dispersal (Humphrey, 1971). Neither absolute numbers of laboratory-confirmed cases in coyotes throughout the United States nor geographic spread ever again reached the extent exemplified by the 1915 western states outbreak. Nevertheless, its message should have prepared public health professionals for a repeat lesson more than 70 years later.

Rabies cases in coyotes were quite few and only sporadically reported in the United States from 1960 through the mid-1980s. For example, a Sonora canine rabies virus variant occasionally would be detected in animals along the west Texas border with Mexico (Rhode *et al.*, 1997). This situation began to change slowly at a focus near the south Texas–Mexico border associated with another rabies virus variant known in coyotes and domestic dogs from the region at least since 1978 (Clark *et al.*, 1994). During 1988, a south Texas county reported 6 confirmed cases of rabies in coyotes and 2 cases in dogs. At the same time, an adjacent county reported 9 cases of rabid dogs. During 1989–1990, 7 coyotes and 65 dogs were reported rabid in these areas. By 1991, the outbreak expanded approximately 160 km north, with a case total of 42 rabid coyotes and 25 dogs over 10 counties. In 1992, it rose to 70 rabid coyotes and 41 dogs from a 12-county area, and by 1993, 71 of the 74 total cases in coyotes and 42 of 130 total cases in dogs reported from the entire United States were from south Texas. By comparison, in that year, no other state reported more than 7 cases in dogs. The risk of artificial spread to other areas was realized during 1993 by identification of the coyote rabies virus variant from a dog infected on a compound in Alabama, where imported coyotes from Texas were released for hunting purposes (Krebs *et al.*, 1994). Over some 18 counties in 1994, the number of coyote rabies cases reached 77, with 32 cases in dogs, and peaked at 80 rabid coyotes, with 36 cases in dogs, in 20 counties during 1995 when an oral vaccination program began to halt its progression (Fearneyhough *et al.*, 1998). Unfortunately, as in Alabama previously, translocation of coyote rabies happened again, this time from Texas to Florida (CDC, 1995). During November and December 1994, rabies was diagnosed in 5 dogs from two associated kennels in Florida. In addition, 2 other dogs at one of the kennels died with suspected but unconfirmed rabies. The rabies virus recovered from these dogs was identified as a rabies virus variant not previously found in Florida but rather the same virus enzootic among coyotes in south Texas. The suspected source of infection was translocation of infected coyotes from Texas to Florida, also used in hunting enclosures. Luckily, cases of rabies in coyotes at the Texas nidus continued to decline each year from 1996–1999, with 19, 4, 4, and 2 reports, respectively. None has been reported to date in 2000.

At least two human cases were associated with the Texas coyote rabies outbreak, in 1991 and 1994, but the history surrounding each exposure was unclear. With the elimination of dog-to-dog transmission in Canada and the United States, this recent coyote rabies saga and the subsequent reemergence of canine rabies should once again impart the sense of wildlife's role in jeopardizing this rather fragile public health success story. Yet, besides the data gained from historical surveillance reports, few research studies concentrate on rabies in coyotes, beyond demonstration of their basic susceptibility to bat rabies virus, aerosol infection, or virologic curiosities (Constantine, 1966a,b,c; Behymer *et al.*, 1974). Explanations as to the dearth of knowledge surrounding rabies in coyotes may be best summed up by the following past opinion: "… although they are a potential hazard as a reservoir or vector of rabies, they do not appear to be of major epidemiologic significance …" (Sikes, 1966).

Given this dearth of information, limited studies were initiated at the CDC during the 1990s in response to the need for development of an oral vaccine in coyotes and necessity for challenge studies of its efficacy. Salivary glands of 43 naturally infected Texas coyotes were removed, and concentrations of rabies virus were obtained. Most glands contained more than 5 logs of rabies virus at a minimum (Fig. 5). Data were interpreted within all the limitations related to

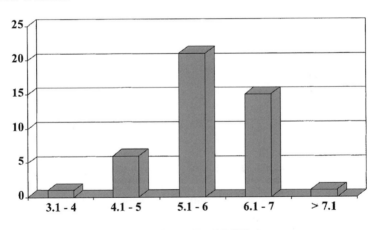

Fig. 5.   Quantity of virus isolated from salivary glands of rabid coyotes. Each symbol represents an individual coyote ($n = 43$). For experimental inoculation, a 10% w/v suspension of a salivary gland homogenate from a naturally infected Texas coyote was prepared and titrated by intracranial inoculation of 4–6-week-old ICR mice. Final dilutions were prepared in 2% horse serum and distilled water. Virus titrations of the salivary glands from the infected coyotes were performed by intracranial inoculation of 4–6-week-old ICR mice.

Day

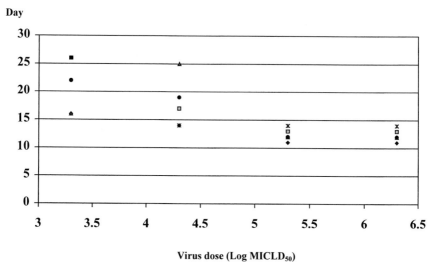

Virus dose (Log MICLD$_{50}$)

Fig. 6. Incubation period of coyotes infected with rabies virus. Each symbol represents an individual coyote (n = 19). A 10% w/v suspension of a salivary gland homogenate from a naturally infected Texas coyote was prepared and titrated by intracranial inoculation of 4–6-week-old ICR mice. Final dilutions were in 2% horse serum and distilled water.

potential viral deterioration from the time of death in the field until the period of harvest in the laboratory. Adult coyotes of equal sexes were maintained in captivity and were inoculated with four serial tenfold dilutions of a homogenized salivary gland from a naturally infected rabid coyote. The virus isolated was representative of the south Texas canine rabies virus variant. All exposed coyotes succumbed to the higher concentrations, and 80% of animals developed fatal illness when exposed to at least 3.3 logs of rabies virus (Fig. 6). Incubation periods ranged from 10–26 days, with a suggestion of an inverse relationship to infectious dose. Frozen sections of salivary glands obtained at necropsy of infected coyotes were examined by immunofluorescent microscopy. Whereas all five sections obtained from animals inoculated with at least 4.3 logs of virus contained evidence of rabies virus antigen, only 2 of 5 and 2 of 4 samples were positive from coyotes inoculated with a higher (5.3) or lower (3.3) concentration of virus, respectively. Clinical signs were characteristic of the paralytic form of the disease and included altered appetite, depression, confusion, anisocoria, excessive salivation, ataxia, and paresis. Only a single animal exhibited aggressive signs and charged its cage at the sight of animal handlers. Morbidity periods typically were 3–4 days. Based on these limited findings, coyotes appear quite susceptible to this particular rabies virus variant (as do domestic dogs). Such data suffer the limitation of all experimental studies, and field outcomes depend in part on the quantity of virus excreted in the saliva over time and the manner in which coyotes actually infect one another. On a minor note, experimental use of this canid rabies virus in coyotes at the CDC did lead to an unanticipated and unprecedented case of nonbite transmission to a laboratory beagle (Rupprecht *et al.*, 1994). This event reemphasized the volatile mix especially implicit with certain lyssaviruses, hosts, and environmental situations and the danger inherent in cavalier attempts to predict the future when surrounded by profound unknowns.

E. Bats

Neither a single chapter nor even a book can deal with the subject of rabies in bats adequately. Surveying the literature, from Constantine's 1962–1986 (Constantine, 1962, 1966a,b,c, 1967, 1975, 1979, 1986; Constantine and Woodall, 1964, 1966; Constantine *et al.*, 1968a,b, 1972, 1979) pioneering studies to a recent book review (Brass, 1994), more questions than answers flow. At first glance, greater time and attention seem to have been paid to rabies in carnivores than in bats, based on past accounts in the published literature. This is due in no small part to the magnitude of the problem in dogs, observer bias, the domestication of carnivores, and the relative difficulty in adapting some bats to captivity. However, over the last century of study, multiple independent lines of laboratory and field inquiry have shown that the natural history and biologic behavior of rabies in the *Chiroptera* and *Carnivora* share many commonalities, including the following points:

1. Based on experimental evidence, bats are neither more nor less susceptible to rabies than are carnivores.

2. The bite route is the fundamental means of rabies transmission among bats.

3. Basic aspects of rabies pathogenesis to and from the CNS of bats are the same as described for other animals.

4. When physiologically active, minimum and maximum incubation periods of rabies in the *Chiroptera* are believed to be no different than those observed in the *Carnivora*.

5. Both aspects of paralytic and furious rabies have been described in bats.

6. Besides virus found in the CNS and salivary glands of rabid bats, a plethora of other tissues, such as brown fat, may contain viral antigen in the end stage of disease.

7. Although a number of viral variants have been described from bats and are believed to be adapted to them, they are known to be infectious for other animals as well.

8. While some of the most ancient references to rabies only mention carnivores, bat rabies is believed to be at least as old as, if not older than, that

in other mammals based on historical references suggestive of vampire rabies in the Americas more than 500 years ago and in deference to the modern distribution and abundance of the disease in the *Chiroptera*.

9. As documented in free-ranging carnivores, such as the mongoose, rabies VNA have been described in bats, suggestive of acquired herd immunity in certain species and under suitable social and environmental conditions.

10. Rumor, conjecture, and previous unconfirmed reports to the contrary, there is no credible evidence for the existence of a carrier state of rabies among bats, in which individuals remain clinically normal while shedding virus in the saliva over prolonged periods of time.

Despite these major similarities, fundamental differences do exist between rabies in bats and the disease in carnivores, such as the following:

1. With the exception of Antarctica, the distribution of rabies in bats is global in nature.

2. The ecologic advantage offered by flight enhances the potential for invasion of new areas and rapid dispersal much more readily than by earthbound carnivores, as illustrated by the discovery of a rabid bat in the United Kingdom.

3. The biodiversity seen in overall species richness is reflected in the relative quantity of *Lyssavirus* variants harbored in both Old and New World bat reservoirs, more so than the relatively few examples identified to date in carnivores worldwide.

4. Given the issue of size alone, one would expect a greater absolute number of rabid bats as a point prevalence, as well as a greater density in space, compared with larger-bodied carnivores.

5. In those species of *Chiroptera* which undergo a true hibernation, the virus can exploit a host mechanism to "overwinter," whereas representatives among the carnivores that might possess this physiologic ability are not significant reservoirs.

6. The observation of a true epizootic of rabies in most bat species does not appear to reflect the same quality of attributes as reflected in the *Carnivora* concerning magnitude in time and space and the percentage positivity rate offered by diagnostic submissions, although surveillance bias may be operative.

7. The phenomenon of aerosol transmission of rabies under field conditions, albeit rare, has only been documented in bats.

8. Considering vampire bats as obligate vertebrate parasites dependent on blood, regular rabies spillover infections to other nonbat species should occur much more frequently than for any present examples in the *Carnivora*.

9. Although occasional spillover of bat rabies virus variants has been detected in carnivores, the converse has not been recorded regarding carnivore rabies viruses in bats, although it is possible in theory.

10. No significant rabies outbreaks have been either initiated or perpetuated by bats in carnivores, and no secondary transmission to humans has been documented from nonbat species infected with bat rabies virus variants (e.g., bat to cat to human).

11. Control methods of bat rabies, such as the successful use of oral vaccination in carnivores, will remain quite challenging.

12. Bats are the most prominent direct source of human rabies in parts of North America (e.g., Canada and the United States), South America (e.g., Chile), western Europe, and Australia, especially where the disease in carnivores has been controlled.

The latter point is especially disturbing because of the great progress made in human rabies prevention over the last century. For example, human rabies in the United States decreased from more than 100 cases annually in the early 1900s (primarily due to rabid dogs) to only 1–2 cases during the last several decades. However, from 1980–2000, most of the indigenous cases of human rabies resulted from infection with bat rabies virus variants. Yet only 2 of these cases had a clear history of a bite, although most patients had obvious bat contact (CDC, 2000c). In most of these cases, a rabies virus variant associated with silver-haired and eastern pipistrelle bats (*Lasionycteris noctivagans* and *pipistrellus subflavus*) was identified. The inability of health professionals to obtain an accurate history on potential human exposures involving bats is problematic. Clearly, some bat rabies virus variants may possess peculiar biologic characteristics that support infectious transmission even under limited bite conditions (Dietzschold *et al.*, 2000). Moreover, circumstances surrounding human exposure to bats frequently are peculiar (Pape *et al.*, 1999). Typically, people may not know that a bat bite is a potential risk for rabies. This may be due in part to the rather limited lesions caused by bats when compared with the teeth and jaws of common carnivores (Fig. 7).

Taken at face value, these points appear as prominent facts. Alternatively, they can be offered as hypotheses in need of testing. From the preceding, several unique opportunities worthy of introspection should be clear for those willing to accept the challenge of the enigma called *bat rabies*.

X. OTHER ANIMALS AS RESERVOIRS

Considering the existence of several robust rabies reservoirs among multiple carnivore examples (e.g., fox, raccoon, skunk, and mongoose), the absence of

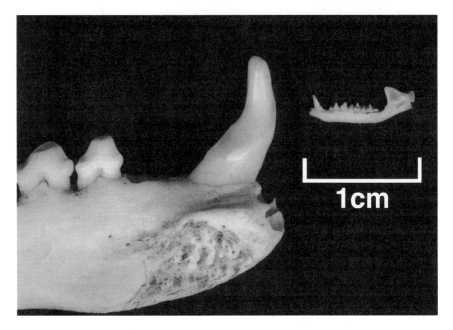

Fig. 7. Comparison of the mandible of a *Myotis* sp. bat with the canine tooth of a raccoon.

others may appear puzzling at first. Yet evolutionary bottlenecks and recent constraints imposed by humans may limit the ability of various species to serve in an ideal host capacity as animal reservoirs. For example, the canids are one of the oldest extant taxa in the group, widely distributed, and usually small to moderate in size. Many are fairly solitary, but even more social examples (e.g., side-striped jackal, African wild dog, bush dog, and small-eared dog) have experienced a recent lowering of population densities and extreme habitat fragmentation (Gascoyne *et al.*, 1993). The introduction of rabies into this already complicated scene can have further deleterious effects on threatened and endangered species, as has been observed with both the gray and the Ethiopian wolf (Chapman, 1978; Ballard and Krausman, 1997; Theberge *et al.*, 1994; Weiler *et al.*, 1995; Sillero-Zubiri *et al.*, 1996). No doubt occasionally these can act as effective vectors, as seems to be the case for blacked-backed and golden jackals in parts of Africa and Asia, almost akin to the New World coyote, but not often as stable reservoirs (Rhodes *et al.*, 1998). Indeed, historically, throughout temperate portions of the Old World, humans attacked by rabid wolves represent some of the highest cases of fatality per event on record (Butzeck, 1987; Ianshin *et al.*, 1979; Shah and Jaswal, 1976; Bahmanyar *et al.*, 1976; Selimov *et al.*, 1978). Nevertheless, it is quite unlikely that these large canids can serve as adequate long-term reservoirs.

No unique rabies virus variants have been acquired from wolves, and those which have been typed appear to be of fox origin.

Rabies has been reported extensively from raccoon dogs (*Nyctereutes procynonoides*), particularly in eastern Europe and the Baltic region, but little is known of the direct role they may play in perpetuation of rabies independent of the red fox. They are highly adaptable canids that originate from eastern Asia but were raised for fur and released in the former Soviet Union between 1928 and 1955. Individuals gradually dispersed westward after their original purposeful human translocation (Cherkasskiy, 1988), and it is questionable if they could sustain rabies for an indefinite period.

As with the restrictions on the *Canidae*, the same could be said for many of the felids, the quintessential predators and one of the most specialized groups in the *Carnivora*. With few exceptions, they exploit a rather solitary existence. Acquisition of a large body size in some groups (e.g., tiger, panther, jaguar, and leopard) has added utility in hunting hoofed stock but does tend to limit absolute numbers. Effective depredations on humans and their domestic animals have resulted in severe population reductions of most wild cat taxa. Nevertheless, rabid felids can be effective vectors. For example, after raccoons, skunks, foxes, and coyotes, the bobcat is the most common wild carnivore found with rabies in the United States, and human cases have resulted from infection by these wild felids. To date, no reservoirs have been described for any feline species. Similar comments could be made about the bears, hyenas, and others. An entirely aquatic existence offered by the cetaceans and other marine mammals such as the dugong and manatee fashion a rather implausible air of likely rabies exposure. Many pinnipeds (i.e., seals, sea lions, and their relatives) do form huge social aggregations during the reproductive season and provide an intermediate link to both infected terrestrial carnivores (such as foxes and skunks) and some bats (such as the vampires), but relatively few rabid specimens have been reported thus far. Besides inadequate veterinary surveillance at remote rookeries, the insulation offered by blubber, the frequent bathing of lesions surrounded by seawater, and deaths in the marine environment from debilitation or active shark consumption are educated guesses as to their absence in rabies statistics.

When one scans the published global literature and surveillance reports from Eurasia, Africa, and the Americas, one is impressed with the zoologic potpourri of cases that have been reported, diverse enough to fill a child's alphabet book. For example, these involve the aardwolf, armadillo, baboon, badger, bison, camel, caracal, chipmunk, civet, duiker, elephant, fox squirrel, genet, honey badger, hyena, hyrax, *Ictonyx*, javelina, kudu, llama, lion, marmoset, *Nasua*, ocelot, opossum, otter, polecat, rabbit, rat, reindeer, roe deer, springbok, suricate, *Taurotragus*, ursids, vole, warthog, weasel, wildcat, *Xerus*, yak, zebra, and a host of others (Batista-Morais *et al.*, 2000; Berry, 1993; Cappucci *et al.*, 1972; CDC, 1990; Dieterich and Ritter, 1982; Dowda and DiSalvo, 1984; Frye and Cucuel, 1968;

Karp et al., 1999; Leffingwell and Neill, 1989; Rausch, 1975; Walroth et al., 1996; Wimalaratne and Kodidara, 1999; Swanepoel et al., 1993; Stoltenow et al., 2000; Taylor et al., 1991). After speculating on the question of diagnostic fidelity and the potential for cross-contamination, bona fide cases do support the contention that practically all mammals are susceptible to rabies within the limitations of niche availability to the virus and adequate human sampling. Almost all occur as single, incidental observations. However, multiple occurrences in a herd or pack can occur with dramatic finality, as illustrated by the thousands of cases reported from kudu (Barnard et al., 1982; Hubschle, 1988), probably enhanced by artificial propagation in game ranching. The tally sheet, however, is simply a record of victims, dead-end infections exposed by those individuals with a combination of evolutionary and ecologic attributes that serve as unfortunate host to one of the oldest infectious diseases. Will this always be the case, and will new reservoirs arise? As suggested by the bats and their multitude of *Lyssavirus* variants, are there new examples yet to be discovered among other small mammals (or nonmammals)?

Despite their ubiquity in distribution and abundance and their diversity as the largest mammalian order, documented cases of rabies in rodents are uncommon (Childs et al., 1997; Moro et al., 1991). To date, there are no known rodent reservoirs nor identified human rabies cases attributable to contact with rabid rodents in the United States. Detection of rabies in rodents depends in part on several variables, including the probability of rodent contact with a reservoir species; the ability of the individual rodent to survive an initial, presumably traumatic, encounter with a naturally infected animal, typically a carnivore; the likelihood that the infected rodent can avoid terminal predation, particularly during the debilitating stages of encephalomyelitis; and the opportunity for human interaction and successful submission and testing at a diagnostic laboratory. Thus it is not surprising that when rabies is diagnosed, large-bodied (>1 kg) rodents, such as woodchucks or beavers, predominate, and significant long-term spatial-temporal patterns may appear gradually when particular hosts or viral variants emerge, especially in areas of high human population density. For example, from 1953–1976, during a period when nonspecific results based on inclusion bodies could have led to false-positive diagnoses, only 3 rabid beavers were recorded, despite their occurrence throughout the continental United States. In contrast, from 1977–1996, 16 rabid beavers were recorded, all within the eastern raccoon rabies enzootic, at a time when laboratory test specificity had improved dramatically. Little is known concerning the pathogenesis and epizootiology of such cases in the beaver or other wild rodents. The issue of relative size may be especially relevant not only as to the opportunity for survival after rabies exposure but also as to the chance for a person to observe an unusual event in an otherwise shy or wary species such as a woodchuck or beaver. The following is illustrative of the point. Since 1990, at least 4 beavers were diagnosed as rabid in North Carolina. All were found near a popular public water source. A brief review of several case histories imparts the sense that they may be even more frequent than expected. Obviously, direct interaction with a rather formidable, large-bodied rodent led to their investigation:

June 1997 — A beaver in Chatham County, Jordan Lake, swam toward a bass boat and tried to board and attack the fishermen. As it entered the boat, it was killed with a paddle.

August 1997 — Another beaver was observed from the same lake as the case in June. It swam into a public swimming area and bit a teenager on the arm. The beaver was scared away a short distance but returned to attack other swimmers. Finally, after being herded into a shallow cove, it was killed.

April 1998 — A beaver was found dead near a pond at the state zoo. It was examined as a curiosity for cause of death, not as a direct public health risk.

April 1998 — A beaver in Cabarrus County left the woods surrounding a trailer park and charged some children playing nearby. It was killed at the site.

Multiple samples from the head of this latter animal were examined for rabies virus antigen (Fig. 8). Immunofluorescent and immunohistochemical tests for rabies

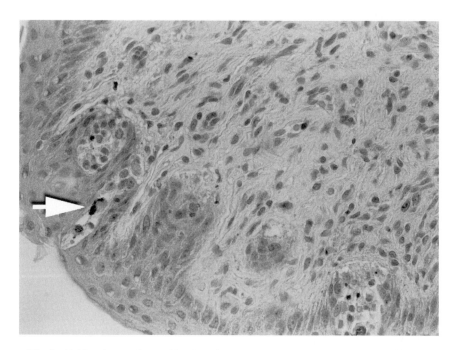

Fig. 8.   Rabies virus nucleocapsid antigen in the epithelium of the dorsal surface of the tongue (papillae) of a naturally infected beaver, stained by immunohistochemistry and the streptavidin-biotin peroxidase system (400 ×).

virus antigen were positive for all tissues examined, including skin, tonsil, tongue, lymph nodes, cranial nerves, and salivary glands. In this case, spillover infection resulted from the rabies virus variant associated with raccoons in the eastern United States. As the largest rodent in North America, with prominent mandibles and incisors, beavers may inflict severe bites. On the basis of these very preliminary results suggesting vector competence, laboratory submission of suspect beavers and other wild rodents should continue to be evaluated on a case-by-case basis, particularly in situations with unprovoked human or domestic animal exposure by an ill animal. Given the diversity of rodent species, global abundance, variety of lifestyles, and proven competence as significant hosts for other viral diseases, one would anticipate that at least one salient example should be found eventually to meet the minimum attributes of a rabies virus reservoir in this group.

XI. CONCLUSIONS

Many unanswered questions remain in a basic understanding of animal rabies. Key facets to basic mammalian susceptibility to rabies still require definition. Adequate explanations to long incubation periods in animals do not yet exist. The site and manner of virus sequestered during this period — within or outside the nervous system — await recognition. Factors that may predispose a neurotropic virus to nonneural sites and the conditions, albeit rare, that may drive toward viremia need identification. A convincing neurochemical mechanism for altered behavior during rabies has not been made. The importance of the nonbite route, including transplacental or aerosol transmission and body fluids such as milk, is unknown. Coherent algorithms should be able to predict when a productive fatal infection is likely to result versus acquired immunity. A melding of applied ecology and virology may permit the elucidation of common features that are important in the definition of an ideal rabies host. Influence of minor genetic changes on phenotypic alterations should be explored, particularly as related to significant biologic outcomes. Use of more realistic disease models could allow rabies reemergence to be anticipated and perhaps even prevented *a priori*.

Clearly, a number of factors influence the biologic outcome of rabies exposure to an individual animal toward the opportunity for primary establishment, spread, and persistence in a population and other communities. Ultimate response depends in part on the virus and mammal in question, as well as individual variables such as age, nutritional state, underlying disease burden, prior exposure, and genetic makeup. Progress has been made in the last decade in understanding primary rabies pathogenesis with advancement in major areas that use molecular techniques such as PCR, *in situ* hybridization, and immunohistochemistry. Undoubtedly, additional features of animal rabies pathobiology also may be more fully elucidated using lyssavirus street isolates of public health relevance, more natural routes of infection, variable exposures to differing concentrations of virus, and a greater diversity of natural host species. Ultimately, such endeavors can result in a better understanding of rabies epizootiology toward renewed prevention and control throughout the next century of inquiry.

REFERENCES

Aitken, T. H., Kowalski, R. W., Beaty, B. J., Buckley, S. M., Wright, J. D., Shope, R. E., and Miller, B. R. (1984). Arthropod studies with rabies-related Mokola virus. *Am. J. Trop. Med. Hyg.* **33**, 945–952.

Allworth, A., Murray, K., and Morgan, J. (1996). A human case of encephalitis due to a *Lyssavirus* recently identified in fruit bats. *Commun. Dis. Intell.* **20**, 504.

Anderson, L. J., Williams, L. P., Jr., Layde, J. B., Dixon, F. R., and Winkler, W. G. (1984). Nosocomial rabies: Investigation of contacts of human rabies cases associated with a corneal transplant. *Am. J. Public Health* **74**, 370–372.

Anonymous. (1990). Compendium of animal rabies control. *J. Am. Vet. Med. Assoc.* **196**, 36–39.

Aranda, M., and Lopez-de, B. L. (1999). Rabies in skunks from Mexico. *J. Wildlife Dis.* **35**, 574–577.

Artois, M., and Aubert, M. F. A. (1985). Behavior of rabid foxes. *Rev. Ecol.* **4**, 171–176.

Aubert, M. F. A. (1992). Epidemiology of fox rabies. In *Wildlife Rabies Control*, K. Bogel, F.-X. Meslin, and M. Kaplan, (eds.), pp. 9–18. Wells Medical, Kent, UK.

Baer, G. M., and Olson, H. R. (1972). Recovery of pigs from rabies. *J. Am. Vet. Med. Assoc.* **160**, 1127–1128.

Baer, G. M., Cleary, W. F., Diaz, A. M., and Perl, D. F. (1977). Characteristics of 11 rabies virus isolates in mice: Titers and relative invasiveness of virus, incubation period of infection, and survival of mice with sequelae. *J. Infect. Dis.* **136**, 336–345.

Bahmanyar, M., Fayaz, A., Nour-Salehi, S., Mohammadi, M., and Koprowski, H. (1976). Successful protection of humans exposed to rabies infection: Postexposure treatment with the new human diploid cell rabies vaccine and antirabies serum. *JAMA* **236**, 2751–2754.

Ballard, W. B., and Krausman, P. R. (1997). Occurrence of rabies in wolves of Alaska. *J. Wildlife Dis.* **33**, 242–245.

Barnard, B. J., Hassel, R. H., Geyer, H. J., and De Koker, W. C. (1982). Non-bite transmission of rabies in kudu (*Tragelaphus strepsiceros*). *Onderstepoort J. Vet. Res.* **49**, 191–192.

Batista-Morais, N., Neilson-Rolim, B., Matos-Chaves, H. H., Brito-Neto, J., and Maria-da-Silva, L. (2000). Rabies in tamarins (*Callithrix jacchus*) in the State of Ceara, Brazil, a distinct viral variant? *Mem. Inst. Oswaldo Cruz* **95**, 609–610.

Beamer, R. D., Mohr, C. O., and Barr, T. R. B. (1960). Resistance of the opossum to rabies virus. *Am. J. Vet. Res.* **21**, 507–510.

Behymer, D. E., Frye, F. L., Riemann, H. P., Franti, C. E., and Enright, J. B. (1974). Observations on the pathogenesis of rabies: Experimental infection with a virus of coyote origin. *J. Wildlife Dis.* **10**, 197–203.

Bell, G. P. (1980). A possible case of interspecific transmission of rabies in insectivorous bats. *J. Mammal.* **61**, 528–530.

Beran, G. W., Nocete, A. P., Elvina, O., Gregorio, S. B., Moreno, R. R., Nakao, J. C., Burchett, G. A., Canizares, H. L., and Macasaet, F. F. (1972). Epidemiological and control studies on rabies in the Philippines. *Southeast Asian J. Trop. Med. Public Health* **3**, 433–445.

Bergeron, J. A., Quinn, W. J., and Stackhouse, L. L. (1981). Rabies in a ewe and a 6-week-old lamb. *Mod. Vet. Pract.* **62**, 784–785.

Berry, H. H. (1993). Surveillance and control of anthrax and rabies in wild herbivores and carnivores in Namibia. *Rev. Sci. Technol.* **12**, 137–146.

Bigler, W. J., Hoff, G. L., Smith, J. S., McLean, R. G., Trevino, H. A., and Ingwersen, J. (1983). Persistence of rabies antibody in free-ranging raccoons. *J. Infect. Dis.* **148**, 610.

Black, D., and Wiktor, T. J. (1986). Survey of raccoon hunters for rabies antibody titers: Pilot study. *J. Fla. Med. Assoc.* **73**, 517–520.

Black, J. G., and Lawson, K. F. (1970). Sylvatic rabies studies in the silver fox (*Vulpes vulpes*): Susceptibility and immune response. *Can. J. Comp. Med.* **34**, 309–311.

Blancou, J. A., Aubert, M. F. A., and Artois, M. (1982). Rage experimentale du furet (*Mustela putorius furo*). *Rev. Med. Vet.* **133**, 553–557.

Blancou, J., Aubert, M. F. A., and Artois, M. (1991). Fox rabies. In *The Natural History of Rabies*, G. M. Baer (ed.), pp. 257–290. CRC Press, Boca Raton, FL.

Bögel, K., Moegle, H., Knorpp, F., Arata, A., Dietz K., and Diethelm, P. (1976). Characteristics of the spread of a wildlife rabies epidemic in Europe. *Bull. WHO* **54**, 433–447.

Boulger, L. R., and Porterfield, J. S. (1958). Isolation of a virus from Nigerian fruit bats. *Transaction* **52**, 421–424.

Bourhy, H., Kissi, B., Lafon, M., Sacramento, D., and Tordo, N. (1992). Antigenic and molecular characterization of bat rabies virus in Europe. *J. Clin. Microbiol.* **30**, 2419–2426.

Brass, D. (1994). *Rabies in Bats*, p. 335. Livia Press, Ridgefield, CT.

Buckley, S. M. (1975). Arbovirus infection of vertebrate and insect cell cultures, with special emphasis on Mokola, Obodhiang, and Kotonkan viruses of the rabies serogroup. *Ann. N.Y. Acad. Sci.* **266**, 241–250.

Butzeck, S. (1987). The wolf, *Canis lupus L.*, as a rabies vector in the 16th and 17th centuries. *Z. Gesamte. Hyg.* **33**, 666–669.

Cappucci, D. T., Jr., Emmons, R. W., and Sampson, W. W. (1972). Rabies in an Eastern fox squirrel. *J. Wildlife Dis.* **8**, 340–342.

Centers for Disease Control (1972). Rabies in a laboratory worker — Texas. *Morb. Mortal. Weekly Rep.* **21**, 113–124.

Centers for Disease Control (1977). Rabies in a laboratory worker — New York. *Morb. Mortal. Weekly Rep.* **26**, 183–184.

Centers for Disease Control and Prevention (1990). Rabies in a llama — Oklahoma. *Morb. Mortal. Weekly Rep.* **39**, 203–204.

Centers for Disease Control and Prevention (1995). Translocation of coyote rabies — Florida, 1994. *Morb. Mortal. Weekly Rep.* **44**, 580–587.

Centers for Disease Control and Prevention (1998). Compendium of animal rabies control, 1998. National Association of State Public Health Veterinarians, Inc. *Morb. Mortal. Weekly Rep.* **47** (RR-9), 1–9.

Centers for Disease Control and Prevention (1999). Human rabies prevention — United States, 1999. Recommendations of the Advisory Committee on Immunization Practices (ACIP). *Morb. Mortal. Weekly Rep.* **48** (RR-1), 1–21.

Centers for Disease Control and Prevention (2000a). Compendium of animal rabies prevention and control, 2000. National Association of State Public Health Veterinarians, Inc. *Morb. Mortal. Weekly Rep.* **49**, 21–30.

Centers for Disease Control and Prevention (2000b). Update: Raccoon rabies epizootic — United States and Canada, 1999. *Morb. Mortal. Weekly Rep.* **49**, 31–35.

Centers for Disease Control and Prevention (2000c). Human Rabies — California, Georgia, Minnesota, New York, and Wisconsin, 2000. *Morb. Mortal. Weekly Rep.* **49**, 1111–1115.

Chapman, R. C. (1978). Rabies: Decimation of a wolf pack in arctic Alaska. *Science* **201**, 365–367.

Charlton, K. M., and Casey, G. A. (1979). Experimental rabies in skunks: Oral, nasal, tracheal and intestinal exposure. *Can. I. Comp. Med.* **43**, 168–172.

Charlton, K. M., Casey, G. A., and Webster, W. A. (1984). Rabies virus in the salivary glands and nasal mucosa of naturally infected skunks. *Can. J. Comp. Med.* **48**, 338–339.

Charlton, K. M., Casey, G. A., and Campbell, J. B. (1987). Experimental rabies in skunks: Immune response and salivary gland infection. *Comp. Immunol. Microbiol. Infect. Dis.* **10**, 227–235.

Charlton, K. M., Webster, W. A., Casey, G. A., and Rupprecht, C. E. (1988). Skunk rabies. *Rev. Infect. Dis.* **10** (Suppl. 4), S626–S628.

Charlton, K. M., Webster, W. A., and Casey, G. A. (1991). Skunk rabies. In *The Natural History of Rabies*, G. M. Baer (ed.), pp. 307–324. CRC Press, Boca Raton, FL.

Charlton, K. M. (1994). The pathogenesis of rabies and other lyssaviral infections: Recent studies. *Curr. Top. Microbiol. Immunol.* **187**, 95–119.

Charlton, K. M., Casey, G. A., Wandeler, A. I., and Nadin-Davis, S. (1996). Early events in rabies virus infection of the central nervous system in skunks (*Mephitis mephitis*). *Acta Neuropathol.* **91**, 89–98.

Charlton, K. M., Nadin-Davis, S., Casey, G. A., and Wandeler, A. I. (1997). The long incubation period in rabies: Delayed progression of infection in muscle at the site of exposure. *Acta Neuropathol.* **94**, 73–77.

Cherkasskiy, B. L. (1988). Roles of the wolf and the raccoon dog in the ecology and epidemiology of rabies in the USSR. *Rev. Infect. Dis.* **10** (Suppl. 4), S634–S636.

Childs, J. E., Trimarchi, C. V., and Krebs, J. W. (1994). The epidemiology of bat rabies in New York State, 1988–1992. *Epidemiol. Infect.* **113**, 501–511.

Childs, J. E., Colby, L., Krebs, J. W., Strine, T., Feller, M., Noah, D., Drenzek, C., Smith, J. S., and Rupprecht, C. E. (1997). Surveillance and spatiotemporal associations of rabies in rodents and lagomorphs in the United States 1985–1994. *J. Wildlife Dis.* **33**, 20–27.

Clark, H. F., and Kritchevsky, D. (1972). Growth and attenuation of rabies virus in cell cultures of reptilian origin. *Proc. Soc. Exp. Biol. Med.* **139**, 1317–1325.

Clark, K. A., Neill, S. U., Smith, J. S., Wilson, P. J., Whadford, V. W., and McKirahan, G. W. (1994). Epizootic canine rabies transmitted by coyotes in south Texas. *J. Am. Vet. Med. Assoc.* **204**, 536–540.

Constantine, D. G. (1962). Rabies transmission by the non-bite route. *Public Health Rep.* **77**, 287–289.

Constantine, D. G. (1966a). Transmission experiments with bat rabies isolates: Reaction of certain *Carnivora*, opossum, and bats to intramuscular inoculations of rabies virus isolated from free-tailed bats. *Am. J. Vet. Res.* **27**, 16–19.

Constantine, D. G. (1966b). Transmission experiments with bat rabies isolates: Bite transmission of rabies to foxes and coyote by free-tailed bats. *Am. J. Vet. Res.* **27**, 20–23.

Constantine, D. G. (1966c). Transmission experiments with bat rabies isolates: Responses of certain *Carnivora* to rabies virus isolated from animals infected by nonbite route. *Am. J. Vet. Res.* **27**, 13–15.

Constantine, D. G. (1967). Bat rabies in the southwestern United States. *Public Health Rep.* **82**, 867–888.

Constantine, D. G. (1975). Rabies virus in bats' brain and salivary glands (Letter). *New Engl. J. Med.* **292**, 51.

Constantine, D. G. (1979). An updated list of rabies-infected bats in North America. *J. Wildlife Dis.* **15**, 347–349.

Constantine, D. G. (1986). Absence of prenatal infection of bats with rabies virus. *J. Wildlife Dis.* **22**, 249–250.

Constantine, D. G., and Woodall, D. F. (1964). Latent infection of Rio Bravo virus in salivary glands of bats. *Public Health Rep.* **79**, 1033–1039.

Constantine, D. G., and Woodall, D. F. (1966). Transmission experiments with bat rabies isolates: Reactions of certain *Carnivora*, opossum, rodents, and bats to rabies virus of red bat origin when exposed by bat bite or by intrasmuscular inoculation. *Am. J. Vet. Res.* **27**, 24–32.

Constantine, D. G., Tierkel, E. S., Kleckner, M. D., and Hawkins, D. M. (1968a). Rabies in New Mexico cavern bats. *Public Health Rep.* **83**, 303–316.

Constantine, D. G., Solomon, G. C., and Woodall, D. F. (1968b). Transmission experiments with bat rabies isolates: Responses of certain carnivores and rodents to rabies viruses from four species of bats. *Am. J. Vet. Res.* **29**, 181–190.

Constantine, D. G., Emmons, R. W., and Woodie, J. D. (1972). Rabies virus in nasal mucosa of naturally infected bats. *Science* **175**, 1255–1256.

Constantine, D. G., Humphrey, G. L., and Herbenick, T. B. (1979). Rabies in *Myotis thysanodes*, *Lasiurus ega*, *Euderma maculatum* and *Eumops perotis* in California. *J. Wildlife Dis.* **15**, 343–345.

Crandell, R. A. (1991). Arctic fox rabies. In *The Natural History of Rabies*, G. M. Baer (ed.), pp. 291–306. CRC Press, Boca Raton, FL.

Crawford-Miksza, L. K., Wadford, D. A., and Schnurr, D. P. (1999). Molecular epidemiology of enzootic rabies in California. *J. Clin. Virol.* **14**, 207–219.

Creel, S., Creel, N. M., Munson, L., Sanderlin, D., and Appel, M. J. G. (1997). Serosurvey for selected viral diseases and demography of African wild dogs in Tanzania. *J. Wildlife Dis.* **33**, 823–832.

Crick, J., Tignor, G. H., and Moreno, K. (1982). A new isolate of Lagos bat virus from the Republic of South Africa. *Trans. R. Soc. Trop. Med. Hyg.* **76**, 211–213.

Dean, D. J., Abelseth, M. K., and Atanasiu, D. P. (1996). The fluorescent antibody test. In *Laboratory Techniques in Rabies*, F. X. Meslin, M. M. Kaplan, and H. Koprowski (eds.), pp. 88–95. World Health Organization, Geneva.

de Mattos, C., de Mattos, C., Loza-Rubio, E., Aguilar-Setien, A., Orciari, L. A., and Smith, J. S. (1999). Molecular characterization of rabies virus isolates from Mexico: Implications for transmission dynamics and human risk. *Am. J. Trop. Med. Hyg.* **61**, 587–597.

Delpietro, H. A., and Russo, R. G. (1996). Ecological and epidemiologic aspects of the attacks by vampire bats and paralytic rabies in Argentina and analysis of the proposals carried out for their control. *Rev. Sci. Technol.* **15**, 971–984.

Dieterich, R. A., and Ritter, D. G. (1982). Rabies in Alaskan reindeer. *J. Am. Vet. Med. Assoc.* **181**, 1416.

Dietzschold, B., Rupprecht, C. E., Tollis, M., Lafon, M., Mattei, J., Wiktor, T. J., and Koprowski, H. (1988). Antigenic diversity of the glycoprotein and nucleocapsid proteins of rabies and rabies-related viruses: Implications for epidemiology and control of rabies. *Rev. Infect. Dis.* **10** (Suppl. 4), S785–S798.

Dietzschold, B., Morimoto, K., Hooper, D. C., Smith, J. S., Rupprecht, C. E., and Koprowski, H. (2000). Genotypic and phenotypic diversity of rabies virus variants involved in human rabies: Implications for postexposure prophylaxis. *J. Hum. Virol.* **3**, 50–57.

Dowda, H., and DiSalvo, A. F. (1984). Naturally acquired rabies in an eastern chipmunk (*Tamias striatus*). *J. Clin. Microbiol.* **19**, 281–282.

Eigen, M., and C. K. Biebricher. (1988). Sequence space and quasispecies distribution. In *RNA Genetics*, Vol. 3: *Variability of RNA Genomes*, E. Domingo, J. J. Holland, and P. Ahlquist (eds.), pp. 211–245. CRC Press, Boca Raton, FL.

Everard, C. O., and Everard, J. D. (1988). Mongoose rabies. *Rev. Infect. Dis.* **10** (Suppl. 4), S610–S614.

Familusi, J. B., Osunkoya, B. O., Moore, D. L., Kemp, G. E., and Fabiyi, A. (1972). A fatal human infection with Mokola virus. *Am. J. Trop. Med. Hyg.* **21**, 959–963.

Familusi, J. B., and Moore, D. L. (1972). Isolation of a rabies related virus from the cerebrospinal fluid of a child with "aseptic meningitis." *Afr. J. Med. Sci.* **3**, 93–96.

Fearneyhough, M. G., Wilson, P .J., Clark, K. A., Smith, D. R., Johnston, D. H., Hicks, B. N., and Moore, G. M. (1998). Results of an oral rabies vaccination program for coyotes. *J. Am. Vet. Med. Assoc.* **212**, 498–502.

Fekadu, M. (1972). A typical rabies in dogs in Ethiopia. *Ethiop. Med. J.* **10**, 79–86.

Fekadu, M., Shaddock, J. H., and Baer, G. M. (1981). Intermittent excretion of rabies virus in the saliva of a dog two and six months after it had recovered from experimental rabies. *Am. J. Trop. Med. Hyg.* **30**, 1113–1115.

Fekadu, M., Shaddock, J. H., and Baer, G. M. (1982). Excretion of rabies virus in the saliva of dogs. *J. Infect. Dis.* **145**, 715–719.

Fekadu, M., Shaddock, J. H., Chandler, F. W., and Baer, G. M. (1983). Rabies virus in the tonsils of a carrier dog. *Arch. Virol.* **78**, 37–47.

Fekadu, M. (1991a). Canine rabies. In *The Natural History of Rabies*, G. M. Baer (ed.), pp. 367–378. CRC Press, Boca Raton, FL.

Fekadu, M. (1991b). Latency and aborted rabies. In *The Natural History of Rabies*, G. M. Baer (ed.), pp. 191–198. CRC Press, Boca Raton, FL.

Field, H., McCall, B., and Barrett, J. (1999). Australian bat *Lyssavirus* infection in a captive juvenile black flying fox. *Emerg. Infect. Dis.* **5**, 438–440.

Flamand, A., Coulon, P., Lafay, F., and Tuffereau, C. (1993). Avirulent mutants of rabies virus and their use as live vaccine. *Trends Microbiol.* **1**, 317–320.

Foggin, C. M. (1982). A typical rabies virus in cats and a dog in Zimbabwe. *Vet. Rec.* **110**, 338.

Foggin, C. M. (1983). Mokola virus infection in cats and a dog in Zimbabwe. *Vet. Rec.* **113**, 115.

Foggin, C. M. (1988). Rabies and rabies-related viruses in Zimbabwe: Historical, virological and ecological aspects. Ph.D. dissertation, University of Zimbabwe, Harare, Zimbabwe.

Foley, H. D., McGettigan, J. P., Siler, C. A., Dietzschold, B., and Schnell, M. J. (2000). A recombinant rabies virus expressing vesicular stomatitis virus glycoprotein fails to protect against rabies virus infection. *Proc. Natl. Acad. Sci. USA* **97**, 14680–14685.

Follmann, E. H., Ritter, D. G., and Beller, M. (1994). Survey of trappers in northern Alaska for rabies antibody. *Epidemiol. Infect.* **113**, 137–141.

Fraser, G. C., Hooper, P. T., Lunt, R. A., Gould, A. R., Gleeson, L. J., Hyatt, A. D., Russell, G. M., and Kattenbelt, J. A. (1996). Encephalitis caused by a *Lyssavirus* in fruit bats in Australia. *Emerg. Infect. Dis.* **2**, 327–331.

Frye, F. L., and Cucuel, J. P. (1968). Rabies in an ocelot. *J. Am. Vet. Med. Assoc.* **153**, 789–790.

Gascoyne, S. C., King, A. A., Laurenson, M. K., Borner, M., Schildger, B., and Barrat, J. (1993). Aspects of rabies infection and control in the conservation of the African wild dog (*Lycaon pictus*) in the Serengeti Region, Tanzania. Onderstepoort *J. Vet. Res.* **60**, 415–420.

George, J. P., George, J., Blancou, J., and Aubert, M. F. A. (1980) Description clinique de la rage du renard. *Rev. Med. Vet.* **131**, 153–160.

Gleeson, L. J. (1997). Australian bat *Lyssavirus*: A newly emerged zoonosis? *Aust. Vet. J.* **75**, 188.

Greenwood, R. J., Newton, W. E., Pearson, G. L., and Schamber, G. J. (1997). Population and movement characteristics of radio-collared striped skunks in North Dakota during an epizootic of rabies. *J. Wildlife Dis.* **33**, 226–241.

Gremillion-Smith, C., and Woolf, A. (1988). Epizootiology of skunk rabies in North America. *J. Wildlife Dis.* **24**, 620–626.

Hamir, A. N., Moser, G., and Rupprecht, C. E. (1996). Clinicopathologic variation in raccoons infected with different street rabies virus isolates. *J. Vet. Diagn. Invest.* **8**, 31–37.

Hanlon, C. A., Ziemer, E. L., Hamir, A. N., and Rupprecht, C. E. (1989). Cerebrospinal fluid analysis of rabid and vaccinia–rabies glycoprotein recombinant, orally vaccinated raccoons (*Procyon lotor*). *Am. J. Vet. Res.* **50**, 364–367.

Hanlon, C. A., and Rupprecht, C. E. (1998). The reemergence of rabies. In *Emerging Infections I*, pp 59–80. ASM Press, Washington, DC.

Hanna, J. N., Carney, I. K., Smith, G. A., Tannenberg, A. E., Deverill, J. E., Botha, J. A., Serafin, I. L., Harrower, B. J., Fitzpatrick, P. F., and Searle, J. W. (2000). Australian bat lyssavirus infection: A second human case, with a long incubation period. *Med. J. Aust.* **172**, 597–599.

Hemachudha, T. (1994). Human rabies: Clinical aspects, pathogenesis, and potential therapy. In *Lyssaviruses*, C. E. Rupprecht, B. Dietzschold, and H. Koprowski (eds.), pp. 121–144. Springer-Verlag, Berlin.

Hill, R. E., Jr., and Beran, G. W. (1992a). Experimental inoculation of raccoons procyonlotor with rabies virus of skunk origin. *J. Wildlife Dis.* **28**, 51–56.

Hill, R. E., Jr., Beran, G. W., and Clark, W. R. (1992b). Demonstration of rabies virus–specific antibody in the sera of free-ranging Iowa raccoons (*Procyon lotor*). *J. Wildlife Dis.* **28**, 377–385.

Hill, R. E., Jr., Smith, K. E., Beran, G. W., and Beard, P. D. (1993). Further studies on the susceptibility of raccoons (*Procyon lotor*) to a rabies virus of skunk origin and comparative susceptibility of striped skunks (*Mephitis mephitis*). *J. Wildlife Dis.* **29**, 475–477.

Hou, L., Martin, L. D., Zhou, Z., and Feduccia, A. (1996). Early adaptive radiation of birds: Evidence from fossils from northeastern China. *Science* **274**, 1164–1167.

Howard, D. R. (1981a). Rabies virus tropism in naturally infected skunks (*Mephitis mephitis*). *Am. J. Vet. Res.* **42**, 2187–2190.

Howard, D. R. (1981b). Rabies virus titer from tissues of naturally infected skunks (*Mephitis mephitis*). *Am. J. Vet. Res.* **42**, 1595–1597.

Howard, D. R. (1981c). Transplacental transmission of rabies virus from a naturally infected skunk. *Am. J. Vet. Res.* **42**, 691–692.

Hubschle, O. J. (1988). Rabies in the Kudu antelope (*Tragelaphus strepsiceros*). *Rev. Infect. Dis.* **10** (Suppl. 4), S629–S633.

Hudson, L. C., Weinstock, D., Jordan, T., and Bold-Fletcher, N. O. (1996a). Clinical features of experimentally induced rabies in cattle and sheep. *J. Vet. Med. Series B* **43**, 85–95.

Hudson, L. C., Weinstock, D., Jordan, T., and Bold-Fletcher, N. O. (1996b). Clinical presentation of experimentally induced rabies in horses. *J. Vet. Med. Series B* **43**, 277–285.

Humphrey, G. L. (1971). Field control of animal rabies. In *Rabies*, Y. Nagano and F. M. Davenport (eds.), pp. 277–342, University Park Press, Baltimore.

Ian'shin, IuM., Voitanik, L. I., Ospanov, K. S., and Abdullin, B. K. (1979). [Therapeutic and preventive vaccination of persons bitten by wolves in the Aktiubinsk region]. *Zh. Mikrobiol. Epidemiol. Immunobiol.* **9**, 87–89 [Russian].

Jackson, A. C. (1994). The fatal neurologic illness of the fourth Duke of Richmond in Canada: Rabies. *Ann. R. Coil. Physicians Surg. Can.* **27**, 40–1.

Jackson, A. C., Phelan, C. C., and Rossiter, J. P. (2000). Infection of Bergmann glia in the cerebellum of a skunk experimentally infected with street rabies virus. *Can. J. Vet. Res.* **64**, 226–228.

Jaussaud, R., Strady, C., Lienard, M., and Strady, A. (2000). Rabies in France: An update. *Rev. Med. Interne* **21**, 679–683.

Jay, M. T., Reilly, K. F., Debess, E. E., Haynes, E. H., Bader, D. R., and Barrett, L. R. (1994). Rabies in a vaccinated wolf-dog hybrid. *J. Am. Vet. Med. Assoc.* **205**, 1729–1732, 1719.

Johnson, R. H. (1995). Rabies vaccination of wolf-dog hybrids. *J. Am. Vet. Med. Assoc.* **206**, 426–427.

Johnston, D. H., and Beauregard, M. (1969). Rabies epidemiology in Ontario. *J. Wildlife Dis.* **5**, 357–370.

Jorgenson, R. D., and Gough, P. M. (1976). Experimental rabies in a great horned owl. *J. Wildlife Dis.* **12**, 444–447.

Karp, B. E., Ball, N. E., Scott, C. R., and Walcoff, J. B. (1999). Rabies in two privately owned domestic rabbits. *J. Am. Vet. Med. Assoc.* **215**, 1824–1827.

Kasempimolporn, S., Saengseesom, W., Lumlertdacha, B., and Sitprija, V. (2000). Detection of rabies virus antigen in dog saliva using a latex agglutination test. *J. Clin. Microbiol.* **38**, 3098–3099.

Kaufmann, J. H. (1982). Raccoon and allies. In *Wild mammals of North America*, J. A. Chapman and G. A. Geldhamer (eds.), pp. 567–785. Johns Hopkins University Press, Baltimore.

Kemp, G. E., Causey, O. R., Moore, D. L., Odelola, A., and Fabiyi, A. (1972). Mokola virus. Further studies on IbAn 27377, a new rabies-related etiologic agent of zoonosis in Nigeria. *Am. J. Trop. Med. Hyg.* **21**, 356–359.

King, A., and Crick, J. (1988). Rabies-related viruses. In *Rabies*, J. B. Campbell (ed.), pp. 177–199. Kluwer Academic Publishers, Boston.

King, A. A., Meredith, C. D., and Thomson, G. R. (1994). The biology of southern Africa lyssavirus variants. In *Lyssaviruses*, C. E. Rupprecht (ed.), pp. 267–296. Springer-Verlag, Berlin.

Krebs, J. W., Strine, T. W., Smith, J. S., Rupprecht, C. E., and Childs, J. E. (1994). Rabies surveillance in the United States during 1993. *J. Am. Vet. Med. Assoc.* **205**, 1695–1709.

Krebs, J. W., Smith, J. S., Rupprecht, C. E., and Childs, J. E. (1999). Rabies surveillance in the United States during 1998. *J. Am. Vet. Med. Assoc.* **215**, 1786–1798.

Krebs, J. W., Rupprecht, C. E., and Childs, J. E. (2000). Rabies surveillance in the United States during 1999. *J. Am. Vet. Med. Assoc.* **217**, 1779–1811.

Lafon, M. (1994). Immunobiology of lyssaviruses: The basis for immunoprotection. In *Lyssaviruses*, C. E. Rupprecht, B. Dietzschold, and H. Koprowski (eds.), pp. 145–160. Springer-Verlag, Berlin.

le Gonidec, G., Rickenbach, A., Robin, Y., and Heme, G. (1978). Isolement d'une souche de virus Mokola au Cameroun. *Ann Microbiol. (Inst. Pasteur)* **129A**, 245–249.

Leffingwell, L. M., and Neill, S. U. (1989). Naturally acquired rabies in an armadillo (*Dasypus novemcinctus*) in Texas. *J. Clin. Microbiol.* **27**, 174–175.

Lewis, V. J., and Thacker, W. L. (1974). Limitations of deteriorated tissue for rabies diagnosis. *Health. Lab. Sci.* **11**, 8–12.

Lodmell, D. L. (1983). Genetic control of resistance to street rabies virus in mice. *J. Exp. Med.* **157**, 451–460.

Lord, R. D. (1992). Seasonal reproduction of vampire bats and its relation to seasonality of bovine rabies. *J. Wildlife Dis.* **28**, 292–294.

Martinez-Burnes, J., Lopez, A., Medellin, J., Haines, D., Loza, E., and Martinez, M. (1997). An outbreak of vampire bat–transmitted rabies in cattle in northeastern Mexico. *Can. Vet. J.* **38**, 175–177.

McLean, R. G. (1975). Raccoon rabies. In *The Natural History of Rabies*, G. M. Baer (ed.), pp. 53–76. Academic Press, New York.

Mallory, L. B. (1915). Campaign against rabies in Modoc and Lassen counties. *CA State Board of Health Monthly Bulletin* **11**, 273–277.

Mebatsion, T., Cox, J. H., and Frost, J. W. (1992a). Isolation and characterization of 115 street rabies virus isolates from Ethiopia by using monoclonal antibodies: Identification of 2 isolates as Mokola and Lagos bat viruses. *J. Infect. Dis.* **166**, 972–977.

Mebatsion, T., Sillero-Zubiri, C., Gottelli, D., and Cox, J. H. (1992b). Detection of rabies antibody by ELISA and RFFIT in unvaccinated dogs and in the endangered Simien jackal (*Canis simensis*) of Ethiopia. *Zentralbl. Veterinarmed.[B]* **39**, 233–235.

Meredith, C. D., Prossouw, A. P., and Koch, H. P. (1971). An unusual case of human rabies thought to be of chiropteran origin. *S. Afr. Med. J.* **45**, 767–769.

Meredith, C. D., and Standing, E. (1981). Lagos bat virus in South Africa. *Lancer* **11**, 832–833.

Meredith, C. D., Nel, L. H., and Von Teichman, B. F. (1996). Further isolation of Mokola virus in South Africa (Letter). *Vet. Rec.* **138**, 119–120.

Moro, M. H., Horman, J. T., Fischman, H. R., Grigor, J. K., and Israel, E. (1991). The epidemiology of rodent and lagomorph rabies in Maryland, 1981 to 1986. *J. Wildlife Dis.* **27**, 452–456.

Muller W. W. (1988) Present status of bat-rabies in Europe. *Parassitologia* **30**, 121–122.

Murphy, F. A., Bell, J. F., Bauer, S. P., Gardner, J. J., Moore, G. J., Harrison, A. K., and Coe, J. E. (1980). Experimental chronic rabies in the cat. *Lab. Invest.* **43**, 231–241.

Murray, K., Rogers, R., Selvey, L., Selleck, P., Hyatt, A., Gould, A., Gleeson, L., Hooper, P., and Westbury, H. (1995). A novel morbillivirus pneumonia of horses and its transmission to humans. *Emerg. Infect. Dis.* **1**, 31–33.

Nathanson, N., and Gonzalez-Scarano, F. (1991). Immune response to rabies virus. In *The Natural History of Rabies*, G. M. Baer (ed.), pp. 145–161. CRC Press, Boca Raton, FL.

Nettles, V. F., Shaddock, J. H., Sikes, R. K., and Reyes, C. R. (1979). Rabies in translocated raccoons. *Am. J. Public Health* **69**, 601–602.

Nichol, S. T., Rowe, J. E., and Fitch, W. M. (1993). Punctuated equilibrium and positive Darwinian evolution in vesicular stomatitis virus (see comments). *Proc. Natl. Acad. Sci. USA* **90**, 10424–10428.

Niezgoda, M., Diehl, D., Hanlon, C. A., and Rupprecht, C. E. (1991). Pathogenesis of street rabies virus in raccoons. Wildlife Disease Association, 40th Annual Conference, Fort Collins, CO, pp. 57–58.

Niezgoda, M., Briggs, D. J., Shaddock, J., Dreesen, D. W., and Rupprecht, C. E. (1997). Pathogenesis of experimentally induced rabies in domestic ferrets. *Am. J. Vet. Res.* **58**, 1327–1331.

Niezgoda, M., Briggs, D. J., Shaddock, J., and Rupprecht, C. E. (1998). Viral excretion in domestic ferrets (*Mustela putorius furo*) inoculated with a raccoon rabies isolate. *Am. J. Vet. Res.* **59**, 1629–1632.

Noah, D. L., Smith, M. G., Gotthardt, J. C., Krebs, J. W., Green, D., and Childs, J. E. (1996). Mass human exposure to rabies in New Hampshire: Exposures, treatment, and cost. *Am. J. Public Health* **86**, 1149–1151.

Nowak, A. (1991). In *Mammals of the World*, Walker (ed.) Johns Hopkins University Press, Baltimore.

Odegaard, O. A., and Krogsrud, J. (1981). Rabies in Svalbard: Infection diagnosed in arctic fox, reindeer and seal. *Vet. Rec.* **109**, 141–142.

Orr, P. H., Rubin, M. R., and Aoki, F. Y. (1988). Naturally acquired serum rabies neutralizing antibody in a Canadian Inuit population. *Arctic Med. Res.* **47**, 699–700.

Overall, K. L. (2000). Rabies vaccine labeling and the wolf hybrid. *J. Am. Vet. Med. Assoc.* **216**, 20.

Pal, S. R., Arora, B., Chhuttani, P. N., Broor, S., Choudhury, S., Joshi, R. M., and Ray, S. D. (1980). Rabies virus infection of a flying fox bat, *Pteropus policephalus*, in Chandigarh, Northern India. *Trop. Geogr. Med.* **32**, 265–267.

Pape, W. J., Fitzsimmons, T. D., and Hoffman, R. E. (1999). Risk for rabies transmission from encounters with bats, Colorado, 1977–1996. *Emerg. Infect. Dis.* **5**, 433–437.

Parker, R. L., and Wilsnack, R. E. (1966). Pathogenesis of skunk rabies virus: Quantitation in skunks and foxes. *Am. J. Vet. Res.* **27**, 33–38.

Perez-Jorda, J. L., Ibanez, C., Munoz-Cervera, M., and Tellez, A. (1995). *Lyssavirus* in *Eptesicus serotinus* (*Chiroptera: Vespertilionidae*). *J. Wildlife Dis.* **31**, 372–377.

Perl, D. P., Bell, J. F., and Moore, G. J. (1977). Chronic recrudescent rabies in a cat. *Proc. Soc. Exp. Biol. Med.* **155**, 540–548.

Rausch, R. L. (1975). Rabies in experimentally infected bears, *Ursus* spp., with epizootiologic notes. *Zentralbl. Veterinarmed.[B]* **22**, 420–437.

Records, E. (1932). Rabies — Its history in Nevada. *Calif. West. Med.* **37**, 90–94.

Rhode, R. E., Neill, S. U., Clark, K. A., and Smith, J. S. (1997). Molecular epidemiology of rabies epizootics in Texas. *Clin. Diagn. Virol.* **8**, 209–217.

Rhodes, C. J., Atkinson, R. P., Anderson, R. M., and Macdonald, D. W. (1998). Rabies in Zimbabwe: Reservoir dogs and the implications for disease control. *Philos. Trans. R. Soc. Lond. [B].* **353**, 999–1010.

Rosatte, R. C., and Gunson, J. R. (1984). Presence of neutralizing antibodies to rabies virus in striped skunks from areas free of skunk rabies in Alberta. *J. Wildlife Dis.* **20**, 171–176.

Rottcher, D., and Sawchuk, A.M. (1978). Wildlife rabies in Zambia. *J. Wildlife Dis.* **14**, 513–517.

Rupprecht, C. E., Hamir, A. N., Johnston, D. H., and Koprowski, H. (1988). Efficacy of a vaccinia–rabies glycoprotein recombinant virus vaccine in raccoons (*Procyon lotor*). *Rev. Infect. Dis.* **10** (Suppl. 4), S803–S809.

Rupprecht, C. E., Gilbert, J., Pitts, R., Marshall, K. R., and Koprowski, H. (1990). Evaluation of an inactivated rabies virus vaccine in domestic ferrets. *J. Am. Vet. Med. Assoc.* **196**, 1614–1616.

Rupprecht, C. E., Nesby, S., Fekadu, M., Orciari, L. A., Shaddock, J. S., Sanderlin, D., Yager, P., Whitfield, and Smith, J. S. (1994). When the "impossible" happens: Non-bite rabies contamination in a laboratory beagle. In *Proceedings of the Vth Annual International Meeting, Advances Towards Rabies Control in the Americas*, Niagara Falls, Ontario, Canada.

Rupprecht, C. E., Smith, J. S., Yager, P. A., Orciari, L. A., Shaddock, J. S., Sanderlin, D., Niezgoda, M., Whitfleld, S., Shoemake, H., Warner, C. K., Gleeson, L., and Murray, K. (1996). Preliminary analysis of a new lyssavirus isolated from an Australian fruit bat. In *Proceedings of the VIIth Annual International Meeting, Advances Towards Rabies Control in the Americas*, Centers for Disease Control and Prevention, Atlanta, GA.

Saluzzo, J.-F., Rollin, P. E., Dauguet, C., Digoutte, J.-P., Georges, A.-J., and Sureau, P. (1984). Premier isolement du virus Mokola a partir d'un rongeur (*Lophuromys sikapusi*). *Ann. Virol. (Inst. Pasteur)* **135E**, 57–66.

Sawchuk, A. M., and Rottcher, D. (1978). Mongoose rabies in Zambia. *J. Wildlife Dis.* **14**, 54–55.

Schneider, L. G., and Burtscher, H. (1967). Studies on the pathogenesis of rabies in fowls after intracerebral infection. *Zentralbl. Veterinarmed.[B].* **14**, 598–624.

Schneider, L. G., Barnard, B. J. H., and Schneider, H. P. (1985). Application of monclonal antibodies for epidemiological investigations and oral vaccination studies. In *Rabies in the Tropics*, pp. 47–53.

Schneider, L. G., and Cox, J. H. (1994). Bat lyssaviruses in Europe. In *Lyssaviruses*, C. E. Rupprecht, B. Dietzschold, and H. Koprowski (eds.), pp. 207–218. Springer-Verlag, Berlin.

Seganti, L., Superti F., Bianchi, S., Orsi, N., Divizia, M., and Pana, A. (1990). Susceptibility of mammalian, avian, fish, and mosquito cell lines to rabies virus infection. *Acta. Virol. (Praha)* **34**, 155–163.

Selimov, M. A., Klyueva, E. V., Aksenova, T. A., Lebedeva, I. R., and Gribencha, L. F. (1978). Treatment of patients bitten by rabid or suspected rabid wolves with inactivated tissue culture rabies vaccine and rabies gammaglobulin. *Dev. Biol. Stand.* **40**, 141–146.

Shah, U., and Jaswal, G. S. (1976). Victims of a rabid wolf in india: Effect of severity and location of bites on development of rabies. *J. Infect. Dis.* **134**, 25–29.

Shannon, L. M., Poulton, J. L., Emmons, R. W., Woodie, J. D., and Fowler, M. E. (1988). Serological survey for rabies antibodies in raptors from California. *J. Wildlife Dis.* **24**, 264–267.

Shope, R. E., Murphy, F. A., Harrison, A. K., Causey, O. R., Kemp, G. E., Simpson, D. I., and Moore, D. L. (1970). Two African viruses serologically and morphologically related to rabies virus. *J. Viral.* **6**, 690–692.

Shope, R. (1975). Rabies virus antigenic relationships. In *The Natural History of Rabies*, G. M. Baer (ed.), Vol. I, pp. 141–152. Academic Press, New York.

Sikes, R. K., and Tierkel, E. S. (1961). Wildlife rabies studies in the southeast. In *Proceedings of the 64th Annual Meeting of the U.S. Livestock Sanitation Association*, Charleston, WV, pp. 268–272.

Sikes, R. K. (1962). Pathogenesis of rabies in wildlife: I. Comparative effect of varying doses of rabies virus inoculated into foxes and skunks. *Am. J. Vet. Res.* **23**, 1041–1047.

Sikes, R. K., and Tierkel, E. S. (1966). Wolf, fox and coyote rabies. In *Proceedings of the National Rabies Symposium*. U.S. Department of Health, Education and Welfare. Public Health Service, Atlanta, GA, pp. 31–33.

Sillero-Zubiri, C., King, A. A., and Macdonald, D. W. (1996). Rabies and mortality in Ethiopian wolves (*Canis simensis*). *J. Wildlife Dis.* **32**, 80–86.

Smart, N. L., and Charlton, K. M. (1992). The distribution of challenge virus standard rabies virus versus skunk street rabies virus in the brains of experimentally infected rabid skunks. *Acta. Neuropathol. (Berl.)* **84**, 501–508.

Smith, J. S., Sumner, J. W., Roumillat, L. F., Baer, G. M., and Winkler, W. G. (1984). Antigenic characteristics of isolates associated with a new epizootic of raccoon rabies in the United States. *J. Infect. Dis.* **149**, 769–774.

Smith, J. S., and Seidel, H. D. (1993). Rabies: A new look at an old disease. *Prog. Med. Virol.* **40**, 82–106.

Smith, J. S. (1996). New aspects of rabies with emphasis on epidemiology, diagnosis, and prevention of the disease in the United States. *Clin. Microbiol. Rev.* **9**, 166–176.

Somayajulu, M. V., and Reddy, G. V. (1989). Live dogs and dead men. *J. Assoc. Phys. India* **37**, 6–17.

Speare, R., Skerratt, L., Foster, R., Berger, L., Hooper, P., Lunt, R., Blair, D., Hansman, D., Goulet, M., and Cooper, S. (1997). Australian bat lyssavirus infection in three fruit bats from north Queensland. *Commun. Dis. Intell.* **21**, 117–120.

Steck, F. (1968). Zoonoses in Britain: Some present and potential hazards to man. Rabies, the European situation. *Vet. Rec.* **83** (Suppl. 15).

Steck, F., and Wandeler, A. (1980). The epidemiology of fox rabies in Europe. *Epidemiol. Rev.* **2**, 71–96.

Steele, J. H., and Fernandez, P. J. (1991). History of rabies and global aspects. In *The Natural History of Rabies*, G. M. Baer (ed.), pp. 1–24. CRC Press, Boca Raton, FL.

Stoltenow, C. L., Shirely, L. A., Jones, T., and Rupprecht, C. E. (1999). Clinical report: Atypical rabies in a cow. *Bovine Pract.* **33**, 4–5.

Stoltenow, C. L., Solemsass, K., Niezgoda, M., Yager, P., and Rupprecht, C. E. (2000). Rabies in an American bison from North Dakota. *J. Wildlife Dis.* **36**, 169–171.

Sureau, P., Germain, M., Herve, J. P., Geoffroy, B., Cornet, J. P., Heme, G., and Robin, Y. (1977). Isolation of the Lagos-bat virus in the Central African Republic. *Bull. Soc. Pathol. Exot. Filiales* **70**, 467–470.

Swanepoel, R., Barnard, B. J. H., Meredith, C. D., Bishop, G. C., Bruckner, G. K., Foggin, C. M., and Hubschle, O. J. B. (1993). Rabies in southern Africa. *Onderstepoort J. Vet. Res.* **60**, 325–346.

Tabel, H., Corner, A. H., Webster, W. A., and Casey, C. A. (1974). History and epizootiology of rabies in Canada. *Can. Vet. J.* **15**, 271–281.

Tan, D. S., Peck, A. J., and Omar, M. (1969). The importance of Malaysian bats in the transmission of oral disease. *Med. J. Malaysia* **24**, 32–35.

Taylor, M., Elkin, B., Maier, N., and Bradley, M. (1991). Observation of a polar bear with rabies. *J. Wildlife Dis.* **27**, 337–339.

Theberge, J. B., Forbes, G. J., Barker, I. K., and Bollinger, T. (1994). Rabies in wolves of the Great Lakes region. *J. Wildlife Dis.* **30**, 563–566.

Tidemann, C. R., Vardon, M. J., Nelson, J. E., Speare, R., and Gleeson, L. J. (1997). Health and conservation implications of Australian bat lyssavirus. *Aust. Zool.* **30**, 369–376.

Tignor, G. H., Murphy, F. A., Clark, H. F., Shope, R. E., Madore, P., Bauer, S. P., Buckely, S. M., and Meredith, C. D. (1977). Duvenhage virus: morphological, biochemical, histopathological, and antigenic relationships to the rabies serogroup. *J. Gen. Virol.* **37**, 595–611.

Toma, B., and Andral, L. (1977). Epidemiology of fox rabies. *Adv. Virus Res.* **21**, 1–36.

Tordo, N. (1996). Characteristics and molecular biology of the rabies virus. In *Laboratory Techniques in Rabies* F. X. Meslin, M. M. Kaplan, and H. Koprowski (eds.), pp. 28–51. World Health Organization, Geneva.

Trimarchi, C. V., and Debbie, J. (1977). Naturally occurring rabies virus and neutralizing antibody in two species of insectivorous bats of New York State. *J. Wildlife Dis.* **13**, 366–369.

Trimarchi, C. V., Rudd, R. J., and Abelseth, M. K. (1986). Experimentally induced rabies in four cats inoculated with a rabies virus isolated from a bat. *Am. J. Vet. Res.* **47**, 777–780.

Vaughn, J. B., Gerhardt, P., and Paterson, J. (1963). Excretion of street rabies virus in saliva of cats. *JAMA* **184**, 705.

Vaughn, J. B., Gerhardt, P., and Newell, K. W. (1965). Excretion of street rabies virus in the saliva of dogs. *JAMA* **193**, 363–368.

Vila, C., Amorim, I. R., Leonard, J. A., Posada, D., Castroviejo, J., Petrucci-Fonseca, F., Crandall, K. A., Ellegren, H., and Wayne, R. K. (1999). Mitochondrial DNA phylogeography and population history of the gray wolf, *Canis lupus*. *Mol. Ecol.* **8**, 2089–2103.

Walroth, R., Brown, N., Wandeler, A., Casey, A., and MacInnes, C. (1996). Rabid black bears in Ontario. *Can. Vet. J.* **37**, 492.

Wandeler, A., Muller, J., Wachendorfer, G., Schale, W., Forster, U., and Steck, F. (1974). Rabies in wild carnivores in central Europe: III. Ecology and biology of the fox in relation to control operations. *Zentralbl. Veterinarmed.[B]*. **21**, 765–773.

Wandeler, A. I. (1980). Epidemiology of fox rabies. In *The Red Fox*, E. Zimen (ed.), pp. 237–249. Kluwer, Boston.

Wandeler, A. I., Nadin-Davis, S. A., Tinline, R. R., and Rupprecht, C. E. (1994). Rabies epizootiology: An ecological and evolutionary perspective. *Curr. Top. Microbiol. Immunol.* **186**, 297–324.

Weiler, G. J., Garner, G. W., and Ritter, D. G. (1995). Occurrence of rabies in a wolf population in northeastern Alaska. *J Wildlife Dis.* **31**, 79–82.

Whitby, J. E., Johnstone, P., and Sillero-Zubiri, C. (1997). Rabies virus in the decomposed brain of an Ethiopian wolf detected by nested reverse transcription-polymerase chain reaction. *J. Wildlife Dis.* **4**, 912–915.

Whitby, J. E., Heaton, P. R., Black, E. M., Wooldridge, M., McElhinney, L. M., and Johnstone, P. (2000). First isolation of a rabies-related virus from a Daubenton's bat in the United Kingdom. *Vet. Rec.* **147**, 385–388.

Wiktor, T. J., and Koprowski, H. (1978). Monoclonal antibodies against rabies virus produced by somatic cell hybridization: Detection of antigenic variants. *Proc. Natl. Acad. Sci. USA* **75**, 3938–3942.

Wilbur, L. A., and Aubert, M. F. A. (1996). The NIH test for potency. In *Laboratory Techniques in Rabies*, F.-X. Meslin, M. M. Kaplan, and H. Koprowski (eds.), 4th ed., pp. 360–368. World Health Organization, Geneva.

Wilkinson, L. (1988). Understanding the nature of rabies: An historical perspective. In *Rabies*, J. B. Campbell and K. M. Charlton (eds.), pp. 1–23. Kluwer Academic Publishers, Boston.

Wimalaratne, O., and Kodikara, D. S. (1999). First reported case of elephant rabies in Sri Lanka. *Vet. Rec.* **144**, 98.

Winkler, W. G., Baker, E. R., and Hopkins, C. C. (1972). An outbreak of non-bite transmitted rabies in a laboratory animal colony. *Am. J. Epidemiol.* **95**, 267–277.

Winkler, W. G. (1975). Fox rabies. In *The Natural History of Rabies*, G. M. Baer (ed.), 2nd., pp. 3–22. Academic Press, New York.

Winkler, W. G., Shaddock, J. S., and Bowman, C. (1985). Rabies virus in salivary glands of raccoons (*Procyon lotor*). *J. Wildlife Dis.* **21**, 297–298.

Winkler, W. G., and Jenkins, S. R. (1991). Raccoon rabies. In *The Natural History of Rabies*, G. M. Baer (ed.), pp. 325–340. CRC Press, Boca Raton, FL.

Xiang, Z. Q., Knowles, B. B., McCarrick, J. W., and Ertl, H. C. J. (1995). Immune effector mechanisms required for protection to rabies virus. *Virology* **214**, 398–404.

Yamaoka, H. (1962). Rabies virus inoculated into the quail. *Ann. Paediatr. Jpn.* **8**, 92–96.

6

Human Disease

ALAN C. JACKSON

Departments of Medicine (Neurology) and Microbiology and Immunology
Queen's University
Kingston, Ontario, K7L 3N6
Canada

I. INTRODUCTION

Since antiquity, rabies has been one of the most feared diseases. Human rabies remains an important public health problem in many developing countries where dog rabies is endemic. Worldwide, there are over 30,000 reported human deaths each year due to rabies (World Health Organization, 2000), and the actual number probably exceeds 50,000. In the 1990s, up to 6 human cases of rabies were diagnosed per year in the United States, and many of these infections were acquired indigenously from unrecognized exposures to insectivorous bats

219

(Noah *et al.*, 1998). A significant number of additional rabies cases probably go unrecognized in the United States and Canada because undiagnosed acute and fatal neurologic illnesses are not uncommon and a history of an animal exposure may not exist.

II. EXPOSURES AND INCUBATION PERIOD

The infectious cycle of rabies virus is perpetuated mainly through animal bites with the deposition of rabies virus–laden saliva into subcutaneous tissues and muscle. With respect to human rabies, worldwide, dogs are by far the most common and important rabies vector; bats are most important in the United States and Canada, although there is also a reservoir in terrestrial animals. Other types of nonbite exposures, including contamination of an open wound, scratch, abrasion, or mucous membrane by saliva or central nervous system (CNS) tissue from an infected animal, occur commonly but are rarely responsible for transmission of rabies virus. Handling and skinning of infected carcasses and perhaps consumption of raw infected meat have resulted in transmission of rabies virus (Tariq *et al.*, 1991; Kureishi *et al.*, 1992; Wallerstein, 1999). Rarely, inhalation of aerosolized rabies virus in caves containing millions of bats (Constantine, 1962) or in laboratories (Winkler *et al.*, 1973; Tillotson *et al.*, 1977b) has resulted in human rabies. At least eight cases of rabies have resulted from transplantation (human-to-human) of rabies virus–infected corneas (Table I). In another report, transmission did not occur after corneal transplantation from a donor with rabies after postexposure prophylactic therapy was initiated (Sureau *et al.*, 1981).

TABLE I

Human Rabies Cases Transmitted by Corneal Transplantation

Location	Year	Age of patient (recipient)	Time to death (days)	Reference
United States	1978	37	50	Houff *et al.*, 1979
France	1979	36	41	Galian *et al.*, 1980
Thailand	1981	41	22	Thongcharoen *et al.*, 1981
Thailand	1981	25	33	Thongcharoen *et al.*, 1981
India	1987	62	15	Gode and Bhide, 1988
India	1988	48	264[a]	Gode and Bhide, 1988
Iran	1994	40	27	Javadi *et al.*, 1996
Iran	1994	35	41	Javadi *et al.*, 1996

[a] Patient received two doses of rabies vaccine about 1 month after the transplant.

Transplantation of other tissues or organs has not been documented to date to be associated with transmission of rabies virus, but it is clear that tissues or organs should never be transplanted from a donor who dies from an undiagnosed neurologic disease. Most other reported cases of human-to-human transmission have not been well documented. Two patients with rabies from Ethiopia were described, and their only known exposure was contact with family members who died of rabies (Fekadu et al., 1996). In this report, a 41-year-old woman died of rabies 33 days after her 5-year-old son died of rabies; he had bitten his mother on her little finger. A 5-year-old boy presented with rabies 36 days after his mother died of rabies; he had repeatedly received kisses from his mother on his mouth during her illness. Sexual transmission of rabies virus is not well documented. Although natural human-to-human transmission of rabies likely occurs very rarely, anyone in direct contact with rabies patients, including family members and health care workers, should employ strict isolation precautions in order to minimize the risk of transmission of the virus via saliva or other secretions (Remington et al., 1985). Evidence of transplacental transmission of rabies virus exists in a single report from Turkey (Sipahioglu and Alpaut, 1985).

Human rabies usually develops 20–90 days after exposure, although occasionally disease develops after only a few days (Anderson et al., 1984), and rare cases have occurred after a year or more following exposure. Three immigrants from Laos, the Philippines, and Mexico developed rabies in the United States due to rabies virus strains from their countries of origin with incubation periods of at least 11 months and 4 and 6 years, which were based on the time of their immigration (Smith et al., 1991). The incubation period (from exposure to onset of disease) in rabies has a greater length and variability than in most other infectious diseases, which may cause considerable emotional stress to the patient. Very long incubation periods raise the possibility of another unrecognized or forgotten exposure, particularly in rabies-endemic areas. Severe multiple bites and facial bites are associated with shorter incubation periods (Warrell and Warrell, 1991), although attempts to find a clear correlation between the site of the bite and the incubation period have not been successful (Dupont and Earle, 1965). There may be no history of a bite exposure because it was either unrecognized, particularly with insectivorous bat bites (Jackson and Fenton, 2001), or forgotten or because no inquiry was made while the patient was still lucid. With known bite exposures from rabid animals, the following has been observed in untreated persons who develop rabies: 50–80% occurrence after head bites, 15–40% after hand or arm bites, and 3–10% after leg bites, and the risk is about 0.1% for contamination of minor wounds with saliva, including scratches (Hattwick, 1974). The biologic bases for this is unclear, but it may be related to a number of factors, including the density of rabies virus receptors in affected tissues, the degree of innervation in tissues in different anatomic locations, the quantity of virus inoculated, and the properties of the rabies virus variant. Some individuals with rabies virus exposures may have inapparent rabies virus infection and develop naturally acquired immunity (Doege and Northrop, 1974). Low titers of rabies virus neutralizing antibodies were present in Canadian Inuit hunters (7 of 20) and their wives (2 of 11) (Orr *et al.*, 1988) and also in 6.6% (15 of 226) of unimmunized students and faculty members of a veterinary medical school at the inception of a rabies vaccine trial (Ruegsegger *et al.*, 1961).

In rabies, nonspecific prodromal symptoms, including fever, chills, malaise, fatigue, insomnia, anorexia, headache, anxiety, and irritability, may last for up to 10 days prior to the onset of neurologic symptoms (Warrell, 1976). About 30–70% of patients develop pain, paresthesias, and/or pruritus at or close to the site of the bite, and the bite wound often has healed by the time that these symptoms develop (Dupont and Earle, 1965; Hattwick, 1974). These local neurologic symptoms are likely more common with bat virus strains than with dog virus strains (Hemachudha, 1997a; Noah *et al.*, 1998). The pruritus may result in severe excoriations from scratching. Retroorbital pain also occurred as an early symptom in some of the patients with transmission by corneal transplantation. Local neurologic symptoms may reflect infection involving local peripheral sensory ganglia (dorsal root or trigeminal ganglia). Weakness also may develop in the bitten extremity, and this may be more common after transmission of rabies virus from bats than from dogs (Hemachudha, 1997a). The initial neurologic symptoms occasionally may occur at a site distant from the bite, although the pathogenic basis for this phenomenon is not clear. This has been described in two patients bitten on their toes who developed severe itching of their ears (Hemachudha, 1994). Tremor also has been described involving the bitten extremity (Warrell, 1976).

III. CLINICAL FORMS OF DISEASE

A. Classic Rabies

About 80% of patients develop a classic or encephalitic (also called *furious*) form of rabies, and about 20% experience a paralytic form of disease. In classic rabies, patients have episodes of generalized arousal or hyperexcitability that are separated by lucid periods (Warrell, 1976), and these features reflect brain involvement with the infection. Intermittent episodes may occur with confusion, hallucinations, agitation, and aggressive behavior, which typically last for periods of 1–5 minutes (Hattwick, 1974; Warrell and Warrell, 1991; Hemachudha, 1997b). The episodes may occur spontaneously or be precipitated by a variety of sensory stimuli (tactile, auditory, visual, or olfactory). Biting behavior of patients with rabies has been described (Dupont and Earle, 1965; Emmons *et al.*, 1973; Warrell, 1976), but it is unusual. Fever is common and may be quite high (over 42°C), and there may be signs of autonomic dysfunction, including hypersalivation, lacrimation, sweating, piloerection (gooseflesh), and dilated pupils. The autonomic dysfunction may result from the infection directly involving the autonomic nervous system in the hypothalamus, spinal cord, and/or autonomic ganglia. Parasympathetic stimulation may increase the production of saliva above the normal volume of about 1 liter per 24 hours. Often patients appear frightened with wide palpebral fissures, dilated pupils, and an open mouth (Nicholson, 1994). Movement disorders have been noted (Warrell, 1976). Seizures, including convulsions, may occur, but they are not common, and they usually occur late in the illness. Cranial nerve signs may be present, including ophthalmoplegia, facial weakness, impaired swallowing, and tongue weakness. There also may be nuchal rigidity, reflecting leptomeningeal inflammation.

About 50–80% of patients develop hydrophobia, which is a characteristic and the most widely recognized manifestation of rabies. Hydrophobia is not a feature of other neurologic diseases. The term *hydrophobia* is derived from the Greek meaning "fear of water." Patients initially may experience pain in the throat or difficulty swallowing. On attempts to swallow, they experience contractions of the diaphragm, sternocleidomastoids, scalenes, and other accessory muscles of inspiration that last for about 5–15 seconds and may be associated with epigastric pain (Fig. 1). These symptoms may be followed by contraction of neck muscles,

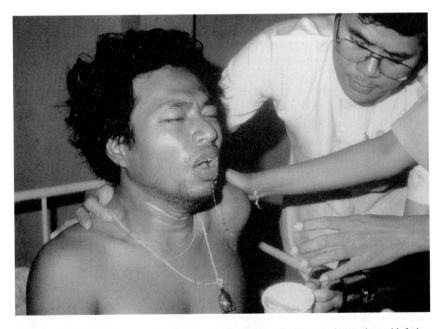

Fig. 1. Hydrophobic spasm of inspiratory muscles associated with terror in a patient with furious rabies encephalitis attempting to swallow water. (*Copyright D. A. Warrell, Oxford, UK*).

resulting in flexion or extension of the neck, and rarely by opisthotonic posturing. There may be associated retching, vomiting, coughing, aspiration into the trachea, grimacing, convulsions, and hypoxia (Editorial, 1975). Patients may die during severe spasms with the development of cardiorespiratory arrest if supportive care measures are not initiated (Warrell and Warrell, 1991). During the spasms, there is an associated feeling of terror, often without associated pain. Patients avoid drinking for long periods of time, often despite intense thirst, resulting in dehydration. Subsequently, the sight, sound, or even mention of water (or liquids) may trigger these spasms, indicating that hydrophobia is reinforced by conditioning (Warrell et al., 1976). Hydrophobic spasms also may occur spontaneously, particularly later in the course of the illness. A draft of air on the skin or the breath of an examiner may have the same effect, which has been termed *aerophobia*, and a number of other stimuli, including water splashed on the skin, attempts by the patient to speak, and stimulation from bright lights or loud sounds, also may precipitate spasms (Warrell, 1976). Patients may wear heavy clothing in order to avoid drafts. The fan test, elicited by fanning a current of air across the face and observing the patient for spasms of the pharyngeal and neck muscles, has been used as a diagnostic test at the bedside to demonstrate the presence of aerophobia (Wilson et al., 1975). Sobbing respiration (like a child who has been crying) with a two-stage (sniff-sniff) inspiration followed by a slow, full expiration has been described (Pearson, 1976). Later these spasms merge with the development of periodic, apneustic, or ataxic breathing as the patient's level of consciousness deteriorates (Warrell et al., 1976). The hydrophobia of rabies is likely due to selective infection of neurons that inhibit the inspiratory motor neurons in the region of the nucleus ambiguus in the brainstem (Warrell et al., 1976; Warrell, 1976). This results in exaggeration of defensive reflexes that protect the respiratory tract. Vocal cord weakness may result in a change in the voice, and patients may make barklike sounds. Increased libido, priapism (painful spontaneous erections), and spontaneous ejaculations occur occasionally in rabies, and they may be early manifestations of the disease (Gardner, 1970; Talaulicar, 1977; Bhandari and Kumar, 1986; Udwadia et al., 1988; Dutta, 1996). There is often progression to severe flaccid paralysis, coma, and multiple organ failure. The paralysis that develops either in association with or after the development of coma should not be confused with paralytic rabies, in which the muscle weakness develops early in the course of the illness (see Sect. IIIB). Rabies is fatal, and death usually occurs within 14 days of the onset of clinical manifestations, although the time of death may be delayed with initiation of intensive care measures. One patient survived for 133 days (Emmons et al., 1973).

A wide variety of medical complications can develop in patients with rabies. Many of these complications occur in critically ill patients with other acute neurological disorders, but some may be related to the widespread infection in the CNS with systemic (extraneural) organ involvement (Jackson et al., 1999).

Cardiopulmonary complications are the most common and important. Respiratory complications include hyperventilation, hypoxemia, respiratory depression with apnea, atelectasis, and aspiration with secondary pneumonia (Hattwick, 1974). Sinus tachycardia is a common cardiac feature, and the degree of the tachycardia is often in excess of that expected for the degree of fever (Warrell *et al.*, 1976). Cardiac arrhythmias (including wandering atrial/nodal pacemaker, sinus brady-cardia, and supraventricular or ventricular ectopic beats), hypotension, heart fail-ure, and cardiac arrest may occur (Hattwick, 1974; Warrell *et al.*, 1976). Cardiac arrhythmias may account for the sudden death of patients who are alert and do not have advanced neurologic signs of rabies. Cardiac manifestations may reflect infection involving the autonomic nervous system or myocardium (Ross and Armentrout, 1962; Cheetham *et al.*, 1970; Raman *et al.*, 1988; Metze and Feiden, 1991; Jackson *et al.*, 1999). Either hyperthermia or hypothermia may be present, likely reflecting hypothalamic involvement of the infection. Gastrointestinal hemorrhage, often including hematemesis, is a common complication (Kureishi *et al.*, 1992). Endocrine complications include both inappropriate secretion of antidiuretic hormone and diabetes insipidus (Hattwick, 1974; Bhatt *et al.*, 1974).

B. Paralytic Rabies

In paralytic rabies, flaccid muscle weakness develops early in the course of the disease, and the weakness is prominent. It is likely that patients frequently are misdiagnosed with this clinical form of the disease, especially if a history of an animal bite is not obtained. The earliest description of paralytic rabies was recorded in 1887 (Gamaleia, 1887). Paralytic rabies also has been called *dumb rabies*. Patients may be literally dumb or mute due to laryngeal muscle weakness, but the term *dumb rabies* usually refers to the quieter clinical features and promi-nent weakness rather than specifically to the presence of anarthria (Editorial, 1978; Mills *et al.*, 1978). The development of paralytic rabies does not appear to be related to the anatomic site of the bite (Tirawatnpong *et al.*, 1989), and the incubation period is similar to that in classic rabies. Patients are alert with a nor-mal mental status at the onset of this clinical form of rabies. The weakness often begins in the bitten extremity and spreads to involve the other extremities, some-times in an ascending pattern. Muscle fasciculations may be present (Phuapradit *et al.*, 1985). Frequently, the facial muscles are weak bilaterally. Associated bilateral deafness has been reported (Phuapradit *et al.*, 1985). Although patients may have local pain, paresthesias, or pruritus at the site of the bite, the sensory examination is usually normal in these patients. The clinical picture may be confused with the Guillain-Barré syndrome, including both the acute inflamma-tory demyelinating polyradiculopathy and the more severe motor–sensory neu-ropathy of acute onset with predominantly axonal lesions (called the *axonal*

Guillain-Barré syndrome) (Feasby *et al.*, 1986; Griffin *et al.*, 1996; Sheikh *et al.*, 1998). Sphincter involvement, especially with urinary incontinence, is common in paralytic rabies, but this is not a feature of the Guillain-Barré syndrome (Asbury and Cornblath, 1990). In addition, pain and sensory disturbances may occur in paralytic rabies. Myoedema has been reported as a sign observed in paralytic rabies but not in classic rabies (Hemachudha *et al.*, 1987). However, myoedema has not been confirmed as an important sign of paralytic rabies in other reports. In myoedema, percussion of a muscle (e.g., deltoid or thigh muscle) with a tendon hammer results in local mounding of the muscle without propagated contractions and with electrical silence; the mounding disappears over a few seconds. Myoedema is thought to be a normal physiologic phenomenon, and its presence does not indicate neuromuscular pathology (Hornung and Nix, 1992). Hence the importance of this sign in rabies needs clarification in the future. Bulbar and respiratory muscles eventually become weak in paralytic rabies, resulting in death. Hydrophobia is more unusual in the paralytic form of the disease, although mild inspiratory spasms are observed commonly (Hemachudha *et al.*, 1988). Survival in paralytic rabies is usually longer (up to 30 days) than in classic rabies. It is unclear if the hydrophobic spasms per se lead to death in the first few days of illness in classic disease (Editorial, 1978) or if they are a reflection of a more life-threatening distribution of the infection in the nervous system.

An unusual human outbreak of rabies affecting over 70 people occurred in Trinidad between 1929 and 1937 with transmission of the virus from vampire bats (Hurst and Pawan, 1931; Pawan, 1939; Waterman, 1959). All patients with rabies in this outbreak had the paralytic form of the disease. This led to diagnostic uncertainty, and initially, poliomyelitis and botulism were suspected. A similar outbreak of paralytic rabies has not been observed elsewhere, although 9 miners died of paralytic rabies transmitted by vampire bats in British Guiana (presently Guyana) in 1953 (Nehaul, 1955). Similarly, 7 children died of paralytic rabies in Surinam in 1973–1974, and vampire bats probably also were the responsible vector (Verlinde *et al.*, 1975). However, rabies virus transmitted by vampire bats does not always produce paralytic rabies. A 1990 outbreak of human rabies in Peru with transmission from vampire bats exclusively produced cases of classic rabies (Lopez *et al.*, 1992). Furthermore, it has been observed that a dog may bite two individuals and one develops classic rabies while the other develops paralytic rabies (Hemachudha *et al.*, 1988; Wilde and Chutivongse, 1988).

The pathogenetic basis for the two different clinical forms of rabies has not been determined. In a small series, there were no marked differences in the regional distribution of rabies virus antigen or in the inflammatory changes (Tirawatnpong *et al.*, 1989). However, at the time of death, the distribution of the viral infection may be much more widespread and not closely reflect the distribution at the time of the patient's presentation with paralytic rabies. It is curious that an earlier serum neutralizing antibody response was observed in patients with classic rabies than in those with paralytic rabies (Hemachudha, 1994). There is evidence that patients with paralytic rabies have defects in immune responsiveness, including lack of lymphocyte proliferative responses to rabies virus antigen (Hemachudha et al., 1988) and lower levels of serum cytokines, including interleukin-6 and the soluble interleukin-2 receptor, than patients with classic rabies (Hemachudha et al., 1993). In contrast, there is evidence from a Chinese case that an immunopathologic attack on rabies virus–infected axons, which was most marked in the ventral spinal nerve roots, may be important in the pathogenesis of paralytic rabies (Sheikh et al., 1998).

IV. INVESTIGATIONS

A. Imaging Studies

Computed tomographic (CT) studies of the brain usually are normal in rabies (Faoagali et al., 1988; Mrak and Young, 1993; White et al., 1994), although hypodense cortical lesions (Sow et al., 1996) and nonenhancing basal ganglia hypodensities (Awasthi et al., 2001) have been described. There have been a few reports of magnetic resonance imaging (MRI) studies of the brain, although both normal findings (Mrak and Young, 1993; Sing and Soo, 1996) and increased signals in gray matter areas have been reported (Hantson et al., 1993; Awasthi et al., 2001). Increased signals were observed on T_2-weighted images in the medulla (Fig. 2) and pons with only minimal gadolinium enhancement in these areas in a patient from California infected by a rabies virus strain associated with Mexican free-tailed bats (Pleasure and Fischbein, 2000). Gadolinium enhancement of cervical nerve roots was described in a patient with paralytic rabies (Laothamatas et al., 1997). Gadolinium enhancement involving the medulla and hypothalamus also was described in the same report in another patient with paralytic rabies. This indicates imaging evidence of brain infection, which has been shown in histopathologic studies at the time of death (Chopra et al., 1980).

B. Laboratory Studies

The electroencephalogram may be normal or show nonspecific abnormalities in human rabies. Slow wave activity has been observed as well as periodic (Komsuoglu et al., 1981) and epileptiform activity. Detailed electrophysiologic studies, including nerve conduction velocities and electromyography, have not been reported to date. Electrophysiologic evidence of a primary axonal neuropathy was found in two patients with paralytic rabies (Prier et al., 1979a,b).

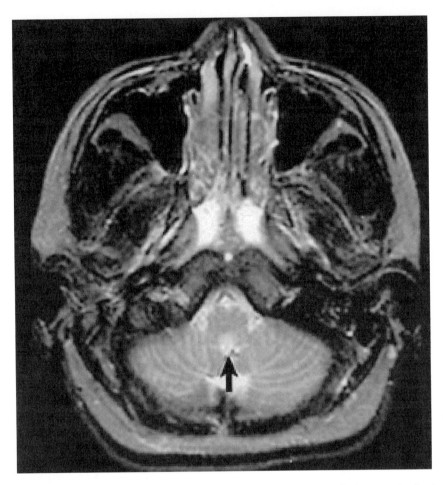

Fig. 2. An axial T_2-weighted magnetic resonance image through the medulla demonstrating focal increased signal in the dorsal midline (*arrow*) (General Electric 1.5-T Signa system; TR, 2500 ms; TE, 80 ms). (*Reproduced with permission from Pleasure and Fischbein, in Archives of Neurology 57: 1765–1769, 2000 Copyright © 2000, American Medical Association.*)

Hematologic and biochemical tests usually are normal, although hyponatremia may occur secondary to inappropriate secretion of antidiuretic hormone. Cerebrospinal fluid (CSF) analysis may be abnormal in human rabies. A CSF pleocytosis (elevated number of white cells) was found in 59% of patients in the first week of illness and in 87% after the first week (Anderson *et al.*, 1984). The white cell count usually is less than 100 cells/μl, and the leukocytes are predominantly mononuclear cells. The CSF protein concentration may be mildly elevated, and glucose is usually in the normal range, although low CSF glucose levels have been reported (Roine *et al.*, 1988; Chotmongkol *et al.*, 1991). Serum neutralizing antibodies against rabies virus usually are not present in unimmunized patients until the second week of the illness, and patients frequently die prior to having a detectable serum antibody level (Hattwick, 1974; Anderson *et al.*, 1984; Kasempimolporn *et al.*, 1991). Antibody had not developed in serum by 10 days after the onset of clinical symptoms in 5 of 18 (28%) patients with rabies in the United States (Noah *et al.*, 1998). One patient who had received interferon therapy had not developed antibodies by the time of death 24 days after the onset of symptoms (Sibley *et al.*, 1981). Rabies virus antibodies develop in the CSF later than in the serum, and the CSF titer is lower. Very high titers of rabies virus antibodies in the CSF have been interpreted as evidence of rabies encephalitis in vaccinated patients (Hattwick *et al.*, 1972; Porras *et al.*, 1976; Tillotson *et al.*, 1977b; Alvarez *et al.*, 1994). Rabies virus occasionally may be isolated from saliva and less commonly from the CSF or urine sediment (Anderson *et al.*, 1984). Viral isolation is more likely during early disease before neutralizing antibodies appear because they can result in "autosterilization" of tissues. Rabies virus antigen may be demonstrated antemortem by using the fluorescent antibody technique in frozen sections from skin biopsies (see Fig. 1C in Chap. 9). Biopsies usually are obtained by using a full-thickness punch biopsy (3–7 mm in diameter) from a hairy area at the nape of the neck (Bryceson *et al.*, 1975; Warrell *et al.*, 1988). Many sections should be examined to ensure thorough evaluation of several hair follicles. Antigen is found in small sensory nerves adjacent to hair follicles. Antigen detection also has been performed on corneal impression smears, but the sensitivity of the method is low, and false-positive results have occurred (Koch *et al.*, 1975; Anderson *et al.*, 1984; Mathuranayagam and Rao, 1984; Warrell *et al.*, 1988; Noah *et al.*, 1998).

1. Detection of Rabies Virus RNA

Small amounts of rabies virus RNA from brain tissue, CSF, or saliva can be amplified using reverse transcriptase–polymerase chain reaction (RT-PCR), making this recently adapted technique a valuable diagnostic tool for rabies. RT-PCR was used initially on CSF specimens and later on saliva to confirm a diagnosis of rabies (Kamolvarin *et al.*, 1993; McColl *et al.*, 1993; Crepin *et al.*, 1998). In a study on both CSF and saliva samples from 9 patients with confirmed rabies, the premortem diagnosis of rabies was confirmed by positive RT-PCR in 5 of 9 patients (56%) in saliva and in only 2 of 9 patients (22%) in CSF (Crepin *et al.*, 1998). In comparison, skin biopsies were positive for rabies virus antigen using the fluorescent antibody technique in 5 of 7 patients (86%). These findings, led to a recommendation that both skin biopsy and saliva specimens be obtained for testing with immunofluorescence and RT-PCR, respectively. Of the 20 human rabies cases diagnosed before death in the United States since 1980, rabies virus

RNA was detected in saliva from all 10 patients who had the test performed, including 3 who had negative viral isolation from saliva (Noah *et al.*, 1998).

2. Brain Tissue

The presence of Negri bodies in neurons is a pathologic hallmark of rabies observed on routine histologic staining, but these characteristic inclusion bodies in the cytoplasm of infected neurons (see Chap. 8) may be absent. The diagnosis of rabies in humans using brain biopsies has not been assessed adequately, but rabies virus antigen was detected successfully in brain tissues obtained by biopsy from 3 of 3 cases in the United States (Noah *et al.*, 1998). Postmortem CNS tissues, which may be obtained by a needle (e.g., Vim-Silverman or trucut needle) aspiration technique through either the orbit or the foramen magnum (Sow *et al.*, 1996; Warrell, 1996; Tong *et al.*, 1999), can be assessed for viral isolation, rabies virus antigen, or rabies virus RNA, although false-negative results may occur. Hence a full autopsy may not be required to confirm a diagnosis of rabies when it is suspected clinically but unconfirmed antemortem. Rabies may not be diagnosed until postmortem neuropathologic examination of the brain is performed because this diagnosis was not considered by the patient's physicians (King *et al.*, 1978; Munoz *et al.*, 1996; Geyer *et al.*, 1997). A range of diagnostic investigations may be performed on postmortem human tissues, including viral isolation, the fluorescent antibody test [on fresh or formalin-fixed and paraffin-embedded (Whitfield *et al.*, 2001) specimens], immunoperoxidase staining for rabies virus antigen or *in situ* hybridization for rabies virus RNA (Jackson and Wunner, 1991), or detection of rabies virus RNA by using RT-PCR amplification (see Sect. IVB1).

V. DIFFERENTIAL DIAGNOSIS

The diagnosis of rabies may be difficult if a history of an exposure has not been obtained. Patients and their relatives may not be able to recall an animal exposure even when questioned directly, especially with bat exposures. There may be a history of recent travel in a rabies-endemic area. Rabies is misdiagnosed most commonly as either a psychiatric or laryngopharyngeal disorder. The disease also may present with bizarre neuropsychiatric symptoms mimicking conditions such as schizophrenic psychosis or acute mania (Goswami *et al.*, 1984).

Patients often become quite fearful about the possibility of developing rabies after an animal bite or exposure. Rabies hysteria is a conversion disorder in which patients exhibit clinical features similar to rabies with unconscious motivation that involves poorly understood neural networks (Wilson *et al.*, 1975; Ron, 2001), which should not be confused with malingering (feigning), in which there is deception by the patient. Rabies hysteria is probably the most difficult differential diagnosis. It is characterized by a shorter incubation period (often a few hours or a day or two) than rabies, an early onset of inability of the patient to communicate, bizarre spasms, spitting out of water taken in the mouth with no actual attempt at swallowing, barking, biting, aggressive behavior directed toward health care workers, lack of fever and neurologic signs, and a long clinical course with recovery. Village practitioners in endemic areas may establish a reputation that they can cure rabies due to their treatment of patients with rabies hysteria (Wilson *et al.*, 1975). However, it should be emphasized that the clinical picture may be so bizarre in patients with rabies that they may be misdiagnosed as having hysteria (Bisseru, 1972).

Other viral encephalitides may show behavioral disturbances with fluctuations in the level of consciousness. However, hydrophobic spasms are not observed, and it is unusual for a conscious patient to have prominent brainstem signs in other encephalitides. Herpes simiae (B virus) encephalomyelitis, which is transmitted by monkey bites, is often associated with a shorter incubation period than that of rabies (e.g., 3–4 days), vesicles may be present at the site of the bite (also in the monkey's oral cavity), and recovery may occur (Palmer, 1987). Two recent cases of rabies in the United States were misdiagnosed as Creutzfeldt–Jakob disease (Geyer *et al.*, 1997). Both these patients had rapidly progressive neurologic illnesses with prominent myoclonus.

Tetanus, a disease caused by the neurotoxin from the bacteria *Clostridium tetani*, may develop due to a dirty wound caused by an animal bite. Tetanus has a shorter incubation period (usually 3–21 days) than rabies and, unlike rabies, is characterized by sustained muscle rigidity involving axial muscles, including paraspinal, abdominal, masseter (trismus), laryngeal, and respiratory muscles, with superimposed brief recurrent muscle spasms (Mayer and Potes, 1987). In tetanus, the mental state is not affected, there is no CSF pleocytosis, and the prognosis is much better than for patients with rabies.

Postvaccinal encephalomyelitis is another important differential diagnosis, particularly in patients who have been immunized with a vaccine derived from neural tissues (e.g., Semple vaccine). Postvaccinal encephalomyelitis usually develops within 2 weeks of initiation of vaccination, and this is helpful to know if the illness develops much later. Local sensory symptoms (paresthesias, pain, and pruritus), alternating intervals of agitation and lucidity, and hydrophobia are clinical features that strongly suggest a diagnosis of rabies rather than postvaccinal encephalomyelits.

Paralytic rabies resembles the Guillain-Barré syndrome, including both acute inflammatory demyelinating polyradiculopathy and acute motor–sensory axonal neuropathy, and in a recent pathologic series of the latter, one patient (case number 1 in the report) subsequently was demonstrated to have paralytic rabies (Griffin *et al.*, 1996; Sheikh *et al.*, 1998). Local symptoms at the site of the bite, piloerection, early or persistent bladder dysfunction, and fever are more suggestive of paralytic rabies. The Guillain-Barré syndrome occasionally may occur as a postvaccinal complication from rabies vaccines derived from neural tissues, particularly the suckling mouse brain vaccine (Toro *et al.*, 1977).

VI. THERAPY

Preventative therapy for rabies after exposures is highly effective if current recommendations are followed (Centers for Disease Control and Prevention, 1999). However, even minor deviations from these recommendations may result in the development of rabies. Unfortunately, treatment of rabies has proved to be very disappointing. Therapy with human leukocyte interferon in three patients with high-dose intraventricular and systemic (intramuscular) administration was not associated with a beneficial clinical effect, but this therapy was not initiated until between 8 and 14 days after the onset of symptoms (Merigan *et al.*, 1984). Similarly, antiviral therapy with intravenous ribavirin (16 patients given doses of 16–400 mg) was unsuccessful in China (Kureishi *et al.*, 1992). An open trial of therapy with combined intravenous and intrathecal administration of either ribavirin (one patient) or interferon-α (three patients) (Warrell *et al.*, 1989) also was unsuccessful. Anti–rabies virus hyperimmune serum of either human or equine origin has been administered intravenously and by the intrathecal route (Emmons *et al.*, 1973; Hattwick *et al.*, 1976; Basgoz and Frosch, 1998), but there was no clear beneficial effect. Therapy is supportive, and adequate sedation and analgesia are very important for palliation. In some cases, survival may be prolonged for a few weeks with intensive care.

VII. RECOVERY FROM RABIES

Survival from rabies has been well documented in only four patients (Table II), and all of these patients received rabies immunization prior to the onset of clinical disease. There is no well-documented case of survival from rabies without prior rabies immunization. The first recovery from rabies, which was the only patient without significant neurologic sequelae, occurred in 1970 (Hattwick *et al.*, 1972). Matthew Winkler, a 6-year-old boy from Ohio, was bitten on his left thumb by a big brown bat (*Eptesicus fuscus*) that was later shown to be rabid. Vaccination was initiated with duck embryo rabies vaccine beginning 4 days after the bite, and shortly after completing the multidose therapy (20 days after the bite), the boy became ill with fever and meningeal signs. His CSF showed 125 white cells/μl (75% mononuclear cells and 25% polymorphonuclear leukocytes), and the CSF protein was elevated. He developed abnormal behavior and later lapsed

TABLE II

Cases of Human Rabies with Recovery

Location	Year	Age of patient	Transmission	Immunization	Outcome	Reference
United States	1970	6	Bat bite	Duck embryo vaccine	Complete recovery	Baer et al., 1982
Argentina	1972	45	Dog bite	Suckling mouse brain vaccine	Mild sequelae	Porras et al., 1976
United States	1977	32	Laboratory (vaccine strain)	Preexposure vaccination	Sequelae	Tillotson et al., 1977a,b
Mexico	1992	9	Dog bite	Postexposure vaccination (combination)	Severe sequelae[a]	Alvarez et al., 1994

[a] Patient died less than 4 years after developing rabies with marked neurological sequelae (L. Alvarez, personal communication).

into a coma. He had focal neurologic signs and seizures and developed cardiac and respiratory complications. He subsequently showed progressive improvement. A brain biopsy was consistent with encephalitis. His serum neutralization titer against rabies virus peaked at 1:63,000 at 3 months. This titer was much higher than has been observed secondary to vaccination. He also had very high titers of neutralizing antibodies in the CSF, which has not been observed with vaccination. Rabies virus was not isolated from brain tissue, CSF, or saliva, probably as a result of the high antibody levels.

The second patient with recovery was a 45-year-old woman who sustained multiple deep bites to her left arm from a dog in Argentina in 1972 (Porras et al., 1976). The dog developed neurologic signs and died 4 days later. The patient received 14 daily doses of suckling mouse brain rabies vaccine beginning 10 days after the bites, which were followed by two booster doses. Twenty-one days after the bites (at the time of her twelfth vaccine dose), the patient developed left arm paresthesias, which subsequently spread and became accompanied by pain; vaccination was continued. She was admitted to hospital with quadriparesis and hyperreflexia 31 days after the bites. She had limb weakness, tremor in her upper extremities (especially on the left), cerebellar signs (asynergia, ataxia, dysmetria, and dysdiadochokinesia), generalized myoclonus, and hyperreflexia in her lower extremities. Prominent cerebellar signs are unusual in rabies, despite the characteristic infection of neurons in the cerebellum, including Purkinje cells and deep cerebellar nuclei. Her CSF showed 5 cells/μl, and CSF protein was mildly elevated at 0.65 g/liter. Her serum neutralization titer against rabies virus peaked at 1:640,000 at about 3 months, and she also had very high titers of neutralizing antibodies in the CSF. Rabies virus was not isolated from her saliva or CSF, and corneal impression smears were negative for rabies virus antigen. Neurologic deterioration occurred shortly after she received each of the two booster doses of rabies vaccine and included altered mental status, generalized seizures, dysphagia, and quadriparesis. She showed neurologic improvement over the next few months. Thirteen months after the onset of her symptoms, her recovery was reported as "nearly complete." However, there was no description of her residual neurologic deficits (Porras et al., 1976). The unusual neurologic features of this patient and the clinical worsening after booster doses of the suckling mouse brain rabies vaccine were administered raise the question of whether encephalomyelitis due to the rabies vaccine played a significant role in this patient's clinical picture.

The third patient was a 32-year-old laboratory technician in New York in 1977 who was preimmunized with duck embryo rabies vaccine (Tillotson et al., 1977a,b). About 5 months prior to his illness, he had a rabies virus neutralizing antibody titer of 1:32. He worked with live rabies virus vaccine strains, and he was likely exposed to an aerosol of rabies virus about 2 weeks prior to the onset of his illness. He experienced initial malaise, headache, fever, chills, nausea, and then lethargy with intermittent delirium. He was admitted to hospital in Albany, New York, 6 days after the onset of his symptoms with expressive aphasia, hyperreflexia, and primitive reflexes. CSF showed 230 white cells/μl (95% mononuclear cells), and his CSF protein was elevated at 1.17 g/liter. The day after admission to hospital, he deteriorated and went into a deep coma. His serum neutralizing antibody titer increased from 1:32 to 1:64,000 and subsequently increased to 1:175,000 over a 10-day period during his illness (Tillotson et al., 1977a). He also developed a high titer of CSF antibodies. Rabies virus antigen was not detectable in a skin biopsy or in corneal impression smears. Four months after the onset of his illness, he was ambulatory, but he had residual aphasia and spasticity (Tillotson et al., 1977a). This was the first report of a case of rabies in a preimmunized individual and only the fourth well-documented case with transmission due to airborne exposure to the virus.

The fourth and most recent case from 1992 occurred in a 9-year-old boy in Mexico (Alvarez et al., 1994). This boy received severe facial bites from a dog and obtained local wound treatment. On the day after the bites, vaccination was initiated with VERO rabies vaccine, but passive immunization with rabies immune globulin was not given. Nineteen days after the bites, the boy developed fever and dysphagia. He subsequently demonstrated a variety of neurologic signs and had convulsions. He never developed hydrophobia or inspiratory spasms. He was admitted to hospital and subsequently became comatose. CSF showed 184 cells/μl (65% mononuclear cells). He required mechanical ventilation for several days. Rabies virus was not isolated from saliva, and rabies virus antigen was not found in either a skin biopsy or corneal impression smears. His peak serum seutralizing antibody titer was 1:34,800 (39 days after the bite), and he had a very high CSF antibody titer. He had severe neurologic sequelae, including quadriparesis and visual impairment. He died almost 4 years later (L. Alvarez, personal communication).

Recovery in the preceding four patients with rabies inspired physicians to manage patients with rabies aggressively in intensive care units. The hope was that if patients, even previously unimmunized, could be maintained through the acute phase of their illness and avoid complications, then perhaps they could clear the viral infection and recover. Unfortunately, this approach has been disappointing because there has not been even a single case with recovery, although the survival period has been markedly prolonged, with a duration of illness lasting up to 133 days after the onset of symptoms (Rubin *et al.*, 1970; Emmons *et al.*, 1973; Bhatt *et al.*, 1974; Lopez *et al.*, 1975; Gode *et al.*, 1976; Udwadia *et al.*, 1989).

VIII. RABIES DUE TO OTHER *LYSSAVIRUS* GENOTYPES

In addition to rabies virus, which is *Lyssavirus* genotype 1, there are six other *Lyssavirus* genotypes, and five have been associated with cases of human rabies: Mokola virus (genotype 3), Duvenhage virus (genotype 4), European bat lyssavirus 1 (genotype 5), European bat lyssavirus 2 (genotype 6), and Australian bat lyssavirus (genotype 7) (see Chaps. 2 and 3). They are commonly called *rabies-like* or *rabies-related viruses*. Lagos bat virus (genotype 2), which was first isolated from fruit-eating bats in Nigeria, is the only genotype that has not been associated with human disease.

A. Duvenhage Virus

In 1970, a 31-year-old man from rural South Africa developed an illness with fever, excessive sweating, hydrophobia, and spasms of his face, arms, and torso that were precipitated by being touched (Meredith *et al.*, 1971). He also exhibited confusion, irritability, and marked aggressiveness. He died after an illness lasting about 5 days. He lived outside the recognized enzootic and epizootic areas for rabies, but he had been bitten on the lip by a bat while sleeping about 4 weeks earlier. The virus isolated from the patient's brain was a new virus and was characterized and named *Duvenhage virus* (genotype 4). This patient's clinical illness was indistinguishable from that caused by rabies virus (genotype 1).

B. Mokola Virus

Mokola virus was isolated from shrews in Nigeria (Shope *et al.*, 1970). In 1968, a 3½-year-old girl from Nigeria presented with a sudden onset of fever and convulsions (Familusi and Moore, 1972). She rapidly made a complete recovery. There were no cells in her CSF, and the CSF protein and glucose were normal. Mokola virus was isolated from her CSF, although the shrew isolate of Mokola virus was handled in the same laboratory during the same time period. Cross-contamination of specimens in the laboratory remains a possible explanation for this viral isolation. The girl's neutralizing antibody titers were very low and disappeared within several months. The febrile convulsion was unlikely related to Mokola virus infection.

A 6-year-old girl died in Nigeria in 1971 after a 6-day illness (Familusi *et al.*, 1972). She presented with drowsiness, confusion, and weakness involving her extremities and trunk and progressed to coma. Her CSF was normal without a pleocytosis. At autopsy, there were large eosinophilic inclusion bodies in the cytoplasm of neurons, and Mokola virus was isolated from her brain. Shrews were known to be plentiful around the house where she lived, although there was no documented evidence that she actually had been bitten. Mokola virus infection was associated with meningoencephalitis in this case without the typical features of brainstem involvement seen in classic rabies.

C. European Bat Lyssavirus 1

In 1985, an 11-year-old girl from Belgorod, Russia, was bitten on the lower lip by an unidentified bat and died with signs of rabies (Selimov *et al.*, 1989). The viral isolate was called *Yuli virus* and classified as European bat lyssavirus type 1 (genotype 5) (Bourhy *et al.*, 1992).

D. European Bat Lyssavirus 2

In 1985, a 30-year-old zoologist from Finland developed numbness in his right arm and neck with leg weakness. His CSF was normal without a pleocytosis. Subsequently, he developed myoclonus of his legs, agitation, hyperexcitability, inspiratory spasms, dysarthria, dysphagia, and hypersalivation. He had a delirium that progressed to coma. Diabetes insipidus occurred, and he died 23 days after the onset of the illness. He had never been vaccinated against rabies and had been bitten by bats in several countries over the previous 5 year period, including an exposure in southern Finland 51 days prior to the onset of his symptoms. A virus was isolated that resembled the enzootic European bat rabies virus isolates and classified as European bat lyssavirus type 2 (genotype 6) (Bourhy *et al.*, 1992). This patient also had a clinical illness that was indistinguishable from that caused by rabies virus (genotype 1).

E. Australian Bat Lyssavirus

In 1996, a 39-year-old woman from Australia died after a 20-day illness (Samaratunga *et al.*, 1998). She cared for fruit bats and had sustained numerous scratches to her left arm over 4 weeks prior to the onset of her illness (Samaratunga *et al.*, 1998), and she also had apparently been bitten by a yellow-bellied sheathtail bat, *Saccolaimus flaviventris* (an insectivorous bat) (Hanna *et al.*, 2000). She developed progressive left arm weakness. Her CSF showed 100 white cells/μl (80% mononuclear cells, 20% polymorphonuclear leukocytes). She deteriorated with diplopia, dysarthria, dysphagia, and ataxia. She later developed progressive limb and facial weakness with reduced deep tendon reflexes and fluctuations in her level of consciousness prior to her death. Small eosinophilic cytoplasmic inclusions were observed in neurons in gray matter areas. RT-PCR amplification of nucleic acids extracted from brain tissue and CSF indicated that she was infected with a virus identical to Australian bat lyssavirus (genotype 7) that had been identified previously in flying foxes, which are fruit-eating bats. This patient had typical brainstem involvement of rabies, which quickly progressed to diffuse brain involvement.

In 1998, a 37-year-old woman from Mackay, Queensland, was admitted to hospital with a 5-day history of fever, paresthesia around the dorsum of her left hand, pain about the left shoulder girdle, and sore throat with difficulty swallowing (Hanna *et al.*, 2000). There were pharyngeal spasms, evidence of autonomic instability, and progressive neurologic deterioration. She died 19 days after onset of the illness. Twenty-seven months prior to the onset of her illness (during 1996), she was bitten at the base of her left little finger by a flying fox (fruit bat) in the course of removing the bat from the back of a young child. She did not receive rabies postexposure prophylaxis. Heminested PCR analyses on multiple tissues and saliva were positive for the flying fox (*Pteropus* sp.) variant of Australian bat lyssavirus (Hanna *et al.*, 2000). Although *Lyssavirus* infections of flying foxes have been recognized only recently in Australia, rabies virus infection was recognized in a gray-head flying fox (*Pteropus poliocephalus*) that died in India in 1978 (Pal *et al.*, 1980) and also in two dog-faced fruit bats (*Cyanopterus brachyotis*) from Thailand (Smith *et al.*, 1967). It is unclear exactly when and how Australian bat lyssavirus obtained its foothold in Australian frugivorous and insectivorous bats, but it is clear that the virus poses a threat to human health in this region.

REFERENCES

Alvarez, L., Fajardo, R., Lopez, E., Pedroza, R., Hemachudha, T., Kamolvarin, N., Cortes, G., and Baer, G. M. (1994). Partial recovery from rabies in a nine-year-old boy. *Pediatr. Infect. Dis. J.* **13**, 1154–1155.

Anderson, L. J., Nicholson, K. G., Tauxe, R. V., and Winkler, W. G. (1984). Human rabies in the United States, 1960 to 1979: Epidemiology, diagnosis, and prevention. *Ann. Intern. Med.* **100**, 728–735.

Asbury, A. K., and Cornblath, D. R. (1990). Assessment of current diagnostic criteria for Guillain-Barré syndrome. *Ann. Neurol.* **27** (Suppl.), S21–S24.

Awasthi, M., Parmar, H., Patankar, T., and Castillo, M. (2001). Imaging findings in rabies encephalitis. *Am. J. Neuroradiol.* **22**, 677–680.

Baer, G. M., Shaddock, J. H., Houff, S. A., Harrison, A. K., and Gardner, J. J. (1982). Human rabies transmitted by corneal transplant. *Arch. Neurol.* **39**, 103–107.

Basgoz, N., and Frosch, M. P. (1998). Case records of the Massachusetts General Hospital: A 32-year-old woman with pharyngeal spasms and paresthesias after a dog bite. *New Engl. J. Med.* **339**, 105–112.

Bhahdari, M., and Kumar, S. (1986). Penile hyperexcitability as the presenting symptom of rabies. *Br. J. Ural.* **58**, 224–233.

Bhatt, D. R., Hattwick, M. A. W., Gerdsen, R., Emmons, R. W., and Johnson, H. N. (1974). Human rabies: Diagnosis, complications, and management. *Am. J. Dis. Child.* **127**, 862–869.

Bisseru, B. (1972). Human rabies. In: *Rabies*, B. Bisseru (ed.), pp. 385–453. William Heinemann Medical Books, London.

Bourhy, H., Kissi, B., Lafon, M., Sacramento, D., and Tordo, N. (1992). Antigenic and molecular characterization of bat rabies virus in Europe. *J. Clin. Microbiol.* **30**, 2419–2426.

Bryceson, A. D. M., Greenwood, B. M., Warrell, D. A., Davidson, N. M., Pope, H. M., Lawrie, J. H., Barnes, H. J., Bailie, W. E., and Wilcox, G. E. (1975). Demonstration during life of rabies antigen in humans. *J. Infect. Dis.* **131**, 71–74.

Centers for Disease Control and Prevention (1999). Human rabies prevention — United States, 1999: Recommendations of the Advisory Committee on Immunization Practices (ACIP). *Morb. Mortal. Weekly Rep.* **48** (RR-1), 1–21.

Cheetham, H. D., Hart, J., Coghill, N. F., and Fox, B. (1970). Rabies with myocarditis: Two cases in England. *Lancet* **1**, 921–922.

Chopra, J. S., Banerjee, A. K., Murthy, J. M. K., and Pal, S. R. (1980). Paralytic rabies: A clinico-pathological study. *Brain* **103**, 789–802.

Chotmongkol, V., Vuttivirojana, A., and Cheepblangchai, M. (1991). Unusual manifestation in paralytic rabies. *Southeast Asian J. Trop. Med. Public Health* **22**, 279–280.

Constantine, D. G. (1962). Rabies transmission by nonbite route. *Public Health Rep.* **77**, 287–289.

Crepin, P., Audry, L., Rotivel, Y., Gacoin, A., Caroff, C., and Bourhy, H. (1998). Intravitam diagnosis of human rabies by PCR using saliva and cerebrospinal fluid. *J. Clin. Microbiol.* **36**, 1117–1121.

Doege, T. C., and Northrop, R. L. (1974). Evidence for inapparent rabies infection. *Lancet* **2**, 826–829.

Dupont, J. R., and Earle, K. M. (1965). Human rabies encephalitis: A study of forty-nine fatal cases with a review of the literature. *Neurology* **15**, 1023–1034.

Dutta, J. K. (1996). Excessive libido in a woman with rabies. *Postgrad. Med. J.* **72**, 554.

Editorial (1975). Diagnosis and management of human rabies. *Br. Med. J.* **3**, 721–722.

Editorial (1978). Dumb rabies. *Lancet* **2**, 1031–1032.

Emmons, R. W., Leonard, L. L., DeGenaro, F., Jr., Protas, E. S., Bazeley, P. L., Giammona, S. T., and Sturckow, K. (1973). A case of human rabies with prolonged survival. *Intervirology* **1**, 60–72.

Familusi, J. B., and Moore, D. L. (1972). Isolation of a rabies related virus from the cerebrospinal fluid of a child with "aseptic meningitis." *Afr. J. Med. Sci.* **3**, 93–96.

Familusi, J. B., Osunkoya, B. O., Moore, D. L., Kemp, G. E., and Fabiyi, A. (1972). A fatal human infection with Mokola virus. *Am. J. Trop. Med. Hyg.* **21**, 959–963.

Faoagali, J. L., De Buse, P., Strutton, G. M., and Samaratunga, H. (1988). A case of rabies. *Med. J. Aust.* **149**, 702–707.

Feasby, T. E., Gilbert, J. J., Brown, W. F., Bolton, C. F., Hahn, A. F., Koopman, W. F., and Zochodne, D. W. (1986). An acute axonal form of Guillain-Barré polyneuropathy. *Brain* **109**, 1115–1126.

Fekadu, M., Endeshaw, T., Alemu, W., Bogale, Y., Teshager, T., and Olson, J. G. (1996). Possible human-to-human transmission of rabies in Ethiopia. *Ethiop. Med. J.* **34**, 123–127.

Galian, A., Guerin, J. M., Lamotte, M., Le Charpentier, Y., Mikol, J., Dureaux, J. B., Gerard, de Lavergne, E., Atanasiu, P., Ravisse, P., and Sureau, P. (1980). Human-to-human transmission of rabies via a corneal transplant — France. *Morb. Mortal. Weekly Rep.* **29**, 25–26.

Gamaleia, N. (1887). Etude sur la rage paralytique chez l'homme. *Ann. Inst. Pasteur (Paris)* **1**, 63–83.

Gardner, A. M. N. (1970). An unusual case of rabies (Letter). *Lancet* **2**, 523.

Geyer, R., Van Leuven, M., Murphy, J., Damrow, T., Sastry, L., Miller, S., Goldoft, M., Grendon, J., Kobayashi, J., and Stehr-Green, P. A. (1997). Human rabies — Montana and Washington, 1997. *Morb. Mortal. Weekly Rep.* **46**, 770–774.

Gode, G. R., and Bhide, N. K. (1988). Two rabies deaths after corneal grafts from one donor (Letter). *Lancet* **2**, 791.

Gode, G. R., Raju, A. V., Jayalakshmi, T. S., Kaul, H. L., and Bhide, N. K. (1976). Intensive care in rabies therapy: Clinical observations. *Lancet* **2**, 6–8.

Goswami, U., Shankar, S. K., Channabasavanna, S. M., and Chattopadhyay, A. (1984). Psychiatric presentations in rabies: A clinicopathologic report from south India with a review of literature. *Trop. Geogr. Med.* **36**, 77–81.

Griffin, J. W., Li, C. Y., Ho, T. W., Tian, M., Gao, C. Y., Xue, P., Mishu, B., Cornblath, D. R., Macko, C., McKhann, G. M., and Asbury, A. K. (1996). Pathology of the motor–sensory axonal Guillain-Barré syndrome. *Ann. Neurol.* **39**, 17–28.

Hanna, J. N., Carney, I. K., Smith, G. A., Tannenberg, A. E. G., Deverill, J. E., Botha, J. A., Serafin, I. L., Harrower, B. J., Fitzpatrick, P. F., and Searle, J. W. (2000). Australian bat lyssavirus infection: A second human case, with a long incubation period. *Med. J. Aust.* **172**, 597–599.

Hantson, P., Guerit, J. M., de Tourtchaninoff, M., Deconinck, B., Mahieu, P., Dooms, G., Aubert-Tulkens, G., and Brucher, J. M. (1993). Rabies encephalitis mimicking the electrophysiological pattern of brain death: A case report. *Eur. Neurol.* **33**, 212–217.

Hattwick, M. A., Corey, L., and Creech, W. B. (1976). Clinical use of human globulin immune to rabies virus. *J. Infect. Dis.* **133** (Suppl. A) A266–A272.

Hattwick, M. A. W. (1974). Human rabies. *Public Health Rev.* **3**, 229–274.

Hattwick, M. A. W., Weis, T. T., Stechschulte, C. J., Baer, G. M., and Gregg, M. B. (1972). Recovery from rabies: A case report. *Ann. Intern. Med.* **76**, 931–942.

Hemachudha, T. (1994). Human rabies: Clinical aspects, pathogenesis, and potential therapy. In: *Lyssaviruses*, C. E. Rupprecht, B. Dietzschold and H. Koprowski (eds.), pp. 121–143. Springer-Verlag, Berlin.

Hemachudha, T. (1997a). Rabies. *Curr. Opin. Neurol.* **10**, 260–267.

Hemachudha, T. (1997b). Rabies. In: *Central Nervous System Infectious Diseases and Therapy*, K. L. Roos (ed.), pp. 573–600. Marcel Dekker, New York.

Hemachudha, T., Panpanich, T., Phanuphak, P., Manatsathit, S., and Wilde, H. (1993). Immune activation in human rabies. *Trans. R. Soc. Trop. Med. Hyg.* **87**, 106–108.

Hemachudha, T., Phanthumchinda, K., Phanuphak, P., and Manutsathit, S. (1987). Myoedema as a clinical sign in paralytic rabies (Letter). *Lancet* **1**, 1210.

Hemachudha, T., Phanuphak, P., Sriwanthana, B., Manutsathit, S., Phanthumchinda, K., Siriprasomsup, W., Ukachoke, C., Rasameechan, S., and Kaoroptham, S. (1988). Immunologic study of human encephalitic and paralytic rabies: Preliminary report of 16 patients. *Am. J. Med.* **84**, 673–677.

Hornung, K., and Nix, W. A. (1992). Myoedema: A clinical and electrophysiological evaluation. *Eur. Neurol.* **32**, 130–133.

Houff, S. A., Burton, R. C., Wilson, R. W., Henson, T. E., London, W. T., Baer, G. M., Anderson, L. J., Winkler, W. G., Madden, D. L., and Sever, J. L. (1979). Human-to-human transmission of rabies virus by corneal transplant. *New Engl. J. Med.* **300**, 603–604.

Hurst, E. W., and Pawan, J. L. (1931). An outbreak of rabies in Trinidad without history of bites, and with the symptoms of acute ascending myelitis. *Lancet* **2**, 622–628.

Jackson, A. C., and Fenton, M. B. (2001). Human rabies and bat bites (Letter). *Lancet* **357**, 1714.

Jackson, A. C., and Wunner, W. H. (1991). Detection of rabies virus genomic RNA and mRNA in mouse and human brains by using *in situ* hybridization. *J. Virol.* **65**, 2839–2844.

Jackson, A. C., Ye, H., Phelan, C. C., Ridaura-Sanz, C., Zheng, Q., Li, Z., Wan, X., and Lopez-Corella, E. (1999). Extraneural organ involvement in human rabies. *Lab. Invest.* **79**, 945–951.

Javadi, M. A., Fayaz, A., Mirdehghan, S. A., and Ainollahi, B. (1996). Transmission of rabies by corneal graft. *Cornea* **15**, 431–433.

Kamolvarin, N., Tirawatnpong, T., Rattanasiwamoke, R., Tirawatnpong, S., Panpanich, T., and Hemachudha, T. (1993). Diagnosis of rabies by polymerase chain reaction with nested primers. *J. Infect. Dis.* **167**, 207–210.

Kasempimolporn, S., Hemachudha, T., Khawplod, P., and Manatsathit, S. (1991). Human immune response to rabies nucleocapsid and glycoprotein antigens. *Clin. Exp. Immunol.* **84**, 195–199.

King, D. B., Sangalang, V. E., Manuel, R., Marrie, T., Pointer, A. E., and Thomson, A. D. (1978). A suspected case of human rabies — Nova Scotia. *Can. Dis. Weekly Rep.* **4**, 49–51.

Koch, F. J., Sagartz, J. W., Davidson, D. E., and Lawhaswasdi, K. (1975). Diagnosis of human rabies by the cornea test. *Am. J. Clin. Pathol.* **63**, 509–515.

Komsuoglu, S. S., Dora, F., and Kalabay, O. (1981). Periodic EEG activity in human rabies encephalitis (Letter). *J. Neurol. Neurosurg. Psychiatry.* **44**, 264–265.

Kureishi, A., Xu, L. Z., Wu, H., and Stiver, H. G. (1992). Rabies in China: Recommendations for control. *Bull. WHO* **70**, 443–450.

Laothamatas, J., Hemachudha, T., Tulyadechanont, S., and Mitrabhakdi, E. (1997). Neuroimaging in paralytic rabies. *Ramathibodi Med. J.* **20**, 149–156.

Lopez, M., Neves, J., Moreira, E. C., Reis, R., Tafuri, W. L., Pittella, J. E., Marinho, R. P., Alvares, J. M., Filho, I. D., Silva, O. S., Foscarini, L. F., Ribeiro, M. B., Campos, G. B., Martins, M. T., Gontijo, M. T., and Marra, U. D. (1975). Human rabies: I. Intensive treatment. *Rev. Inst. Med. Trop. Sao Paulo* **17**, 103–110.

Lopez, R. A., Miranda, P. P., Tejada, V. E., and Fishbein, D. B. (1992). Outbreak of human rabies in the Peruvian jungle. *Lancet* **339**, 408–411.

Mathuranayagam, D., and Rao, P. V. (1984). Antemortem diagnosis of human rabies by corneal impression smears using immunofluorescent technique. *Ind. J. Med. Res.* **79**, 463–467.

Mayer, R. F., and Potes, E. (1987). Biological toxins. In: *Current Therapy in Neurologic Disease*, R. T. Johnson (ed.), 2nd ed., pp. 270–274. B.C. Decker, Toronto.

McColl, K. A., Gould, A. R., Selleck, P. W., Hooper, P. T., Westbury, H. A., and Smith, J. S. (1993). Polymerase chain reaction and other laboratory techniques in the diagnosis of long incubation rabies in Australia. *Aust. Vet. J.* **70**, 84–89.

Meredith, C. D., Rossouw, A. P., and Koch, H. v. P. (1971). An unusual case of human rabies thought to be of chiropteran origin. *S. Afr. Med. J.* **45**, 767–769.

Merigan, T. C., Baer, G. M., Winkler, W. G., Bernard, K. W., Gibert, C. G., Chany, C., Veronesi, R., and Collaborative Group (1984). Human leukocyte interferon administration to patients with symptomatic and suspected rabies. *Ann. Neurol.* **16**, 82–87.

Metze, K., and Feiden, W. (1991). Rabies virus ribonucleoprotein in the heart (Letter). *New. Engl. J. Med.* **324**, 1814–1815.

Mills, R. P., Swanepoel, R., Hayes, M. M., and Gelfand, M. (1978). Dumb rabies: Its development following vaccination in a subject with rabies. *Central Afr. J. Med.* **24**, 115–117.

Mrak, R. E., and Young, L. (1993). Rabies encephalitis in a patient with no history of exposure. *Hum. Pathol.* **24**, 109–110.

Munoz, J. L., Wolff, R., Jain, A., Sabino, J., Jacquette, G., Rapoport, M., Lieberman, J., Baisley, C. C., Ward, B. H., Brown, C. R., Stolte, P. M., Crowley, A. B., Hastings, H., Cartter, M. L., Hadler, J. L., French, T. W., Kreindel, S., Knowlton, R., Birkhead, G. S., Debbie, J. G., Hanlon, C. A., Trimarchi, C. V., and Morse, D. L. (1996). Human rabies — Connecticut, 1995. *Morb. Mortal. Weekly Rep.* **45**, 207–209.

Nehaul, B. B. G. (1955). Rabies transmitted by bats in British Guiana. *Am. J. Trop. Med. Hyg.* **4**, 550–553.

Nicholson, K. G. (1994). Human rabies. In: *Handbook of Neurovirology*, R. R. McKendall and W. G. Stroop (eds.), pp. 463–480. Marcel Dekker, New York.

Noah, D. L., Drenzek, C. L., Smith, J. S., Krebs, J. W., Orciari, L., Shaddock, J., Sanderlin, D., Whitfield, S., Fekadu, M., Olson, J. G., Rupprecht, C. E., and Childs, J. E. (1998). Epidemiology of human rabies in the United States, 1980 to 1996. *Ann. Intern. Med.* **128**, 922–930.

Orr, P. H., Rubin, M. R., and Aoki, F. Y. (1988). Naturally acquired serum rabies neutralizing antibody in a Canadian Inuit population. *Arctic Med. Res.* **47** (Suppl. 1), 699–700.

Pal, S. R., Arora, B., Chhuttani, P. N., Broor, S., Choudhury, S., Joshi, R. M., and Ray, S. D. (1980). Rabies virus infection of a flying fox bat, *Pteropus poliocephalus*, in Chandigarh, northern India. *Trop. Geogr. Med.* **32**, 265–267.

Palmer, A. E. (1987). B virus, *Herpesvirus simiae*: Historical perspective. *J. Med. Primatol.* **16**, 99–130.

Pawan, J. L. (1939). Paralysis as a clinical manifestation in human rabies. *Ann. Trop. Med. Parasitol.* **33**, 21–29.

Pearson, C. A. (1976). Rabies (Letter). *Lancet* **1**, 206.

Phuapradit, P., Manatsathit, S., Warrell, M. J., and Warrell, D. A. (1985). Paralytic rabies: Some unusual clinical presentations. *J. Med. Assoc. Thai.* **68**, 106–110.

Pleasure, S. J., and Fischbein, N. J. (2000). Correlation of clinical and neuroimaging findings in a case of rabies encephalitis. *Arch. Neurol.* **57**, 1765–1769.

Porras, C., Barboza, J. J., Fuenzalida, E., Adaros, H. L., Oviedo, A. M., and Furst, J. (1976). Recovery from rabies in man. *Ann. Intern. Med.* **85**, 44–48.

Prier, S., Gibert, C., Bodros, A., and Krymolieres, F. (1979a). Neurophysiological changes in non-vaccinated rabies patients (Letter). *Lancet* **1**, 620.

Prier, S., Gibert, C., Bodros, A., Vachon, F., Atanasiu, P., and Masson, M. (1979b). Les neuropathies de la rage humaine: etude clinique et electrophysiologique de deux cas [Human rabies neuropathies: Clinical and electrophysiological study in two cases (author's translation), French]. *Rev. Neurol.* **135**, 161–168.

Raman, G. V., Prosser, A., Spreadbury, P. L., Cockcroft, P. M., and Okubadejo, O. A. (1988). Rabies presenting with myocarditis and encephalitis. *J. Infect.* **17**, 155–158.

Remington, P. L., Shope, T., and Andrews, J. (1985). A recommended approach to the evaluation of human rabies exposure in an acute-care hospital. *JAMA* **254**, 67–69.

Roine, R. O., Hillbom, M., Valle, M., Haltia, M., Ketonen, L., Neuvonen, E., Lumio, J., and Lahdevirta, J. (1988). Fatal encephalitis caused by a bat-borne rabies-related virus: Clinical findings. *Brain* **111**, 1505–1516.

Ron, M. (2001). Explaining the unexplained: understanding hysteria (Editorial). *Brain* **124**, 1065–1066.

Ross, E., and Armentrout, S. A. (1962). Myocarditis associated with rabies: Report of a case. *New Engl. J. Med.* **266**, 1087–1089.

Rubin, R. H., Sullivan, L., Summers, R., Gregg, M. B., and Sikes, R. K. (1970). A case of human rabies in Kansas: Epidemiologic, clinical, and laboratory considerations. *J. Infect. Dis.* **122**, 318–322.

Ruegsegger, J. M., Black, J., and Sharpless, G. R. (1961). Primary antirabies immunization of man with HEP Flury virus vaccine. *Am. J. Public Health* **51**, 706–716.

Samaratunga, H., Searle, J. W., and Hudson, N. (1998). Non-rabies lyssavirus human encephalitis from fruit bats: Australian bat lyssavirus (pteropid lyssavirus) infection. *Neuropathol. Appl. Neurobiol.* **24**, 331–335.

Selimov, M. A., Tatarov, A. G., Botvinkin, A. D., Klueva, E. V., Kulikova, L. G., and Khismatullina, N. A. (1989). Rabies-related Yuli virus: Identification with a panel of monoclonal antibodies. *Acta Virol.* **33**, 542–546.

Sheikh, K. A., Jackson, A. C., Ramos-Alvarez, M., Li, C. Y., Ho, T. W., Asbury, A. K., and Griffin, J. W. (1998) Paralytic rabies: Immune attack on nerve fibers containing axonally transported viral proteins (Abstract). *Neurology* **50** (Suppl. 4), A183.

Shope, R. E., Murphy, F. A., Harrison, A. K., Causey, O. R., Kemp, G. E., Simpson, D. I. H., and Moore, D. L. (1970). Two African viruses serologically and morphologically related to rabies virus. *J. Virol.* **6**, 690–692.

Sibley, W. A., Ray, C. G., Petersen, E., Ryan, K., Graham, A. R., Gibbs, M. A., Feinberg, W., Minnick, L., Habek, T. J., Merigan, T. C., Budinich, M. L., Rodriguez-Torres, J. G., Porter, B. W., and Sacks, J. J. (1981). Human rabies acquired outside the United States from a dog bite. *Morb. Mortal. Weekly Rep.* **43**, 537–540.

Sing, T. M., and Soo, M. Y. (1996). Imaging findings in rabies. *Australas. Radiol.* **40**, 338–341.

Sipahioglu, U., and Alpaut, S. (1985). Transplacental rabies in a human [Turkish]. *Mikrobiyol. Bul.* **19**, 95–99.

Smith, J. S., Fishbein, D. B., Rupprecht, C. E., and Clark, K. (1991). Unexplained rabies in three immigrants in the United States: A virologic investigation. *New Engl. J. Med.* **324**, 205–211.

Smith, P. C., Lawhaswasdi, K., Vick, W. E., and Stanton, J. S. (1967). Isolation of rabies virus from fruit bats in Thailand. *Nature* **216**, 384.

Sow, P. S., Diop, B. M., Ndour, C. T. Y., Soumare, M., Ndoye, B., Faye, M. A., Gonzalez, J., Badiane, S., and Collseck, A. M. (1996). Occipital cerebral aspiration ponction: Technical procedure to take a brain specimen for postmortem virological diagnosis of human rabies in Dakar. *Med. Malad. Infect.* **26**, 534–536.

Sureau, P., Portnoi, D., Rollin, P., Lapresle, C., and Chaouni-Berbich, A. (1981). [Prevention of inter-human rabies transmission after corneal graft] [French]. *C. R. Seances Acad. Sci. Serie III* **293**, 689–692.

Talaulicar, P. M. S. (1977). Persistent priapism in rabies. *Br. J. Urol.* **49**, 462.

Tariq, W. U. Z., Shafi, M. S., Jamal, S., and Ahmad, M. (1991). Rabies in man handling infected calf (Letter). *Lancet* **337**, 1224.

Thongcharoen, P., Wasi, C., Sirikavin, S., Boonthai, P., Bedavanij, A., Dumavibhat, P., Chantarakul, N., Eungprabbanth, V., Puthavathana, P., Chavanich, L., and Tantawachakit, S. (1981). Human-to-human transmission of rabies via corneal transplant — Thailand. *Morb. Mortal. Weekly Rep.* **30**, 473–474.

Tillotson, J. R., Axelrod, D., and Lyman, D. O. (1977a). Follow-up on rabies — New York. *Morb. Mortal. Weekly Rep.* **26**, 249–250.

Tillotson, J. R., Axelrod, D., and Lyman, D. O. (1977b). Rabies in a laboratory worker — New York. *Morb. Mortal. Weekly Rep.* **26**, 183–184.

Tirawatnpong, S., Hemachudha, T., Manutsathit, S., Shuangshoti, S., Phanthumchinda, K., and Phanuphak, P. (1989). Regional distribution of rabies viral antigen in central nervous system of human encephalitic and paralytic rabies. *J. Neurol. Sci.* **92**, 91–99.

Tong, T. R., Leung, K. M., and Lam, A. W. S. (1999). Trucut needle biopsy through superior orbital fissure for diagnosis of rabies. *Lancet* **354**, 2137–2138.

Toro, G., Vergara, I., and Roman, G. (1977). Neuroparalytic accidents of antirabies vaccination with suckling mouse brain vaccine: Clinical and pathologic study of 21 cases. *Arch. Neurol.* **34**, 694–700.

Udwadia, Z. F., Udwadia, F. E., Katrak, S. M., Dastur, D. K., Sekhar, M., Lall, A., Kumta, A., and Sane, B. (1989). Human rabies: Clinical features, diagnosis, complications, and management. *Crit. Care Med.* **17**, 834–836.

Udwadia, Z. F., Udwadia, F. E., Rao, P. P., and Kapadia, F. (1988). Penile hyperexcitability with recurrent ejaculations as the presenting manifestation of a case of rabies. *Postgrad. Med. J.* **64**, 85–86.

Verlinde, J. D., Li-Fo-Sjoe, E., Versteeg, J., and Dekker, S. M. (1975). A local outbreak of paralytic rabies in Surinam children. *Trop. Geogr. Med.* **27**, 137–142.

Wallerstein, C. (1999). Rabies cases increase in the Philippines. *Br. Med. J.* **318**, 1306.

Warrell, D. A. (1976). The clinical picture of rabies in man. *Trans. R. Soc. Trop. Med. Hyg.* **70**, 188–195.

Warrell, D. A., Davidson, N. M., Pope, H. M., Bailie, W. E., Lawrie, J. H., Ormerod, L. D., Kertesz, A., and Lewis, P. (1976). Pathophysiologic studies in human rabies. *Am. J. Med.* **60**, 180–190.

Warrell, D. A., and Warrell M. J. (1991). Rabies. In: *Infections of the Central Nervous System,* H. P. Lambert (ed.), pp. 317–328. B.C. Decker, Philadelphia.

Warrell, M. J. (1996). Rabies. In: *Manson's Tropical Diseases,* G. C. Cook (ed.), pp. 700–720. W.B. Saunders, London.

Warrell, M. J., Looareesuwan, S., Manatsathit, S., White, N. J., Phuapradit, P., Vejjajiva, A., Hoke, C. H., Burke, D. S., and Warrell, D. A. (1988). Rapid diagnosis of rabies and post-vaccinal encephalitides. *Clin. Exp. Immunol.* **71**, 229–234.

Warrell, M. J., White, N. J., Looareesuwan, S., Phillips, R. E., Suntharasamai, P., Chanthavanich, P., Riganti, M., Fisher-Hoch, S. P., Nicholson, K. G., Manatsathit, S., Vannaphan, S., and Warrell, D. A. (1989). Failure of interferon-α and tribavirin in rabies encephalitis. *Br. Med. J.* **299**, 830–833.

Waterman, J. A. (1959). Acute ascending rabic myelitis: Rabies — Transmitted by bats to human beings and animals. *Carib. Med. J.* **21**, 46–74.

White, M., Davis, A., Rawlings, J., Neill, S., Hendricks, K., Simpson, D., Gann, W., Jones, B., Rountree, S., Vuong, D., Berry, D., McChesney, T., Simmons, J., Ferris, K., Wise, F., Reardon, J., Brunner, W., Walker, W., Rosenberg, J., Emmons, R., Jackson, R. J., Rutherford, G. W., Resendiz, P. E. R., and Echeverri, G. B. (1994). Human rabies — Texas and California, 1993. *Morb. Mortal. Weekly Rep.* **43**, 93–96.

Whitfield, S. G., Fekadu, M., Shaddock, J. H., Niezgoda, M., Warner, C. K., and Messenger, S. L. (2001). A comparative study of the fluorescent antibody test for rabies diagnosis in fresh and formalin-fixed brain tissue specimens. *J. Virol. Methods* **95**, 145–151.

Wilde, H., and Chutivongse, S. (1988). Rabies: current management in Southeast Asia. *Med. Prog.* **15**, 14–23.

Wilson, J. M., Hettiarachchi, J., and Wijesuriya, L. M. (1975). Presenting features and diagnosis of rabies. *Lancet* **2**, 1139–1140.

Winkler, W. G., Fashinell, T. R., Leffingwell, L., Howard, P., and Conomy, J. P. (1973). Airborne rabies transmission in a laboratory worker. *JAMA* **226**, 1219–1221.

World Health Organization (2000). *World Survey of Rabies No. 34 for the Year 1998.* World Health Organization, Geneva.

7

Pathogenesis

ALAN C. JACKSON

Departments of Medicine (Neurology) and Microbiology and Immunology
Queen's University
Kingston, Ontario K7L 3N6
Canada

I. INTRODUCTION

Rabies virus is a highly neurotropic virus that causes an acute infection of the central nervous system (CNS). Most of what is known about the events that take place during rabies has been learned from experimental models using animals. Fixed laboratory strains of rabies virus and rodent models have been used commonly, although the events in these models may not closely mimic the disease under natural conditions either in humans or in animals. There are a number of sequential steps that occur after peripheral inoculation of rabies virus via an animal bite, which is the most common mechanism of transmission (Fig. 1). The steps include replication in peripheral tissues, spread along peripheral nerves and the spinal cord to the brain, dissemination within the CNS, and centrifugal spread along nerves to various organs, including the salivary glands. Each of the pathogenetic steps will be discussed individually below. In addition, mechanisms of brain dysfunction in rabies will be addressed.

II. EVENTS AT THE SITE OF EXPOSURE

Early studies in rabies pathogenesis, which were performed in order to establish the pathways and rate of viral spread, involved amputation of the tail or leg of an animal proximal to the site of inoculation with a fixed or "street" strain of rabies virus. Amputation was found to be capable of preventing the development of rabies, and the timing of the procedure was important. In later studies, neurectomy of the sciatic nerve was performed instead of amputation, and similar results were observed (Baer *et al.*, 1965, 1968). These experiments clearly demonstrated that there was an incubation period in rabies during which there was time-dependent movement of virus along peripheral nerves from the site of inoculation to the CNS, and models using street rabies virus supported the idea that the virus remains at or near the site of entry for most of the long incubation period (Baer and Cleary, 1972). However, the time periods in which the procedures were life-saving in rodents infected with fixed rabies virus strains generally were very short (Dean *et al.*, 1963; Baer *et al.*, 1965), suggesting a different mechanism of viral entry than in natural rabies.

Under natural conditions, human and animals may experience long and variable incubation periods following a bite exposure that are likely biologically important in maintaining enzootic rabies. In humans, the incubation period is usually between 20 days and 3 months, although incubation periods rarely may be longer than 1 year (Smith *et al.*, 1991). There is uncertainty about the events that occur during this incubation period. There has been speculation that macrophages may sequester rabies virus *in vivo* because persistent *in vitro* infection of human and murine monocytic cell lines and of primary murine bone marrow

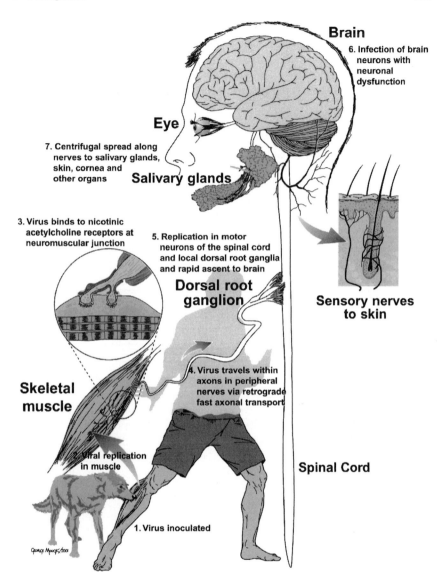

Brain

6. Infection of brain
   neurons with
   neuronal
   dysfunction

Eye

7. Centrifugal spread along
   nerves to salivary glands,
   skin, cornea and
   other organs   **Salivary glands**

3. Virus binds to nicotinic
   acetylcholine receptors at   5. Replication in motor
   neuromuscular junction   neurons of the spinal cord
                                       and local dorsal root ganglia
                                       and rapid ascent to brain

**Dorsal root
ganglion**   **Sensory nerves
                                       to skin**

**Skeletal
muscle**   4. Virus travels within
                              axons in peripheral
                              nerves via retrograde
                              fast axonal transport

2. Viral replication
   in muscle   **Spinal Cord**

1. Virus inoculated

George Mpoojs/2001

Fig. 1.   Schematic diagram showing the sequential steps in the pathogenesis of rabies after an animal bite.

macrophages have been demonstrated with different rabies virus strains (Ray *et al.*, 1995), but this has not yet been demonstrated in a natural animal model. The best experimental animal studies to date examining the events that take place during the incubation period were performed in striped skunks using a Canadian isolate of street rabies virus obtained from skunk salivary glands (Charlton *et al.*, 1997). Studies performed using reverse transcriptase–polymerase chain reaction (RT-PCR) amplification showed that viral genomic RNA frequently was present in the inoculated muscle (found in 4 of 9 skunks) but not in either spinal ganglia or the spinal cord when skunks were sacrificed 62–64 days after inoculation. Immunohistochemical studies performed prior to the development of clinical disease showed evidence of infection of extrafusal muscle fibers and occasional fibrocytes at the site of inoculation. Although it is unclear, the infection of muscle fibers may be a critical pathogenetic step for the virus to gain access to the peripheral nervous system. In a highly susceptible host after intramuscular inoculation, rabies virus–infected suckling hamsters showed early infection of striated muscle cells near the site of inoculation, and shortly afterward, neuromuscular and neurotendinal spindles became infected near the site of inoculation, which was followed by evidence of infection of small nerves within muscles, tendons, and adjoining connective tissues (Murphy *et al.*, 1973a). However, these events occurred within a few days of inoculation and do not mimic the situation with long incubation periods seen in natural infections.

In mouse models, early infection of muscle or other extraneural tissues was not observed following inoculation of fixed rabies virus strains (Johnson, 1965; Coulon *et al.*, 1989). Virus-specific RNA was not detected with RT-PCR amplification in the masseter muscle of adult mice between 6 and 30 hours after inoculation of CVS in the muscle, although viral RNA was identified in trigeminal ganglia at 18 hours and in the brainstem at 24 hours after inoculation (Shankar *et al.*, 1991). These studies suggest that rabies virus is capable of direct entry into peripheral nerves without a replicative cycle in extraneural cells and that the incubation period can be short. This likely occurs frequently in rodent models using fixed strains of rabies virus and accounts for the short period of time that amputation or neurectomy is protective after peripheral inoculation of fixed rabies virus (Dean *et al.*, 1963; Baer *et al.*, 1965). Unfortunately, these models provide little information about events that take place during the long incubation period of natural rabies.

A. Nicotinic Acetylcholine Receptor

The nicotinic acetylcholine receptor was the first identified receptor for rabies virus (Lentz *et al.*, 1982). Rabies virus antigen was detected at sites coincident with the nicotinic acetylcholine receptor in infected cultured chick myotubes from chicken embryos and also shortly after immersion of mouse diaphragms in a suspension of rabies virus. It was evident from these studies that the distribution of viral antigen detected by fluorescent antibody staining at sites in neuromuscular junctions corresponded to the distribution of nicotinic acetylcholine receptors. The receptors were stained with rhodamine-conjugated α-bungaro-toxin. Pretreatment of myotubes with either the nicotinic cholinergic antagonist α-bungarotoxin (irreversible binding) or *d*-tubocurarine (reversible binding) reduced the number of myotubes that became infected with rabies virus. Further studies in other laboratories showed that pretreatment of cultured rat myotubes with α-bungarotoxin had an inhibitory effect on infection (Tsiang *et al.*, 1986). Binding of radiolabeled rabies virus to purified *Torpedo* acetylcholine receptor also was inhibited by nicotinic antagonists but not by atropine (a muscarinic antagonist) (Lentz *et al.*, 1986). Monoclonal antibodies raised against a peptide containing residues 190–203 of the rabies virus glycoprotein also inhibited bind-ing of the rabies virus glycoprotein and α-bungarotoxin to the acetylcholine recep-tor (Bracci *et al.*, 1988). Further studies have shown that both rabies virus and neurotoxins bind to residues 173–204 of the α_1 subunit of the acetylcholine recep-tor and that the highest-affinity virus-binding determinants are located within residues 179–192 (Lentz, 1990). These studies have provided strong evidence that rabies virus binds to nicotinic acetylcholine receptors in neuromuscular junctions.

Snake venom neurotoxins are polypeptides that bind with high affinity to nico-tinic acetylcholine receptors and competitively block the depolarizing action of acetylcholine. When the amino acid sequence of the rabies virus glycoprotein was compared with that of snake venom neurotoxins, a significant sequence similar-ity was found between a segment (residues 151–238) of the rabies virus glyco-protein and the entire long neurotoxin sequence (71–74 residues) (Lentz *et al.*, 1984). The glycoprotein showed identity with residues at the end of loop 2 of the long neurotoxin (the "toxic loop"), which is a long central loop projecting from the molecule that is highly conserved among all the neurotoxins (Fig. 2). This suggests that this region of the rabies virus glycoprotein is likely a recognition site for the acetylcholine receptor (Lentz, 1985).

Lentz and coworkers indicated that binding of rabies virus to acetylcholine receptors would localize and concentrate the virus on postsynaptic cells, which would facilitate subsequent uptake and transfer of virus to peripheral motor nerves (Lentz *et al.*, 1982). Speculation was offered that attachment of rabies virus also would cross-link receptors and induce endocytosis and internalization of the virus (Lentz *et al.*, 1986). Studies performed in chick spinal cord–muscle cocultures confirmed this notion by showing that CVS and tracers colocalized at neuromuscular junctions and nerve terminals, which provided evidence that the neuromuscular junction is the major site of entry into neurons (Lewis *et al.*, 2000). Subsequently, colocalization with endosome tracers indicated that the virus resides in an early endosome compartment. There is also supporting ultra-structural evidence that rabies virus particles enter nerve terminals by endocyto-sis (Iwasaki and Clark, 1975; Charlton and Casey, 1979b). The acidic interior of the endosome triggers fusion of the viral membrane with the endosome mem-brane, which allows the viral nucleocapsid to escape into the cytoplasm.

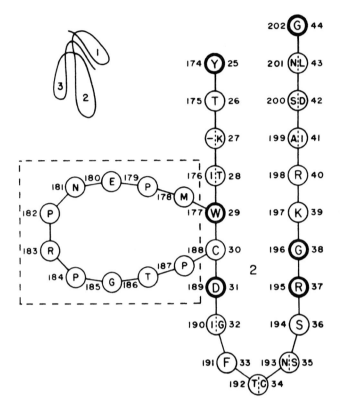

Fig. 2. A model showing the similarity of the rabies virus glycoprotein with the "toxic" loop of the neurotoxins. The segment of the glycoprotein (residues 174–202) corresponding to loop 2 of the long neurotoxins (Karlsson positions 25–44) is positioned in relationship to a schematic representation of loop 2. Within circles, residues or gaps in the glycoprotein are shown on the left and those in the neurotoxin on the right. One letter is shown where the glycoprotein and toxin are identical. Bold circles are residues highly conserved or invariant among all the neurotoxins. A 10-residue insertion in the glycoprotein is enclosed in the box. The rabies virus sequence is of the CVS strain, and the neurotoxin sequence is *Ophiophagus hannah*, toxin b. (*Inset*) Schematic of neurotoxin structure showing positions of loops 1, 2, and 3. (*Reproduced with permission from Lentz et al., in Science 226: 847–848, 1984. Copyright 1984 by American Association for the Advancement of Science.*)

Although rabies virus infection with fixed strains is restricted to a small number of cell types *in vivo*, fixed viruses can infect a much larger variety of cell types *in vitro*. L8 cells are rat skeletal muscle cells that differentiate from myoblasts without acetylcholine receptors to myotubes that elaborate high-density acetylcholine receptors. Unexpectedly, L8 myoblasts were fully susceptible to rabies virus infection, yet they failed to demonstrate significant binding of radiolabeled α-bungarotoxin (Reagan and Wunner, 1985). Four cell lines (BHK-21 cells, CER cells, mouse neuroblastoma cells, and *Aedes albopictus* clone C6/36), which are known to be susceptible to rabies virus infection *in vitro*, also did not demonstrate significant binding of α-bungarotoxin (Reagan and Wunner, 1985). Hence the α-bungarotoxin binding sites of the nicotinic acetylcholine receptor are clearly not necessary for attachment and infection of cells *in vitro*, and different structures may serve as rabies virus receptors in different cell types. Attachment of rabies virus to other cell surface constituents likely uses different domains of the viral glycoprotein than those used for binding to the acetylcholine receptor (Lentz, 1985). There is evidence that carbohydrate moieties, phospholipids, and highly sialylated gangliosides contribute to the cellular membrane receptor structure for rabies virus (Superti *et al.*, 1984; Superti *et al.*, 1986; Conti *et al.*, 1986). Viral penetration, which occurs subsequent to viral attachment, is very important in determining host cell range and cellular tropism (Lentz, 1985).

Variations in animal susceptibility to rabies virus infection have been recognized for many years. When infected by intramuscular inoculation, foxes are highly sensitive to rabies virus infection, dogs are less sensitive, and opossums are highly resistant (Baer *et al.*, 1990a). The difference in susceptibility between the red fox and the opossum could reflect the quantity of acetylcholine receptors in muscle (Baer *et al.*, 1990b). A striking difference in the muscle content B_{max} of nicotinic acetylcholine receptors was found with 180.5 fmol/mg protein present in red foxes and only 11.4 fmol/mg protein present in opossums, which was a highly significant difference ($p < 0.001$). No difference was observed in the binding affinity K_d. In addition, radiolabeled rabies virus bound much better to fox muscles than to opossum muscles. Hence the susceptibility of different animal species to rabies virus may, at least in part, be related to the quantity of nicotinic acetylcholine receptors in their muscles.

B. Superficial and Nonbite Exposures

The vast majority of human rabies cases that occur without a history of an exposure are thought to be due to unrecognized or forgotten bites, and molecular characterization of the rabies virus strains has indicated that they are most frequently from the strain found in silver-haired bats and eastern pipistrelle bats in the United States (Noah *et al.*, 1998). Experimental studies on the silver-haired bat virus indicate that the virus replicates well at lower than normal body temperatures (34°C) and is associated with higher infectivity in cell types present in the dermis, including fibroblasts and epithelial cells, than with coyote street virus (Morimoto *et al.*, 1996). Hence the silver-haired bat virus may have been selected for efficient local replication in the dermis, which could explain the success of this strain. However, after superficial exposures, it is unclear how or at precisely what sites the virus invades peripheral nerves in the skin or subcutaneous tissues.

Humans rarely have been infected by the airborne route in caves containing millions of bats (Constantine, 1962) and in laboratory accidents with aerosolized rabies virus (Winkler *et al.*, 1973; Tillotson *et al.*, 1977). Viral entry by the olfactory and oral routes is much less common than by bites. Relatively little experimental work has been done with routes of viral entry other than one simulating a bite exposure (using inoculation techniques). The nasal mucosa has been shown to act as a site of viral entry by suckling guinea pigs that have inhaled street rabies virus (Hronovsky and Benda, 1969). Rabies virus antigen was found initially in nasal mucosa cells 6 days later. Early brain infection was prominent in the olfactory bulbs, suggesting that rabies virus spread into the brain by an olfactory pathway. Similar results were obtained using a variety of rabies virus strains in mice and hamsters (Fischman and Schaeffer, 1971). Rabies virus antigen has been observed in olfactory receptor cells of naturally infected Mexican free-tailed bats obtained from a cave, suggesting that the nasal mucosa is a portal of entry in natural infection of bats by airborne rabies virus in caves (Constantine *et al.*, 1972). Experimental studies showing transmission of rabies to a variety of species of carnivorous animals caged in a cave containing millions of bats supported infection by the airborne route (Constantine, 1962). However, it is thought that the presence of very large numbers of bats in an unventilated area is necessary for airborne transmission of rabies virus.

Oral transmission of rabies virus might occur naturally by consumption of carcasses of rabid animals by wildlife and also may be important when humans eat raw dog meat (Wallerstein, 1999). Low susceptibility was observed when mice (Charlton and Casey, 1979a) and skunks (Charlton and Casey, 1979c) were given CVS or street rabies virus either by the oral route or by intestinal instillation. Mice, hamsters, guinea pigs, and rabbits of different ages were infected with CVS either orally or by gastric tube administration (Fischman and Ward, 1968). In CVS-infected weanling mice and hamsters that were infected by this route, rabies virus antigen was not observed in intestinal mucosal cells but was found in neurons in Auerbach's and Meissner's plexuses of the stomach and intestine (Fischman and Schaeffer, 1971). These findings suggest that viral entry by the oral route likely occurs via breaks in the integrity of the gastrointestinal mucosa. However, the importance of oral transmission in natural rabies of animals remains uncertain.

III. SPREAD TO THE CNS

Centripetal spread of rabies virus to the CNS occurs within motor and perhaps also sensory axons of peripheral nerves. Colchicine, a microtubule-disrupting agent active for tubulin-containing cytoskeletal structures, is an effective inhibitor of fast axonal transport in the sciatic nerve of rats (Tsiang, 1979). Colchicine was applied locally to the sciatic nerve using elastomer cuffs in order to obtain high local concentrations of the drug and avoid adverse systemic effects. Propagation of rabies virus was prevented, providing strong evidence that rabies virus spreads from sites of peripheral inoculation to the CNS by retrograde fast axonal transport. Human dorsal root ganglia neurons in a compartmentalized cell culture system were used to show that viral retrograde transport occurs at a rate of between 50 and 100 mm/d (Tsiang et al., 1991). More recent preliminary evidence has shown that the rabies virus phosphoprotein, which is a member of the ribonucleocapsid complex (see Chap. 2), interacts with dynein light chain 8 (LC8). Dynein LC8 is a component of both cytoplasmic myosin V and dynein that are involved in actin-based transport (important in early steps of viral entry) and microtubule-based transport (for fast axonal transport) in neurons, respectively (Jacob et al., 2000; Raux et al., 2000). Others used mouse and hamster models to demonstrate early and at least near-simultaneous involvement of motor neurons in the spinal cord and primary sensory neurons in dorsal root ganglia (Johnson, 1965; Murphy et al., 1973a; Jackson and Reimer, 1989; Coulon et al., 1989). In addition, after inoculation of mice in the masseter muscle with CVS, early infection was found in trigeminal ganglia (Shankar et al., 1991; Jackson, 1991b). Studies using RT-PCR amplification showed that infection was detectable in trigeminal ganglia (18 hours after inoculation) before the brainstem (24 hours after inoculation) (Shankar et al., 1991). However, elegant new transneuronal tracer methods using CVS in rats (Tang et al., 1999) and studies in rhesus monkeys (Kelly and Strick, 2000) have not shown early infection of primary sensory neurons. Two days after inoculation of CVS into the bulbospongiosus muscle of rats, the distribution of rabies virus antigen was limited to ipsilateral bulbospongiosus motor neurons in the spinal cord (Tang et al., 1999). One day later (3 days after inoculation), there was evidence of transfer of antigen to interneurons in the dorsal gray commissure, intermediate zone, and sacral parasympathetic nucleus and also to external urethral sphincter motor neurons; at this time there was no labeling of primary sensory neurons in local dorsal root ganglia. This study indicates that a motor pathway rather than a sensory pathway is important in the spread of rabies virus to the CNS. It is unclear if the different results obtained in earlier studies are due to differences in the animal models and in particular to different species of animals used in the studies.

IV. SPREAD WITHIN THE CNS

Once CNS neurons (usually in the spinal cord) become infected in rodent models, there is rapid dissemination of rabies virus infection along neuroanatomic pathways. Rabies virus also spreads within the CNS, as in the peripheral nervous system, by fast axonal transport. Evidence was provided for axonal transport using stereotaxic brain inoculation in rats (Gillet *et al.*, 1986) and by the administration of colchicine, which inhibited virus transport within the CNS (Ceccaldi *et al.*, 1989, 1990). Studies on cultured rat dorsal root ganglia neurons showed that anterograde fast axonal transport of rabies virus is in the range of 100–400 mm/d (Tsiang *et al.*, 1989). However, the importance of this is unclear because transneuronal tracing studies with CVS in rhesus monkeys have indicated that the spread of rabies virus occurs exclusively by retrograde axonal transport, with transsynaptic transport of rabies virus also occurring exclusively in the retrograde direction (Kelly and Strick, 2000). Ultrastructural studies in a skunk model indicated that most viral budding occurs on synaptic or adjacent plasma membranes of dendrites, with less prominent budding from the plasma membrane of the perikaryon (Charlton and Casey, 1979b). Most virions were found partially engulfed by an invaginated membrane of an adjacent axon terminal, indicating transneuronal dendroaxonal transfer of virus. Virions also occasionally were observed budding freely into the intercellular space.

After footpad inoculation of mice with CVS, there was early involvement of neurons in the brainstem tegmentum and deep cerebellar nuclei (Jackson and Reimer, 1989). Subsequently, the infection spread to involve cerebellar Purkinje cells and neurons in the diencephalon, basal ganglia, and cerebral cortex. Rabies virus, like Borna disease virus (Carbone *et al.*, 1987), spread to the hippocampus relatively late after peripheral inoculation. Rabies virus predominantly infected pyramidal neurons of the hippocampus, with relative sparing of neurons in the dentate gyrus in adult mice (Jackson and Reimer, 1989). Although rabies virus is highly neuronotropic, skunk rabies virus has been observed to infect Bergmann glia in the cerebellum more prominently than Purkinje cells in experimentally infected skunks (Jackson *et al.*, 2000). In street virus–infected skunks, initial infection was present in the lumbar spinal cord, and transit to the brain occurred via a variety of long ascending and descending fiber tracts, including rubrospinal, corticospinal, spinothalamic, spino-olivary, vestibulospinal/spinovestibular, reticulospinal/spinoreticular, cerebellospinal/spinocerebellar, and dorsal column pathways (Charlton *et al.*, 1996).

V. SPREAD FROM THE CNS

Centrifugal spread or viral spread from the CNS to peripheral sites along neuronal routes is essential for transmission of rabies virus to its natural hosts. Salivary gland infection is necessary for the transfer of infectious oral fluids by rabid vectors. The salivary glands receive parasympathetic innervation by the facial (via the submandibular ganglion or Langley's ganglion in some animals) and glossopharyngeal (via the otic ganglion) nerves, sympathetic innervation via the superior (or cranial) cervical ganglion, and afferent (sensory) innervation (Emmelin, 1967). Unilateral excision of a portion of the lingual nerve and the cranial cervical ganglion of dogs and foxes resulted in very low viral titers in denervated salivary glands compared with contralateral salivary glands after street rabies virus infection (Dean *et al.*, 1963). Evidence of widespread infection of salivary gland epithelial cells is a result of viral spread along multiple terminal axons rather than spread between epithelial cells (Charlton *et al.*, 1983). Rabies virus antigen was found concentrated in the apical region of mucous acinar cells, and ultrastructural studies showed that viral matrices were present in the basal region and that there was viral budding on the apical plasma membrane into the acinar lumen and into the intercellular canaliculi and, occasionally, onto membranes of secretory granules (Balachandran and Charlton, 1994). Viral titers in salivary glands may be higher than in CNS tissues (Dierks, 1975).

In addition to salivary gland infection, evidence was found in a suckling hamster model of centrifugal spread involving the central, peripheral, and autonomic nervous systems in many peripheral sites (Murphy *et al.*, 1973b). Infection was observed in the ganglion cell layer of the retina and in corneal epithelial cells, which are innervated by sensory afferents via the trigeminal nerve. Epithelial cells in both superficial and deep layers of the cornea were found to be infected (Balachandran and Charlton, 1994). Detection of rabies virus antigen in corneal impression smears has been used as a diagnostic test for human rabies (Koch *et al.*, 1975), and rabies virus has been transmitted by corneal transplantation in humans (see Chap. 6). Infection is found in free sensory nerve endings of tactile hair, and skin biopsies are one of the best diagnostic methods of confirming an antemortem diagnosis of rabies in humans (see Chap. 6). Antigen may be demonstrated in small nerves around hair follicles or in epithelial cells of hair follicles in the skin, which is taken from the nape of the neck (rich in hair follicles). Widespread infection may be observed in sensory nerve end organs, in the oral and nasal cavities, including the olfactory epithelium and taste buds in the tongue.

Studies in both natural and experimental rabies have demonstrated infection involving neurons in a variety of extraneural organs, including the adrenal medulla, cardiac ganglia, and plexuses in the luminal gastrointestinal tract, major salivary glands, liver, and exocrine pancreas (Debbie and Trimarchi, 1970; Balachandran and Charlton, 1994; Jackson *et al.*, 1999). In addition, there is infection involving a variety of nonneuronal cells, including acini in major salivary glands in rabies vectors, epithelium of the tongue, cardiac and skeletal muscle, hair follicles, and even pancreatic islets (Debbie and Trimarchi, 1970; Murphy *et al.*, 1973b; Balachandran and Charlton, 1994; Jackson *et al.*, 1999). There are a few reports of myocarditis in human cases of rabies (Ross and Armentrout, 1962; Cheetham *et al.*, 1970; Araujo *et al.*, 1971).

VI. ANIMAL MODELS OF RABIES VIRUS NEUROVIRULENCE

Viral *neurovirulence* can be defined as the capacity of a virus to cause disease of the nervous system, especially the CNS. Analysis of neurovirulence usually is approached in experimental models by comparing infections in a host with closely related viruses (e.g., different rabies virus strains or a parent rabies virus and a variant) (Jackson, 1991a). The ability of a virus to spread to the CNS from a peripheral site, or *neuroinvasiveness*, is an important component of neurovirulence after natural routes of viral entry. The route of inoculation is often very important in evaluating neurovirulence experimentally. Intracerebral inoculation is used commonly for convenience, and a number of peripheral sites also have been used in different models, including footpad, intramuscular, intraperitoneal, and intraocular inoculation. Species, age, and the immune status of the host also have proved to be important factors in neurovirulence (Flamand *et al.*, 1984).

Monoclonal antibody–resistant (MAR) variant viruses were selected *in vitro* from CVS and ERA laboratory strains of rabies virus with neutralizing antiglycoprotein antibodies (Dietzschold *et al.*, 1983; Seif *et al.*, 1985). Mutations involving antigenic site III are located between amino acid residues 330 and 338 of the CVS and ERA glycoprotein. Variants with a single-amino-acid change at position 333 with loss of either arginine (Dietzschold *et al.*, 1983; Seif *et al.*, 1985) or lysine (Tuffereau *et al.*, 1989) have diminished virulence in mice after intracerebral inoculation, whereas variants with amino acid changes at other positions remain neurovirulent. Comparisons of avirulent variants with their parent viruses in mouse and rat models after different routes of inoculation have been a useful approach in understanding the biologic basis of rabies virus neurovirulence. Both MAR variants RV194-2 (Dietzschold *et al.*, 1983) and Av01 (Coulon *et al.*, 1982) have substitution of a glutamine for the arginine of CVS at position 333 of the glycoprotein.

A. Events at the Site of Exposure

A virulent rabies virus variants, but not the parent CVS strain, have been shown to cause infection in extraneural sites close to the site of inoculation in different models. For example, the MAR variant Av01 infected the anterior epithelium of the lens after inoculation into the anterior chamber of the eye in rats (Kucera *et al.*, 1985) (Fig. 3). Similarly, the MAR variant RV194-2 inoculated into the tongue of mice and rats produced local infection involving epithelial tissues, glandular cells, and muscles (Torres-Anjel *et al.*, 1984). In these models, the variant viruses demonstrated less restricted cellular tropism than CVS, which is a highly neuronotropic parental strain.

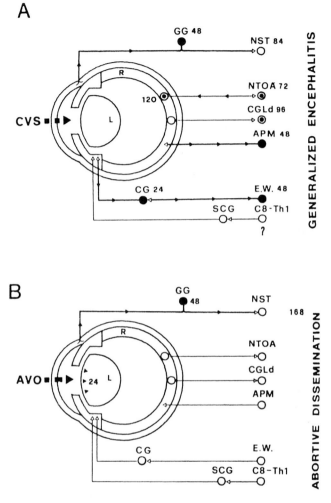

Fig. 3. Propagation of CVS (*A*) and avirulent variant rabies virus strains AVO (*B*) through the trigeminal (*top*), visual (*center*), and autonomic (*bottom*) interconnections between the eye and brain. *Symbols*: Open arrows, direction of neurotransmission; closed arrows, direction of propagation of the virus; circles, peripheral and central neuronal somata infected primarily (closed), secondarily (dots), and not infected (open) at each interval of time, indicated in hours after inoculation. APM, area praetectalis medialis; C8-Th 1, spinal preganglionic sympathetic neurons; CG, ciliary ganglion; CGLd, lateral geniculate body (dorsal part); E.W., Edinger-Westphal nucleus; GG, trigeminal (gasserian) ganglion; L, lens; NST, terminal trigeminal sensory nucleus; NTOA, terminal nuclei of the accessory optic system; R, retina; SCG, superior cervical sympathetic ganglion. (*Reproduced with permission from Kucera et al., in Journal of Virology 55: 158–162, 1985.*)

B. Spread to the CNS

After inoculation of the MAR variant Av01 and parent CVS into forelimb muscles of mice, the spinal cord and dorsal root ganglia neurons were examined for the presence of rabies virus antigen (Coulon *et al.*, 1989). Both viruses infected ventral horn cells and dorsal root ganglia at similar rates and efficiencies. After CVS and RV194-2 were inoculated into the masseter muscle of mice, both viruses spread to the ipsilateral motor nucleus of the trigeminal nerve in the pons at similar rates (Jackson, 1991b). RVl94-2 but not CVS spread to the ipsilateral trigeminal ganglion during the first 2 days after inoculation. There was no restriction in the pathways taken by the variants to the CNS in either of the models, and the variants did not demonstrate any impairment of their neuroinvasive properties.

An excellent model was developed for studying the pathways of viral spread to the brain by inoculating rabies virus into the anterior chamber of the eye in rats (Kucera *et al.*, 1985). There are six potential neural pathways for viral spread to occur between the eye and brain (see Fig. 3). Rabies virus was localized in tissues using immunofluorescent staining. After inoculation of CVS, viral antigen was detected initially at 24 hours in the ipsilateral ciliary ganglion and later in the Edinger–Westphal nucleus of the oculomotor nerve (parasympathetic pathway). At 48 hours, virus also spread to the ipsilateral ganglion of the trigeminal nerve (an afferent sensory pathway) and to neurons of the contralateral area praetectalis medialis, which projects to the retina via preopticoretinal fibers. In contrast, the Av01 variant propagated in the trigeminal pathway but not in either parasympathetic or preopticoretinal fibers. Neurons in the trigeminal ganglion also were infected at 48 hours, indicating a similar rate of spread. Thus the avirulent MAR variant spreads to the brain in this model using more limited pathways than its virulent parent virus.

C. Spread within the CNS

Studies performed using masseter muscle (Jackson, 1991b) and intranasal (Lafay *et al.*, 1991) inoculation of virus in mice indicate that the rate of spread of virus variants within the CNS is similar to that of the virulent parent virus, suggesting that they use the same fast axonal transport mechanism. The topographic distribution of virus in the CNS infections after inoculation of CVS and RV194-2 in the masseter muscle was quite similar (Jackson, 1991b). The infections were widespread and involved major regions of the CNS, including the cerebral cortex, hippocampus, brainstem, cerebellum, and spinal cord. The same neuronal cell types were infected, although fewer neurons were infected by RV194-2 and viral spread was less efficient. After intranasal instillation of CVS and Av01, Av01 was observed to produce infection of fewer olfactory neurons than CVS (Lafay *et al.*, 1991).

Intracerebral inoculation is a crude technique in which the inoculum spreads throughout the cerebrospinal fluid (CSF) spaces, including the ventricular system and subarachnoid space (Mims, 1960). A stereotaxic apparatus can deliver an inoculum into a precise location in the brain. Both Av01 and RV194-2 surprisingly were found to be neurovirulent after stereotaxic inoculation into the neostriatum or cerebellum of adult mice (Yang and Jackson, 1992), although Av01 infected fewer neurons and deaths occurred later than after stereotaxic inoculation with CVS (Jackson, 1994). After inoculation of Av01 into the striatum, the infection was widespread in the brain, and there were morphologic changes of apoptosis in neurons (A.C. Jackson, unpublished observations) as well as infiltration with inflammatory cells. Serum neutralizing antibodies against rabies virus were produced later and in smaller quantities than after intracerebral inoculation. Av01 is likely neurovirulent after stereotaxic brain inoculation because this route produces both a direct site of viral entry into the CNS and a low level of immune stimulation.

Studies performed with rabies virus glycoprotein gene-deficient recombinant rabies virus showed limited spread in the brains of mice after intracerebral inoculation (Etessami *et al.*, 2000). After stereotaxic inoculation of the recombinant into the rat striatum, infection remained restricted to initially infected neurons, and there was no evidence of transsynaptic spread to secondary neurons. Hence the rabies virus glycoprotein is necessary for transsynaptic spread of rabies virus from one neuron to another.

D. Spread from the CNS

Since centrifugal spread of CVS is limited, comparisons of the spread of CVS and variants from the CNS have not been as useful as for spread to the CNS and within the CNS. In the model of Kucera *et al.* (1985) using intraocular inoculation of rats, CVS spread from the nuclei of the accessory optic system to ganglionic cells of the retina in both eyes (see Fig. 3). Av01 did not show evidence of centrifugal spread in this model. In contrast, both CVS and RV194-2 infected trigeminal ganglia bilaterally after inoculation in a masseter muscle, indicating centrifugal spread to contralateral ganglia (Jackson, 1991b). In general, CVS does not spread to extraneural organs after either intracerebral or peripheral routes of inoculation (A. C. Jackson, unpublished observations).

E. Summary

Analysis of avirulent (MAR) variants of CVS has given important insights into the mechanisms of rabies virus neurovirulence. Changes in cellular tropisms of variants have been observed close to the site of inoculation. Variants remain neu-roinvasive, although there may be restrictions in their pathways to the CNS. Once variants reach the CNS, they spread widely, although interneuronal spread is inef-ficient, fewer neurons become infected than with CVS, and cellular tropisms are unchanged in the CNS. Variants are also capable of spreading centrifugally, but in general, this is very limited for both variants and CVS. The rate of viral spread centrally and peripherally is similar for variants and CVS, indicating that the fast axonal transport mechanism probably is not different. A single amino acid change in the rabies virus glycoprotein clearly has dramatic effects on rabies virus neu-rovirulence. In the future it will be challenging to determine the mode of action of specific viral gene products in the host that affect neurovirulence.

VII. RABIES VIRUS RECEPTORS

A. Nicotinic Acetycholine Receptor

The nicotinic acetylcholine receptor was the first rabies virus receptor identi-fied, and this receptor is felt to be important for the spread of the virus from the neuromuscular junction at peripheral sites in order to gain access to the CNS along peripheral nerves (Lentz et al., 1982). Although strongly suspected, it is unclear if the nicotinic acetylcholine receptor is also an important receptor in the CNS. Binding of rabies virus to nicotinic acetylcholine receptors in the brain could cause neuronal dysfunction. An anti–rabies virus glycoprotein monoclonal antibody was used to generate (by immunization) an anti-idiotypic antibody, B9, that selectively binds to nicotinic acetylcholine receptors (Hanham et al., 1993). Immunostaining of neuronal elements in the brains of rabies virus–infected mice with the B9 antibody was reduced greatly. This suggests that rabies virus binds to nicotinic acetylcholine receptors in the brain, but the pathogenetic significance of this binding in producing neuronal dysfunction in rabies has not yet been estab-lished. During 1998, there were reports from two independent research groups identifying another two putative rabies virus receptors: the neural cell adhesion molecule (NCAM) (Thoulouze et al., 1998) and the low-affinity p75 neurotrophic receptor (Tuffereau et al., 1998).

B. Neural Cell Adhesion Molecule Receptor

All cell lines susceptible to rabies virus infection appear to contain NCAM, which is a cell adhesion glycoprotein of the immunoglobulin superfamily, on their cell surface; NCAM was not found on the surface of resistant cell lines (Thoulouze et al., 1998). Incubation of susceptible cells with rabies virus decreased surface expression of NCAM and had no effect on other integral proteins of the cell membrane, whereas a control virus, vaccinia virus, did not affect surface NCAM. These findings are consistent with internalization of virus–NCAM complexes during viral entry by adsorptive endocytosis. Infection was inhibited when NCAM was blocked with heparan sulfate, which is a natural ligand physiologically, or either a polyclonal or monoclonal antibody directed against NCAM. In addition, soluble NCAM neutralized rabies virus infection, indicating that occupation of the receptor site on virus particles prevented binding to the rabies virus receptors on target cells. When resistant L cells were transfected with NCAM cDNA, the cells became susceptible to rabies virus infection. Hence there is very strong *in vitro* evidence that NCAM is a rabies virus receptor.

Primary cortex cultures were prepared from NCAM-deficient (knockout) and their wild-type littermate mice (Thoulouze *et al.*, 1998). After infection with CVS, a significantly lower mean number of cells became infected in NCAM-deficient cultures ($7.8 \pm 3.9\%$) than in wild-type cultures ($18.6 \pm 8.9\%$) ($p < 0.005$). After inoculation of CVS into the masseter muscle of NCAM-deficient and wild-type mice, significantly less rabies virus antigen was found in the brainstem/cerebellum, diencephalon, and cerebral cortex in NCAM-deficient than in wild-type mice, indicating that viral spread was less efficient without NCAM. After inoculation of CVS in hindlimb muscles, the mean survival of NCAM-deficient mice was 13.6 days compared with 10.2 days in wild-type mice ($p = 0.002$), indicating a slower progression of disease without NCAM. The absence of NCAM *in vivo* only mildly delayed death of the mice. This suggests that although NCAM is biochemically important, there must be other functionally important rabies virus receptors in the CNS in addition to NCAM. Possibilities include the nicotinic acetylcholine receptor, the low-affinity p75 neurotropic receptor, and one or more as yet unidentified receptors (Reagan and Wunner, 1985; Superti *et al.*, 1986).

C. Low-Affinity p75 Neurotrophic Receptor

A recent report that the low-affinity p75 neurotrophic receptor (p75[NTR]) is a receptor for street rabies virus further suggests multiple candidates for the rabies virus receptor (Tuffereau *et al.*, 1998). A random-primed cDNA library from the mRNA of neuroblastoma cells (NG108) was used to transfect COS7 cells. A single plasmid was identified after subcloning in which transfected BSR cells bound soluble rabies virus glycoprotein. The 1.3-kb insert of this plasmid showed high homology with both rat and human p75[NTR]. Most cell lines of non-neuronal cell origin are not permissive for street rabies virus infection. BSR cells with stable expression of p75[NTR] were isolated, and they were found to bind soluble rabies virus glycoprotein. A fox street rabies virus isolate was able to infect p75[NTR]-expressing BSR cells but relatively few control BSR cells. p75[NTR]-expressing BSR cells were only slightly more susceptible to infection with CVS, and p75[NTR]-expressing BSR cells were 3 to 10 times more susceptible to CVS infection than control BSR cells in the presence of 10% serum. Since CVS, like street rabies virus strains, is highly neuronotropic *in vivo*, one would expect that CVS probably also would use the same receptors as street rabies viruses *in vivo*. In addition, evaluation of nonadapted street rabies virus infection of mice would be difficult. For example, a high incidence of spontaneous recovery with neurologic sequelae has been observed after peripheral inoculation of mice with a fox isolate of street virus (Jackson *et al.*, 1989). When p75[NTR]-deficient mice were infected intracerebrally with CVS, similar clinical features of disease and pathologic changes were observed in the brain as in mice expressing p75[NTR] (Jackson and Park, 1999). These findings raise questions about the importance of the p75[NTR] in the pathogenesis of rabies, although one cannot exclude the possibility that the repertoire of receptors used by street and fixed rabies virus strains are completely different *in vivo*.

VIII. BRAIN DYSFUNCTION IN RABIES

Despite the dramatic and severe clinical neurologic signs in rabies, the neuropathologic findings usually are quite mild (Perl and Good, 1991). This suggests that neuronal dysfunction must occur in rabies without detectable morphologic changes. Studies performed *in vitro* have shown that rabies virus has little or no inhibitory effect on cellular RNA and protein synthesis (Madore and England, 1977; Ermine and Flamand, 1977; Tuffereau and Martinet-Edelist, 1985). However, *in vivo* studies using CVS-24–infected rats showed that there was progressive reduction in the expression of the noninducible housekeeping gene that encodes glyceraldehyde-3-phosphate dehydrogenase and also the late response gene that encodes proenkephalin, possibly due to the global suppression of cellular protein synthesis related to extensive synthesis of rabies virus mRNA (Fu *et al.*, 1993). This occurred in association with induction of immediate-early-response genes (*erg-1, junB,* and *c-fos*) in the hippocampus and cerebral cortex, where there was colocalization of expression of these genes with viral mRNA expression. In another study, infection of mice with CVS-N2c resulted in down regulation of about 90% of genes in the normal brain at more than four-fold lower levels by using subtraction hybridization (Prosniak *et al.*, 2001). Only about 1.4% of genes became upregulated, including genes involved in regulation of cell metabolism, protein synthesis, and growth and differentiation. Although the basis of the neuronal dysfunction in rabies at the cellular level is unknown, a few of the leading hypotheses explaining neuronal dysfunction will be discussed.

A. Defective Neurotransmission

1. Acetylcholine

One hypothesis, that defective cholinergic neurotransmission might be the basis for neuronal dysfunction in rabies, led to the investigation of specific binding to muscarinic acetylcholine receptors in CVS-infected rat brains with an ^{3}H-labeled antagonist, quinuclidinyl benzylate (QNB) (Tsiang, 1982). This showed that binding of ^{3}H-labeled QNB to infected brain homogenates was decreased by 96 hours after infection compared with controls and that the binding was decreased markedly at 120 hours, which was 10–20 hours before death was expected to occur. The greatest reduction in binding was found in the hippocampus, and smaller reductions were observed in the cerebral cortex and in the caudate nucleus.

When cholinergic neurotransmission was examined in CVS-infected and uninfected control mice, the enzymatic activities of choline acetyltransferase and acetylcholinesterase, which are required for the synthesis and degradation of acetylcholine, respectively, were similar in the cerebral cortex and hippocampus of moribund CVS-infected and control mice (Jackson, 1993). In contrast to the findings in infected rats, binding to muscarinic acetylcholine receptors, which was assessed with ^{3}H-labeled QNB using Scatchard plots, was not significantly different in the cerebral cortex or hippocampus of CVS-infected and uninfected control mice. These findings cast doubt on the importance of rabies virus binding to muscarinic acetylcholine receptors in the brain. However, it is possible that differences in the species (mouse versus rat) or in the route of inoculation (peripheral versus intracerebral) account for the differences in the results of the two studies.

Reduced specific binding of ^{3}H-labeled QNB in the hippocampus (35% reduction) and brainstem (27% reduction), but not in other brain regions, was reported in naturally infected rabid dogs in Thailand compared with uninfected control dogs (Dumrongphol *et al.*, 1996). The results were similar with both the furious and dumb forms of clinical disease. K_d values were increased, indicating a decrease in receptor affinity, and B_{max} values, reflecting receptor content, were unchanged in rabid dogs. Curiously, increased K_d values were found to be similar in the hippocampus whether or not rabies virus antigen was detectable at that site. These findings argue against alteration of muscarinic receptor binding as a specific consequence of rabies virus infection of neurons. They suggest an unknown indirect mechanism for altered receptor affinity that is not related to clinical manifestations of disease or the local viral load.

2. Serotonin

Defective neurotransmission involving neurotransmitters other than acetylcholine could be important in the pathogenesis of rabies, and serotonin has received the most attention. Serotonin has a wide distribution in the brain, and it is important in the control of sleep and wakefulness, pain perception, memory, and a variety of behaviors (Julius, 1991). Alterations of sleep stages have been recognized in experimental rabies in mice (see Sect. VIIIB). Ligand binding to serotonin (5-HT) receptor subtypes was studied in the brains of CVS-infected rats (Ceccaldi *et al.*, 1993). Binding to 5-HT_1 receptor sites using $[^3\text{H}]5\text{-HT}$ was not affected in the hippocampus, but there was a marked decrease in maximum binding B_{max} in the cerebral cortex 5 days after inoculation of CVS into the masseter muscles. $[^3\text{H}]5\text{-HT}$ binding assessed in the presence of drugs masking 5-HT_{1A}, 5-HT_{1B}, and 5-HT_{1C} receptors was reduced by 50% in the cerebral cortex 3 days after inoculation, whereas binding of ligands specific for 5-HT_{1A} and 5-HT_{1B} receptor sites was not affected. These results suggest that rabies virus infection specifically affects 5-HT_{1D}-like receptors in the cerebral cortex. Furthermore, the reduced binding was demonstrated before rabies virus antigen was detected in the cerebral cortex. Hence the effect of rabies virus on receptor binding is unlikely due to either direct or indirect effects of viral replication in cortical neurons. There are important serotonergic projections from the dorsal raphe nuclei in the brainstem to the cerebral cortex that can lead to early infection of the midbrain raphe nuclei in experimental rabies in skunks (Smart and Charlton, 1992). It is possible that the reduced binding to 5-HT_{1D}-like receptors is an indirect effect of the infection at noncortical sites by unknown mechanisms or that it is part of a physiologic response to the stress produced by the infection. In support of impaired serotonergic neurotransmission in rabies, decreased (31%) potassium-evoked release of $[^3\text{H}]5\text{-HT}$ synaptosomes from the cerebral cortex of CVS-infected rats was found compared with controls (Bouzamondo *et al.*, 1993). Hence there is evidence of both impaired release and binding of serotonin, which might play an important role in producing the neuronal dysfunction in rabies.

3. γ-Amino-n-Butyric Acid

Impairments of both release and uptake of γ-amino-*n*-butyric acid (GABA) have been found in CVS-infected primary rat cortical neuronal cultures (Ladogana *et al.*, 1994). A 45% reduction of $[^3\text{H}]\text{GABA}$ uptake was found 3 days after infection, which coincided with the time of peak viral growth in the cultures. Kinetic analysis revealed major reductions in V_{max}, indicating a decrease in the number of fully active GABA transport sites. There were no significant changes in K_m in infected cultures in comparison with controls, reflecting the affinity of the GABA transport system. Potassium- and veratridine-induced $[^3\text{H}]\text{GABA}$ release was increased in infected cultures by 98% and 35%, respectively, compared with controls. The importance of these abnormalities in both the uptake and release of GABA on rabies pathogenesis *in vivo* has yet to be determined.

B. Electrophysiologic Alterations

In addition to effects on neurotransmission, viruses may have important effects on the electrophysiologic properties of neurons. Electroencephalographic (EEG) recordings of mice infected with CVS showed that the initial changes were alterations of sleep stages, including the disappearance of rapid-eye-movement (REM) sleep and the development of pseudoperiodic facial myoclonus (Gourmelon et al., 1986). Later, there was a generalized EEG slowing (at 2–4 cycles per second), and terminally, there was an extinction of hippocampal slow activity with flattening of cortical activity. Brain electrical activity terminated about 30 minutes before cardiac arrest, indicating that cerebral death in experimental rabies occurs prior to failure of vegetative functions. Street virus–infected mice showed progressive disappearance of all sleep stages with a concomitant increase in the duration of waking stages (indicating insomnia), and these changes occurred before the development of clinical signs of rabies (Gourmelon et al., 1991). There was an absence of EEG abnormalities in street virus–infected mice that lasted through the preagonal phase of the disease. Since pathologic changes are more marked in neurons infected with fixed rabies viruses than street rabies virus strains, these observations are consistent with the idea that functional impairment of brain neurons is much more important in street rabies virus infection than in infection with fixed rabies virus strains.

C. Ion Channels

Defective neurotransmission is not the only potential explanation for functional impairment of neurons in rabies. Viral infections might have important effects on ion channels of neurons. Studies were performed in vitro using rabies virus (RC-HL strain) infection of mouse neuroblastoma NA cells and the whole-cell patch clamp technique (Iwata et al., 1999). The infection reduced the functional expression of voltage-dependent sodium channels and inward rectifier potassium channels, and there was a decreased resting membrane potential reflecting membrane depolarization. There was no change in the expression of delayed rectifier potassium channels, indicating that nonselective dysfunction of ion channels had not occurred. The reduction in sodium channels and inward rectifier potassium channels could prevent infected neurons from firing action potentials and generating synaptic potentials, resulting in functional impairment.

Rabies virus (RC-HL strain) infection of NG108-15 cells in vitro was not found to alter the functional expression of voltage-dependent calcium ion channels (Iwata et al., 2000). NGl08-15 cells express both α_2-adrenoreceptors and muscarinic receptors. Induced voltage-dependent calcium ion channel current inhibition with noradrenaline (α_2-adrenoreceptors) was decreased significantly in rabies virus infection, whereas carbachol (muscarinic receptors) inhibition remained unchanged. Since α_2-adrenoreceptor-mediated inhibition of voltage-dependent calcium ion current serves as a brake mechanism to keep neurons from releasing their neurotransmitters beyond physiologic requirements, the impaired modulation by α_2-adrenoreceptors could possibly contribute to clinical features of rabies, including hyperexcitability and aggressive behavior (Iwata *et al.*, 2000).

D. Apoptosis

Apoptosis is a process by which cells undergo physiologic cell death in response to diverse stimuli. It is a normal process in embryonic development, maturation of the immune system, and normal tissue turnover (Buja *et al.*, 1993; Thompson, 1995). Morphologically, apoptosis is characterized by nuclear and cytoplasmic condensation of single parenchymal cells followed by fragmentation of the nuclear chromatin and subsequent formation of multiple fragments of condensed nuclear material and cytoplasm (Buja *et al.*, 1993). Phagocytosis of this material occurs, although an inflammatory reaction normally is absent. In contrast, cellular death due to necrosis is characterized by preservation of cell outlines, and there is variable swelling of the cell and of organelles. Cellular fragmentation occurs as a late event in necrosis. There are derangements in energy and substrate metabolism in necrosis that result in breaks in the plasma membrane and organellar membranes. Apoptosis is associated with endonuclease-mediated cleavage of the DNA of nuclear chromatin, resulting in DNA fragments with sizes in multiples of a single nucleosome length (180 bp). The internucleosomal cleavage of the DNA results in a "ladder" appearance on agarose gel electrophoresis, whereas in necrosis there is less specific degradation of DNA into a "smear" containing fragments of different sizes.

Apoptotic cell death likely plays an important pathogenetic role in a wide variety of viral infections, including a large number of RNA and DNA viruses (Razvi and Welsh, 1995; Hardwick, 1997). There have been a few reports of virus infections associated with apoptosis in the CNS of experimental animals (Fairbairn *et al.*, 1994; Lewis *et al.*, 1996; Pekosz *et al.*, 1996; Oberhaus *et al.*, 1997; Tsunoda *et al.*, 1997; Jackson and Rossiter, 1997b). There is also evidence that apoptosis is important in a variety of human CNS infections, including HIV encephalitis (Petito and Roberts, 1995), HTLV-1–associated myelopathy (HAM)/tropical spastic paraparesis (Umehara *et al.*, 1994), and subacute sclerosing panencephalitis (McQuaid *et al.*, 1997).

In recent studies, strong evidence of apoptotic cell death was found in both cultured cells and neurons in experimental rabies models in mice produced by intracerebral inoculation of fixed rabies virus strains (Jackson and Rossiter, 1997a; Jackson and Park, 1998; Jackson, 1999). *In vitro* studies in CVS infected cultured rat prostatic adenocarcinoma (AT3) cells showed striking morphologic changes of apoptosis at both the levels of light and electron microscopy, whereas AT3 cells transfected with the *bcl-2* gene (an antiapoptosis gene) did not demonstrate apoptotic changes (Jackson and Rossiter, 1997a). Terminal deoxynucleotidyltransferase-mediated dUTP–digoxigenin nick end labeling (TUNEL) staining was demonstrated in infected AT3 cells, indicating evidence of oligonucleosomal DNA fragmentation typical of apoptosis. *In vitro* infection of mouse neuroblastoma cells (N18) with CVS also was particularly associated with apoptosis (Theerasurakarn and Ubol, 1998). *In vitro* studies also have shown that the ERA strain of fixed rabies virus replicates and induces apoptosis in mouse spleen lymphocytes and the human T-lymphocyte cell line Jurkat (Thoulouze *et al.*, 1997) and that cell death was concomitant with expression of the viral glycoprotein.

In adult mice infected intracerebrally with CVS, morphologic changes of apoptosis were observed in neurons, particularly in pyramidal neurons of the hippocampus and cortical neurons, and there was positive TUNEL staining in the same regions (Jackson and Rossiter, 1997a) (Fig. 4). Double-labeling studies indicated that infected neurons actually underwent apoptosis. Increased expression of the Bax protein was observed in neurons in areas in where apoptosis was prominent (Jackson and Rossiter, 1997a). However, all infected neurons (e.g., Purkinje cells) did not demonstrate morphologic features of apoptosis or positive TUNEL staining.

CVS-infected suckling mice (6 days old) showed even more extensive infection, with a greater number of neurons demonstrating positive immunostaining for rabies virus antigen, more widespread and severe morphologic changes of apoptosis, and greater TUNEL staining (Jackson and Park, 1998) (Fig. 5). In this suckling mouse model, uninfected neurons in the external granular layer of the cerebellum also underwent apoptosis (see Fig. 5*B*,*C*) due to indirect mechanisms. Adult mice immunosuppressed with cyclophosphamide also developed massive apoptosis in the brain that was similar to immunocompetent mice, indicating that immune mechanisms may not be important in the pathogenesis of rabies virus–induced apoptosis of neurons (Theerasurakarn and Ubol, 1998).

Bax-deficient mice and their wild-type littermates also were studied to determine the importance of the *bax* gene in this model. Markedly less severe morphologic features of apoptosis were observed in the cerebral cortex, hippocampus, and cerebellum after intracerebral inoculation of suckling *bax*-deficient (knockout) mice with variant RV194-2 (avirulent in adult mice) than were found in the same regions in wild-type mice, although the infections were fatal in both groups (Jackson, 1999). Although the Bax protein plays an important role in modulating rabies virus–induced apoptosis under specific experimental conditions, this study indicates that other modulators are likely more important than Bax. The extent of apoptosis and pathogenicity were studied in primary neuron cultures infected with two stable variants of CVS-24, CVS-B2c

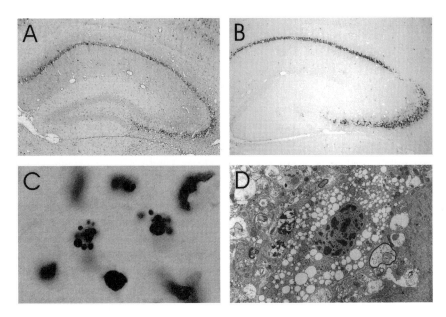

Fig. 4. Immunostaining for rabies virus antigen in the hippocampus of a mouse 7 days after intracerebral inoculation with CVS showing antigen in pyramidal neurons and in cortical neurons; neurons in the dentate gyrus do not demonstrate staining (*A*). TUNEL staining in the hippocampus of a mouse 7 days after intracerebral inoculation with CVS showing marked staining is present in pyramidal neurons but not in neurons of the dentate gyrus (*B*). Note the similarity in the distribution of TUNEL staining (*B*) and rabies virus antigen (*A*). Neurons in the cerebral cortex 8 days after inoculation with CVS showing multiple condensations of nuclear chromatin in two cells (*arrowheads*) (*C*). Hippocampal pyramidal neuron showing a pattern of irregular chromatin condensation and marked cytoplasmic vacuolation (*D*). (*A*: immunoperoxidase–hematoxylin; *B*: TUNEL staining; *C*: cresyl violet staining; *D*: transmission electron microscopy; magnifications: *A, B,* × 27; *C,* × 1220; *D,* × 4870.) (*Adapted with permission from Jackson and Rossiter, in Journal of Virology 71:5603–5607, 1997.*)

and CVS-N2c (Morimoto *et al.*, 1999). The authors found that the extent of apoptosis actually was lower in primary neuron cultures infected with the more pathogenic variant CVS-N2c than with the less pathogenic variant CVS-B2c in adult mice. However, *in vivo* studies examining apoptosis were not performed in mice with these variant strains.

The occurrence and importance of apoptosis in rabies under natural conditions (i.e., street rabies virus infection in a natural host) has not yet been established. Adult mice were infected experimentally by the intracerebral route (S. Ubol, personal communication) with dog and bat isolates of street rabies virus (Ubol and Kasisith, 2000). Strong TUNEL staining was observed in the cerebrum and cerebellum, but the involved neural cell types were not identified in this report. Upregulation of Nedd-2 (caspase 2) mRNA was observed in the brains of both

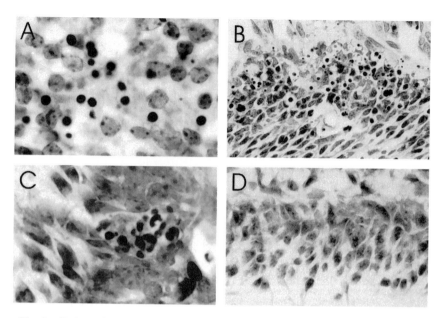

Fig. 5. Brain sections after intracerebral inoculation with CVS-11 of 6-day-old mice. Multiple neurons in the dentate gyrus of the hippocampus showing chromatin condensations involving entire nuclei (A). The external granular layer of the cerebellum of a CVS-infected mouse showing many cells with condensations of nuclear chromatin (B). Nuclear chromatin condensations in multiple cells in the external granular layer of the cerebellum in an infected mouse (C). External granular layer of the cerebellum of an uninfected mouse of the same age showing the absence of typical apoptotic morphology (D). (A–D: cresyl violet staining; magnifications: A, C, × 880; B, × 400; D, × 490.) (*Adapted with permission from Jackson and Park, in Acta Neuropathologica 95:159–164, 1998.*)

infected adult and suckling mice. Nedd-2 is a developmentally downregulated apoptosis gene, and reactivation of this gene may be important in rabies virus–induced apoptosis. There is a report demonstrating evidence of apoptosis in a single human rabies case (Adle-Biassette *et al.*, 1996). It is possible that the mechanisms that are important in inducing apoptosis in experimental models are also important in producing the neuronal dysfunction in natural rabies.

E. Nitric Oxide

Nitric oxide is a short-lived gaseous radical that acts as a biologic mediator for diverse cell types. It is produced by many different cells and mediates a variety of functions, including vasodilation, neurotransmission, immune cytotoxicity, production of synaptic plasticity in the brain, and neurotoxicity (Nathan, 1992; Lowenstein *et al.*, 1994). Nitric oxide is released by the enzyme nitric oxide synthase (NOS), which also produces other reactive oxides of nitrogen (Nathan, 1992). There are three isoforms of NOS: neuronal NOS (nNOS, also NOS-l), inducible NOS (iNOS, also NOS-2), and endothelial NOS (eNOS, also NOS-3). nNOS is constitutively expressed and inducible with cytokines, including IFN-γ, TNF-α, and IL-12, whereas iNOS is inducible with lipopolysaccharides, IFN-γ, and TNF-α.

Nitric oxide plays a variety of roles in different viral infections (Reiss and Komatsu, 1998). In some viral infections (e.g., Sindbis virus infection), inhibition of NOS results in increased mortality of infected mice, suggesting that nitric oxide plays a protective role in the pathogenesis of the viral infection (Tucker *et al.*, 1996). The human immunodeficiency virus type 1 coat protein, gp120, is neurotoxic in primary cortical cultures, and nitric oxide likely contributes to the neurotoxicity (Dawson *et al.*, 1993). Nitric oxide mediates much of the antimicrobial activity of mouse macrophages against a variety of bacterial, fungal, protozoal and helminthic pathogens (Nathan and Hibbs, 1991). Nitric oxide also has antiviral activity. Replication of herpes simplex virus type 1 in the mouse RAW macrophage cell line, which is transformed with Abelson leukemia virus, was inhibited by IFN-γ and bacterial lipopolysaccharide, which induce nitric oxide production (Croen, 1993). Competitive and noncompetitive inhibitors of NOS substantially reduced the antiviral effect of activated RAW macrophages. An exogenous donor of nitric oxide, *S*-nitroso-L-acetyl penicillamine (SNAP), reduced herpes simplex virus replication in a variety of cell lines, including RAW macrophages, and the antiviral effect of SNAP did not appear to be due to a cytotoxic effect of nitric oxide. The ability of IFN-γ to inhibit replication of ectromelia, vaccinia, and herpes simplex virus type 1 in mouse RAW macrophages correlated with the cellular production of nitric oxide, and viral replication was restored with exposure to NOS inhibitors (Karupiah *et al.*, 1993). Karupiah *et al.* also showed that a competitive inhibitor of iNOS, *N*-methyl-L-arginine, converted resolving ectromelia virus infection in mice into fulminant mousepox. During infection with vesicular stomatitis virus (a rhabdovirus), nitric oxide has been shown to inhibit viral replication and promote viral clearance and recovery of infected mice (Komatsu *et al.*, 1996).

Induction of iNOS mRNA occurred in mice infected experimentally with street rabies virus (Koprowski *et al.*, 1993). iNOS mRNA was detected using RT-PCR amplification in the brains of three of six paralyzed mice 9–14 days after inoculation of rabies virus in the masseter muscle. iNOS mRNA expression was induced rapidly in the brains of the rabid mice. Koprowski *et al.* speculated that nitric oxide and/or other endogenous neurotoxins may mediate the neuronal dysfunction in rabies and other infectious diseases (Koprowski *et al.*, 1993; Zheng *et al.*, 1993). The onset of clinical signs in rabies virus–infected rats and the clinical progression of disease correlated with increasing quantities of nitric oxide in the brain to levels up to 30-fold more than in controls, which was determined using spin trapping of nitric oxide and electron paramagnetic resonance spectroscopy (Hooper *et al.*, 1995). iNOS was detected by immunostaining in CVS-infected rats in many cells throughout the brain near blood vessels, which were identified as microglia and macrophages (Van Dam *et al.*, 1995). CVS-24–infected rats developed a reduction in nNOS activity with reductions in nNOS mRNA and nNOS immunoreactivity and an increase in iNOS activity in the brain in a time-dependent manner (Akaike *et al.*, 1995). Choline acetyltransferase activity in the brain remained unchanged, indicating that the decrease in nNOS activity did not reflect generalized neuronal loss. The nitric oxide produced by macrophages may be neurotoxic because its reaction with superoxide anion O_2^- leads to the formation of peroxynitrate, which is a reactive oxidizing agent capable of causing tissue damage (Akaike *et al.*, 1995). Ubol *et al.* (2001) found that treating with the iNOS inhibitor aminoguanidine (AG) delayed the death of CVS-11–infected mice by 1.0–1.6 days (depending on the dose). A delay in rabies virus replication was observed in the AG-treated mice. The role of nitric oxide in rabies pathogenesis clearly needs further study because it exerts both beneficial and detrimental effects, and complex mechanisms are involved.

F. Bases for Behavioral Changes

The neuroanatomic bases for the behavioral changes in animals with rabies have not yet been well characterized. Limbic system infection and dysfunction are suspected to play an important role in the behavioral changes, including alertness, loss of natural timidity, aberrant sexual behavior, and aggressiveness (Johnson, 1971). However, experimental rabies studies in these models have not been particularly helpful in giving insights into the neuroanatomic substrate for behavioral changes because these changes normally are not observed in rodent models, and hippocampal infection actually occurs relatively late after peripheral routes of inoculation (Jackson and Reimer, 1989). The neural mechanisms of aggressive behavior are not well understood. Aggressive behavior is associated with lesions in a variety of locations in the brain, including the posterior olfactory bulbs, the ventromedial nucleus of the hypothalamus, and the septal area (Isaacson, 1989). Offensive aggression, which often is impulsive and seemingly unprovoked, has been associated with low CNS serotonergic activity as well as increased testosterone in humans and animal studies (Kalin, 1999). Aggressive behavior is essential in most rabies vectors for horizontal transmission of the virus to other hosts by biting. Early and selective brainstem infection in rabies would allow centrifugal spread of the virus to salivary glands as well as involvement of the serotonergic system in the raphe nuclei, resulting in aggressive behavior of animals with adequate cognitive and motor function in order to execute successful viral transmission by biting. Few studies have been performed in natural models of rabies in which aggressive behavior is exhibited. Striped skunks inoculated peripherally with a skunk isolate of street rabies virus were compared with skunks infected with CVS (Smart and Charlton, 1992). The street virus–infected skunks exhibited aggressive responses to presentation of a stick in their cages, and this behavior was not observed in CVS-infected skunks. Heavy accumulations of viral antigen were found in the midbrain raphe nuclei, red nucleus, dorsal motor nucleus of the vagus, and hypoglossal nucleus in street virus–infected skunks but not in CVS-infected skunks. Impaired serotonin neurotransmission from the raphe nuclei in the brainstem may account for the development of aggressive behavior in natural vectors of rabies.

IX. RECOVERY FROM RABIES AND CHRONIC RABIES VIRUS INFECTION

Although rabies usually is considered a uniformly fatal disease, it has been recognized that animals sometimes may recover from rabies. Recovery from rabies also has been called *abortive rabies*, which can occur either with or without neurologic sequelae (Bell, 1975). There have been a large number of reports of survival after the development of neurologic illness, particularly in experimental animals (Jackson, 1997). Because of limitations on laboratory diagnostic tests performed during life, a conclusive diagnosis of rabies is only rarely made in natural cases that recover. Animals clinically suspected of having rabies usually are killed, and they do not have an opportunity to recover. In a series of five reports from the Pasteur Institute of Southern India, the unusual case of a chronically infected dog was described (Veeraraghavan et al., 1967a,b, 1968, 1969, 1970). A 14-year-old boy died with hydrophobia 48 days after he stepped on a dog and was bitten in November 1965 (Veeraraghavan et al., 1967a). The dog was observed at the Pasteur Institute until it died in February 1969 (Veeraraghavan et al., 1970). During that period, rabies virus was isolated from daily saliva samples taken from the dog on 13 occasions between January and May 1966 (Veeraraghavan et al., 1967b) and once in January 1967 after the dog was given a course of prednisolone (Veeraraghavan et al., 1968). Rabies virus was not isolated postmortem from the dog's brain, spinal cord, or salivary glands, although fluorescent antibody staining showed rabies virus antigen in its brain and spinal cord (Veeraraghavan et al., 1970). No anti–rabies virus antibodies were found in the dog's blood at any time (Veeraraghavan et al., 1967b, 1968, 1969, 1970). This is an extremely interesting and unusual series of reports. It is unlikely that this seronegative dog excreted a virulent rabies virus that was responsible for the boy's death. The boy may have become infected from an undocumented rabies exposure months or even years earlier (Smith et al., 1991). There was a poor correlation of this laboratory's results with viral isolation and antigen detection in saliva samples and in CNS tissues from the dog. This could be explained by the presence of neutralizing antibodies in tissues, but this should not have been possible because the dog was seronegative. The viral isolations from saliva samples could have been due to contamination in the laboratory. Because of a number of inconsistencies, there remains uncertainty about the validity of this series of reports.

In another report, five dogs in Ethiopia are described that remained healthy for up to 72 months after the first isolation of rabies virus from their saliva (Fekadu, 1972, 1975). However, exposures from these dogs did not result in any human cases of rabies. Excretion of rabies virus was documented in the saliva of a dog experimentally infected with an Ethiopian strain of dog rabies virus for up to 6 months after its recovery from rabies (Fekadu et al., 1981).

Early studies on rabies pathogenesis in vampire bats, which were performed in Trinidad, suggested that bats might be chronically infected with rabies virus and secrete infectious rabies virus over periods lasting up to several months (Pawan, 1936). These early studies were performed before modern virologic methods became available and suffered from inadequate diagnostic evaluations, which largely were limited to examination of tissues for Negri bodies. Infections with a variety of other bat viruses, including Rio Bravo virus, may have been misdiagnosed as rabies virus (Moreno and Baer, 1980; Constantine, 1988). More recent experimental studies have shown that vampire bats have variable incubation periods lasting up to 4 weeks and then develop an acute disease with excretion of virus in the saliva that is not prolonged (Moreno and Baer, 1980). Hence there is little support for the concept of a carrier state in these bats; the outcome of rabies virus infection in bats is felt to be similar to that in terrestrial animals.

Remarkable cases of experimental rabies in two cats were reported (Murphy et al., 1980). Cat 1 developed paralysis, most marked in its hindlimbs, 17 days after inoculation of a rabies virus strain isolated from a big brown bat. The cat showed slow progressive recovery until 100 weeks after inoculation, when it developed progressive neurologic deterioration with aggressive behavior and weakness and atrophy; it was killed for further study 136 weeks after inoculation. Cat 2 remained well until 120 weeks after inoculation, when it developed progressive neurologic deterioration; it was also killed at 136 weeks after inoculation. There were high titers of neutralizing antibody in the serum and CSF of both cats. Rabies virus was not isolated from the saliva or tissue suspensions from these cats except from the brain of cat 2 by explant culture techniques. Rabies virus antigen was detected at multiple sites in the CNS, and viral inclusions were found in neurons at four sites in the brain of cat 2. Degenerative neuronal changes were noted, and there were extensive inflammatory changes in both cats. Perl et al. (1977) also reported a similar recrudescent form of rabies in a cat infected experimentally with a bat rabies virus isolate. At necropsy, there were features of a chronic encephalitis. Rabies virus could not be isolated from CNS tissues, probably because of the presence of neutralizing antibodies. These well-documented extraordinary cases indicate that chronic rabies virus infection may occur rarely, at least under experimental conditions. However, it is unclear if chronic rabies infections have any significance in the natural history of rabies, including a role in perpetuation of rabies in natural reservoirs. If animals with chronic rabies are unable to transmit the virus and are incompetent vectors, then this chronic state may not have any biologic importance in nature.

X. SUMMARY

Rabies is a normally fatal viral infection of the nervous system in humans and animals with characteristic clinical manifestations. Considerable progress has been made in understanding the pathogenesis of rabies. Rabies virus is highly neurotropic. It binds to the nicotinic acetylcholine receptor at the neuromuscular junction, and it spreads by axonal transport via peripheral nerves to the CNS, where it produces causes widespread infection of neurons within the CNS. The combination of virus-induced behavioral changes in rabies vectors and centrifugal spread of the virus to salivary glands allows efficient transmission of the infection.

An understanding of the basis of rabies virus neurovirulence is emerging from studies on variants using a variety of animal models. A single amino acid change in the rabies virus glycoprotein at position 333 has dramatic effects on the outcome of infection, and it affects the efficiency and pathways of viral spread and cellular tropisms.

The precise events at the site of viral entry during the long incubation period of rabies remain poorly understood. The fundamental basis for neuronal dysfunction in rabies has not yet been determined, although there are several hypotheses under active study at the present time. A better understanding of rabies pathogenesis hopefully will lead to advances in the treatment of rabies and other viral diseases.

REFERENCES

Adle-Biassette, H., Bourhy, H., Gisselbrecht, M., Chretien, F., Wingertsmann, L., Baudrimont, M., Rotivel, Y., Godeau, B., and Gray, F. (1996). Rabies encephalitis in a patient with AIDS: A clinicopathological study. *Acta Neuropathol.* **92**, 415–420.

Akaike, T., Weihe, E., Schaefer, M., Fu, Z. F., Zheng, Y. M., Vogel, W., Schmidt, H., Koprowski, H., and Dietzschold, B. (1995). Effect of neurotropic virus infection on neuronal and inducible nitric oxide synthase activity in rat brain. *J. Neurovirol.* **1**, 118–125.

Araujo, M. D. F., de Brito, T., and Machado, C. G. (1971). Myocarditis in human rabies. *Rev. Inst. Med. Trop. Sao Paulo* **13**, 99–102.

Baer, G. M., Bellini, W. J., and Fishbein, D. B. (1990a). Rhabdoviruses. In *Virology*, Vol. 1, B. N. Fields, D. M. Knipe, R. M. Chanock, M. S. Hirsch, J. L. Melnick, T. P. Monath, and B. Roizman (eds.), pp. 883–930. Raven Press, New York.

Baer, G. M., and Cleary, W. F. (1972). A model in mice for the pathogenesis and treatment of rabies. *J. Infect. Dis.* **125**, 520–527.

Baer, G. M., Shaddock, J. H., Quirion, R., Dam, T. V., and Lentz, T. L. (1990b). Rabies susceptibility and acetylcholine receptor (Letter). *Lancet* **335**, 664–665.

Baer, G. M., Shantha, T. R., and Bourne, G. H. (1968). The pathogenesis of street rabies virus in rats. *Bull. WHO* **38**, 119–125.

Baer, G. M., Shanthaveerappa, T. R., and Bourne, G. H. (1965). Studies on the pathogenesis of fixed rabies virus in rats. *Bull. WHO* **33**, 783–794.

Balachandran, A., and Charlton, K. (1994). Experimental rabies infection of non-nervous tissues in skunks (*Mephitis mephitis*) and foxes (*Vulpes vulpes*). *Vet. Pathol.* **31**, 93–102.

Bell, J. F. (1975). Latency and abortive rabies. In *The Natural History of Rabies*, G. M. Baer (ed.), pp. 331–354. Academic Press, New York.

Bouzamondo, E., Ladogana, A., and Tsiang, H. (1993). Alteration of potassium-evoked 5-HT release from virus-infected rat cortical synaptosomes. *Neuroreport* **4**, 555–558.

Bracci, L., Antoni, G., Cusi, M. G., Lozzi, L., Niccolai, N., Petreni, S., Rustici, M., Santucci, A., Soldani, P., Valensin, P. E., and Neri, P. (1988). Antipeptide monoclonal antibodies inhibit the binding of rabies virus glycoprotein and alpha-bungarotoxin to the nicotinic acetylcholine receptor. *Mol. Immunol.* **25**, 881–888.

Buja, L. M., Eigenbrodt, M. L., and Eigenbrodt, E. H. (1993). Apoptosis and necrosis: Basic types and mechanisms of cell death. *Arch. Pathol. Lab. Med.* **117**, 1208–1214.

Carbone, K. M., Duchala, C. S., Griffin, J. W., Kincaid, A. L., and Narayan, O. (1987). Pathogenesis of Borna disease in rats: Evidence that intra-axonal spread is the major route for virus dissemination and the determinant for disease incubation. *J. Virol.* **61**, 3431–3440.

Ceccaldi, P.-E., Ermine, A., and Tsiang, H. (1990). Continuous delivery of colchicine in the rat brain with osmotic pumps for inhibition of rabies virus transport. *J. Virol. Methods* **28**, 79–84.

Ceccaldi, P.-E., Fillion, M.-P., Ermine, A., Tsiang, H., and Fillion, G. (1993). Rabies virus selectively alters 5-HT$_1$ receptor subtypes in rat brain. *Eur. J. Pharmacol.* **245**, 129–138.

Ceccaldi, P.-E., Gillet, J. P., and Tsiang, H. (1989). Inhibition of the transport of rabies virus in the central nervous system. *J. Neuropathol, Exp. Neurol.* **48**, 620–630.

Charlton, K. M., and Casey, G. A. (1979a). Experimental oral and nasal transmission of rabies virus in mice. *Can. J. Comp. Med.* **43**, 10–15.

Charlton, K. M., and Casey, G. A. (1979b). Experimental rabies in skunks: Immunofluorescence light and electron microscopic studies. *Lab. Invest.* **41**, 36–44.

Charlton, K. M., and Casey, G. A. (1979c). Experimental rabies in skunks: Oral, nasal, tracheal and intestinal exposure. *Can. J. Comp. Med.* **43**, 168–172.

Charlton, K. M., Casey, G. A., and Campbell, J. B. (1983). Experimental rabies in skunks: Mechanisms of infection of the salivary glands. *Can. J. Comp. Med.* **47**, 363–369.

Charlton, K. M., Casey, G. A., Wandeler, A. I., and Nadin-Davis, S. (1996). Early events in rabies virus infection of the central nervous system in skunks (*Mephitis mephitis*). *Acta Neuropathol.* **91**, 89–98.

Charlton, K. M., Nadin-Davis, S., Casey, G. A., and Wandeler, A. I. (1997). The long incubation period in rabies: Delayed progression of infection in muscle at the site of exposure. *Acta Neuropathol.* **94**, 73–77.

Cheetham, H. D., Hart, J., Coghill, N. F., and Fox, B. (1970). Rabies with myocarditis: Two cases in England. *Lancet* **1**, 921–922.

Constantine, D. G. (1988). Transmission of pathogenic organisms by vampire bats. In *Natural History of Vampire Bats*, A. M. Greenhall and U. Schmidt (eds.), pp. 167–189. CRC Press, Boca Raton, FL.

Constantine, D. G. (1962). Rabies transmission by nonbite route. *Public Health Rep.* **77**, 287–289.

Constantine, D. G., Emmons, R. W., and Woodie, J. D. (1972). Rabies virus in nasal mucosa of naturally infected bats. *Science* **175**, 1255–1256.

Conti, C., Superti, F., and Tsiang, H. (1986). Membrane carbohydrate requirement for rabies virus binding to chicken embryo related cells. *Intervirology* **26**, 164–168.

Coulon, P., Derbin, C., Kucera, P., Lafay, F., Prehaud, C., and Flamand, A. (1989). Invasion of the peripheral nervous systems of adult mice by the CVS strain of rabies virus and its avirulent derivative Av01. *J. Virol.* **63**, 3550–3554.

Coulon, P., Rollin, P., Aubert, M., and Flamand, A. (1982). Molecular basis of rabies virus virulence: I. Selection of avirulent mutants of the CVS strain with anti-G monoclonal antibodies. *J. Gen. Virol.* **61**, 97–100.

Croen, K. D. (1993). Evidence for an antiviral effect of nitric oxide: Inhibition of herpes simplex virus type 1 replication. *J. Clin. Invest.* **91**, 2446–2452.

Dawson, V. L., Dawson, T. M., Uhl, G. R., and Snyder, S. H. (1993). Human immunodeficiency virus type 1 coat protein neurotoxicity mediated by nitric oxide in primary cortical cultures. *Proc. Natl. Acad. Sci. USA* **90**, 3256–3259.

Dean, D. J., Evans, W. M., and McClure, R. C. (1963). Pathogenesis of rabies. *Bull. WHO* **29**, 803–811.

Debbie, J. G., and Trimarchi, C. V. (1970). Pantropism of rabies virus in free-ranging rabid red fox *Vulpes fulva. J. Wildlife Dis.* **6**, 500–506.

Dierks, R. E. (1975). Electron microscopy of extraneural rabies infection. In *The Natural History of Rabies*, G. M. Baer (ed.), pp. 303–318. Academic Press, New York.

Dietzschold, B., Wunner, W. H., Wiktor, T. J., Lopes, A. D., Lafon, M., Smith, C. L., and Koprowski, H. (1983). Characterization of an antigenic determinant of the glycoprotein that correlates with pathogenicity of rabies virus. *Proc. Natl. Acad. Sci. USA* **80**, 70–74.

Dumrongphol, H., Srikiatkhachorn, A., Hemachudha, T., Kotchabhakdi, N., and Govitrapong, P. (1996). Alteration of muscarinic acetylcholine receptors in rabies viral-infected dog brains. *J. Neurol. Sci.* **137**, 1–6.

Emmelin, N. (1967). Nervous control of salivary glands. In *Handbook of Physiology*, Sect. 6, Vol. II, C. F. Code (ed.), pp. 595–632. American Physiological Society, Washington, DC.

Ermine, A., and Flamand, A. (1977). RNA syntheses in BHK_{21} cells infected by rabies virus. *Ann. Microbiol.* **128**, 477–488.

Etessami, R., Conzelmann, K. K., Fadai-Ghotbi, B., Natelson, B., Tsiang, H., and Ceccaldi, P. E. (2000). Spread and pathogenic characteristics of a G-deficient rabies virus recombinant: An *in vitro* and *in vivo* study. *J. Gen. Virol.* **81**, 2147–2153.

Fairbairn, D. W., Carnahan, K. G., Thwaits, R. N., Grigsby, R. V., Holyoak, G. R., and O'Neill, K. L. (1994). Detection of apoptosis induced DNA cleavage in scrapie-infected sheep brain. *FEMS Microbiol. Lett.* **115**, 341–346.

Fekadu, M. (1972). Atypical rabies in dogs in Ethiopia. *Ethiop. Med. J.* **10**, 79–86.

Fekadu, M. (1975). Asymptomatic non-fatal canine rabies (Letter). *Lancet* **1**, 569.

Fekadu, M., Shaddock, J. H., and Baer, G. M. (1981). Intermittent excretion of rabies virus in the saliva of a dog two and six months after it had recovered from experimental rabies. *Am. J. Trop. Med. Hyg.* **30**, 1113–1115.

Fischman, H. R., and Schaeffer, M. (1971). Pathogenesis of experimental rabies as revealed by immunofluorescence. *Ann. N.Y. Acad. Sci.* **177**, 78–97.

Fischman, H. R., and Ward, F. E. (1968). Oral transmission of rabies virus in experimental animals. *Am. J. Epidemiol.* **88**, 132–138.

Flamand, A., Coulon, P., Pepin, M., Blancou, J., Rollin, P., and Portnoi, D. (1984). Immunogenic and protective power of avirulent mutants of rabies virus selected with neutralizing monoclonal antibodies. In *Modern Approaches to Vaccines: Molecular and Chemical Basis of Virus Virulence and Immunogenicity*, R. M. Chanock and R. A. Lerner (eds.), pp. 289–294. Cold Spring Harbor Laboratory, Cold Spring Harbor, NY.

Fu, Z. F., Weihe, E., Zheng, Y. M., Schafer, M.-H., Sheng, H., Corisdeo, S., Rauscher, F. J., Koprowski, H., and Dietzschold, B. (1993). Differential effects of rabies and Borna disease viruses on immediate-early- and late-response gene expression in brain tissues. *J. Virol.* **67**, 6674–6681.

Gillet, J. P., Derer, P., and Tsiang, H. (1986). Axonal transport of rabies virus in the central nervous system of the rat. *J. Neuropathol. Exp. Neurol.* **45**, 619–634.

Gourmelon, P., Briet, D., Clarencon, D., Court, L., and Tsiang, H. (1991). Sleep alterations in experimental street rabies virus infection occur in the absence of major EEG abnormalities. *Brain Res.* **554**, 159–165.

Gourmelon, P., Briet, D., Court, L., and Tsiang, H. (1986). Electrophysiological and sleep alterations in experimental mouse rabies. *Brain Res.* **398**, 128–140.

Hanham, C. A., Zhao, F., and Tignor, G. H. (1993). Evidence from the anti-idiotypic network that the acetylcholine receptor is a rabies virus receptor. *J. Virol.* **67**, 530–542.

Hardwick, J. M. (1997). Virus-induced apoptosis. *Adv. Pharmacol.* **41**, 295–336.

Hooper, D. C., Ohnishi, S. T., Kean, R., Numagami, Y., Dietzschold, B., and Koprowski, H. (1995). Local nitric oxide production in viral and autoimmune diseases of the central nervous system. *Proc. Natl. Acad. Sci. USA* **92**, 5312–5316.

Hronovsky, V., and Benda, R. (1969). Development of inhalation rabies infection in suckling guinea pigs. *Acta Virol.* **13**, 198–202.

Isaacson, R. L. (1989). The neural and behavioural mechanisms of aggression and their alteration by rabies and other viral infections. In *Progress in Rabies Control: Proceedings of the Second International IMVI ESSEN/WHO Symposium on "New Developments in Rabies Control", Essen, 5–7 July 1988, and, Report of the WHO Consultation on Rabies, Essen, 8 July 1988, WHO Consultation on Rabies*, O. Thraenhart, H. Koprowski, K. Bögel and P. Sureau (eds.), pp. 17–23. Wells Medical, Royal Tunbridge Wells, Kent, UK.

Iwasaki, Y., and Clark, H. F. (1975). Cell-to-cell transmission of virus in the central nervous system: II. Experimental rabies in mouse. *Lab. Invest.* **33**, 391–399.

Iwata, M., Komori, S., Unno T., Minamoto, N., and Ohashi, H. (1999). Modification of membrane currents in mouse neuroblastoma cells following infection with rabies virus. *Br. J. Pharmacol.* **126**, 1691–1698.

Iwata, M., Unno, T., Minamoto, N., Ohashi, H., and Komori, S. (2000). Rabies virus infection prevents the modulation by α_2-adrenoceptors, but not muscarinic receptors, of Ca^{2+} channels in NG108-15 cells. *Eur. J. Pharmacol.* **404**, 79–88.

Jackson, A. C. (1991a). Analysis of viral neurovirulence. In *Molecular Genetic Approaches to Neuropsychiatric Diseases*, J. Brosius and R. T. Fremeau (eds.), pp. 259–277. Academic Press, San Diego.

Jackson, A. C. (1991b). Biological basis of rabies virus neurovirulence in mice: Comparative pathogenesis study using the immunoperoxidase technique. *J. Virol.* **65**, 537–540.

Jackson, A. C. (1993). Cholinergic system in experimental rabies in mice. *Acta Virol.* **37**, 502–508.

Jackson, A. C. (1994). Animal models of rabies virus neurovirulence. In *Current Topics in Microbiology and Immunology*, Vol. 187: *Lyssaviruses*, C. E. Rupprecht, B. Dietzschold, and H. Koprowski (eds.), pp. 85–93. Springer-Verlag, Berlin.

Jackson, A. C. (1997). Rabies. In *Viral Pathogenesis*, N. Nathanson, R. Ahmed, F. Gonzalez-Scarano, D. E. Griffin, K. Holmes, F. A. Murphy, and H. L. Robinson (eds.), pp. 575–591. Lippincott-Raven, Philadelphia.

Jackson, A. C. (1999). Apoptosis in experimental rabies in *bax*-deficient mice. *Acta Neuropathol.* **98**, 288–294.

Jackson, A. C., and Park, H. (1998). Apoptotic cell death in experimental rabies in suckling mice. *Acta Neuropathol.* **95**, 159–164.

Jackson, A. C., and Park, H. (1999). Experimental rabies virus infection of p75 neurotrophin receptor–deficient mice. *Acta Neuropathol.* **98**, 641–644.

Jackson, A. C., Phelan, C. C., and Rossiter, J. P. (2000). Infection of Bergmann glia in the cerebellum of a skunk experimentally infected with street rabies virus. *Can. J. Vet. Res.* **64**, 226–228.

Jackson, A. C., and Reimer, D. L. (1989) Pathogenesis of experimental rabies in mice: An immuno-histochemical study. *Acta Neuropathol.* **78**, 159–165.

Jackson, A. C., Reimer, D. L., and Ludwin, S. K. (1989). Spontaneous recovery from the encephalomyelitis in mice caused by street rabies virus. *Neuropathol. Appl. Neurobiol.* **15**, 459–475.

Jackson, A. C., and Rossiter, J. P. (1997a). Apoptosis plays an important role in experimental rabies virus infection. *J. Virol.* **71**, 5603–5607.

Jackson, A. C., and Rossiter, J. P. (1997b). Apoptotic cell death is an important cause of neuronal injury in experimental Venezuelan equine encephalitis virus infection of mice. *Acta Neuropathol.* **93**, 349–353.

Jackson, A. C., Ye, H., Phelan, C. C., Ridaura-Sanz, C., Zheng, Q., Li, Z., Wan, X., and Lopez-Corella, E. (1999). Extraneural organ involvement in human rabies. *Lab. Invest.* **79**, 945–951.

Jacob, Y., Badrane, H., Ceccaldi, P. E., and Tordo, N. (2000). Cytoplasmic dynein LC8 interacts with lyssavirus phosphoprotein. *J. Virol.* **74**, 10217–10222.

Johnson, R. T. (1965). Experimental rabies: Studies of cellular vulnerability and pathogenesis using fluorescent antibody staining. *J. Neuropathol. Exp. Neurol.* **24**, 662–674.

Johnson, R. T. (1971). The pathogenesis of experimental rabies. In *Rabies,* Y. Nagano and F. M. Davenport (eds.), pp. 59–75. University Park Press, Baltimore.

Julius, D. (1991). Molecular biology of serotonin receptors. *Annu. Rev. Neurosci.* **14**, 335–360.

Kalin, N. H. (1999). Primate models to understand human aggression. *J. Clin. Psychiatry* **60** (Suppl. 15), 29–32.

Karupiah, G., Xie, Q., Buller, M. L., Nathan, C., Duarte, C., and MacMicking, J. D. (1993). Inhibition of viral replication by interferon-gamma-induced nitric oxide synthase. *Science* **261**, 1445–1448.

Kelly, R. M., and Strick, P. L. (2000). Rabies as a transneuronal tracer of circuits in the central nervous system. *J. Neurosci. Methods* **103**, 63–71.

Koch, F. J., Sagartz, J. W., Davidson, D. E., and Lawhaswasdi, K. (1975). Diagnosis of human rabies by the cornea test. *Am. J. Clin. Pathol.* **63**, 509–515.

Komatsu, T., Bi, Z., and Reiss, C. S. (1996). Interferon-γ induced type I nitric oxide synthase activity inhibits viral replication in neurons. *J. Neuroimmunol.* **68**, 101–108.

Koprowski, H., Zheng, Y. M., Heber-Katz, E., Fraser N., Rorke, L., Fu, Z. F., Hanlon, C., and Dietzschold, B. (1993). *In vivo* expression of inducible nitric oxide synthase in experimentally induced neurologic disease. *Proc. Natl. Acad. Sci. USA* **90**, 3024–3027.

Kucera, P., Dolivo, M., Coulon, P., and Flamand, A. (1985). Pathways of the early propagation of virulent and avirulent rabies strains from the eye to the brain. *J. Virol.* **55**, 158–162.

Ladogana, A., Bouzamondo, E., Pocchiari, M., and Tsiang, H. (1994). Modification of tritiated γ-amino-*n*-butyric acid transport in rabies virus–infected primary cortical cultures. *J. Gen. Virol.* **75**, 623–627.

Lafay, F., Coulon, P., Astic, L., Saucier, D., Riche, D., Holley, A., and Flamand, A. (1991). Spread of the CVS strain of rabies virus and of the avirulent mutant AvO1 along the olfactory pathways of the mouse after intranasal inoculation. *Virology* **183**, 320–330.

Lentz, T. L. (1985). Rabies virus receptors. *Trends Neurosci.* **8**, 360–364.

Lentz, T. L. (1990). Rabies virus binding to an acetylcholine receptor α-subunit peptide. *J. Mol. Recognit.* **3**, 82–88.

Lentz, T. L., Benson, R. J. J., Klimowicz, D., Wilson, P. T., and Hawrot, E. (1986). Binding of rabies virus to purified *Torpedo* acetylcholine receptor. *Mol. Brain Res.* **387**, 211–219.

Lentz, T. L., Burrage, T. G., Smith, A. L., Crick, J., and Tignor, G. H. (1982). Is the acetylcholine receptor a rabies virus receptor? *Science* **215**, 182–184.

Lentz, T. L., Wilson, P. T., Hawrot, E., and Speicher, D. W. (1984). Amino acid sequence similarity between rabies virus glycoprotein and snake venom curaremimetic neurotoxins. *Science* **226**, 847–848.

Lewis, J., Wesselingh, S. L., Griffin, D. E., and Hardwick, J. M. (1996). Alphavirus-induced apoptosis in mouse brains correlates with neurovirulence. *J. Virol.* **70**, 1828–1835.

Lewis, P., Fu, Y., and Lentz, T. L. (2000). Rabies virus entry at the neuromuscular junction in nerve–muscle cocultures. *Muscle Nerve* **23**, 720–730.

Lowenstein, C. J., Dinerman, J. L., and Snyder, S. H. (1994). Nitric oxide: A physiologic messenger. *Ann. Intern. Med.* **120**, 227–237.

Madore, H. P., and England, J. M. (1977). Rabies virus protein synthesis in infected BHK-21 cells. *J. Virol.* **22**, 102–112.

McQuaid, S., Mcmahon, J., Herron, B., and Cosby, S. L. (1997). Apoptosis in measles virus-infected human central nervous system tissues. *Neuropathol. Appl. Neurobiol.* **23**, 218–224.

Mims, C. A. (1960). Intracerebral injections and the growth of viruses in the mouse brain. *Br. J. Exp. Pathol.* **41**, 52–59.

Moreno, J. A., and Baer, G. M. (1980). Experimental rabies in the vampire bat. *Am. J. Trop. Med. Hyg.* **29**, 254–259.

Morimoto K., Hooper, D. C., Spitsin, S., Koprowski, H., and Dietzschold, B. (1999). Pathogenicity of different rabies virus variants inversely correlates with apoptosis and rabies virus glycoprotein expression in infected primary neuron cultures. *J. Virol.* **73**, 510–518.

Morimoto, K., Patel, M., Corisdeo, S., Hooper, D. C., Fu, Z. F., Rupprecht, C. E., Koprowski, H., and Dietzschold, B. (1996). Characterization of a unique variant of bat rabies virus responsible for newly emerging human cases in North America. *Proc. Natl. Acad. Sci. USA* **93**, 5653–5658.

Murphy, F. A., Bauer, S. P., Harrison, A. K., and Winn, W. C. (1973a). Comparative pathogenesis of rabies and rabies-like viruses: Viral infection and transit from inoculation site to the central nervous system. *Lab. Invest.* **28**, 361–376.

Murphy, F. A., Bell, J. F., Bauer, S. P., Gardner, J. J., Moore, G. J., Harrison, A. K., and Coe, J. E. (1980). Experimental chronic rabies in the cat. *Lab. Invest.* **43**; 231–241.

Murphy, F. A., Harrison, A. K., Winn, W. C., and Bauer, S. P. (1973b). Comparative pathogenesis of rabies and rabies-like viruses: Infection of the central nervous system and centrifugal spread of virus to peripheral tissues. *Lab. Invest.* **29**, 1–16.

Nathan, C. (1992). Nitric oxide as a secretory product of mammalian cells. *FASEB J.* **6**, 3051–3064.

Nathan, C. F., and Hibbs, J. B. (1991). Role of nitric oxide synthesis in macrophage antimicrobial activity. *Curr. Opin. Immunol.* **3**, 65–70.

Noah, D. L., Drenzek, C. L., Smith, J. S., Krebs, J. W., Orciari, L., Shaddock, J., Sanderlin, D., Whitfield, S., Fekadu, M., Olson, J. G., Rupprecht, C. E., and Childs, J. E. (1998). Epidemiology of human rabies in the United States, 1980 to 1996. *Ann. Intern. Med.* **128**, 922–930.

Oberhaus, S. M., Smith, R. L., Clayton, G. H., Dermody, T. S., and Tyler, K. L. (1997). Reovirus infection and tissue injury in the mouse central nervous system are associated with apoptosis. *J. Virol.* **71**, 2100–2106.

Pawan J. L. (1936). Rabies in the vampire bat of Trinidad, with special reference to the clinical course and the latency of infection. *Ann. Trop. Med. Parasitol.* **30**, 401–422.

Pekosz, A., Phillips, J., Pleasure, D., Merry, D., and Gonzalez-Scarano, F. (1996). Induction of apoptosis by La Crosse virus infection and role of neuronal differentiation and human *bcl*-2 expression in its prevention. *J. Virol.* **70**, 5329–5335.

Perl, D. P., Bell, J. F., Moore, G. J., and Stewart, S. J. (1977). Chronic recrudescent rabies in a cat. *Proc. Soc. Exp. Biol. Med.* **155**, 540–548.

Perl, D. P., and Good, P. F. (1991). The pathology of rabies in the central nervous system. In *The Natural History of Rabies*, G. M. Baer (ed.), pp. 163–190. CRC Press, Boca Raton, FL.

Petito, C. K., and Roberts, B. (1995). Evidence of apoptotic cell death in HIV encephalitis. *Am. J. Pathol.* **146**, 1121–1130.

Prosniak, M., Hooper, D. C., Dietzschold, B., and Koprowski, H. (2001). Effect of rabies virus infection on gene expression in mouse brain. *Proc. Natl. Acad. Sci. USA* **98**, 2758–2763.

Raux, H., Flamand, A., and Blondel, D. (2000). Interaction of the rabies virus P protein with the LC8 dynein light chain. *J. Virol.* **74**, 10212–10216.

Ray, N. B., Ewalt, L. C., and Lodmell, D. L. (1995). Rabies virus replication in primary murine bone marrow macrophages and in human and murine macrophage-like cell lines: Implications for viral persistence. *J. Virol.* **69**, 764–772.

Razvi, E. S., and Welsh, R. M. (1995). Apoptosis in viral infections. *Adv. Virus Res.* **45**, 1–60.

Reagan, K. J., and Wunner, W. H. (1985). Rabies virus interaction with various cell lines is independent of the acetylcholine receptor: Brief report. *Arch. Virol.* **84**, 277–282.

Reiss, C. S., and Komatsu, T. (1998). Does nitric oxide play a critical role in viral infections? *J Virol.* **72**, 4547–4551.

Ross, E., and Armentrout, S. A. (1962). Myocarditis associated with rabies: Report of a case. *New Engl. J. Med.* **266**, 1087–1089.

Seif, I., Coulon, P., Rollin, P. E., and Flamand, A. (1985). Rabies virulence: Effect on pathogenicity and sequence characterization of rabies virus mutations affecting antigenic site III of the glycoprotein. *J. Virol.* **53**, 926–935.

Shankar, V., Dietzschold, B., and Koprowski, H. (1991). Direct entry of rabies virus into the central nervous system without prior local replication. *J. Virol.* **65**, 2736–2738.

Smart, N. L., and Charlton, K. M. (1992). The distribution of challenge virus standard rabies virus versus skunk street rabies virus in the brains of experimentally infected rabid skunks. *Acta Neuropathol.* **84**, 501–508.

Smith, J. S., Fishbein, D. B., Rupprecht, C. E., and Clark, K. (1991). Unexplained rabies in three immigrants in the United States: A virologic investigation. *New Engl. J. Med.* **324**, 205–211.

Superti, F., Hauttecoeur, B., Morelec, M. J., Goldoni, P., Bizzini, B., and Tsiang, H. (1986). Involvement of gangliosides in rabies virus infection. *J. Gen. Virol.* **67**, 47–56.

Superti, F., Seganti, L., Tsiang, H., and Orsi, N. (1984). Role of phospholipids in rhabdovirus attachment to CER cells: Brief report. *Arch. Virol.* **81**, 321–328.

Tang, Y., Rampin, O., Giuliano, F., and Ugolini, G. (1999). Spinal and brain circuits to motoneurons of the bulbospongiosus muscle: Retrograde transneuronal tracing with rabies virus. *J. Comp Neurol.* **414**, 167–192.

Theerasurakarn, S., and Ubol, S. (1998). Apoptosis induction in brain during the fixed strain of rabies virus infection correlates with onset and severity of illness. *J. Neurovirol.* **4**, 407–414.

Thompson, C. B. (1995). Apoptosis in the pathogenesis and treatment of disease. *Science* **267**, 1456–1462.

Thoulouze, M. I., Lafage, M., Montano-Hirose, J. A., and Lafon, M. (1997). Rabies virus infects mouse and human lymphocytes and induces apoptosis. *J. Virol.* **71**, 7372–7380.

Thoulouze, M. I., Lafage, M., Schachner, M., Hartmann, U., Cremer, H., and Lafon, M. (1998). The neural cell adhesion molecule is a receptor for rabies virus. *J. Virol.* **72**, 7181–7190.

Tillotson, J. R., Axelrod, D., and Lyman, D. O. (1977). Rabies in a laboratory worker — New York. *Morb. Mort. Weekly Rep.* **26**, 183–184.

Torres-Anjel, M. J., Montano-Hirose, J., Cazabon, E. P. I., Oakman, J. K., and Wiktor, T. J. (1984). A new approach to the pathobiology of rabies virus as aided by immunoperoxidase staining. *Am. Assoc. Vet. Lab. Diagn.* **27**, 1–26.

Tsiang, H. (1979). Evidence for an intraaxonal transport of fixed and street rabies virus. *J. Neuropathol. Exp. Neurol.* **38**, 286–296.

Tsiang, H. (1982). Neuronal function impairment in rabies-infected rat brain. *J. Gen. Virol.* **61**, 277–281.

Tsiang, H., Ceccaldi, P. E., and Lycke, E. (1991). Rabies virus infection and transport in human sensory dorsal root ganglia neurons. *J. Gen. Virol.* **72**, 1191–1194.

Tsiang, H., de la Porte, S., Ambroise, D. J., Derer, M., and Koenig, J. (1986). Infection of cultured rat myotubes and neurons from the spinal cord by rabies virus. *J. Neuropathol. Exp. Neurol.* **45**, 28–42.

Tsiang, H., Lycke, E., Ceccaldi, P.-E., Ermine, A., and Hirardot, X. (1989). The anterograde transport of rabies virus in rat sensory dorsal root ganglia neurons. *J. Gen. Virol.* **70**, 2075–2085.

Tsunoda, I., Kurtz, C. I., and Fujinami, R. S. (1997). Apoptosis in acute and chronic central nervous system disease induced by Theiler's murine encephalomyelitis virus. *Virology* **228**, 388–393.

Tucker, P. C., Griffin, D. E., Choi, S., Bui, N., and Wesselingh, S. (1996). Inhibition of nitric oxide synthesis increases mortality in Sindbis virus encephalitis. *J. Virol.* **70**, 3972–3977.

Tuffereau, C., Benejean, J., Blondel, D., Kieffer, B., and Flamand, A. (1998). Low-affinity nerve-growth factor receptor (P75NTR) can serve as a receptor for rabies virus. *EMBO J.* **17**, 7250–7259.

Tuffereau, C., Leblois, H., Benejean, J., Coulon, P., Lafay, F., and Flamand, A. (1989). Arginine or lysine in position 333 of ERA and CVS glycoprotein is necessary for rabies virulence in adult mice. *Virology* **172**, 206–212.

Tuffereau, C., and Martinet-Edelist, C. (1985). Shutoff of cellular RNA after infection with rabies virus. *C. R. Acad. Sci.* **300**, 597–600.

Ubol, S., and Kasisith, J. (2000). Reactivation of Nedd-2, a developmentally downregulated apoptotic gene, in apoptosis induced by a street strain of rabies virus. *J. Med. Microbiol.* **49**, 1043–1046.

Ubol, S., Sukwattanapan, C., and Maneerat, Y. (2001). Inducible nitric oxide synthase inhibition delays death of rabies virus–infected mice. *J. Med. Microbiol.* **50**, 238–242.

Umehara, F., Nakamura, A., Izumo, S., Kubota, R., Ijichi, S., Kashio, N., Hashimoto, K., Usuku, K., Sato, E., and Osame, M. (1994). Apoptosis of T-lymphocytes in the spinal cord lesions in HTLV-I–associated myelopathy: A possible mechanism to control viral infection in the central nervous system. *J. Neuropathol. Exp. Neural.* **53**, 617–624.

Van Dam, A. M., Bauer, J., Manahing, W. K. H., Marquette, C., Tilders, F. J. H., and Berkenbosch, F. (1995). Appearance of inducible nitric oxide synthase in the rat central nervous system after rabies virus infection and during experimental allergic encephalomyelitis but not after peripheral administration of endotoxin. *J. Neurosci. Res.* **40**, 251–260.

Veeraraghavan, N., Gajanana, A., and Rangasami, R. (1967a). Hydrophobia among persons bitten by apparently healthy animals. In *The Pasteur Institute of Southern India, Coonoor: Annual Report of the Director 1965 and Scientific Report 1966*, pp. 90–91. Diocesan Press, Madras.

Veeraraghavan, N., Gajanana, A., Rangasami, R., Kumari, C., Saraswathi, K. C., Devaraj, R., and Hallan, K. M. (1967b). Studies on the salivary excretion of rabies virus by the dog from Surandai. In *The Pasteur Institute of Southern India, Coonoor: Annual Report of the Director 1965 and Scientific Report 1966*, pp. 91–97. Diocesan Press, Madras.

Veeraraghavan, N., Gajanana, A., Rangasami, R., Oonnunni, P. T., Saraswathi, K. C., Devaraj, R., and Hallan, K. M. (1969). Studies on the salivary excretion of rabies virus by the dog from Surandai. In *The Pasteur Institute of Southern India, Coonoor: Annual Report of the Director 1967 and Scientific Report 1968*, pp. 68–70. Diocesan Press, Madras.

Veeraraghavan N., Gajanana, A., Rangasami, R., Oonnunni, P. T., Saraswathi, K. C., Devaraj, R., and Hallan, K. M. (1970). Studies on the salivary excretion of rabies virus by the dog from Surandai. In *The Pasteur Institute of Southern India, Coonoor: Annual Report of the Director 1968 and Scientific Report 1969*, p. 66. Diocesan Press, Madras.

Veeraraghavan, N., Gajanana, A., Rangasami, R., Saraswathi, K. C., Devaraj, R., and Hallan, K. M. (1968). Studies on the salivary excretion of rabies virus by the dog from Surandai. In *The Pasteur Institute of Southern India, Coonoor: Annual Report of the Director 1966 and Scientific Report 1967*, pp. 71–78. Diocesan Press, Madras.

Wallerstein, C. (1999). Rabies cases increase in the Philippines. *Br. Med. J.* **318**, 1306.

Winkler, W. G., Fashinell, T. R., Leffingwell, L., Howard, P., and Conomy, J. P. (1973). Airborne rabies transmission in a laboratory worker. *JAMA* **226**, 1219–1221.

Yang, C., and Jackson, A. C. (1992). Basis of neurovirulence of avirulent rabies virus variant Av01 with stereotaxic brain inoculation in mice. *J. Gen. Virol.* **73**, 895–900.

Zheng, Y. M., Schafer, M. K.-H., Weihe, E., Sheng, H., Corisdeo, S., Fu, Z. F., Koprowski, H., and Dietzschold, B. (1993). Severity of neurological signs and degree of inflammatory lesions in the brains of rats with Borna disease correlate with the induction of nitric oxide synthase. *J. Virol.* **67**, 5786–5791.

8

Pathology

YUZO IWASAKI and MUNESHIGE TOBITA

Miyagi National Hospital
Yamamoto-cho, Watari-gun
Miyagi 989-2202, Japan

I. INTRODUCTION

In the majority of rabies cases, the pathologic manifestation in the central nervous system (CNS) is acute encephalomyelitis. Macroscopic findings in the brain of acute rabies encephalitis usually are unremarkable. The brain may be slightly swollen, and meningeal and parenchymal vessels are moderately congested, largely reflecting terminal respiratory and cardiac failures. Hemorrhage or tissue necrosis is not a usual feature of rabies encephalitis (Jackson, 1997, Mrak and Young, 1994).

283

A normal gross appearance of the brain with a paucity of inflammatory cell reaction is common in other forms of acute viral encephalitis, such as Japanese encephalitis, with a relatively short clinical course. Unique to rabies, however, are the pathologic changes that remain inconspicuous even in cases with long incubation periods, suggesting virus persistence in extraneural organs and/or a lack of host immune responses during the incubation period.

On the other hand, in cases of paralytic or dumb rabies with early and prominent paralysis, the spinal cord is preferentially involved. In such cases, the brain also may be involved, and inflammatory changes are prominent in the brainstem (Hurst and Pawan, 1932, Chopra *et al.*, 1980).

Vigorous postexposure treatments with immunoglobulin, rabies vaccine, and life-sustaining measures may modify the pathology considerably, but essential features of rabies, including the presence of Negri bodies and glial nodules, are well retained (Anonymous, 1998).

II. HISTOPATHOLOGY OF RABIES ENCEPHALOMYELITIS

Microscopic findings are not paralleled by the severity of the clinical illness. Although the severity of histopathologic changes is variable from case to case, the changes generally are subtle and inconspicuous. Sporadic occurrence of pyknotic or necrotic neurons and mild perivascular and subarachnoidal inflammatory cell infiltration usually are the main pathologic changes in hematoxylin and eosin–stained sections of infected brain.

Thus, if Negri bodies, a classic hallmark of the disease, are absent, then histopathologic diagnosis of rabies cannot be made, and immunohistochemical demonstration of rabies virus antigens and/or detection of viral RNA by polymerase chain reaction amplification is mandatory for confirmation of the diagnosis (see Chap. 9).

A. Degeneration of Neurons

In natural rabies, either pyknotic or chromatolytic neurons are seen throughout the CNS but are found most frequently in the brainstem, particularly in the floor of the fourth ventricle and periaqueductal gray matter. The region of neuronal degeneration may extend down to the gray matter of the cervical spinal cord and up to the thalamus and, less frequently, to the cerebral cortex (Dupont and Earle, 1965). In general, these degenerative neurons do not harbor Negri bodies but are positive for viral antigens by immunostaining and may be accompanied by inflammatory reactions (Iwasaki *et al.*, 1985).

In comparison with natural infections with a "street" virus, fixed rabies virus infections exert more severe cytopathic effects in both cell cultures and animals. In experimental animal infections with fixed virus, chromatin condensation is a constant finding in infected neurons, whereas discrete Negri bodies usually are not found. Thus, Atanasiu (1975) stated, "The histologic lesions of rabies are of two types: Negri bodies in street virus infection and nuclear alterations in fixed rabies virus infection."

In light of recent studies on apoptotic neurons in experimental infections with fixed rabies virus using intracerebral inoculation (Jackson and Rossiter, 1997, Jackson and Park, 1998, Jackson, 1999), many, but not all, classic descriptions of chromatin condensation in fixed virus–infected neurons could be reflecting the process of apoptosis. Apoptosis may occur with or without viral antigen expression, and the mechanism of apoptosis could be related directly or indirectly to virus replication.

Of particular interest is the infection in the *bax*-deficient mouse. Apoptosis in *bax*-deficient mice was less severe in the cerebral cortex, hippocampus, and cerebellum than that in wild-type mice, whereas it was moderate to severe in the brainstem in both strains of mice (Jackson, 1999). Thus the regional difference in the severity of neuronal degeneration and selective cellular vulnerability in rabies virus infection (Johnson, 1965) can be explained in part by the inducibility of bax protein, a pro-apoptotic protein, in host cells.

B. Inflammatory Reactions

Perivascular and parenchymal collections of inflammatory cells once were thought to be specific for rabies (Babes, 1892), but they are neither unique nor specific for rabies. Perivascular infiltrates are composed of lymphocytes and monocytes intermingled with small numbers of polymorphonuclear and plasma cells, depending on the stage and severity of the infection.

The phenotype of inflammatory cells is not well studied, but in one case of human rabies with a clinical disease of 17 days' duration, 50–70% of mononuclear cells in the perivascular spaces were CD3-positive T-lymphocytes, and more than one-third of CD3 cells were CD4 helper T-lymphocytes. CD20-positive B-lymphocytes were negligible, and the rest were CD68-positive monocyte/macrophage lineage cells (Iwasaki *et al.*, 1993). The same study also showed that more than half the CD3 cells at the site of inflammation distributed outside the perivascular spaces.

As in other viral encephalitides, neuronophagia and glial nodules, namely, aggregates of monocyte/macrophage lineage cells around a single or a group of infected neurons, often are seen in the areas where neuronal degeneration and inflammatory cell infiltration are conspicuous (Fig. 1). They are readily identified

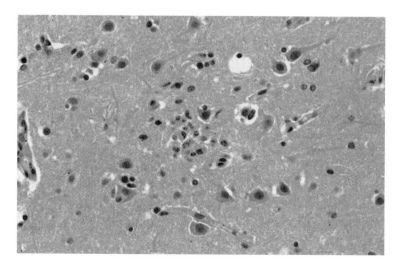

Fig. 1.   A glial nodule in the parietal cortex. Note an aggregate of macrophages associated with necrotic neurons: human rabies hematoxylin and eosin stain; (magnification × 100).

by labeling with anti-CD68 antibody and other markers for monocytes or microglia. Babes (1892) was the first to note focal collections of "embryonal cells", monocyte/macrophage lineage cells, surrounding degenerating neurons, and coined the term *rabidic tubercules*. Thus glial nodules in rabies are often referred to as *Babes' nodules*.

Topographic dissociation between the site of inflammatory reactions and that of the Negri body has been reported (Dupont and Earle, 1965). In a study of 49 autopsy cases, inflammatory changes were found in the medulla and pons in 38.1% of cases, in the spinal cord in 35.7%, in the thalamus in 28.6%, and in the cerebellum and hippocampus in 14.3% (each). Negri bodies were found rarely in these inflammatory lesions. On the other hand, Negri bodies were seen in 59.5% of cases in the cerebellum, in 42.9% of cases in the hippocampus, and only in 14.3% of cases in the medulla and 11.9% in the pontine nuclei. In the lesions with Negri bodies, inflammatory changes usually were inconspicuous.

C. Negri and Lyssa Bodies

The discovery of eosinophilic intracytoplasmic inclusion bodies in rabies is credited to Adelchi Negri, an Italian pathologist, who published beautiful illustrations of the inclusions (Negri, 1903). Negri bodies can be recognized readily in hematoxylin and eosin–stained paraffin sections when preservation of the tissue is adequate (Fig. 2). With hematoxylin and eosin staining, they are glassy

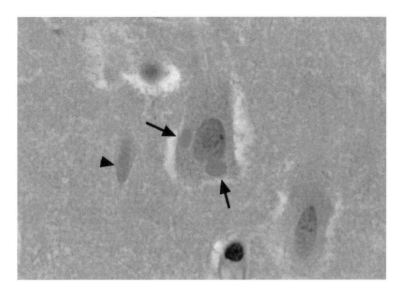

Fig. 2. A neuron with two intracytoplamic inclusions called *Negri bodies* (*arrows*). Also note an extracellular mass on the left side of the neuron (*arrowhead*). Ammon's horn, human rabies, hematoxylin and eosin stain; (magnification × 300).

eosinophilic cytoplasmic masses with a clear boundary but have no distinct halo like the cytoplasmic inclusions in subacute sclerosing panencephalitis. They are round, oval, or spindle-shaped and have dimensions of 1–20 μm. The size may depend on animal species. They are large in cattle (Acton and Harvey, 1911) and small in rabbits (Goodpasture, 1925). Most of them are homogeneously stained with eosin, but small pale or dark spots can be seen within the eosinophilic mass on hematoxylin and eosin staining. The presence of more than two inclusions in a single cell is not unusual. With Seller's methylene blue–fuchsin stain, a commonly used technique for rapid diagnosis by impression or smear, the Negri body is defined as an inclusion with inner basophilic granules, heterogeneous matrix, magenta tinge, and relatively less refractile than other viral inclusions (Dupont and Earle, 1965).

Based on observation of street virus–infected dog and rabbit brains using the Mann staining method with methylene blue and eosin, Negri (1903) described "*innere Körperchen*," or an inner body, a small basophilic granule within the inclusions. Thus presence of an inner body has been used for definitive identification of a Negri body.

Later, Goodpasture (1925) coined the term *lyssa body* in reference to inclusions without an inner body after an experimental study that was designed to prove a neural transmission of rabies virus in rabbits inoculated with a street virus of dog origin. Goodpasture identified distinct neuronal inclusions without an inner body by a new staining method with carbol aniline fuchsin and stated that the presence of Negri bodies is the result of the action of the virus on the cell and is not an essential feature of the disease, although it is an indicator of the infection. He thought of neurofibrils as a cellular substrate for the acidophilic mass of the lyssa body, which is analogous to neurofibrillary degeneration in Alzheimer disease.

In rabid brains, lyssa bodies are more numerous than Negri bodies. It has been claimed that lyssa bodies lack specificity because similar eosinophilic inclusions also can be found in normal animals. For example, eosinophilic thalamic inclusions are indistinguishable from lyssa bodies. They are found in normal aged humans and animals, and the number increases in certain metabolic disorders such as thiamine deficiency (Aikawa et al., 1983). Moreover, Goodpasture (1925) himself cast doubt on the specificity of lyssa bodies because Lentz (1909) had described intracellular and extracellular masses in dog brains of "Staupe" (canine distemper), and their morphology and staining properties were identical to lyssa bodies.

The specificity of the inclusions in rabies was first established by demonstration of rabies virus antigens in the inclusions by an immunofluorescence technique (Goldwasser and Kissling, 1958). In later studies on experimental animals, immunohistochemistry for viral antigens did not discriminate between the inclusions with or without an inner body. Both are similarly positive for viral antigens. Ultrastructurally, Negri and lyssa bodies are composed of similar viral components (Matsumoto, 1963; Miyamoto and Matsumoto, 1965). Thus the term *Negri body* generally refers to inclusions both with and without an inner body.

Within the CNS, rabies virus infection occurs almost exclusively in nerve cells, and the Negri body is found solely in neurons. However, ultrastructural evidence for the involvement of astrocytes has been reported in the mouse (Matsumoto, 1963; Iwasaki and Clark, 1975), in the dog (Fekadu et al., 1982), and in the monkey (Perl et al., 1972). In addition, the frequent occurrence of viral antigens, but not of inclusions, was described in both astrocytes and oligodendroglia in human rabies (Feiden et al., 1985). Rabies virus antigens also have been demonstrated in ependymal cells of mouse brains after an intracerebral inoculation with a large dose of fixed virus but not after footpad inoculation (Jackson and Reimer, 1989).

In addition to intracytoplasmic inclusions, similar eosinophilic masses are seen occasionally in the neuropil (see Fig. 2). These extraneuronal inclusions may correspond to the antigenic masses disclosed by immunohistochemistry in the neuropil (Fig. 3) and the ultrastructural observation of viral matrices and virions in dendritic processes of neurons. Indeed, ultrastructural studies always disclose wider dissemination of virus matrix and virions in both intracytoplasmic and extracellular locations than light microscopy.

Eosinophilic intranuclear inclusions have been reported in hamster brains inoculated with arctic rabies virus (Crandell, 1965), but this report has not been confirmed by other studies. Since rabies virus replication in culture cells does not require a nuclear phase, a viral nature of intranuclear inclusions is unlikely.

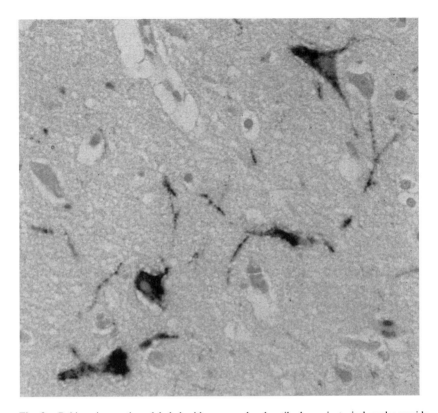

Fig. 3. Rabies virus antigen labeled with a monoclonal antibody against viral nucleocapsids. Distinct reaction products are detected in both neurons and their long processes distant from the perikaryon. Note a lack of inflammatory reactions. Parietal cortex, human rabies (magnification × 100).

Although the incidence of Negri bodies in the CNS varies widely, partly due to the examination protocol and definition of the inclusion, the inclusions have been seen in 50% (Herzog, 1945) to 71% (Dupont and Earle, 1965) of natural infections in humans. In one report, the number of inclusions was correlated with the duration of clinical disease (Sandhyamani *et al.*, 1981). The distribution of Negri bodies differs from one case to another, but the hippocampus has been thought to be the best place to encounter the inclusion. However, a higher incidence of inclusions was found in the cerebellum (59.5%) versus the hippocampus (42.9%) (Dupont and Earle, 1965). Moreover, ubiquitous distribution of the inclusions throughout the gray matter of the brain has been reported repeatedly (Gonzalez-Angulo *et al.*, 1970; Sung *et al.*, 1976; Feiden *et al.*, 1985; Perl and Good, 1991).

In summary, two points are worth noting: (1) the inclusions are absent in fixed virus infections, and (2) in street virus infections, inclusions are found rarely in degenerating neurons in acute inflammatory lesions, particularly in the lower brainstem, whereas distinct inclusions are more likely to be found in larger neurons in normal-appearing tissues with little inflammatory reactions. Pyramidal cells in the Ammon horn of the hippocampus and the Purkinje cells in the cerebellar cortex are examined most frequently for diagnostic purposes, and a high incidence of inclusions is reported in these regions. Undoubtedly, the Negri body is a histopathologic hallmark of rabies and has great diagnostic value, but the pathognomonic significance should be interpreted with reservation.

III. INVOLVEMENT OF THE PERIPHERAL NERVOUS SYSTEM

The peripheral nervous system (PNS) is inevitably involved during the centripetal and centrifugal spread of rabies virus with passage from the site of virus entry to the CNS and dissemination of progeny virus from the CNS to extraneural organs, respectively. All the motor nerve endings, sensory end organs, somatic and autonomic nerves and ganglia potentially are involved in rabies. Among these, ganglionic lesions have been studied most extensively from an early era of rabies investigation.

A. Ganglionic Lesions in Natural Infection

Nepveu (1872) first described the proliferation of satellite cells in the Gasserian ganglion of a human victim of rabies. Van Gehuchten and Nelis (1900) made important observations in cranial nerve and spinal ganglia of rabid animals, and ganglionic changes in rabies often are referred to as the *Van Gehuchten and Nelis lesion* or *Van Gehuchten nodule*. The main features of the lesion are the proliferation of capsular (satellite) cells around chromatolytic neurons and interstitial infiltration of lymphocytes (Fig. 4). The diagnostic value of Van Gehuchten lesions in ganglion nodosum (inferior ganglion of the vagus nerve) in rabies was emphasized (Herzog, 1945). The lesion was found in all 52 cases studied (human and animals), whereas Negri bodies were detected in only half the cases (Herzog, 1945).

Pathologic changes of the PNS also were reported in nine autopsy cases of rabies encephalomyelitis (Tangchai and Vejjajiva, 1971). These authors found chromatolysis and fine cytoplasmic vacuolation of neurons in the dorsal root ganglia of five cases, and this was accompanied by proliferation of capsular cells and interstitial and epineurial fibrosis. Perivenous infiltration of lymphocytes and monocytes also was seen in three of the cases. Disintegration of axons and severe demyelination of peripheral nerves were evident in seven cases, five of which were accompanied by proliferation of Schwann cells. Edematous widening of epineurial and perineurial spaces was seen in three cases. However, the authors did not find any inclusions.

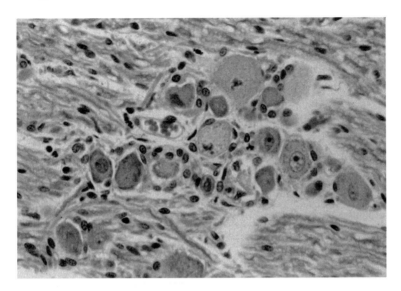

Fig. 4. Van Gehuchten nodule in the rat trigeminal ganglion developed after the intraneural inoculation of street virus into the ipsilateral mental nerve. Note a group of chromatolytic neurons accompanied by proliferation of satellite cells and infiltration of a few lymphocytes, hematoxylin and eosin stain; (magnification × 100).

In two cases of human rabies, the occurrence of Negri bodies in the trigeminal ganglion cells and of matrices and virions in the nerve were described, but there was no comment on inflammatory changes (Garcia-Tamayo *et al.*, 1972). Moreover, infiltration of lymphocytes and plasma cells and proliferation of satellite cells were reported in the cervical and lumbar spinal ganglia and paravertebral sympathetic ganglia of a patient who died 2½ months after a cat bite involving a finger (Sung *et al.*, 1976). Cytoplasmic inclusions were abundant in dorsal ganglia, but few were present in sympathetic ganglia. These authors also described patchy or diffuse perineurial and/or endoneurial lymphocyte and plasma cell infiltration and perivascular cell infiltration in the brachial plexus and femoral and obturator nerves. Others noted the occurrence of peripheral neuritis in two of six autopsy cases (Sandyamani *et al.*, 1981). In a more recent autopsy case, numerous Negri bodies also were observed in a dorsal root ganglion corresponding to the site of a dog bite, where neuronal loss and extensive inflammatory cell infiltration also were evident (Anonymous, 1998).

B. Ganglionic Lesions in Experimental Infections

The development of viral antigens in dorsal ganglia was seen after footpad inoculation in 4-day-old hamsters (Murphy *et al.*, 1973). As early as 60–72 hours after footpad inoculation, viral antigens were detected in ipsilateral dorsal ganglia of the lower lumbar cord and by day 3 in ventral root ganglia. By day 5, the distribution of antigen-positive ganglia extended to the cervical region. Virus titer in the CNS increased as early as 3 days after inoculation. In antigen-positive neurons, there was an accumulation of matrix, and a small number of budding viruses were present without appreciable cytopathic effects. Satellite cells were negative for viral antigens. The Van Gehuchten and Nelis lesion was absent.

Ganglionic changes also were reported in an adult skunk inoculated intramuscularly with street virus (Charlton and Casey, 1979). In this study, the development of viral antigen in the lumbar dorsal root ganglia occurred 10 days after inoculation concomitant with that in the spinal cord. The authors found chromatolysis of neurons, neuronophagia, and perivascular and interstitial mononuclear cell infiltration in the affected ganglia, but proliferation of satellite cells was not mentioned.

IV. INVOLVEMENT OF EXTRANEURAL ORGANS

Infection of extraneural organs mostly takes place secondary to centrifugal spread of the virus from the CNS. In a study on naturally infected red foxes, an immunofluorescence technique revealed the presence of viral antigens in submaxillary and parotid salivary glands, skeletal muscle, esophagus, stomach, intestine, pancreas, thyroid, thymus, lung, heart, adrenal glands, kidney, ureter, bladder, prostate, urethra, and testicles (Debbie and Trimarchi, 1970). Virus replication occurred in epithelial tissue of the salivary glands, brown fat, and cornea, whereas in other nonnervous organs the infection was confined to ganglion cells, nerve fibers, or nerve plexuses within the affected organs (reviewed by Dierks, 1975). Severe degenerative changes of mucous acini with mononuclear cell infiltration also were described in the submaxillary salivary glands of the fox (Dierks, 1975).

More recently, a detailed report was made on antigen distribution in extraneural organs of 14 autopsy cases of human rabies (Jackson *et al.*, 1999). Examination of major salivary glands in 4 cases disclosed moderate focal inflammation in 3 cases, but viral antigens were localized solely to nerve plexuses within the glands, whereas in minor salivary glands of the tongue, the antigens were detected in acini in 3 of 7 cases. In addition, the viral antigens were found in nerve plexuses of the gastrointestinal tract in nearly half the cases and of adrenal glands in 6 of 8 cases. In the heart, the viral antigens were detected in the parasympathetic ganglion cells in 4 of 8 cases and in cardiac muscle fibers in 3 of 8 cases. The antigens also were positive in the tongue muscle in all 7 cases. In the skin, the epithelial cells and cells surrounding hair follicles were positive for the antigen. The infection of extraneural organs sometimes was accompanied by an inflammatory reaction.

V. PATHOLOGY OF PARALYTIC RABIES

An outbreak of paralytic rabies occurred in Trinidad in 1929 and 1930. Since no rabid dogs existed on the island at the time of the outbreak, poliomyelitis was first suspected, but subsequent animal inoculation studies and epidemiologic survey confirmed the diagnosis of rabies with transmission by vampire bats. The pathology of the disease in three autopsy cases was reported (Hurst and Pawan, 1932). Two of the cases had a history of vampire bat bites. The incubation periods were estimated to be 1 month. The patients died within a week after the onset of acute ascending paralysis.

The pathology of the three cases was similar. The spinal cord was congested and soft, and the brain also was congested but not soft. Cardinal histopathologic changes were intense inflammation in the spinal cord and parts of the lower brainstem. Many of perivascular spaces in the parenchyma were filled with lymphocytes and a few polymorphonuclear leukocytes, although meningitis was subtle. Microglial proliferation was conspicuous, and glial nodules were abundant. Chromatolysis of neurons was seen commonly, and neuronophagia was encountered occasionally. Unlike poliomyelitis, both anterior and posterior horns were equally involved. At a few levels in the middle and lower thoracic cord, every neuron was involved, and polymorphonuclear leukocytes were numerous. The lumbar cord was not examined. The lowest part of the medulla was similarly involved in the inflammation, but the inflammation was largely confined to the dorsal half in the pons. The cerebellum was normal. In the cerebral cortex, mild perivascular infiltration and chromatolysis in the large pyramidal cells were seen. No Negri bodies were observed. The Ammon horn was not available for examination in any of the three cases. Lymphocyte infiltration was described in the sciatic nerve.

Interestingly, neuropathologic description of the monkey intracerebrally inoculated with the brain homogenate from one of the victims was very similar to that of human rabies encephalitis, where Negri bodies were present and neuronal degeneration was encountered occasionally, but inflammatory changes were absent or mild.

The pathology of 11 cases of paralytic rabies was reported from India (Chopra et al., 1980). A history of animal bite was obtained in 9 of the 11 cases, 8 by a dog and 1 by a cat. The mean incubation period was 49 days (7–90 days). The interval between the onset of the disease and death was 8.4 days (7–11 days). All patients ultimately developed quadriplegia. Similar to the cases reported earlier (Hurst and Pawan, 1932), the main pathologic changes were severe inflammation and degeneration and loss of neurons in the spinal cord, which was accentuated in the lumbar and lower thoracic segments. The medulla also was involved, but less severely. The inflammation was characterized by dense perivascular infiltration by lymphocytes and proliferation of microglial cells. Intracytoplasmic inclusions were found in Purkinje cells in the cerebellum and pyramidal cells in the hippocampus. They also were seen in the cerebral cortex of 3 cases and in the dorsal root ganglion of 1 case. Of particular interest in the report was a high incidence of segmental demyelination and remyelination in peripheral nerves relative to the incidence of axonal loss.

Thus the virus had reached the brain by the time of death in paralytic rabies. The infection, however, might be terminated prematurely before the development of encephalitic disease by a loss of vital functions due to neuronal degeneration associated with an extraordinary inflammation in the lower brainstem.

The pathogenetic basis of paralytic rabies has not yet been elucidated. The causative agents may be different from those producing encephalitic rabies, but no supportive data for this notion are available. On the other hand, similarity of the pathology of a monkey inoculated with a Trinidad isolate to that of encephalitic rabies suggests that the isolate also had the potential to produce encephalitic rabies. Clearly, the severe inflammation in paralytic rabies is mediated by host immune responses that were induced by rabies virus antigens prior to the onset of clinical disease. At least, in an experimental infection, foot-pad inoculation of a temperature-sensitive variant of the CVS strain of rabies virus induced paralytic disease with severe necrosis of the spinal cord in immunocompetent mice, whereas the same virus induced encephalitis when the host immune reactions were compromised (Iwasaki et al., 1977). Therefore, this suggests that induction of early immune responses by the host immune system is a key issue in paralytic rabies.

VI. ULTRASTRUCTURAL OBSERVATIONS

In the 1960s and early 1970s, most of the electron microscopic studies on rabies were concerned with elucidation of inclusion bodies and morphogenesis of the virus in cultured cells. Later, the focus shifted to replication and spread of the virus *in vivo*.

A. Ultrastructure of Negri Bodies

Ultrastructure of Negri bodies has been examined in both humans (Morecki and Zimmerman, 1969; Gonzalez-Angulo et al., 1970; Leech, 1971; Perl et al., 1972; DeBrito et al., 1973; Sung et al., 1976) and experimental animals (Hottle et al., 1951; Matsumoto, 1963; Miyamoto and Matsumoto, 1965). The ultrastructure of inclusion bodies is essentially the same in humans and animals (Fig. 5).

At first, Morecki and Zimmerman (1969) reported the absence of virions within Negri bodies but the presence of submicroscopic minute clusters of virions in the cytoplasm of neurons. Later, others described the occurrence of virus particles as a component of Negri bodies as well as small clusters confined to the cellular

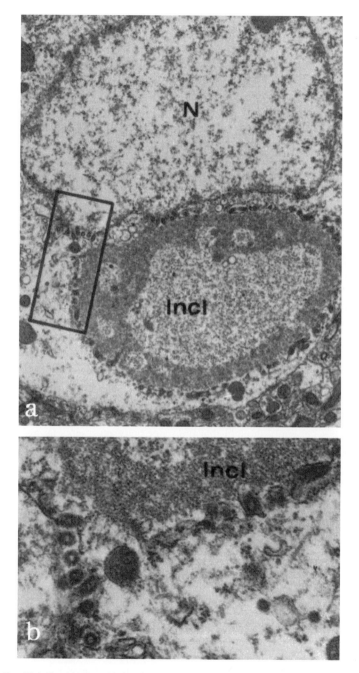

Fig. 5. (A) A Negri body and intracytoplasmic maturation of rabies virus in a pyramidal cell of the hippocampus in the mouse inoculated with street virus (magnification × 10,000). (B) A high- power view of the area indicated with a rectangle in Part A. Note an array of bullet-shaped particles within the endoplasmic reticulum surrounding the inclusion magnification × 33,000. N, nucleus; incl, inclusion.

processes in the neuropil (Gonzalez-Angulo *et al.*, 1970). In addition, a fibrillary matrix and bullet-shaped particles and two other cylindrical or rod-shaped structures were described as components of the inclusion (Sung *et al.*, 1976).

Since autolytic changes and fixation artifacts are inherent in autopsy materials, the fine structure of the Negri body was best studied by experimental infections in animals. An extensive study was made on street virus–infected mice (Matsumoto 1963; Miyamoto and Matsumoto, 1965) that demonstrated conclusively by alternative thick and thin sectioning of tissues that the Negri body is composed of fibrillary virus matrix and virus particles. Three types of particles are seen to be associated with the matrix. The first type is 120–130 nm in diameter and has a single membrane, and the second type is 110–120 nm in diameter and bounded by a double membrane. Branching and segmentation may occur in both types, and they are always found within the cytoplasm. The third type takes the form of a bullet-shaped particle, 75–80 nm wide and 180 nm long, and is limited by a double membrane. Bullet-shaped particles bud off from the plasma membrane into the endoplasmic reticulum or from the cell surface into extracellular spaces. Budding takes place mostly in a close proximity to matrix but also in the absence of matrix. Only the third type is considered to be an infectious virus.

The first and second types are seen commonly in street virus infection, but they also can be seen in fixed virus–infected culture cells at a later stage of infection (Hummeler *et al.*, 1967; Iwasaki *et al.*, 1973). Murphy (1975) commented on the nature of first and second types as follows: (1) they are "physically defective anomalous forms," (2) "permanently bound to intracytoplasmic membrane and trapped," and (3) "thermally denatured after slow accumulation over a protracted course of central nervous system infection."

The ultrastructural counterpart of the basophilic inner body is questionable. Although it is generally thought that the inner body represents an aggregate of virions within a matrix, this may not be the case. Virus matrix occasionally is surrounded by numerous virions (see Fig. 5). If aggregated virions give a basophilic tinge, some inclusions should be encircled by a basophilic rim, but such a rim has never been verified. On the other hand, invagination of cytoplasmic components into inclusions is seen occasionally under the electron microscope. Thus an alternative explanation could be that the inner body represents a small number of free ribosomes and rough endoplasmic reticulum entrapped by inclusions. Therefore, the presence of an inner body may well be indicative of distortion of host cell structures, but it cannot be an essential feature of viral inclusions.

B. Virus Replication in Cultured Cells

Virus entry into host cells may occur in two ways: Most of virus particles are taken up by the process of pinocytosis or viropexis, followed by the molecular dissociation of virions within pinocytotic vesicles. Less commonly, fusion of the viral envelope with the host cell membrane can be seen at the cell surface and at the wall of pinocytotic vesicles (Hummeler *et al.*, 1967; Iwasaki *et al.*, 1973). A release of bullet-shaped progeny virus occurs by budding into the endoplasmic reticulum and extracellular spaces. A minute accumulation of tubular structures called *matrix* usually is found in the vicinity of the site of virus budding. The matrix is largely formed by nucleocapsids of the virus (Hummeler *et al.*, 1967).

Fixed rabies virus grows in a variety of nonneural cells in culture. When virus yield is high, cytopathic effects, sometimes leading to the complete destruction of host cells, can be seen, but there is a time lag between the peak production of progeny virus and the development of cytopathology (Murphy, 1975). In a kinetic study with a high multiplicity of infection in BHK-21 cells with fixed virus, either Flury HEP or ERA strain (Iwasaki *et al.*, 1973), virus entry into host cells took place as early as 5 minutes after inoculation but not after 1 hour. Both engulfment of the inoculum by pinocytosis and subsequent degradation of virus particles within pinocytotic vesicles and fusion of viral envelope with host cell membrane were observed. The first evidence of virus replication was the development of fine cytoplasmic granules, which were distributed randomly in the cytoplasm and faintly labeled with a fluorescent anti-rabies virus antibody 4 hours after virus inoculation. Formation of minute aggregates of nucleocapsids, less than 1 μm in a diameter, was seen at 5 hours. The release of progeny virus was first seen 6 hours after infection. During the first 24 hours of virus infection, virus budding occurred exclusively at the surface of cells without any significant cytopathic changes. This phenomenon coincided with the yield of the highest virus titer in the supernatant of the culture fluid 18–24 hours after infection. Virus budding from the cell surface was not necessarily associated with the accumulation of nucleocapsids. Twenty hours after infection, in addition to budding from the cell surface, budding into the endoplasmic reticulum also was noted. Forty-eight hours after infection, numerous anomalous particles were accumulated within the cytoplasm. Cellular changes were inconspicuous in the earlier stages of the infection, but many of the cells were lysed by 96 hours.

Virus release from the cell surface was further confirmed by an observation of rabies virus–infected neuroblastoma cells with scanning electron microscopy (Iwasaki and Clark, 1977). In the same experiment, a remarkable increase in the number of microvilli occurred concomitant with or prior to expression of viral antigens on the cell surface and budding of progeny virus. Therefore, the observation of relatively subtle cellular changes in the earlier stage of the infection in thin sections could be deceptive.

Rabies virus infection also can be maintained in cell cultures for more than 2 years without any noticeable changes in thymidine and uridine uptake or cytopathic effects (Wiktor and Clark, 1975). Ultrastructural changes in such endosymbiotic infections have not been studied.

C. Replication and Spread of Virus within the CNS

Rabies virus has been thought to mature exclusively within the cytoplasm in the CNS, although virus budding from cell surface has been observed in mucogenic cells of the salivary gland (Dierks *et al.*, 1969) and in the skeletal muscle (Murphy *et al.*, 1973).

The evidence of virus budding from the surface of neuronal perikarya and neurites was first demonstrated in the street virus–infected suckling hamster brain (Murphy *et al.*, 1973). It was demonstrated in fixed virus–infected suckling mouse brain (Iwasaki *et al.*, 1975), as well as in street virus–infected suckling and adult mice (Iwasaki and Clark, 1975), street virus–infected skunks (Charlton and Casey, 1979), and finally, in the human brain (Iwasaki *et al.*, 1985). Virus budding in the olfactory bulb is also shown in a victim of airborne infection with a vaccine strain of rabies virus (Conomy *et al.*, 1977).

In the fixed virus–infected suckling mouse brain, virus budding from the cell surface occurred concomitant with an increase in virus titer in the tissue, and the number of virions in the intercellular spaces was 100 times more than that in the cytoplasm in the early stage of the infection (Iwasaki *et al.*, 1975). Thus the virus released from the cell surface might play a major role in early dissemination of the virus within the CNS in this highly permissive animal model.

In the street virus infection, intracytoplasmic maturation of virus was common. Budding from the cell surface also was seen in both suckling and adult mice, but it was less frequent in street virus infection than in fixed virus infection. It is noteworthy that in both mouse and human brains, virus budding from the cell surface is not necessarily associated with formation of matrix or Negri bodies. Thus the budding site may not be identified using light or fluorescence microscope.

Although all available data support the centripetal spread of rabies virus by axonal transport in peripheral nerves from the site of entry to the CNS (Tsiang, 1979), the mode of virus spread within the CNS appears more complex (Iwasaki, 1991). At present, three potential pathways are postulated: (1) virus dissemination within extracellular spaces, (2) transfer of the virus by fast axonal transport, and (3) cell-to-cell transmission of the virus between contiguous cells and their processes (see Figs. 6–8).

Once virus is released into the extracellular spaces (Fig. 6), it disseminates widely in bulk flow of cerebrospinal fluid in intercellular spaces and the ventricular system. This is an efficient and rapid mechanism of virus dissemination within the CNS. In fact, the width of intercellular spaces is much wider than that once thought (Van Harreveld *et al.*, 1965), and it would be sufficient to allow transit of the virus. This route could be playing a major role in rapid progression of fixed virus infections within the CNS because the virus release from the cell surface precedes the intracellular maturation of the virus in earlier stages of fixed virus infection.

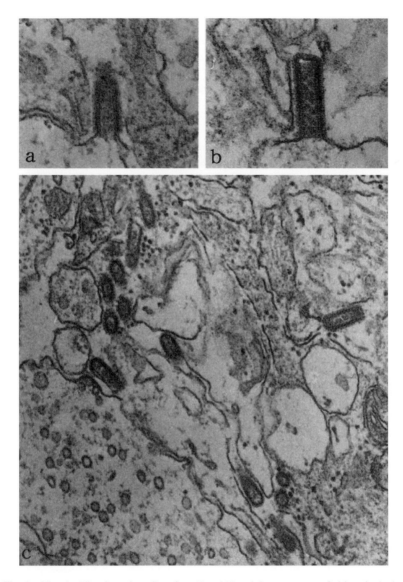

Fig. 6. Virus budding from the cell surface (*A* and *B*) and the occurrence of virions in the inter-cellular space (*C*) in the hippocampus of a suckling mouse intracerebrally inoculated with fixed virus. (magnifications: *A, B*: × 80,000, *C*: × 45,000).

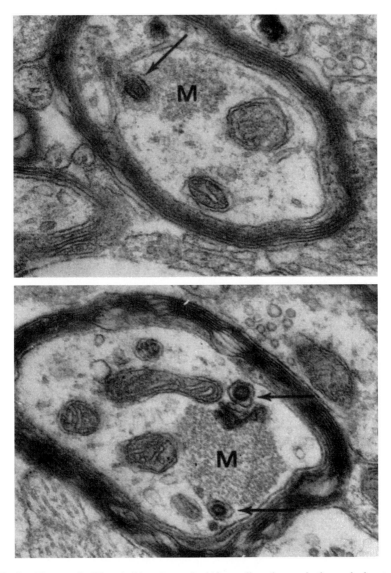

Fig. 7. Virus matrix (*M*) and virions (*arrows*) within myelinated axons in the cerebral cortex of an adult mouse intracerebrally inoculated with street virus (magnification × 40,000).

Transit by axonal transport, on the other hand, may be important in the protracted progression of the infection with street virus because the incidence of virus budding from the cell surface is much lower in street virus infection than in fixed virus infection except in immature animals. Moreover, the presence of virions

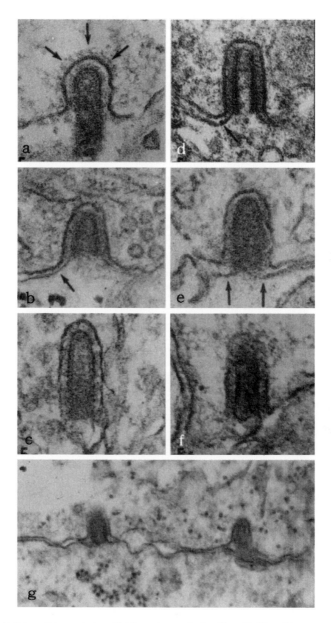

Fig. 8. Cell-to-cell transmission of virions at synaptic junctions (A–F) and between neighboring cells (G) in mouse brains. (A, F, and G) Fixed virus infection. (B, C, D, and E) Street virus infection. Arrows indicate the continuity of viral envelope with host cell membrane (B and E) and formation of receiving membrane (A) (magnification × 100,000).

and matrices is observed repeatedly within both dendrites and axons (Fig. 7). The transit of the virus within the axon also may allow it to circumvent the host immune responses. If this is the case, the infection can progress without recognition of the virus by the host immune system, as suspected in natural infection. In support of this view, the importance of long ascending and descending tracts as a route of virus spread within the CNS was determined after detailed immunohistochemical study on skunks inoculated with street virus into the footpad (Charlton et al., 1996).

Cell-to-cell transmission of virus between contiguous cells and their processes has been observed frequently (Fig. 8), particularly at synaptic junctions in both street and fixed virus infections (Iwasaki and Clark, 1975; Charlton and Casey, 1979) and less frequently in human rabies (Iwasaki et al., 1985). This type of transit not only facilitates virus spread between adjacent cells but also is important in transsynaptic transmission of the virus conveyed from distant sites by axonal transport and may well play a decisive role in the entry of the virus conveyed by peripheral nerves to the CNS (Charlton and Casey, 1979).

D. Virus Replication in Extraneural Tissues

The release of progeny virus from the cell surface was first described in the apical plasma membrane of mucogenic cells in the salivary gland of the fox (Dierks et al., 1969). In red foxes intramuscularly infected with street virus, budding of large numbers of virions into intercellular caniculi and the acinar lumen was observed in contrast to the virus maturation in the CNS, which was seen solely in the cytoplasm of neurons in the same animals. The release of virus from the surface of mucogenic cells into the intercellular caniculus space also was seen in striped skunk and spotted skunk (Dierks, 1975). In the salivary gland, virus maturation occurs mostly at the cell surface, and intracytoplasmic maturation is rare. Moreover, it is not associated with inclusions discernible under a microscope.

In the striated muscle of the suckling hamster, virus was observed budding into the sarcoplasmic reticulum but more often from the surface of myocytes to the extracellular spaces (Murphy et al., 1973). The virus budding occurred with or without accumulation of nucleocapsids, and the host cells showed little or no cytopathology.

VII. CONCLUSIONS

Although main pathologic features of rabies virus infection were described around the turn of nineteenth century, introduction of the electron microscopic and immunohistochemical techniques in the latter half of the twentieth century made it possible to achieve significant progress in understanding rabies pathogenesis and pathology.

Contributions of electron microscopy to rabies research are twofold. First, it confirmed the viral nature of Negri bodies following the demonstration of viral antigens in the inclusions by immunofluorescence. Second, it elucidated the mode of maturation and spread of rabies virus within the nervous system. Ample evidence for virus budding from the surface of neural cells and their processes, particularly at synaptic junctions, has accumulated. Now it can be assumed safely that budding from the host cell surface may precede or coincide with the intracellular maturation of progeny virus in both neural and extraneural tissues. Both transit within intercellular spaces and cell-to-cell transmission between neighboring cells and their processes may be principal events in the CNS, although axonal transport remains crucial in virus transit in the PNS.

ACKNOWLEDGMENT

This chapter is dedicated to Dr. Hilary Koprowski on the occasion of his 85th birthday.

REFERENCES

Acton, C. H. W., and Harvey, M. W. F. (1911). The nature and specificity of Negri bodies. *Parasitology* **4**, 255–272.

Aikawa, H., Suzuki, K., and Iwasaki, Y. (1983). Ultrastructural observation on the thalamic neuronal inclusions in the young mice. *Acta Neuropathol.* **59**, 316–318.

Anonymous (1998). Case records of MGH: Weekly clinicopathological exercises. Case 21-1998. *New Eng. J. Med.* **339**, 105–112.

Atanasiu, P. (1975). Animal inoculation and the Negri body. In *The Natural History of Rabies*, G. M. Baer (ed.), 1st. ed., pp. 374–400. Academic Press, New York.

Babes, V. (1892). Sur certains caracteres des lessions histologiques de la rage. *Ann. Inst. Pasteur* **6**, 209–223.

Charlton, K. M., and Casey, G. A. (1979). Experimental rabies in skunks: Immunofluorescence light and electron microscopic studies. *Lab. Invest.* **41**, 36–44.

Charlton, K. M., Casey, G. A., Wandeler, A. I., and Nadin-Davis, S. (1996). Early events in rabies virus infection of the central nervous system in skunks (*Mephitis mephitis*). *Acta Neuropathol.* **91**, 89–98.

Chopra, J. B., Banerjee, Murphy, J. M. K., and Pal, S. R. (1980). Paralytic rabies: A clinicopathological study. *Brain* **103**, 789–802.

Conomy, J. P., Leibowitz, A., McCombs, W., and Stinson, J. (1977). Airborne rabies encephalitis: Demonstration of rabies virus in the human central nervous system. *Neurology* **27**, 67–69.

Crandell, R. A. (1965). Laboratory investigation of arctic strains of rabies virus. *Acta Pathol. Microbiol. Scand.* **63**, 587–596.

Debbie, J. G., and Trimarchi, C. V. (1970). Pantropism of rabies virus in free-ranging rabid red fox, *Vulpes fulva. J. Wildlife Dis.* **6**, 500–506.

DeBrito, T., DeFantima, M., and Tiriba, A. (1973). Ultrastructure of the Negri body in human rabies. *J. Neurol. Sci.* **20**, 363–372.

Dierks, R. E. (1975). Electron microscopy of extraneural rabies infection. In *The Natural History of Rabies*, G. M. Baer (ed.), 1st. ed., pp. 303–318. Academic Press, New York.

Dierks, R. E., Murphy, F. A., and Harrison, A. K. (1969). Extraneural rabies virus infection: Virus development in fox salivary gland. *Am. J. Pathol.* **54**, 251–273.

Dupont, J. R., and Earle, K. M. (1965). Human rabies encephalitis: A study of forty-nine fatal cases with a review of the literature. *Neurology* **15**, 1023–1034.

Feiden, W., Feiden, U., Gerhardt, L., Reinhardt, V., and Wandeler, A. (1985). Rabies encephalitis: Immunohistochemical investigations. *Clin. Neuropathol.* **4**, 156–164.

Fekadu, M., Chandler, F. W., and Harrison, A. K. (1982). Pathogenesis of rabies in dogs inoculated with an Ethiopian rabies virus strain: Immunofluorescence, histologic and ultrastructural studies of the central nervous system. *Arch. Virol.* **71**, 109–126.

Garcia-Tamayo, J., Avila-Mayor, A., and Anzola-Perez, E. (1972). Rabies virus neuronitis in humans. *Arch. Pathol.* **94**, 11–15.

Goldwasser, R. A., and Kissling, R. E. (1958). Fluorescent antibody staining of street and fixed rabies virus antigens. *Proc. Soc. Exp. Biol. Med.* **98**, 219–223.

Gonzalez-Angulo, A., Marquez-Monter, H., Feria-Velasco, A., and Zavala, B. (1970). The ultrastructure of Negri bodies in Purkinje neurons in human rabies. *Neurology* **20**, 323–328.

Goodpasture, E. W. (1925). A study of rabies, with reference to a neural transmisson of the virus in rabbits, and the structure and significance of Negri bodies. *Am. J. Pathol.* **1**, 547–581.

Herzog, E. (1945). Histologic diagnosis of rabies. *Arch. Pathol.* **39**, 279–280.

Hottle, G. A., Morgan, G., Peers, J. H., and Wyckoff, R. W. G. (1951). The electron microscopy of rabies inclusion (Negri) bodies. *Proc. Soc. Exp. Biol. Med.* **77**, 721–723.

Hummeler, K., Koprowski, H., and Wiktor, T. J. (1967). Structure and development of rabies virus in tissue culture. *J. Virol.* **1**, 152–170.

Hurst, E. W., and Pawan, J. L. (1932). A further account of the Trinidad outbreak of acute rabic myelitis: Histology and experimental disease. *J. Pathol. Bacteriol.* **35**, 301–321.

Iwasaki, Y. (1991). Spread of virus within the central nervous system. In *The Natural History of Rabies*, G. M. Baer (ed.), 2d ed., pp. 121–132. CRC Press, Boca Raton, FL.

Iwasaki, Y., and Clark, H. F. (1975). Cell-to-cell transmission of virus in the central nervous system: II. Experimental rabies in mouse. *Lab. Invest.* **33**, 391–399.

Iwasaki, Y., and Clark, H. F. (1977). Rabies virus infection in mouse neuroblastoma cells. *Lab. Invest.* **36**, 578–584.

Iwasaki, Y., Wiktor, T. J., and Koprowski, H. (1973). Early events of rabies virus replication in tissue cultures: An electron microscopic study. *Lab. Invest.* **28**, 142–148.

Iwasaki, Y., Ohtani, S., and Clark, H. F. (1975). Maturation of rabies virus by budding from neuronal cell membrane in suckling mouse brain. *J. Virol.* **15**, 1020–1023.

Iwasaki, Y., Gerhard, W., and Clark, H. F. (1977). Role of host immune response in the development of either encephalitic or paralytic disease after experimental rabies infection in mice. *Infect. Immun.* **18**, 220–225.

Iwasaki, Y., Liu, D. S., Yamamoto, T., and Konno, H. (1985). On the replication and spread of rabies virus in the human central nervous system. *J. Neuropathol. Exp. Neurol.* **44**, 185–195.

Iwasaki, Y., Sako, K., Tsunoda, I., and Ohara, Y. (1993). Phenotypes of mononuclear cell infiltrates in human central nervous system. *Acta Neuropathol.* **85**, 653–657.

Jackson, A. C. (1997). Rabies. In *Viral Pathogenesis*, N. Nathanson, R. Ahmed, F. Gonzalez-Scarano, D. E. Griffin, K. Holmes, F. A. Murphy, and H. L. Robinson HL (eds.), pp. 575–591. Lippincott-Raven, Philadelphia.

Jackson, A. C. (1999). Apoptosis in experimental rabies in *bax*-deficient mice. *Acta Neuropathol.* **98**, 288–294.

Jackson, A. C., and Reimer, D. L. (1989). Pathogenesis of experimental rabies in mice. *Acta Neuropathol.* **78**, 159–165.

Jackson, A. C., and Rossiter, J. P. (1997). Apoptosis plays an important role in experimental rabies virus infection. *J. Virol.* **71**, 5603–5607.

Jackson, A. C., and Park, H. (1998). Apoptotic cell death in experimental rabies in suckling mice. *Acta Neuropathol.* **95**, 159–164.

Jackson, A. C., Ye, H., Phelan, C. C., Ridaura-Sanz, C., Zhen, Q., Wan, X., and Lopez-Corella, E. (1999). Extraneural organ involvement in human rabies. *Lab. Invest.* **79**, 945–951.

Johnson, R. T. (1965). Experimental rabies: Studies of cellular vulnerability and pathogenesis using fluorescent antibody staining. *J. Neuropathol. Exp. Neurol.* **24**, 662–674.

Leech, R. W. (1971). Electron microscopic study of the inclusion body in human rabies. *Neurology* **21**, 91–94.

Lentz, O. (1909). Über spezifisches Veränderungen.an den Ganglien Zellen Wut-und Staupekranker Tieren. Ein Beitrag zu unseren Kenntnissen über die Bedeutung und Entstehung der Negrischen Köperchen. *Z. Hyg. Infektionskr.* **62**, 63–94.

Matsumoto, S. (1963). Electron microscopic studies of rabies virus in mouse brain. *J. Cell Biol.* **19**, 565–591.

Miyamoto, K., and Matsumoto, S. (1965). The nature of the Negri body. *J Cell Biol.* **27**, 677–682.

Morecki, R., and Zimmerman, H. M. (1969). Human rabies encephalitis: Fine structure study of cytoplasmic inclusions. *Arch. Neurol.* **20**, 599–604.

Mrak, R. E., and Young, L. (1994). Rabies encephalitis in humans: Pathology, pathogenesis and pathophysiology. *J. Neuropathol. Exp. Neurol.* **53**, 1–10.

Murphy, F. A. (1975). Morphology and morphogenesis. In *The Natural History of Rabies*, G. M. Baer (ed.), 1st. ed., pp. 33–61. Academic Press, New York.

Murphy, F. A., Bauer, S. P., Harrison, A. K., and Winn, W. C. (1973). Comparative pathogenesis of rabies and rabies-like viruses: Viral infection and transit from inoculation site to the central nervous system. *Lab. Invest.* **28**, 361–376.

Negri, A. (1903). Beitrag zum Studium der Aetiologie der Tollwuth. *Z. Hyg. Infektionskr.* **43**, 507–528.

Nepveu, M. (1872). Un cas de rage. *C. R. Soc. Biol.* **4**, 133–138.

Perl, D. P., and Good, P. F. (1991). The pathology of rabies in the central nervous system. In *The Natural History of Rabies*, G. M. Baer (ed.), 2d ed., pp. 163–190. CRC Press, Boca Raton, FL.

Perl, D. P., Callaway, C. S., and Hicklin, M. (1972). An ultrastructural study of Negri bodies in experimental rabies following prolonged incubation period (Abstract). *J. Neuropathol. Exp. Neurol.* **31**, 172.

Sandhyamani, S., Roy, S., Gode, G. R., and Kalla, G. N. (1981). Pathology of rabies: A light and electronmicroscopical study with particular reference to the change in cases with prolonged survival. *Acta Neuropathol.* **54**, 247–251.

Sung, J. H., Hayano, M., Mastri, A. R., and Okagaki, T. (1976). A case of human rabies and ultra-structure of the Negri body. *J. Neuropathol. Exp. Neurol.* **35**, 541–549.

Tangchai, P., and Vejjajiva, A. (1971). Pathology of the peripheral nervous system in human rabies. *Brain* **94**, 299–306.

Tsiang, H. (1979). Evidence for an intraaxonal transport of fixed and street rabies virus. *J. Neuropathol. Exp. Neurol.* **38**, 286–299.

Van Gehuchten, A., and Nelis, C. (1900). Les lesions histologiques de la rage chez les animaux et chez l'homme. *Bull. Acad. R. Med. Belg.* **14**, 31–66.

Van Harreveld, A., Crowell, H., and Malhotra, S. K. (1965). A study of extracellular space in central nervous tissue by freeze-substitution. *J. Cell Biol.* **25**, 117.

Wiktor, T. J., and Clark, H. F. (1975). Growth of rabies virus in cell culture. In *The Natural History of Rabies*, G. M. Baer (ed.), 1st. ed., pp. 155–179. Academic Press, New York.

9

Diagnostic Evaluation

CHARLES V. TRIMARCHI

Rabies Laboratory, Wadsworth Center
New York State Department of Health
Albany, New York 12201-0509

JEAN S. SMITH

Rabies Section
Centers for Disease Control and Prevention
Atlanta, Georgia 30333

RABIES

I. INTRODUCTION

A. Utility of Rabies Diagnosis

Rabies diagnostic procedures are performed most frequently for the post-mortem examination of animals that have bitten a person or have otherwise potentially caused human exposure to the disease. These examinations comprise the most important diagnostic contributions to the control and prevention of rabies. Evidence of rabies infection, based on positive diagnostic tests, prompts administration of rabies prophylaxis for exposed persons, preventing onset of the incurable and fatal infection. Demonstration of rabies infection also initiates proper management of exposed domestic animals, including booster vaccination of previously immunized animals and euthanasia or quarantine of unvaccinated animals. Prompt and reliable negative results, on the other hand, can be used to prevent the initiation of unnecessary postexposure prophylaxis (PEP) in humans.

An extremely valuable but less obvious source of investigation in these examinations is the surveillance data revealing the distribution of rabies in domestic and wild mammal populations. These data provide the foundation for good decisions regarding PEP for bites from animals not available for observation or testing (Trimarchi, 2000), and they permit proper targeting of vaccination programs and other rabies control activities in the region.

Because the diagnosis of rabies in animals can now be completed in a reliable manner in less than 1 day, the physician's decision to initiate or withhold PEP is often based on postmortem examination of the biting animal. This practice imposes the highest possible standards of sensitivity on the performance of the test, since the consequences of false-negative reports can be expected to include human mortality. Specificity of the test is also critical because false-positive results can lead not only to unnecessary PEP but also to misleading epizootiologic data.

Tests to detect evidence of rabies infection are also applied to the ante- and postmortem diagnosis of rabies in humans afflicted by an encephalitis of unknown etiology. Furthermore, rabies diagnostic methods support studies of rabies pathobiology, the production of vaccines and vaccine potency testing, and surveillance programs for evaluation of the success of wildlife vaccination campaigns.

B. Range of Diagnostic Methods

Making a reliable diagnosis of rabies based on clinical presentation is very difficult because there are no truly pathognomonic symptoms or signs. Clinically, rabies in animals can be difficult to distinguish from encephalitic conditions caused by other viral infections, including canine distemper. In humans, rabies can be confused with Guillain-Barré syndrome, poliomyelitis, and other viral encephalitides (Plotkin, 2000) (see Chap. 6). Specific histopathologic changes, namely, Negri bodies, in the central nervous system (CNS) can provide microscopic evidence of rabies virus infection but only with a low degree of sensitivity. While the Negri body has been the hallmark of the pathogenesis of rabies for the past 100 years, with recent technological developments, more definitive evidence of rabies virus infection can now be demonstrated by detection of the entire virion, its proteins, or its genome RNA in tissue samples. This can be accomplished by direct visualization of virus particles, detection of viral proteins by visualization of reaction with labeled antibodies, cultivation of infectious virus, or detection of viral RNA in tissue samples. Methods employed include electron microscopy (EM), direct fluorescent antibody (DFA) and indirect fluorescent antibody (IFA) tests, virus cultivation *in vivo* and *in vitro*, immunohistochemistry, enzyme immunoassay, molecular hybridization with labeled nucleic acid (genetic) probes, and reverse transcription–polymerase chain reaction (RT-PCR). Indirect evidence of rabies virus infection can be inferred by the demonstration of rabies-specific virus neutralizing antibody in the serum of an unvaccinated individual or antibody in cerebrospinal fluid (CSF).

II. POSTMORTEM DIAGNOSIS OF RABIES IN ANIMALS

Because of the unique pathogenesis of rabies, it is impossible to diagnose the disease during most of its long and variable incubation period. During this early phase of rabies development, neither the virus nor its antigens or RNA can be identified reliably because their distribution in the host is unpredictable during this period. Also, there is generally no rise in titer of circulating antibodies until a week or more into the clinical phase (Crepin *et al.*, 1998). Consequently, the diagnosis of rabies can only be achieved with 100% certainty by the postmortem examination of brain tissue where rabies virus replicates to high titer. Fortunately, the viral ascent to the brain is restricted to the nervous system and strictly retrograde from the peripheral site of exposure to the CNS (Charlton, 1988) (see Chap. 7). Only after its replication in the CNS does the rabies virus spread centrifugally to the salivary glands and other tissues. This pathogenic pattern permits reliable prediction of the antemortem presence of virus in the saliva of a biting animal. Because several replication cycles of the virus occur in the brain prior to clinical manifestations (Kaplan, 1985), detection of nascent viral antigen in the brain is possible prior to the onset of signs of the disease. Therefore, when an animal bites a human, the attacking animal is quickly sacrificed and tested for the potential of rabies virus transmission. It is never necessary to delay euthanasia for the sake of further development of the disease to achieve a reliable diagnosis.

Microscopic examination of brain tissue stained with the DFA test has become the standard by which the value of all other rabies diagnostic tests or methods are measured and assessed. The DFA test is applied in a wide variety of other rabies-related laboratory functions; specifically, to indicate residual virus in the mouse inoculation and tissue culture virus isolation tests, for the examination of infected cell monolayers in tissue culture neutralization tests for serum antibody, and in research applications such as evaluation of the nonneural tropisms of rabies virus. We will cover this method in more detail and then discuss confirmatory methods and the advantages and disadvantages of other primary tests.

A. Public Health Laboratory Testing

1. Indications for Testing

Not all animals that bite or scratch a person need to be killed and tested for rabies. In countries with strong rabies control programs, rabies is relatively uncommon in domestic animals. The early signs and clinical progression of rabies in companion animals have been described in numerous experimental studies and are recognized easily. Biting incidents involving healthy dogs, cats, and ferrets are common but have never been implicated in North America in a human death from rabies. The public health recommendation drawn from these observations is that in most circumstances an apparently healthy dog, cat, or ferret that has bitten a person can be confined and observed daily for 10 days. Unless the animal develops signs suggestive of rabies during this period, it need not be killed and tested for rabies, and no antirabies biologicals are required for the person bitten. In areas where rabies is poorly controlled in domestic animals, antirabies treatment often is begun at the time of the bite exposure but terminated if the biting animal remains healthy during the observation period.

A 10-day confinement is not sufficient or appropriate for domestic animals showing signs of a neurologic illness and is also not reliable for wild and exotic species due to inadequate opportunity for observations of virus shedding. In these situations, if rabies is suspected, the animal immediately should be humanely euthanized, if necessary, and tested promptly. For many situations, if testing can be arranged within 48 hours of the potential exposure, initiation of PEP can await laboratory results. However, if delay in testing is unavoidable and for high-risk exposures, PEP can be initiated and discontinued if a reliable laboratory examination excludes a diagnosis of rabies.

Rabies control efforts can benefit from a specimen acceptance policy that recognizes the value of testing for a wide range of purposes. In addition to those animals which have potentially exposed a human or a domestic animal to the disease, consideration should be given to testing in the absence of reported contacts for (1) bats captured after close indoor encounters that may meet new aggressive treatment guidelines pertaining to situations where a bat bite may be expected to go unrecognized (Debbie and Trimarchi, 1997; Centers for Disease Control and Prevention, 2000), (2) domestic animals that die or are euthanized with signs that would include rabies in the differential diagnosis, (3) mammalian species not normally suspected of rabies infection (such as bear, deer, and beaver) that present with signs of a neurologic disorder in areas affected by terrestrial rabies cycles, (4) symptomatic rabies vector species captured outside the known geographic distribution of terrestrial rabies outbreak, and (5) rabies vector species in areas of enhanced surveillance conducted for the evaluation of effectiveness of wildlife rabies control strategies such as oral vaccination. These combined data, generated by this broad range of rabies surveillance, are used to define the epizootiologic patterns that establish the appropriate animal bite management decisions when the biting animal is not available for observation or testing.

The natural host range of rabies virus and all other lyssavirus species is limited to mammals. It is therefore not necessary to test species of other classes such as insects, reptiles, and birds. In North America, small rodents, including mice, rats, chipmunks, and squirrels, are essentially free of rabies infection, precluding the need for routine testing of these species (Childs *et al.*, 1997) (see Chaps. 4 and 5). Larger rodents such as woodchucks, muskrats, and beaver are exceptions, as are the smaller rodents that display unusual behavior or are involved in unprovoked bites to humans.

2. Biosafety

Rabies virus is categorized as a biosafety level II pathogen in diagnostic settings (Centers for Disease Control and Prevention, 1993). In certain research and vaccine-production settings, it is elevated to biosafety level III status. All activities related to the handling of animals and samples for rabies diagnosis should be performed following the appropriate standard guidelines and practices to avoid direct contact with potentially infectious fluids or tissues (Kaplan, 1996). Particular attention should be directed at avoiding percutaneous injuries from contaminated instruments, mucous membrane contamination with infectious fluids, and the production and exposure to aerosols of infectious materials. All persons working in rabies diagnostic activities and those capturing, handling, or decapitating rabies-suspect animals should receive rabies preexposure immunization with regular serologic assay of antibody titer and booster injections as necessary (Centers for Disease Control and Prevention, 1999a).

3. Collection, Preservation, and Submission of Specimens

An animal can be euthanized for rabies testing by any humane means that does not damage the head, including barbiturate and nonbarbiturate injectables or gases. The carcass should be refrigerated immediately following death to retard decomposition and autolysis of the brain. Because the animal species, site of exposure, variant of rabies virus, and time and cause of death can all affect the terminal distribution of rabies virus in the brain of infected animals, multiple areas of two to three regions of the brain must be examined to achieve reliable results. Consequently, the intact head of the animal constitutes the ideal specimen for most species. The entire body of bats should be submitted to avoid risk of loss of brain during decapitation of these very small animals and to facilitate identification of the bat species for important epizootiologic considerations. For large livestock such as cattle and horses, shipping of the entire head to a diagnostic laboratory/center poses special problems. For these animals, portions of the brainstem and cerebellum can be removed by the veterinary clinician through the foramen magnum following decapitation at the occipitoaxial juncture (Debbie and Trimarchi, 1992).

The specimen should be preserved by refrigeration during transport to the laboratory. Glycerol as a transport medium has been demonstrated to reduce immunofluorescence intensity even with subsequent washing (Lennette *et al.*, 1965), particularly when used in conjunction with standard acetone fixation (Andrulonis and Debbie, 1976). A single freezing will not deleteriously affect the DFA test or virus isolation, but freezing can delay diagnosis and exacerbate certain dissection problems. Repeated freeze–thaw cycles, on the other hand, can seriously affect sensitivity of diagnostic procedures. While decomposition or mutilation of the CNS may affect diagnostic potential, especially for reliable negative results, laboratory personnel cannot judge suitability of the specimen based solely on a verbal description of the condition of the carcass. Therefore, unless it is clear that the carcass is in advanced stages of decomposition or has been mutilated to the extent that there is no intact CNS, important specimens should be submitted, and an evaluation for suitability will be ascertained at the laboratory (Trimarchi and Briggs, 1999).

To achieve prompt results that will facilitate treatment and to avoid deterioration of tissues, specimen transport to the laboratory should be direct and immediate. Samples shipped to the laboratory by commercial parcel carriers must be packaged properly to avoid exposure hazards. Containment should include double bagging of the specimen in heavy (4 mil), sealed plastic bags, a Styrofoam inner box, and an outer waxed-cardboard box of adequate strength. If brain tissue is removed by the clinician prior to shipping, first it should be contained in a vial or other firm plastic container to protect it from being crushed or macerated during handling. Several hard-frozen gel cold packs of appropriate size should be included to properly refrigerate the contents for several days. Wet ice should be avoided because after thawing water can leak and potentially cause contamination. An envelope containing, if available, a fully completed standard rabies specimen history form should be attached to the outside of the container. If no form is available, all significant information should be provided, including the names, addresses, and telephone numbers of the owner, complainant, and all humans and animals in contact. Information on the clinical observations, date of death or means of euthanasia, exact location of capture, and the person or agency to receive the report also should be provided.

4. Laboratory Reporting Practices and Emergency Examinations

Public health rabies diagnostic laboratories typically operate, for routine examinations, on a traditional 5-day work week. Examination of specimens arriving early on a work day usually is completed the same day, and those arriving late in the day or during weekends and holidays are completed on the next regular work day. Emergency off-hour examinations generally can be arranged by contacting the laboratory or through the local public health agency's epidemiologic unit. Criteria justifying off-hour emergency diagnosis include animals strongly suspected of rabies virus infection that actually have bitten a person and for which a physician is awaiting test results before PEP.

Reports of rabies-positive specimens generally are made immediately to the physician or local public health authority by telephone, either directly from the laboratory or through the epidemiologic branch of the agency. Follow-up written reports of positive findings and routine negative reports generally are issued by mail or facsimile transmission. Submitters should never assume negative findings because they do not receive a report; the specimen may not have been received at the laboratory or the specimen may have been unsatisfactory for reliable examination. Because reporting practices vary widely, the submitter should ascertain local practice.

B. Immunofluorescence on Brain Tissue

Immunoglobulin molecules that attach specifically to epitopes on target antigens can be labeled by a firm chemical attachment of a fluorescent tag to produce a fluorescent antibody conjugate. This conjugate is allowed to react with specimen tissue prepared as smears, impressions, sections, or cultured cell monolayers. During incubation for an appropriate period, the specific antigen–antibody reaction occurs, binding the specific antibody molecule with the attached fluorochrome tag to the desired protein. Washing the specimen slides removes all conjugate components, except for specifically bound molecules. Examination of the slides is performed with a microscope using illuminating light that is rich in wavelengths that stimulate the fluorochrome to emit radiation in the visible spectrum, permitting visualization and localization of the target protein in the tissue preparation. The DFA test may have no more valuable efficacious application in biomedical science than its use for the diagnosis of rabies in postmortem brain samples of rabies-suspect animals.

1. Necropsy and Dissection

After the intact animal head is received for examination, brain removal and dissection are required. The flesh and muscle are removed from the dorsal aspect of the skull, and anterior and lateral cuts are made through the cranium with hammer and chisel, power saw, or scissors and forceps, depending on the species, size, and age of the specimen. After the meninges are dissected away, the exposed brain can be removed intact. Alternatively, the dissection of areas to be examined can be performed in the base of the skull. Another method has been described (Barrat, 1996; Willis, 2000) that employs a soda straw, pipette body, or other hollow tube that is forced through the foramen magnum anteriorly through the brain. After extraction of the tube from the head, the core of tissue is extruded from the tube. Priorities in the necropsy procedure include biocontainment and technician safety, proper accessioning and identification of each specimen, and strict avoidance of potential cross-contamination of specimens.

Areas of the brainstem, such as the medulla and pons, provide the most valuable samples for the demonstration of rabies virus infection in most specimens. This is not surprising given the general model of the virus' route to the CNS from sites of peripheral exposure (see Chap. 7). While it has been suggested that examination of the brainstem alone is adequate (Lee and Becker, 1972; Ito *et al.*, 1985), others have demonstrated the added value of examination of more than one area of the brain (Robinson and DiSalvo, 1980; Masserang and Leffingwell, 1981; Trimarchi *et al.*, 1986). The cerebellum may be the next area of diagnostic value. The hippocampus, once a prime rabies diagnostic sample area because of its role in the demonstration of Negri bodies in the histologic examination for the disease, may be of limited additional value when brainstem and cerebellum can be examined. Sampling of more than one area of the cerebellum and brainstem may improve the sensitivity and reliability of the diagnostic method further in animals that were killed just before onset of rabies or very early during the clinical phase.

2. Fluorescent Conjugate Selection, Preparation, and Evaluation

Because rabies virus nucleoprotein (N protein) is present in infected cells as microscopically recognizable, discrete intracytoplasmic inclusions, antibody preparations specific for the viral N protein are used for diagnostic reagent production (Flamand *et al.*, 1980). The fluorochrome used most frequently in rabies immunofluorescence testing is fluorescein isothiocyanate (FITC), selected because it is stable and produces a characteristic bright apple-green fluorescence that is unlike most autofluorescences produced by animal tissues and cells (Kissling, 1975). The conjugate also may contain a counterstain such as Evans blue for background staining of cellular structures (Rudd and Trimarchi, 1997).

The source of the immunoglobulin molecules for immunofluorescence reagents can be sera of hyperimmunized animals or monoclonal antibodies. Hamsters, rabbits, or horses immunized with fixed laboratory or vaccine strains of rabies virus have been used most often for immune serum reagents. Highly specific anti-rabies N protein–specific antibodies with the desired characteristics of specificity, fluorochrome labeling potential, and panspecific reaction with rabies virus (genotype 1) and other lyssavirus species (genotypes 2–7) have been produced as monoclonal reagents (Wiktor *et al.*, 1980; Bourhy *et al.*, 1992; Fraser *et al.*, 1996). Conjugates produced from cocktails (mixtures) of two or more labeled monoclonal antibodies recognizing different epitopes on the N protein provide highly specific reagents with uniform staining reactions and can be far more consistent from lot to lot than antisera-based reagents. While immune–serum antibody reagents can contain extraneous antibodies and be potentially cross-reactive, monoclonal antibody reagents risk overspecificity and weak affinity for some virus variants (Smith, 2000). It is beneficial in the interpretation of atypical immunofluorescence patterns to have two diagnostic reagents available for comparison and verification of findings.

The determination of the optimal working dilution of the diagnostic reagent is critical to sensitivity and specificity of the test and to economic conjugate use. If the reagent is too concentrated in routine tests, background fluorescence may be too bright, deleteriously affecting contrast of specific stained inclusions, and any nonspecific staining problems will be exacerbated. When the conjugate is too dilute, specific staining intensity may be weak, making specific staining difficult to recognize, particularly on suboptimal specimens due to death early in the clinical phase of the disease, tissue decomposition, or repeated freeze–thaw cycles of the sample. The highest dilution providing very bright green immunofluorescence and the full range of characteristic staining patterns is considered the end-point dilution. In routine testing, the conjugate is used one dilution more concentrated to provide a margin of precaution in the direction of optimal sensitivity. Rabies-positive control slides are used to determine a conjugate's working dilution and must be identical in type and preparation to those used in routine specimen testing. Because there is some variability in the affinity of commercial reagents to the many variants of naturally occurring "street" rabies virus, this important titration should be performed in duplicate on at least two different rabies virus variants.

3. *Immunofluorercence Test Protocol*

Touch impressions or slip smears from each area of brain sampled are made on clean glass microscope slides. For research applications and examination of nonneural tissues, frozen sections are prepared using a cryostat. Duplicate sets of slides are prepared and stored frozen for potential repeat tests on identical slides to evaluate perplexing or uncharacteristic staining patterns. At the same time as the slides are prepared for immunofluorescence examination, a brain suspension can be made in appropriate diluents from the same areas of brain tissue for isolation of virus by *in vivo* or *in vitro* virus cultivation or for RT-PCR for confirmatory testing. Unused tissue samples from diagnostic areas of the brain of each specimen are held at −70°C for additional analysis.

After air drying, the slides are fixed for a period of 1 hour to overnight in acetone at −20°C. Fixation enhances permeability of the cells to labeled antibodies and improves tissue adherence to the slide. Very short fixation periods and a microwave fixation procedure, as an alternative to acetone (Neill *et al.*, 1998) have been described. After removal from acetone, the slides are thoroughly air dried. The diagnostic reagent at working dilution is applied dropwise to each slide, which is then incubated in a moist chamber at 37°C for 30 minutes. The slides then receive multiple washes in buffered saline and are air dried. Each slide must be identified carefully. Application of the staining reagent, fixation, and washing steps all are performed avoiding communal baths and slide-to-slide contact to prevent any potential for contamination between specimens. Coverslips are mounted with a buffered glycerol mountant. Selection of mountant buffer, pH, glycerol concentration, and other components is critical to persistence and intensity of immunofluorescence in the preparations (Smith, 1986). Slides should be read promptly or stored prior to examination for periods of greater than 2 hours at 4°C or overnight and longer at −20°C or colder.

The slides are examined on a standard, incident-light fluorescence microscope fitted with a xenon or mercury vapor lamp. Excitation and barrier filter systems are selected for excitation in the blue or ultraviolet spectrum. The performance of illumination-collecting lenses and mirrors, fluorescence objective lenses, and filter combinations of the recent-generation fluorescence microscopes dramatically improves the brightness and contrast over earlier models. Specific staining appears as a bright apple-green fluorescence against a dark background. Examination is performed at 150× to 450× magnification, and about 25–50 fields are examined for each slide. Ideally, more than one slide is evaluated for each tissue, and all slides from specimens representing possible human exposure to rabies are read by two experienced microscopists.

4. Interpretation of Results and Tests for Specificity

The recruitment and retention of properly trained, experienced microscopists are essential to the interpretation of slides and for maintaining the highest standards of sensitivity and specificity of the test (Trimarchi, 2000). The characteristic apple-green FITC color and bright intensity identify specific staining. The common morphologic structure of the intracytoplasmic inclusions (comprised of N protein) is a three-dimensional round or oval shape with smooth margins and a brighter emission in the periphery (Fig. 1A). In smears or touch impressions, labeled rabies virus N antigen also appears as fine particles and occasionally in long strands, possibly the result of the slide preparation process. Inclusions are seen in large numbers in the cell bodies and dendrites of neurons, particularly in the Purkinje cells of the cerebellum and the large neurons of the brainstem. Rabies-specific antigen occasionally may be present in glial and other nonneuronal cells of the brain (Jackson *et al.*, 2000). Inclusions and particulate fluorescence generally are widespread throughout the CNS of infected animals beginning up to several days before the onset of clinical signs of rabies and before infection of salivary glands is evident by the same method. Occasionally, distribution of antigen may be limited and appear sporadically in some areas of the CNS, especially when the animal is euthanized prior to or very early in the clinical phase. This situation occurs more often in large livestock and particularly in horses (Smith, 1995).

Rabies virus antigen–specific staining generally can be distinguished easily from the yellow, white, and gold autofluorescences of tissue constituents based on the very characteristic color of FITC emission. Granular nonspecific staining can result from drying of the conjugate on the slide during the staining process or from precipitation of aggregates of free FITC in improperly reconstituted, stored, or clarified reagents. Nonspecific staining also can be the result of adherence of labeled IgG elements in the conjugate to Fc receptors on contaminating grampositive cocci in the sample or on immune cells infiltrating the brain in response to an infection other than rabies in the animal (e.g., distemper). Diffuse background staining can be the result of an inappropriate conjugate working dilution or overly high fluorochrome–protein ratios in the reagent.

Unexpected outcomes, unusual antigen distributions, and noncharacteristic morphology of staining patterns require validation of the specificity of the observed reaction. This can be accomplished when using antisera-based reagents by repeating the staining procedure with an aliquot of the conjugate that has been absorbed with rabies virus to remove all rabies-specific labeled IgG. All fluorescence appearing with this preparation is due to nonspecific factors. This procedure is not applicable to conjugates made with monoclonal antibodies because these reagents contain only antibodies directed to viral proteins. Nonspecific staining with monoclonal antibody reagents can be recognized as nonspecific when similar staining appears when test slides are stained with a conjugate made with monoclonal antibodies of the same isotype and at the same concentration as the rabies reagent but specific for a different agent. The cause of repeated nonspecific staining problems should be ascertained as soon as possible and eliminated because it could mask the few specifically stained areas of a very weakly positive specimen.

318

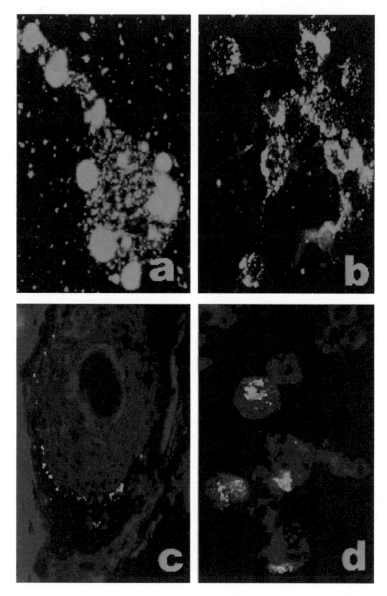

Fig. 1. (*A*) Purkinje cell from the cerebellum of a rabies viruses–infected bovine with large intra-cytoplasmic inclusions and smaller particulate antigen demonstrated with the DFA method (slip smear; ×540 magnification). (*B*) Rabies virus–infected monolayer of murine neuroblastoma cells (DFA method with Evans blue counterstain; ×250 magnification). (*C*) Human hair follicle from nuchal skin biopsy. Nerve cells surrounding follicle are disclosed by specific fluorescence associated with presence of rabies antigen (DFA method on frozen section, Evans blue counterstain; ×250 magnification). (*D*) Human corneal impression with several infected epithelial cells containing inclusions of specifically labeled rabies antigen (DFA method with Evans blue counterstain; ×360 magnification).

A major constraint on the sensitivity of the rabies DFA method is the condition of the brain sample (Lewis and Thacker, 1974). Decomposition and denaturation by heat, repeated freeze–thaw cycles, and exposure to chemicals can contribute to reduced sensitivity. Decomposition will affect the sensitivity of all rabies diagnostic procedures. Immunofluorescence tests may remain positive for a period after virus isolation is no longer possible (Rudd and Trimarchi, 1989). A characteristic positive DFA test result on decomposed or mutilated tissue fragments may support a valid rabies-positive report, confirmed with the appropriate test for specificity or by virus isolation, immunohistochemistry, or molecular methods. One of the most difficult decisions confronting the public health rabies laboratory is determining when a reliable negative result can be issued on a specimen received in a partially decomposed condition or otherwise compromised sample in which no evidence of immunofluorescence is observed. Certainly, once decomposition has advanced in the tissue to a foul smelling, discolored, or liquefied condition due to putrefaction, negative results are invalid. When mutilation or submission of inappropriate samples precludes proper examination of recognizable samples of brainstem and either cerebellum or hippocampus, negative results may not be reliable.

C. Quality Assurance and Quality Control in the Rabies DFA Test

Despite the importance of test results for the medical management of human exposures, postmortem examination of animals is not considered a human clinical examination. Therefore, it has not been regulated for stringent adherence to established standard methods by acts such as the U.S. Clinical Laboratory Improvement Amendment of 1988. Comparison of methods employed reveals many exceptions to accepted practices (Smith, 1995). Observations of the critical importance of seemingly minor test components, such as composition of coverslip mounting medium to immunofluorescence persistence (Smith, 1986; Rudd, personal communication), emphasize the value of the recommendation that uniform procedures be adopted (Hanlon et al., 1999). For example, a recent observation with one of the commercial rabies-specific conjugates has revealed that high concentrations of glycerol and low pH in coverslip mounting media can contribute to very rapid disappearance of specific fluorescence with certain combinations of reagent and virus variant (Chemicon International, 2000). Voluntary rabies proficiency testing programs were conducted in the United States in 1973 and 1992 and annually since 1994. The performance of diagnostic laboratories enrolled in the recent programs has been excellent in the evaluation of positive and negative test slides using the DFA method. Consensus has been best on strongly positive and negative slides. Discrepancies have occurred primarily with very weakly positive specimens (Powell, 1997).

Important factors in the avoidance of false-negative results in rabies diagnosis include strict adherence to a uniform methodology, the use of proper scientific controls for all procedures, diagnostic conjugate quality and proper dilution, and optimization of the microscope lamp and instrument performance. False-positive results are avoided by implementing procedures that reduce the possibility of cross-contamination of negative samples with strong positive samples and by optimizing conjugate diluents and staining and washing conditions to eliminate nonspecific fluorescence. The laboratory can use a selected application of tests for specificity of observed fluorescence, including paired staining with two different diagnostic reagents, with virus-absorbed and sham-absorbed conjugates, and staining with FITC-labeled IgG conjugate specific for another antigen. Every DFA test on a public health sample requires scientific controls by performance of identical procedures on known rabies-positive and rabies-negative slides. Acceptance of tests depends on positive control slides with consistently bright, characteristically distributed immunofluorescence and the expected range of size and morphology of inclusions. Negative controls must display an absence of fluorescence that mimics or could obscure specific fluorescence. Whenever unexpected outcomes are observed, the findings should be confirmed using the DFA test with another rabies reagent or with another test or by a corroborative test at a regional or national reference laboratory. Unexpected outcomes include sporadic antigen distribution in brain tissues or rabies-positive results on a specimen unlikely to have been rabid due to species type (small rodent), location of capture (rabies-free area), or history (vaccinated and no clinical signs of rabies). Good quality control of the DFA test requires that unused brain material, taken from internal portions of areas tested, should be held in reserve for additional testing (Smith, 2000). It bears repeating that practice has demonstrated that microscopists experienced in examination of rabies DFA slides are essential to the proper interpretation of these tests.

Rabies DFA is comparable in sensitivity with *in vivo* and *in vitro* virus isolation methods. There have been no recorded human rabies cases in North America arising from bites of animals that were diagnosed negative for rabies by DFA. Despite its proven reliability, the consequences of a false report for decisions of postexposure management are so unacceptable that some confirmatory tests are required to validate individual negative reports and to maintain confidence in the procedure. This can be accomplished in the same public health laboratories where DFA tests are performed by an alternative backup test performed on each sample or on selected samples, such as highly suspect human exposure cases. Alternatively, confirmation of DFA results can be arranged by collaboration with a national or regional reference laboratory.

Constant vigilance at the laboratory is required to avoid cross-contamination, especially during rabies epizootics that result in extraordinarily large numbers of rabid animals being processed within the laboratory. An active state health department laboratory identified 2745 rabid animals among a total 11,896 animals processed and examined during the course of 1 year (Trimarchi, 1994). Special steps during necropsy must be taken to ensure that instruments, examination gloves, work surfaces, and all other materials that come into contact with the specimen are either disposable and replaced after each specimen or are disinfected thoroughly by boiling or autoclaving and washed after each use. Great care also must be taken during the slide fixation, staining, washing, and coverslip mounting processes to avoid contamination from positive controls or from specimen to specimen (Smith *et al.*, 1996). The standards of avoiding a false-positive outcome as a result of cross-contamination are even greater when molecular methods are employed (see Sect. IVB).

D. Other Methods for Detection of Viral Proteins in Brain Tissue

Although the speed and reliability of the DFA test have made it the stalwart of rabies diagnosis, other antigen detection methods are also applied, and some have advantages for certain testing applications. Tests that can be applied to formalin-fixed tissues benefit from freedom from sample preservation concerns and risks associated with transporting and processing samples containing infectious virus. A potential limitation of the procedure to work with formalin-fixed preparations is the inability to cultivate and proliferate the virus from an inactivated sample. Immunofluorescence methods applied to formalin-fixed tissues and immunohistochemical methods, such as immunoperoxidase staining of formalin-fixed, paraffin-embedded sections, were previously significantly less sensitive than the DFA method on fresh brain tissue. With recent modifications to achieve better immunofluorescence (Warner *et al.*, 1997) and immunohistochemistry on brain sections (Hamir, 1995) and brain impressions (Niezgoda, 1999), these procedures may now be approaching comparable sensitivity to DFA on fresh tissue. The methods have benefited from three major improvements: (1) digestion of the tissue sections with enzymes such as proteinase prior to staining to expose antigenic sites that formerly were masked by bonds resulting from fixation, (2) selection of particularly well-suited monoclonal antibodies as the primary antibody in IFA tests improving sensitivity and specificity, (3) avidin–biotin amplification in the staining process to increase the signal. However, further evaluation and validation of negative test results may be necessary before these tests can be employed regularly to make decisions to withhold rabies postexposure treatment (PET) for potentially exposed humans.

Enzyme-linked immunosorbent assays (ELISA) are showing promise of improved sensitivity as a result of avidin–biotin amplification and are employed for rapid and simple diagnosis of other viral infections. A similar method has been developed for the detection of rabies antigen (Bourhy and Perrin 1996). The method offers the benefit of sensitivity when applied to poorly preserved specimens and manual or automated reading, making them well suited for use in field conditions. While these methods can be used for confirmatory testing to back up the DFA test, they are not used widely in public health laboratories for primary diagnosis. Delays in shipping to the few laboratories that perform these tests and in the processing of the samples presently limit their application for decisions of postexposure management.

E. Histologic Examination

Historically, microscopic examination of histologic preparations was the primary means of identifying evidence of rabies infection in postmortem samples from animals and humans. Fresh brain smears or microtome-cut sections of formalin-fixed, paraffin-embedded tissue were stained with combinations of basic fuchsin and methylin blue (Tierkel and Atanasiu, 1996) or with hematoxylin and eosin (Lepine and Atanasiu, 1996). Histopathologic evidence of encephalitis includes signs of inflammatory response, such as perivascular cuffing and cellular infiltrations (see Chap. 8). The presence of acidophilic intracytoplasmic inclusions, called *Negri bodies*, found prominently in the Purkinje cells of the cerebellum and the pyramidal cells of the hippocampus, is virtually pathognomonic for the disease. When reported by an experienced pathologist, this provides a reliable diagnosis of the disease. Negri bodies detected during routine postmortem examinations of tissue following deaths attributed to encephalitis of unknown etiology continue to disclose occasional human rabies cases that were not suspected antemortem or at the time of death (Centers for Disease Control and Prevention, 1993). Unfortunately, the presence, distribution, and size of Negri bodies are related to the species of animal, variant of rabies virus, and duration of the clinical period prior to death. The sensitivity and reliability of the method are poor, with numerous surveys indicating that 25% or more of animals have no demonstrable Negri bodies (Pert and Good, 1991). The method is therefore of limited value for public health purposes.

III. VIRUS ISOLATLON

The most common confirmatory tests are cultivation of virus by inoculation of animals or cell culture. An asset of either isolation procedure is the availability of cultivated virus for further propagation and characterization by antigenic or genetic analysis (see Chap. 3). The mouse inoculation test (MIT) (Webster and Dawson, 1935) is a sensitive and reliable procedure (Surreau *et al.*, 1991). A small piece of each area of the brain examined by DFA is combined into one homogenized suspension made with mortar and pestle or tissue grinders in a buffered saline diluent containing protein stabilizer and antibiotics. Five weanling laboratory mice are inoculated intracerebrally for each specimen and observed for signs of rabies for 30 days. Mice that develop signs of illness are sacrificed immediately and tested by the DFA method. Favorable attributes of the MIT as a backup test procedure are its applicability to partially decomposed specimens, its high sensitivity in weakly positive specimens, and its technical simplicity. Its main drawback, besides the inherent environmental and ethical issues with the use of live animals in the laboratory, is the typical 7- to 20-day interval between inoculation and onset of observable signs of infection. The period can be shortened by inoculating families of neonatal mice and sacrificing individual neonates daily beginning 5 days after inoculation and examining their brains by DFA. However, this technique requires a larger number of mice per sample and increases the labor-intensive nature of the MIT.

The unpredictable and problematic delay associated with *in vivo* virus isolation (i.e., MIT) can be reduced greatly by inoculation and detection of virus in continuous cell culture. Cell culture medium is used as the diluent for the tissue suspension preparation. After clarification of the suspension preparation by light centrifugation, the sample is inoculated onto cell monolayers or added to cells in suspension. A murine neuroblastoma cell line that is susceptible to rabies virus infection generally is selected (Rudd and Trimarchi, 1987; Umoh and Blenden, 1983). Tissue culture flasks or 96-well plates are seeded with host cells, and the cells are incubated from one to several days before they are examined by DFA for evidence of rabies virus infection. Evidence of infection is found with appearance of intracytoplasmic inclusions in clusters of infected cells (fluorescent foci) in the monolayer (see Fig. 1*B*). Sensitivity, which can be enhanced by the addition of DEAE–dextran to the cell culture medium (Kaplan *et al.*, 1987), rivals that of the IFA test and MIT (Webster and Casey, 1996). With results available in a fixed period of only a few days, cell culture isolation has a much greater practical value than the MIT for prompt initiation of PET in the advent of a weakly positive specimen that was not detected by the original DFA test (Rudd and Trimarchi, 1980).

IV. DETECTION OF VIRAL RNA BY MOLECULAR METHODS

A. Applications, Advantages, and Disadvantages of Molecular Methods

Molecular methods of diagnosis use hybridization or amplification to detect nucleic acid (RNA or DNA) in a test sample and are most useful when serologic or culture methods are unavailable, insensitive, or lack specificity. Nucleic acid–based tests are rapidly supplanting other methods for the diagnosis of herpesvirus and some arbovirus infections of the CNS (Huang *et al.*, 1999).

For many infectious diseases, however, conventional methods are sufficiently sensitive. Such is the case for diagnostic tests of fresh brain tissue for rabies encephalitis.

DFA tests for rabies lack neither rapidity, sensitivity, nor specificity. Almost all samples for rabies diagnosis are taken from animals in the terminal stages of their infection when rabies virus is present at a high copy number in brain tissue and can be detected easily and quickly by DFA. Detection failures (false-negative tests) are potentially a greater problem with nucleotide-based reagents than with tests like the DFA that are based on antigen–antibody reactions. Amino acid sequence homology is higher among lyssavirus samples than is nucleotide homology (Bourhy *et al.*, 1993), and new lyssavirus isolates are more likely to share sufficient antigenic sites with known samples and be detected by immunologic reagents than they are to share regions of high nucleotide sequence homology and be detected by genetic methods.

Nucleic acid–based methods can be a more sensitive test than DFA with brain tissue samples that are too decomposed for direct examination (Heaton *et al.*, 1997), and they can detect viral RNA in such tissues as saliva and CSF that are unsuitable for DFA testing (Crepin *et al.*, 1998; Noah *et al.*, 1998). However, even molecular methods have sensitivity limits, and neither conventional antigen–antibody or genetic methods can rule out a diagnosis of rabies in an animal contact unless samples are taken appropriately and tests are controlled rigorously.

If used appropriately, molecular methods are valuable adjuncts to traditional methods for rabies diagnosis. With their greater sensitivity and applicability to a wider range of tissue samples, nucleic acid–based methods have detected evidence of rabies successfully in cases where conventional methods could not be applied (Centers for Disease Control and Prevention, 1997). Genetic tests also can be useful for the periodic confirmatory tests of DFA that are required for good laboratory practice and often are more sensitive than traditional confirmatory tests such as virus isolation (Whitby, 1997). Genetic tests also are faster than traditional tests, and results can be obtained in less than 24 hours, making these tests useful for the confirmation of unexpected or unusual DFA test observations.

B. Detection of *Lyssavirus* RNA by Hybridizatlon with Nucleic Acid Probes

The first molecular tests for rabies used labeled DNA or RNA probes (synthetic oligonucleotides complementary to the virus RNA) and hybridization methods to detect RNA in tissues (*in situ* hybridization) or RNA extracted from tissues and blotted onto membranes (slot or dot-blot hybridization). Although applications exist for probe hybridization methods in pathogenesis studies, probe-based methods of detection of lyssavirus genomic RNA or mRNA are not used often as diagnostic tests (Ermine *et al.*, 1989; Jackson *et al.*, 1989; Jackson, 1991).

Commercial kits are available for labeling of probes, but no commercial source exists for probes that can be used in rabies diagnosis. Given the genetic diversity among lyssaviruses, multiple probes might be needed to achieve an adequately sensitive detection across the genus. Detection methods based on *in situ* hybridization require lengthy tissue fixation, blocking, and sectioning to prepare samples for examination. The numerous incubation periods and blocking steps required for both *in situ* and blot detection of viral RNA do not permit as rapid a diagnosis as DFA. Hybridization sensitivity also may be lower than the sensitivity of antigen detection methods. Jackson and Rintoul (1992) attributed the loss of signal during postmortem autolysis to the effects of the agonal state, degradation of RNA by ribonucleases, and diffusion of RNA out of cells prior to fixation.

In situ hybridization has the greatest utility in the diagnostic laboratory as a confirmatory test of observations made by DFA examination of fixed tissues (Warner *et al.*, 1999). Blot hybridization also can serve as a check on specificity for PCR (Whitby *et al.*, 1997; Sabouroud *et al.*, 1999) and can increase the sensitivity of the PCR (Whitby *et al.*, 1997).

C. Amplification Methods for Detection of *Lyssavirus* RNA (RT-PCR)

The nucleic acid amplification method used most often as a diagnostic test is the polymerase chain reaction (PCR). PCR is based on the ability of a thermostable DNA polymerase to copy (transcribe) DNA by elongation of a complementary strand (cDNA). Transcription is initiated by priming with a pair of closely spaced oligonucleotides (forward and reverse primers). The PCR product (the amplicon) is double-stranded DNA of a length defined by the spacing of the primer pair. Repeated cycles of denaturation of the amplicon by heating, hybridization with the primer pair at a lower temperature, and copying of DNA by the polymerase for a short period of time produce a million-fold amplification of the target DNA sequence. Because lyssaviruses have an RNA genome, *Lyssavirus* PCR must be preceded by reverse transcription of RNA to cDNA (RT-PCR).

As the number of rabies laboratories performing RT-PCR increases, so has the diversity of reagent mixtures, PCR primer sets, and thermocycling programs used for amplification reactions increased. The customization of protocols for the full range of viral genes and genotypes that are submitted for testing partly reflects the importance of optimization advised in the early days of PCR applications (Saiki, 1989). In reality, the standard PCR protocols provided with commercial kits will work for many applications without customization (Kuno, 1998). Two laboratories have published detailed protocols for RT-PCR using mostly commercial reagents (Tordo *et al.*, 1995; Nadin-Davis, 1998) and this information will not be reproduced here. The following is a more general discussion of primer selection and sensitivity and specificity controls for RT-PCR of *Lyssavirus* RNA.

1. Primer Design

Samples submitted for rabies testing may originate anywhere in the world. The most important factor limiting the utility of RT-PCR as a diagnostic test is the selection of primers that will efficiently amplify all members (genotypes) of the *Lyssavirus* genus. The genomic sequence encoding the N protein, the most conserved of the five viral proteins (Bourhy *et al.*, 1995), was the target of most amplifications, but no one pair of N gene complementary primers was shown to amplify all *Lyssavirus* samples equally well. A pairwise comparison between the two most divergent viruses in the genus, rabies virus (genotype 1) and Mokola virus (genotype 3), reveals an overall nucteotide sequence homology of less than 80% for the N protein gene. Fortunately, some primer mismatch is tolerated in both the initial reverse transcription and subsequent PCR. With the large amounts of RNA usually found in the brains of rabid animals, even an inefficient amplification with a 4-bp mismatch between primer and template yields a detectable product (Fig. 2A). Primer binding and amplification efficiency become more important when the quantity or quality of viral RNA is less than ideal either because of the stage of the rabies infection, the type of sample available for testing, or inappropriate handling of the sample. In situations where RNA is limited or degraded, assay efficiency can be increased by using more closely spaced primers and decreasing the size of the resulting amplicon (Table I) and by using mixtures of primers or degenerate primers (primers with a mixture of nucleotides at some positions) to compensate for primer–template mismatch. There are over 80 published papers from laboratories performing RT-PCR for rabies diagnosis or virus typing. Tables II through VI compare some of the commonly used primers for homology with representative lyssaviruses.

Most protocols for RT-PCR begin with reverse transcription of virus genomic RNA using primers complementary to the 5′ start of the nucleoprotein mRNA (e.g., N7 and 10g in Table II). Data for representative lyssaviruses suggest stronger sequence conservation for the region complementary to the primer N7 (Bourhy *et al.*, 1993), which has no more than three primer–template mismatches with any lyssavirus species. Published sequence data also suggest that the efficiency of primer N7 might be increased by the addition of two conserved nucleotides to its 3′ end and the substitution of inosine for thymidine at nucleotide residue 65 (i.e., the consensus primer in Table II).

In most protocols, the reverse transcription primer is also used as one of the two primers for amplification. The second primer is chosen from upstream sequence, either in the N gene or in the phosphoprotein (P) gene. Early sequence comparisons and successful amplifications suggested RNA conservation around

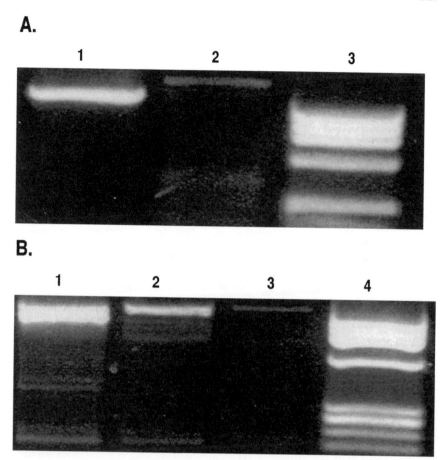

Fig. 2. (*A*) Ethidium bromide–stained agarose gel of amplicons from RT-PCR of Australian bat lyssavirus RNA with primer sets N7 and 304 (lane 1) or N7 and N8 (lane 2). Lane 3 depicts molecular weight markers. Primers are identified in Tables II and III. (*B*) Ethidium bromide–stained agarose gel of amplicons from RT-PCR of dilutions of brain tissue identified in Table I. lane 1, 10^{-3} dilution; lane 2, 10^{-4} dilution; lane 3, 10^{-5} dilution. Lane 4 depicts molecular weight markers. RT-PCR was performed with primers 10g and 1312NBdeg described in Tables II and VI.

the N-terminal amino acid and stop codons of the N protein gene (Smith *et al.*, 1991). These regions are now known to be highly variable (see Fig. 4 in Chap. 3) and are no longer used as primer sequences. Greater success was obtained when the sequence for the second primer was based on the mRNA initiation site for the P gene (Nadin-Davis *et al.*, 1994; primer 304 in Table III) or on a relatively conserved region upstream in the P gene (Bourhy *et al.*, 1993; primer N8 in Table III). Primer 304 will amplify all variants of rabies virus known in the United States and some other lyssavirus species, but amplification of

TABLE I

Comparison of Assay Sensitivity[a]

Sample dilution	Amount of brain tissue	Infectious centers	Amplification reactions (amplicon size)		
			(1336 bp) Primary PCR	(245 bp) Primary PCR	(245 bp) Nested PCR
10^{-1}	2 mg	500 (estimated)	Positive	Positive	ND
10^{-2}	0.2 mg	52	Positive	Positive	ND
10^{-3}	20 µg	5	Positive	Positive	ND
10^{-4}	2 µg	0	Positive	Positive	ND
10^{-5}	0.2 µg	ND	±	Positive	Positive
10^{-6}	20 ng	ND	Negative	Positive	Positive
10^{-7}	2 ng	ND	Negative	Negative	Negative

[a]Sensitivity of comparative assays for rabies virus (unpublished data, Rabies Laboratory, CDC). A 20% suspension of brain tissue (20 mg/100 µl of media) from a naturally infected skunk was clarified by centrifugation, serially diluted, and dispensed in 100-µl aliquots. Aliquots were assayed for infectious virus by incubation with 1×10^6 mouse neuroblastoma cells in an eight-well culture slide. The number of infectious centers per slide was counted at 40 hours after staining by DFA. RNA was extracted from one aliquot of each dilution and resuspended to 100 µl. A 5-µl aliquot of each RNA was reverse transcribed and amplified by PCR with the primers listed in Tables II, V, and VI. The 1336-bp product was produced with primers 10g:1312Nbdeg (see Table VI). The 245-bp primary PCR product was produced with primers 1087NFdeg:1312Nbdeg (see Tables V and VI, respectively). The 245-bp nested PCR product was produced by reamplification of the 10g:1312NBdeg reaction with primers 1087NFdeg:1312NBdeg. Amplicons were detected by electrophoresis in 2% agarose gels with ethidium bromide. ND, not determined.

Mokola and Lagos bat viruses is very inefficient. Primer N8 amplifies Mokola and Lagos bat viruses more efficiently but amplifies Australian bat lyssavirus and some rabies viruses in the United States inefficiently (see Fig. 2A). The region complementary to primer N8 is better conserved than the region complementary to primer 304 in published sequences for lyssaviruses; however, reaction efficiency and the utility of primer N8 might be further increased by the deletion of the highly variable nucleotide at the 3' end and the use of inosine, adenosine, and guanine (degeneracy) at residues 1570, 1576, and 1582 (i.e., the consensus primer in Table III).

The long amplicon produced by an N gene–P gene primer pair is an advantage for virus typing by methods of digestion with restriction enzymes. N gene–P gene primer pairs are less useful, however, for samples with only small amounts of viral RNA or for poorly handled samples with degraded RNA (see Table I). In these situations, the sensitivity of the RT-PCR can be increased by using primers for sequences from internal regions of the N protein gene to produce a smaller

TABLE II

Primers for Reverse Transcription and Amplification of lyssavirus RNA from Nucleotide Sequence at the Start of the Nucleoprotein Gene[a]

	55	82	GenBank accession no./ref.
Primer N7	ATGT AACACCTCTACA ATG		Bourhy et al., 1993
Primer 10g		CTACA ATGGATGCCG AC	Smith et al., 1991
Consensus primer	ATGT AACACCiCTACA ATGGA		
RABV (Pasteur vaccine)	--- ------t-----	--	M13215
RABV (CVS laboratory)	--- ------c-----	--	D42112
RABV (RCHL vaccine)	--- ------t-----	--	AB009663
RABV (fox, polar regions)	--- ------t-----	--	L20673
RABV (raccoon, U.S.)	--- ------t-----	--	U27218
RABV (many)	--- ------------	--	Kissi et al., 1995
RABV (silver-haired bat, U.S.)	------a-	-a-	Unpublished
RABV (red bat, U.S.)	-------	-g	Unpublished
RABV (big brown bat, U.S.)	----a--	--	Unpublished
RABV (yellow bat, U.S.)	--a----	--	Unpublished
ABLV (frugivorous bat)	----gt-t-	-t	AF006497
ABLV (insectivorous bat)	----gt-t-	-t	AF081020
DUV	----t--	-a	U22848
EBLV1	-----tta	--	U22845
EBLV2	-----t--	--	U22846
LAGV (Ethiopia)	----ta---a- ----t-g-	-a	Mebatsion et al., 1993
LAGV (Nigeria)	----t-a-	-a	U22842
MOKV (Ethiopia)	----tc---- ----gt-t-	--	Mebatsion et al., 1993
MOKV (Zimbabwe)	---- ----tc---- ----gt-t-	--	Y09762

[a] Sequence for the initial methionine codon is underlined. Genomic sequence for representative lyssavirus isolates is presented as a DNA positive strand. Primers are oriented as genomic-sense strand for reverse transcription and amplification reactions. Unpublished data, Rabies Laboratory, CDC. Nucleotide position is based on sequence of the Pasteur vaccine strain of rabies virus (Genbank accession no. M13215; Tordo et al., 1986).

TABLE III

Primers for Reverse Amplification of lyssavirus cDNA from Nucleotide Sequence at the Start of the Phosphoprotein (P)[a]

	1514	1534		GenBank accession no./ref.
Primer 304	ATGAGCAAGA TCTTTGTCAA		1568 1585	Smith, 1995
Primer N8			GAGATG GCTGAAGAGA CT	Bourhy et al., 1993
Consensus primer		A	GArATG GCiGAAGArA C	
Consensus sequence	ATGAGCAAGA TCTTTGTCAAA		GAGATG GCTGAAGAGA CT	GenBank accession no./ref.
RABV (CVS11 laboratory)	---------- ----------		------ --------a- --	X55727
RABV (ERA vaccine)	---------- ----------		------ --------a- --	X55728
RABV (PM laboratory)	---------- ----------		------ --------a- --	X55729
RABV (SADB19 vaccine)	---------- ----------		------ --------a- --	M31046
RABV (Pasteur vaccine)	---------- ----------		------ --------a- --	M13215
RABV (RCHL vaccine)	---------- ----c-----		------ ---------- --	AB009663
RABV (CVS laboratory)	---------- --------t-		------ --c------- --	X57783
ABLV (frugivorous bat)	---------- ----------		--a--- --a--g---- --	AF006497
ABLV (insectivorous bat)	---------- ----------		--a--- --a--g---- --	AF081020
DUVV (V008)	---------- -t---a----		------ ---------- -c	AF049115
DUVV (V268)	---------- -t---a----		------ ---------- -c	AF049120
EBLV1 (V002)	---------- ----------		------ -----g---- -a	AF049113
EBLV1 (V023)	---------- ----------		------ -----g---- -a	AF049117
EBLV2 (V286)	---------- ----------		------ --g------- -g	AF049121
LAGV (V267)	--------g ggc-ca-ac-		--a--- --a--g---- --	AF049119
LAGV (V006)	--------g ga--aa-ac-		------ ----g--a- --	AF049114
MOKV (V020)	--------g a-c----gc-		--a--- --a-----a- -c	AF049116
MOKV (V241)	-------ag at--a--ac-		--a--- ---------- --	AF049118
MOKV Zimbabwe	-------ag at--g--gc-		--a--- --a------- --	Y09762

[a]The initial methionine codon of the P gene is underlined. Genomic sequence for representative lyssavirus isolates is presented as a DNA positive strand. Primers should be reoriented as message-sense strand for amplification of N gene sequence. Nucleotide position is based on sequence of the Pasteur vaccine strain of rabies virus (GenBank accession no. M13215; Tordo et al., 1986).

amplicon. Primer sequences for two internal regions have been used (Heaton et al., 1999; Mcquiston et al., 2001), but amplification efficiency is reduced by poor sequence conservation in both regions (see Tables IV through VI).

The primers described in Table IV (Heaton et al., 1999) failed to amplify isolates of several lyssavirus species even with viral RNA extracted from cell culture passaged virus. Nested and heminested RT-PCR was used to increase test sensitivity, but the added expense of reamplification and the increased risks of cross-contamination in reamplifying from DNA (Kwok and Higuchi, 1989; Cooper and

TABLE IV

Primers for Amplification of lyssavirus RNA from Nucleotide Sequence in the Midregion of the Nucleoprotein (N) gene[a]

	641		660	GenBank accession no./ref.
Primer JW6-DPL	-----	---------G	--T--	Heaton et al., 1999
Primer JW6-M	--T--	G-----C---	-----	Heaton et al., 1999
Primer JW6-E	-----	G-------C	-----	Heaton et al., 1999
Consensus primer	CAyAA	rATGTGyGCi	AAyTG	
Consensus sequence	CACAA	AATGTGTGCT	AACTG	
RABV (many)	--y--	r--------i	--y--	Kissi et al., 1995
RABV (dog, Africa)	--t--	------c--c	--t--	U22649
RABV (dog, Thailand)	-----	g-----c---	--t--	U22653
RABV (raccoon, U.S.)	-----	------c---	-----	U27218
RABV (mongoose, S.Afr.)	--t--	g---------	--t--	U22628
RABV (pallid bat, U.S.)	--t--	g-----c---	-----	Unpublished
RABV (red bat, U.S.)	----g	--------c	-----	Unpublished
ABLV (insectivorous bat)	-----	--------g	--t--	AF081020
ABLV (frugivorous bat)	--t--	g-------a	-----	AF006497
DUVV	-----	--------g	--t--	U22848
EBLV1	-----	g-------c	-----	U22845
EBLV2	-----	g-----c--c	-----	U22846
LAGV (Nigeria)	-----	--------a	--t--	U22842
LAGV (Ethiopia)	-----	------c--a	-----	Mebatsion et al., 1993
Mokola (Zimbabwe)	--t--	g-----c---	-----	Y09762
Mokola (Ethiopia)	-----	g-------c	--t--	Mebatsion et al., 1993

[a]Genomic sequence for representative lyssavirus isolates is presented as a DNA positive strand. Primers are oriented as genomic-sense strand for amplification reactions with P gene primers or as message-sense strand for amplification reactions with primers from the N gene start sequence. Unpublished data, Rabies Laboratory, CDC. Nucleotide position is based on sequence of the Pasteur vaccine strain of rabies virus (GenBank accession no. M13215; Tordo et al., 1986).

Poinar, 2000) limit the universal applicability of these PCR primers. Sequence data for this region of the N protein gene suggest that the efficiency of the JW6 primer set could be increased by substitution of inosine for the thymidine residue at position 655 and introduction of degeneracy at nucleotides 645 and 658 (i.e., the consensus primer in Table IV). The increased efficiency mediated by these changes should eliminate a need for reamplification by nested PCR for most samples.

Small amplicons were produced successfully from all DFA-positive rabies virus samples tested to date with the primers listed in Tables V and VI (McQuiston

TABLE V

Primers for Reverse Transcription and Amplification of lyssavirus cDNA from Nucleotide Sequence at the End of the Nucleoprotein Gene[a]

	1157	1176	GenBank accession no./ref.
Primer 1087NFdeg	GAGAARGAAC	TTCARGAATA	Mcquiston *et al.*, 2001
Consensus primer	GAGAArGAAC	TTCArGAiTA	
Consensus sequence	GAGAAAGAAC	TTCAAGAATA	
RABV (many)	- - - - - - - - - -	- - - - - - - - - -	Kissi *et al.*, 1995
RABV (E. pipistrelle bat, U.S.)	- - - - - g - - - -	- - - - - - - - - -	Unpublished
RABV (big brown bat, U.S.)	- - - - - - - - - -	- - - - g - - - - -	Unpublished
RABV (silver-haired bat, U.S.)	- - - - - g - - - -	- - - - g - - - - -	Unpublished
RABV (mongoose, S. Afr.)	- - - - - - - - - -	- - - - - - - g - -	U22628
RABV (skunk, SC U.S.)	- - - - - g - g - -	- - - - g - - - - -	Unpublished
RABV (skunk, SC U.S.)	- - - - - g - - g -	- - - - g - - - - -	Unpublished
RABV (skunk, SC U.S.)	- - - - - g - - - -	- - - - g - - g - -	Unpublished
RABV (raccoon, U.S.)	- - - - - g - - - -	- - - - g - - c - -	Unpublished
RABV (free-tail bat, U.S.)	- - - - - g - - g -	- - - - g - - - - -	Unpublished
RABV (big brown bat, U.S.)	- - - - - - - - - -	- g - - g - - - - -	Unpublished
RABV (skunk, CA, U.S.)	- - - - - - - - - -	- - - - - - - - c -	Unpublished
RABV (skunk, CA, U.S.)	- - - - - - - - - -	- - - - - - - - - t	Unpublished
RABV (skunk, CA, U.S.)	- - - - - - - - - -	- c - - - - - gc -	Unpublished
RABV (skunk, CA, U.S.)	- - - - - - - - - -	- c - g - - - gc -	Unpublished
RABV (dog, Thailand)	- - - - - g - - - -	- c - - g - - g - -	U22653
RABV (big brown bat, U.S)	- - - - - - - - - -	- g - - g - - g - -	Unpublished
RABV (fox, AZ, U.S.)	- - a - - - - - g -	- - - - - - - - - -	Unpublished
RABV (dog 2, Africa)	- - a - - - - - - -	- c - - - - - - - -	U22488
ABLV (insectivorous bat)	- - - - - - - - - -	- - - - g - - t - -	AF081020
ABLV (frugivorous bat)	- - - - - - - - - -	- g - - - - - t - -	AF006497
DUVV	- - - - - - - - g -	- g - - - - - c - -	U22848
EBLV1	- - - - - - - - gt	- a - - g - - t - -	U22845
EBLV2	- - - - gg - - - -	- - gc - - - gc -	U22846
LAGV (Nigeria)	- - - - - - - - - a	- g - - - - - t - -	U22842
LAGV (Ethiopia)	- - - - - - - - ga	- g - - - - - t - -	Mebatson *et al.*, 1993
MOKV (Zimbabwe)	- a - - - - - - ga	- g - - - - - t - -	Y09762
MOKV (Ethiopia)	- - - - - - - - - a	- g - - - - - t - -	Mebatson *et al.*, 1993

[a]Genomic sequence for representative lyssavirus isolates is presented as a DNA positive strand. Primers are oriented as genomic-sense strand for reverse transcription and amplification.
Unpublished data, Rabies Laboratory, CDC. Nucleotide position is based on sequence of the Pasteur vaccine strain of rabies virus (GenBank accession no. M13215; Tordo, *et al.*, 1986).

TABLE VI

Primers for Amplification of lyssavirus cDNA from Nucleotide Sequence at the End of the Nucleoprotein Gene[a]

	1382	1401	GenBank accession no./ref.
Primer 1312NBdeg	TTYGCTGART	TTYTAAACAA	Mcquiston *et al.*, 2001
Consensus primer	TTyGCiGArT	TTyTAAACAA	
Consensus sequence	TTCGCTGAGT	TTCTAAACAA	
RABV (many)	----------	----------	Kissi *et al.*, 1995
RABV (fox, AZ, U.S.)	--t-------	----------	Unpublished
RABV (fox, TX, U.S.)	--t--c--a-	--t-------	Unpublished
RABV (dog, Africa)	--y-------	-yy-------	Kissi *et al.*, 1995
RABV (dog 2, Africa)	--t--c----	--t-g-----	U22488
RABV (raccoon, U.S.)	--t--y--a-	----------	Unpublished
RABV (red bat, U.S.)	--------a-	--t-------	Unpublished
RABV (free-tail bat, U.S.)	--t-----a-	--t-------	Unpublished
RABV (fox, Europe)	--t-----t-	----------	AF033905
RABV (fox, polar regions)	--t--y----	-------y--	Nadin-Davis *et al.*, 1993
RABV (dog-coyote, U.S.–Mexico)	-----a----	----------	Unpublished
RABV (skunk, NC U.S.)	-----c----	----------	Unpublished
RABV (skunk, SC U.S.)	--y-------	-------t--	Unpublished
RABV (skunk, CA, U.S.)	-----c----	--y-g-----	Unpublished
RABV (mongoose, S. Afr.)	--t--c----	----------	U22628
RABV (yellow bat, U.S.)	--t-------	-yt-------	Unpublished
RABV (E. pipestrelle bat, U.S.)	----------	--t-g-----	Unpublished
RABV (red bat, U.S.)	--------a-	--t-g-----	Unpublished
RABV (big brown bat, U.S.)	-----y----	--y----y--	Unpublished
RABV (big brown bat, U.S.)	----------	------gt--	Unpublished
RABV (big brown bat, U.S.)	-----a----	--t-------	Unpublished
RABV (mytosis bat, U.S.)	-----c----	--t-------	Unpublished
ABLV (insectivorous bat)	--t-----a-	-c-------	AF081020
ABLV (frugivorous bat)	--t--g----	----c-----	AF006497
DUVV	--t--a----	-c--c-----	U22848
EBLV1	--t--a----	----c-----	U22845
EBLV2	--t--a--a-	-ct-g-----	U22846
LAGV (Nigeria)	--t--a--a-	-c--c-----	U22842
LAGV (Ethiopia)	--t--a--a-	-t--c-----	Mebatsion *et al.*, 1993
MOKV (Zimbabwe)	--t--a--a-	-ct-------	Y09762
MOKV (Ethiopia)	--t--c--a-	-ct-------	Mebatsion *et al.*, 1993

[a]Genomic sequence for representative lyssavirus isolates is presented as a DNA positive strand. Primers should be reoriented as message-sense strand for amplification reactions. Nucleotide position is based on sequence of the Pasteur vaccine strain of rabies virus (GenBank accession no. M13215; Tordo *et al.*, 1986).

et al., 2001). However, the efficiency of amplification varied with the degree of mutation in an individual variant and in some individual samples of a particular variant. Sequence data for this region of the N protein gene suggest that the efficiency of primer 1087NFdeg might be increased by substitution of inosine for the adenosine residue at position 1174 (i.e., the consensus primer in Table V). The efficiency of primer 1312NBdeg might be increased by substitution of inosine for the thymidine residue at position 1387 (i.e., the consensus primer in Table VI). Even with these changes, poor recognition can be expected for lyssaviruses other than rabies virus (genotype 1).

Most diagnostic laboratories maintain several sets of primers. In laboratories where multiple genetic analyses must be conducted from limited samples (e.g., CSF for diagnosis of encephalitis of unknown etiology), random sequences of six nucleotides (hexamers) can be used in place of a virus-specific oligonucleotide for priming of reverse transcription (Huang *et al.*, 1999). In U.S. rabies laboratories, primers related to N7 and 304 or N8 (see Tables II and III) can be expected to amplify almost all DFA-positive samples. Positive but weak reactions with these primers can be enhanced, if necessary, by retesting with primer sets for smaller amplicons, either with degenerate positions for broad recognition of all variants or with sequences specific for the most common variant in a given geographic area (see Tables V and VI).

2. *Controls for Sensitivity and Specificity*

The sensitivity of RT-PCR is influenced by the size of the targeted RNA sequence, the number of amplification cycles, and the method used to detect the amplified sequence. Regardless of sample handling and RNA extraction method, short pieces of RNA always will be more abundant in test samples than long pieces of RNA, and the shorter the target, the more efficient will be the transcription and amplification reactions (see Table I). Reamplification (nested and heminested PCR) is 10- to 100-fold more sensitive than primary amplification, and hybridization probes are 10- to 100-fold more sensitive than ethidium bromide for detecting amplicons (Heaton *et al*, 1999). RT-PCR can detect rabies-specific RNA in decomposed samples where no evidence of infection is found by DFA (Heaton *et al.*, 1997) and in samples diluted 100- to 1000-fold beyond the level of detection by virus isolation in cell culture (see Table I).

High test sensitivity provokes questions about specificity and the significance of a positive diagnosis of rabies by RT-PCR in animals found negative by all conventional methods. In nucleic acid–based tests, false-positive reactions may be the result of mispriming and amplification of a nontarget sequence to produce an amplicon of the expected size (nonspecific reaction) or, as is more common, contamination of test samples with low levels of target sequences from another sample (specific reaction). False-positive reactions that result from nonspecific priming are identified easily by probe hybridization, restriction digestion, or nucleotide sequencing of the amplicon. Unfortunately, there is no simple method for identifying a contaminating lyssavirus introduced into the test sample from another sample handled during necropsy, a contaminating RNA introduced into an extraction from other extractions, or a contaminating cDNA amplicon introduced into a PCR from previous amplifications. Contamination must be prevented by instituting strict controls on sample handling. Failure to recognize the possibility of false-positive reactions can only lead to an increasing number of unsubstantiated, unusual, and exceptional diagnoses. Two recent well-publicized rabies diagnoses described below illustrate this point. The most likely explanation in both cases was an initial false-positive reading of nonspecific staining in a DFA test compounded by errors of interpretation of confirmatory tests.

In August 1999, a bear cub in a petting zoo in Clermont, Iowa, was diagnosed with rabies based on positive tests by DFA at a university laboratory (Centers for Disease Control and Prevention, 1999b). A primary PCR to confirm the diagnosis was negative, but reamplification by nested PCR produced an amplicon of the expected size for a rabies gene product. An estimated 150 persons received the rabies vaccination series for exposure to the suspected rabid bear. The positive DFA test could not be confirmed at the state public health laboratory or at the national reference laboratory at the Centers for Disease Control and Prevention (CDC), and repeat tests of the sample by both primary and nested PCR at the CDC were negative. Subsequent to these negative findings, the amplicon from the initial nested PCR was sequenced and found not to contain a rabies gene product.

In July 1997, after two bats in a Denmark zoo were diagnosed with rabies, a colony of 40 apparently healthy bats was killed and tested (Ronsholt et al., 1998). Three bats in the colony showed evidence of localized rabies encephalitis on brain smears, and one of these was culture-positive for a lyssavirus; however, 34 of 40 bats had evidence of a rabies encephalitis in tests by PCR (Schaftenaar, 1998). The case investigation prompted speculation about the risk to humans in persistent, subclinical lyssavirus infections in captive bats, and colonies of captive bats in both Denmark and the Netherlands were exterminated. While it is possible that these cases represent a new phenomenon in rabies (a lyssavirus adapted to live commensally with a bat species), other explanations are much more plausible. Nonspecific immunologic reactions can be confused with lyssavirus-specific staining (see Sect. IIB4). Of 30 newborn mice that died after an inoculation with brain material from the rabies-positive zoo bats, only one mouse showed a positive reaction to lyssavirus-specific staining, and the weak reaction observed in the sample was considered atypical by the reporting laboratory. No mention was made in the report of whether RT-PCR or any other test was used to confirm that the death of the inoculated mouse was the result of a lyssavirus infection. Although nucleotide sequencing of a virus isolate from one of the two initial bat cases identified European bat lyssavirus (EBLV), no mention was made of amino acid mutations in the nucleocapsid of the virus that would explain the poor recognition of the agent by DFA. Control mice inoculated with EBLV showed strong and widely disseminated rabies-specific staining in brain smears, as would be expected for animals dying of a rabies encephalitis. The busy diagnostic laboratory had numerous opportunities to contaminate reagents and equipment with positive samples; in the summer of 1997, Denmark was experiencing a 26% increase in confirmed bat rabies cases.

These cases illustrate the problems that accompany inconsistent primary and confirmatory test results. Because clinical signs of rabies appear only after lyssavirus replication in the CNS, brain tissue of rabies-suspected animals should contain ample amounts of virus for detection by both DFA and conventional confirmatory tests. A primary RT-PCR with a sensitivity equivalent to that of conventional methods of virus isolation in cell culture or animals is adequate because these methods, like PCR, amplify the target agent. A single infectious virus particle may not be detected in cell culture or may not kill an inoculated animal, but multiplication during the incubation period produces detectable levels of virus [a focus (infectious center) of infected cells or paralysis and death of an inoculated mouse]. Discordant results obtained by different testing methods should be investigated thoroughly to determine whether the problem is one of insensitivity (inadequate sampling, poor quality reagents and equipment, technical error, or inexperience on the part of laboratory personnel) or one of oversensitivity (cross-contamination of the reaction with virus, viral RNA, or amplicons from other test samples).

Care must be taken during necropsy and during the RNA extraction procedure to avoid cross-contamination of negative brain tissue with brain tissue from strongly positive samples tested earlier. As little as 20 ng of contaminating brain material can produce a false-positive reaction (see Table I). RNA in the protected environment of brain tissue is remarkably stable. RNA from brains left at 37°C for 15 days has been amplified successfully (Heaton *et al.*, 1997). Samples for RNA extraction should be taken with a sterile, disposable scalpel from an interior, untouched portion of brain stem or cerebellum. Negative brain tissue should be carried through all steps of the extraction and amplification as a control for sample handling. Rigorous procedural and quality-control practices are necessary to prevent the possibility of false-positive results due to carryover contamination from positive PCR reactions of other samples. Work areas and equipment for pre- and postamplification must be separate spatially.

Comparison of test samples with dilutions of positive control material around the end point for detection by RT-PCR will convey some sense of the quantity of RNA amplified from the test samples (Fig. 2*B*). When the results for a test sample indicate that the number of starting templates is very low, it may be impossible to exclude sporadic contamination as the source of the positive results. Novel or unexpected results such as DFA-negative, RT-PCR-positive samples of fresh brain material should be confirmed in a second laboratory. Intralaboratory contamination can only be discounted when separate samples of a specimen are sufficiently large that a repeat RNA extraction and RT-PCR can be performed on unsectioned portions.

Warnings about false-positive results appeared 1 year after PCR was first described (Kwok and Higuchi, 1989), and criteria have been established for quality control of molecular tests (Cooper and Poinar, 2000). The routine good practices required to minimize cross-contamination are expensive and time-consuming; however, laboratories that conduct tests and publish results that cannot be substantiated bring disrepute to all of diagnostic virology. Additionally, false-positive tests for rabies result in inappropriate use of vaccines and misuse of biologicals such as immune serum that often are in short supply.

V. DIAGNOSIS OF RABIES IN HUMANS

A. Antemortem Testing

A diagnosis of rabies should be considered in any patient who presents with encephalopathy of unknown cause. The first signs and symptoms of rabies are often nonspecific. Without a clear history of animal bite, rabies often is not suspected until late in the clinical illness. A delayed diagnosis may increase the number of persons potentially exposed to rabies by contact with the patient. An early diagnosis may eliminate the expense and discomfort of unnecessary diagnostic tests and medical treatment of the patient.

Once considered, a diagnosis of rabies is not always easy to confirm. Antemortem diagnosis of rabies is one of the most difficult procedures attempted by a laboratory and should be performed only by experienced laboratories. The risks of performing a brain biopsy are unacceptable for the routine use of these samples for diagnosis. Methods for rabies diagnosis rely on the demonstration of antibody in serum or CSF or detection of virus, viral antigen, or viral RNA in peripheral nerves and tissues. If rabies is suspected, a complete set of samples should be collected for testing by all currently used diagnostic procedures. Because of the implications of a positive test, a finding of rabies must be confirmed in more than one tissue or sample. Because antibody is produced late in a lyssavirus infection, and virus may be absent or present at very low levels in peripheral nerves and tissues, samples taken for antemortem diagnosis cannot definitively rule out rabies. If a suspicion of rabies persists despite negative findings, repeated sampling may be necessary.

B. Sample Collection

Clinicians suspecting rabies in a patient should consult with a state health department or with the Rabies Laboratory at the CDC in Atlanta, GA. The course of the illness, additional history, and laboratory tests for other more common etiologies can determine if samples specific for rabies should be collected. All samples should be considered as potentially infectious. Test tubes and other sample containers must be sealed securely. Tape around the cap will ensure that the containers do not open during transit. If immediate shipment is not possible, samples should be stored frozen at $-20°C$ or below. Samples should be shipped frozen on dry ice by an overnight courier in watertight primary containers and leakproof secondary containers that meet the guidelines of the International Air Transport Association. The laboratory should be telephoned at the time of shipment and given information on the mode of shipment, expected arrival time, and courier tracking number.

1. Saliva

Saliva should be collected with a sterile eyedropper pipette and placed in a small sterile container that can be sealed securely. No preservatives or additional material should be added. Laboratory tests to be performed include detection of lyssavirus RNA by RT-PCR of extracted nucleic acids and isolation of infectious virus in cell culture. Tracheal aspirates and sputum are not suitable for rabies tests.

2. Neck Skin Biopsy

A section of skin 5–6 mm in diameter should be taken from the posterior region of the neck at the hairline. The biopsy specimen should contain a minimum of 10 hair follicles and be of sufficient depth to include the cutaneous nerves at the base of the follicle. The specimen should be placed on a piece of sterile gauze moistened with sterile water or saline in a sealed container. Preservatives or additional fluids should not be added. Neck biopsy samples are tested by RT-PCR on extracted RNA and by immunofluorescence staining for viral antigen in frozen sections of the biopsy. The antigen generally is present in the nerve cells surrounding the base of hair follicles (see Fig. 1C).

3. Serum and CSF

At least 0.5 ml of serum (not whole blood) is needed to test for antibody by indirect immunofluorescence and virus neutralization. If no vaccine or rabies immune serum has been given, the presence of antibody to the challenge virus standard rabies virus in the serum is diagnostic, and tests of CSF are unnecessary. If collected, at least 0.5 ml of CSF should be sent for testing by RT-PCR and neutralization tests. *Lyssavirus*-specific antibody in the CSF, regardless of the immunization history, suggests a rabies encephalitis.

4. Corneal impressions

While positive for lyssavirus antigen in some patients, corneal epithelium is difficult to sample correctly, especially from comatose patients. Because of the risk of permanent damage to the cornea, samples should be taken only by an ophthalmologist after consultation with the rabies testing laboratory (Zaidman and Billingsley, 1998). The sample is collected by vigorously rubbing a flat surface of a clean microscope slide on each cornea. Corneal impression slides are tested by RT-PCR and by immunofluorescence staining for viral antigen. The antigen appears characteristically as round to oval intracytoplasmic inclusions in corneal epithelial cells (see Fig. 1D).

5. Brain Biopsy

The rarity of human rabies and the lack of an effective treatment make routine brain biopsy unwarranted; however, biopsy samples negative in other tests should be tested for evidence of lyssavirus infection. The biopsy is placed in a sterile sealed container without preservatives or additional fluids. Laboratory tests to be performed include RT-PCR and immunofluorescent staining for viral antigen in touch impressions or frozen sections.

C. Significance of Positive and Negative Findings

In a study of antemortem test results for human rabies deaths in the United States between 1980 and 1997 (Noah *et al.*, 1998) and updated with data for more recent cases in Table VII, RT-PCR of RNA extracted from saliva was the most reliable diagnostic test. Positive results were obtained for 15 of 15 cases; however, nested PCR was required in almost all cases to compensate for the often extremely limited amount of RNA in antemortem samples. In a similar study of a smaller number of cases, Crepin *et al.* (1998) diagnosed rabies in 4 of 9 cases by RT-PCR of saliva but did not use nested PCR.

Virus isolation from saliva was positive in 9 of the 15 cases in which this diagnostic method was applied (see Table VII). Successful virus isolation was related to the antibody status of the patient, suggesting that virus is cleared from salivary glands by the immune response to infection. Virus was isolated from 13 of 15 serial saliva samples from antibody-negative patients. Virus isolation methods were negative in 17 of 17 serial saliva samples from antibody-positive patients.

Frozen sections of skin biopsies were positive by DFA in 15 of 20 cases in which this diagnostic method was applied (see Table VII). Observation of 20 or more sections was needed in most cases to reliably detect areas of positive staining. Crepin *et al.* (1998) diagnosed rabies in 5 of 9 patients with this method.

TABLE VII

Summary of Antemortem Diagnostic Test Results for 27 Human Rabies Cases in the United States, 1981–2000

Case	Detection of antigen			Isolation of virus	Detection of RNA	Detection of antibodies	
	Cutaneous nerve	Corneal epithelium	Brain biopsy	Oral secretions		Serum	CSF
2 81AZ	**d8+**	d8−	ns	d11+ d15+	nt	d8 to d24−	d8 to d24+
3 83MA	**d6+** d11+	d6− d18−	d8+	d6− d9 to d13+ d16 to d25−	nt	d6 to d14− d16 to d27+	d8 to d19−
4 83MI	d17− d21−	ns	ns	d17−	nt	**d17+** d22+ d26+	d17− d22− d26+
5 84TX	ns	ns	d17+	d18−	nt	d11− d18+	**d15+**
6 84PA	**d7+**	ns	ns	**d7+**	nt	d7−	d7−
11 90TX	d6−	ns	ns	d6−	nt	d6−	d6−
12 91TX	d6− d14+	ns	ns	**d6+**	**d6+**	d6−	d6−
15 92CA	d4− **d8+** d14−	d3−	ns	d8− d12− d14− d17 nt	**d8+** d12+ d14+ d17+	d3− **d8+** d17+	d14−
17 93TX	ns	ns	ns	ns	ns	d7−	ns
18 93CA	**d6+**	d6 to d10−	ns	**d6+**	**d6+**	d6 to d10−	d9−
22 94WV	**d5+**	ns	d8+	d5−	**d5+**	**d5+**	ns
23 94TN	ns	**d15+**	ns	ns	ns	ns	ns
24 94TX	**d11+**	ns	ns	**d11+**	**d11+**	d11−	d11−
25 95WA	**d8+**	ns	ns	**d8+** d10+	**d8+**	ns	ns

continued

Case	Detection of antigen			Isolation of virus	Detection of RNA	Detection of antibodies	
	Cutaneous nerve	Corneal epithelium	Brain biopsy	Oral secretions		Serum	CSF
26 95CA	d6−	d6−	ns	ns	ns	d6− **d12+**	d5−
27 95CT	ns	d14+	ns	d10−	d10+	**d8+** d12+	d11−
29 96FL	**d9+**	ns	ns	**d9+**	**d9+**	d8−	ns
30 96NH	d5− d6−	ns	ns	**d5+** d6 nt	**d5+** d6 nt	d5− d6+	d5−
31 96KY	ns	ns	ns	ns	ns	**d13+**	ns
32 96MT	d9−	ns	ns	d9 nt	**d9+**	**d9+**	ns
35 97TX	ns	ns	ns	ns	ns	d10−	ns
36 97NJ	**d6+**	ns	ns	d6 nt	**d6+**	d6−	d6−
37 98VA	**d7+**	ns	ns	ns	**d7+**	d8+ d15+	d8+
38 00CA	**d4+**	**d4+**	ns	?	d4 nt	ns	ns
39 00NY	**d6+**	d6−	ns	?	d6 nt	ns	ns
41 00WI	ns	ns	ns	ns	ns	d6−	ns
42 00MN	**d12+**	ns	ns	ns	**d12+**	ns	ns
Number of cases with samples submitted for testing	20	9	3	15	15	22	15
Number of diagnoses	15	3	3	9	15	11	3

[a]d, day of clinical illness; bold text, day of first positive sample; ns, no sample submitted; nt, samples not tested.

Serum was more likely to be positive when taken late in the clinical course (see Table VII; Crepin *et al.*, 1998) but was absent as late as day 24 in one case. Antibody was present in the CSF of only 3 patients. Corneal impressions were the least satisfactory as a diagnostic sample. A positive DFA test was made in only 3 of 9 cases where this sample was taken (see Table VII).

Although a nested PCR of saliva was positive in the 15 of 15 cases in which the test was applied, conventional methods often are equally reliable and can produce a diagnosis within a few hours of receipt in the laboratory. Positive tests were obtained by serology or DFA on skin biopsy in 20 of 25 patients for whom these samples were available (see Table VII).

D. Postmortem Testing of Autopsy Samples

In 15 of 42 human rabies cases reported in the United States since 1980, samples were not obtained specifically for rabies testing before the patient's death. The clinical history in 7 patients was sufficiently suggestive of rabies that fresh brain material obtained during autopsy was submitted immediately for DFA testing. In the remaining patients, however, a diagnosis was delayed for 3 weeks to 6 months after autopsy when findings suggestive of rabies were noted in histologic examination of formalin-fixed brain material. Formalin-fixed brain material from humans is tested as indicated for animal brains in Sect. IID.

VI. RABIES ANTIBODY ASSAYS

Serologic tests for lyssavirus-specific antibody can provide an estimate of vaccine efficacy, an indication of disease prevalence in areas of enzootic rabies, and an antemortem diagnosis in human rabies cases. The different methods used to measure lyssavirus-specific antibody can be described as antigen-binding assays, antibody-function assays, or antigen-function assays (Smith, 1991).

A. Antigen-Binding Assays

Antigen-binding assays measure the attachment of antibody to a lyssavirus or lyssavirus-specific proteins attached to a substrate, typically a slide, microtiter plate, or bead. Bound antibody is detected with antiantibody or Fc-binding protein (staphylococcal protein A or streptococcal protein G) labeled with an enzyme that is detected in the ELISA or labeled with FITC, which is detectable in the IFA. The specificity of antigen-binding assays is determined by the choice of antigen (whole virion versus purified protein) (Cliquet *et al.*, 2000) or by using a labeled control antibody specific for a particular protein in a competitive binding or blocking (Sugiyama *et al.*, 1997; Cleaveland *et al.*, 1999).

Because vaccine efficacy is closely tied to the generation of virus-neutralizing antibodies directed to specific epitopes on the virus glycoprotein, antigen-binding assays involving the viral glycoprotein have not been suitable for estimating immune response to vaccination. Although good correlation has been reported in some studies (Piza *et al.*, 1999), laboratories in the United States are required by the Advisory Committee on Immunization Practices (ACIP) to use virus neutralization tests in assaying antibody titers in persons immunized against rabies (Centers for Disease Control and Prevention, 1999).

Microtiter plate ELISA methods can be simple, inexpensive, and reliable surveys for the presence of rabies antibody in animals in areas of enzootic rabies (Cleaveland *et al.*, 1999; Cliquet *et al.*, 2000). Although species-specific antisera are required for some samples, Fc-binding proteins allow testing of a wide variety of animal sera. Although not commonly used in seroconversion surveys, IFA also can be used to test for antibody-positive animals if FITC-labeled antiantibodies or Fc-binding proteins are available (Hill *et al.*, 1992). IFA is especially valuable for antemortem evaluation of suspected rabies in humans because the test is done easily and results can be obtained quickly.

B. Antibody-Function Assays

Antibody-function assays are based on detection of a non-virus-related function (e.g., complement fixation or hemagglutination) performed by an antibody after an interaction with an antigen. Antigen-function assays were among the earliest serologic methods to be developed but are no longer in wide use.

C. Antigen-Function Assays

Antigen-function assays measure the capacity of antibody to block a specific viral function. Neutralization of virus infectivity is the most widely used antigen-function assay. In all virus neutralization assays, dilutions of heat-inactivated serum are incubated with a constant amount of virus. Although early tests depended on animal inoculation to measure residual virus infectivity after incubation with serum, levels of residual virus are now determined almost exclusively by inoculating cell cultures.

Most of the variation in virus neutralization tests stems from the precision with which the amount of residual infectious virus is measured. The most precise measurement is made by plaque-reduction tests (PRT) in which each infectious unit of virus is counted (Wiktor and Clark, 1973). Because 5–7 days are required

344 Charles V. Trimarchi and Jean S. Smith

for infectious foci (plaques) to reach detectable size, PRT is unsuitable for most diagnostic applications. A more rapid method of measuring antibody present in serum, with many of the advantages of PRT, uses FITC-labeled antibody to detect residual virus. The amount of residual virus is estimated by counting all infectious foci (tissue culture infectious doses, or TCID) within a single well or chamber or by estimating the amount of virus by finding the point at which 50% of inoculated chambers contain virus ($TCID_{50}$) after 3–4 days of incubation.

Several laboratories have modified fluorescent methods of calculating residual virus by increasing the amount of challenge virus and thereby decreasing the length of time required for the virus to reach detectable levels. Although less precise, these methods are suitable as tests of vaccine efficacy, serosurveys, and antemortem serum samples. The rapid fluorescent focus inhibition test (RFFIT) (Smith *et al.*, 1996) determines a $TCID_{50}$ as the dilution of virus at which 50% of observed microscopic fields contain one or more infected cells after a 20-hour incubation period. Tests are performed either in multichamber slides (one chamber per serum dilution) or in microtiter plates (one or two wells per serum dilution). In the fluorescent antibody virus neutralization (FAVN) test (Cliquet *et al.*, 1998), each serum dilution is placed in four wells of a microtiter plate, and each well is simply scored as having virus present or no virus after a 40-hour incubation period. In both methods, test results are reported as International Units by comparison with a reference standard serum. No statistical difference was found between results obtained by the two tests (Briggs *et al.*, 1998). The main differences between the two methods are the time to completion (24 versus 40 hours), the volume of infectious material created in a single test dilution (0.4 ml versus 0.8 ml), and the time required to read the test results (evaluation of 20 microscope fields in one chamber versus a thorough scan of four wells). Additionally, manipulation and reading of microtiter plates in the FAVN are easily automated (Hostnik, 2000).

REFERENCES

Andrulonis, J. A., and Debbie, J. G. (1976). Effect of acetone fixation on rabies immunofluorescence in glycerin-preserved tissues. *Health Lab. Sci.* **47**, 207–209.

Barrat, J. (1996). Simple technique for the collection and shipment of brain specimens for rabies diagnosis. In *Laboratory Techniques in Rabies*, F. X. Meslin, M. M. Kaplan, and H. Koprowski (eds.), 4th ed., pp. 425–432. World Health Organization, Geneva.

Bourhy, H., Kissi, B., Lafon, M., Sacramento, D., and Tordo, N. (1992). Antigenic and molecular characterization of bat rabies virus in Europe. *J. Clin. Microbiol.* **30**, 2419–2426.

Bourhy, H., Kissi, B., and Tordo, N. (1993). Molecular diversity of the *Lyssavirus* genus. *Virology* **194**, 70–81.

Bourhy, H., Kissi, B., Tordo, N., Badrane, H., and Sacramento, D. (1995). Molecular epidemiological tools and phytogenetic analysis of bacteria and viruses with special emphasis on lyssaviruses. *Prevent. Vet. Med.* **25**, 161–181.

Bourhy, H., and Perrin, P. (1996). Rapid rabies enzyme immunodiagnosis (RREID) for rabies antigen detection. In *Laboratory Techniques in Rabies*, F. X. Meslin, M. M. Kaplan, and H. Koprowski (eds.), 4th ed., pp. 105–112. World Health Organization, Geneva.

Briggs, D. J., Smith, J. S., Mueller, F. L., Schwenke, J., Davis. R. D., Gordon, C. R., Schweitzer, K., Orciari, L. A., Yager, P. A., and Rupprecht, C. E. (1998). A comparison of two serological methods for detecting the immune response after rabies vaccination in dogs and cats being exported to rabies-free areas. *Biologicals* **26**, 347–355.

Centers for Disease Control and Prevention (1993). *Biosafety in Microbiological and Biomedical Laboratories*. U.S. Government Printing Office, Washington, D.C.

Centers for Disease Control and Prevention (1993). Human rabies — New York, 1993. *Morbid. Mortal. Weekly Rep.* **42**, 799–806.

Centers for Disease Control and Prevention (1997). Human rabies — Kentucky and Montana, 1996. *Morbid. Mortal. Weekly Rep.* **46**, 397–400.

Centers for Disease Control and Prevention (1999a). Human rabies prevention — United States, 1999 Recommendations of the Advisory Committee on Immunization Practices (ACIP). *Morbid. Mortal. Weekly Rep.* **48** (RR-1).

Centers for Disease Control and Prevention (1999b). Public health response to a potentially rabid bear cub–Iowa, 1999. *Morbid. Mortal. Weekly Rep.* **48**, 971–973.

Centers for Disease Control and Prevention (2000). Human rabies — California, Georgia, Minnesota, New York, and Wisconsin, 2000. *Morbid. Mortal. Weekly Rep.* **49**, 1111–1115.

Charlton, K. M. (1988). The pathogenesis of rabies. In *Rabies*, J. B. Campbell, and K. M. Charlton (eds.), pp. 101–150. Kluwer Academic Publishers, Norwell, MA.

Chemicon International (2000). *Notification on Light Diagnostics Rabies Reagent*. Temecula, CA.

Childs, J. E., Colby, L., Krebs, J. W., Strine, T., Feller, M., Noah, D., Drenzek, C., Smith, J. S., and Rupprecht, C. E. (1997). Surveillance and spatiotemporal associations of rabies in rodents and lagomorphs in the United States, 1985–1994. *J. Wildlife Dis.* **33**, 20–27.

Cleaveland, S., Barrat, J., Barrat, M. J., Selve, M., Kaare, M.. and Esterhuysen, J. (1999). A rabies serosurvey of domestic dogs in rural Tanzania: Results of a rapid fluorescent focus inhibition test (RFFIT) and a liquid-phase blocking ELISA used in parallel. *Epidemiol. Infect.* **123**, 157–164.

Cliquet, F., Aubert, M., and Sagne, L. (1998). Development of a fluorescent antibody virus neutralisation test (FAVN test) for the quantitation of rabies-neutralising antibody. *J. Immunol. Methods* **212**, 79–87.

Cliquet, F., Sagne, L., Schereffer, J. L., and Auhert, M. F. A. (2000). ELISA test for rabies antibody titration in orally vaccinated foxes sampled in the fields. *Vaccine* **18**, 3272–3279.

Cooper, A., and Poinar, H. N. (2000) Ancient DNA: Do it right or not at all. *Science* **289**, 1139.

Crepin, P., Audry, L., Rotivel, Y., Gacoin, A., Caroff, C., and Bourhy, H. (1998). Intravitam diagnosis of human rabies by PCR using saliva and cerebrospinal fluid. *J. Clin. Microbiol.* **36**, 1117–1121.

Davis, C., Neill, S., and Raj, P. (1998). Microwave fixation of rabies specimens for fluorescent antibody testing. *J. Virolog. Methods* **68**, 177–182.

Debbie, J. G., and Trimarchi, C. V. (1992). Rabies. In *Veterinary Diagnostic Virology*, A. E. Castro and W. P. Heuschele (eds.), pp. 116–120. Mosby–Year Book, St. Louis, MO.

Debbie, J. G., and Trimarchi, C. V. (1997). Prophylaxis for suspected exposure to bat rabies. *Lancet* **350**, 1790–1791.

Ermine, A., Tordo, N., and Tsiang, H. (1988). Rapid diagnosis of rabies infection by means of a dot hybridization assay. *Mol. Cell. Probes* **2**, 75–82.

Flamand, A., Wiktor, T. J., and Koprowski, H. (1980). Use of monoclonal antibodies in the detection of antigenic differences between rabies virus and rabies-related virus proteins: I. The nucleocapsid protein. *J. Gen. Virol.* **48**, 105–109.

Fraser, G. C., Hooper, P. T., Lunt, R. A., Gould, A. R., Gleeson. L. J., Hyatt, A. D., Russell, G. M., and Kattenbelt, J. A. (1996). Encephalitis caused by a *Lyssavirus* in fruit bats in Australia. *Emerg. infect. Dis.* **2**, 327–330.

Hamir, A. N., Moser, Z. F., Fu, F.. Dietzschold, B., and Rupprecht, C. E. (1995). Immuno-histochemical test for rabies: Identification of a diagnostically superior monoclonal antibody. *Vet. Rec.* **136**, 295–296.

Hanlon, C., Smith, J., Anderson, G., Trimarchi, C. V., and Schnurr, D. (1999). Laboratory diagnosis of rabies: report of the National Working Group on Prevention and Control of Rabies. *J. Am. Vet. Med. Assoc.* **215**, 1444–1446.

Heaton, P. R., Johnstone, P., McElhinney, L. M., Cowley, R., O'Sullivan, E., and Whitby, J. E. (1997). Heminested PCR assay for detection of six genotypes of rabies and rabies-related viruses. *J. Clin. Microbiol.* **35**, 2762–2766.

Heaton, R. R., McElhinney. L. M., and Lowings, J. P. (1999). Detection and identification of rabies and rabies-related viruses using rapid-cycle PCR. *J. Virol. Methods* **81**, 63–69.

Hill, R. E., Jr., Beran, G. W., and Clark, W. R. (1992). Demonstration of rabies virus-specific antibody in the sera of free-ranging Iowa raccoons (*Procyon lotor*). *J. Wildlife Dis.* **28**, 377–385.

Hooper, D. C., Moromoto, K., Bette, M., Weihe, E., Koprowski, H., and Dietzschold, B. (1998). Collaboration of antibody and inflammation in clearance of rabies virus from the central nervous system. *J. Virol.* **72**, 3711–3719.

Hostnik, P. (2000). The modification of fluorescent antibody virus neutralization (FAVN) test for the detection of antibodies to rabies virus. *J. Vet. Med. S. B.* **47**, 423–427.

Huang, C., Chatterjee, N. K., and Grady, L. J. (1999). Diagnosis of viral infections of the central nervous system (Letter). *New Engl. J. Med.* **340**, 483–484.

Ito, F. H., Vasconcellos, S. A., Erbolato, E. B., Macruz, R., and Cortes, J. A. (1985). Rabies virus in different segments of brain and spinal cord of naturally and experimentally infected dogs. *Int. J. Zoonoses* **38**, 98–105.

Jackson, A. C., Reimer, D. L., and Wunner, W. H. (1989). Detection of rabies virus RNA in the central nervous system of experimentally infected mice using *in situ* hybridization with RNA probes. *J. Virol. Methods* **25**, 1–11.

Jackson, A. C., and Wunner, W. H. (1991). Detection of rabies virus genomic RNA and mRNA in mouse and human brains by using *in situ* hybridization. *J. Virol.* **65**, 2839–2844.

Jackson, A. C., and Rintoul, N. E. (1992). Effects of postmortem autolysis on the detection of rabies virus genomic RNA and mRNA in mouse brain by using in situ hybridization. *Mol. Cell. Probes* **6**, 231–235.

Jackson, A. C., Phelan, C. C., and Rossiter, J. P. (2000). Infection of Bergmann glia in the cerebellum of a skunk experimentally infected with street rabies virus. *Can. J. Vet. Res.* **64**, 226–228.

Kaplan, M. M., Wiktor, T. J., Maes, R. F., Campbell, J. B., and Koprowski, H. (1967). Effect of polyions on the infectivity of rabies virus in tissue culture: Construction of a single-cycle growth curve. *J. Virol.* **1**, 145–151.

Kaplan, M. M. (1996). Safety precautions in handling rabies virus. In *Laboratory Techniques in Rabies*, F. X. Meslin, M. M. Kaplan, and H. Koprowski (eds.), 4th ed., pp. 105–112. World Health Organization, Geneva.

Kissi, B., Tordo, N., and Bourhy, H. (1995). Genetic polymorphism in the rabies virus nucleoprotein gene. *Virology* **209**, 526–537.

Kissling, R. E. (1975). The fluorescent antibody test in rabies. In *The Natural History of Rabies*, G. M. Baer (ed.), Vol. 1, pp. 401–416. Academic Press, New York.

Kuno, G. (1998). Universal diagnostic RT-PCR protocol for arboviruses. *J. Virol. Methods* **72**, 27–41.

Kwok, S., and Higuchi, R. (1989). Avoiding false positives with PCR. *Nature* **339**, 237–238.

Lee, T. K., and Becker, M. E. (1973). Validity of spinal cord examination as a substitute procedure for routine rabies diagnosis. *Public Health Lab.* **31**, 149–164.

Lennette, E. H., Woodie, J. D., Nakamura, K., and Magoffin, R. L. (1965). The diagnosis of rabies by the fluorescent antibody method (FRA) employing immune hamster serum. *Health Lab. Sci.* **2**, 24–34.

Lepine. P., and Atanasiu, P. (1996). Histopathological diagnosis. In *Laboratory Techniques in Rabies*, F. X. Meslin, M. M. Kaplan, and H. Koprowski (eds.), 4th ed., pp. 66–79. World Health Organization, Geneva.

Lewis, V. J., and Thacker, W. L. (1974). Limitations of deteriorated tissues for rabies diagnosis. *Health Lab. Sci.* **11**, 8–12.

Maserang, D. L., and Leffingwell, L. (1981). Single-site localization of rabies virus: Impact on laboratory reporting policy. *Am. J. Public Health* **71**, 428–429.

McQuiston, J. H., Yager, P. A., Smith, J. S., and Rupprecht, C. R., (2001). Epidemiologic characteristics of rabies virus variants in dogs and cats in the United States during 1999. *J. Ver. Med. Asso.* (in press).

Mebatsion, T., Cox, J. H., and Conzelmann, K. K. (1993). Molecular analysis of the rabies-related viruses from Ethiopia. *Onderstepoort J. Vet. Res.* **60**, 289–294.

Nadin-Davies, S. A., Casey, G. A., and Wandeler, A. I. (1993). Identification of regional variants of the rabies virus within the Canadian province of Ontario. *J. Gen. Virol.* **74**, 829–837.

Nadin-Davis, S. A., Casey, G. A., and Wandeler, A. I. (1994). A molecular epidemiological study of rabies virus in central Ontario and western Quebec. *J. Gen. Virol.* **75**, 2575–2583.

Nadin-Davis, S. A. (1998). Polymerase chain reaction protocols for rabies virus discrimination. *J. Virol. Methods* **75**, 1–8.

Niezgoda, M., and Rupprecht, C. E. (1999). Towards the development of another rabies diagnostic test, 10th Annual Rabies in the Americas Meeting, San Diego, CA.

Noah, D. L., Drenzek, C. L., Smith, J. S. Krebs, J. W., Orciari, L. A., Shaddock, J., Sanderlin, D., Whitefield, S., Fekadu, M., Olson, J. G., Rupprecht, C. E., and Childs, J. E. (1998). Epidemiology of human rabies in the United States, 1980 to 1996. *Ann. Intern. Med.* **128**, 922–930.

Perl, D. P., and Good, P. F. (1991). The pathology of rabies in the central nervous system. In *The Natural History of Rabies*, G. M. Baer (ed.), pp. 163–190. CRC Press, Boca Raton, FL.

Piza, A. S., Santos, J. L., Chaves, L. B., and Zanetti, C. R. (1999). An ELISA suitable for the detection of rabies virus antibodies in serum samples from human vaccinated with either cell culture vaccine or suckling mouse brain vaccine. *Rev. Inst. Med. Trop. Sao Paulo* **41**, 39–43.

Powell, J. (1997). Proficiency testing in the rabies diagnostic laboratory. Abstracts of the Eighth Annual Rabies in the Americas Conference, November 2–6, 1997, Kingston, Ontario.

Plotkin, S. A. (2000) Rabies. *Clin. Infect. Dis.* **30**, 4–12.

Robinson, S. J., and DiSalvo, A. F. (1980). Rabies in South Carolina: 1969–1979. *Public Health Lab.* **38**, 315–321.

Ronsholt, L., Sorensen, K. J., Bruschke, C. J. M., Wellenberg, G. J., van Oirschot, J. T., Johnstone, P., Whitby, J. E., and Bourhy, H. (1998). Clinically silent rabies infection in (zoo) bats. *Vet. Rec.* **142**, 519–520.

Rys, P. N., and Persing, D. H. (1993) Preventing false positive: Quantitative evaluation of three protocols for inactivation of polymerase chain reaction amplification products. *J. Clin. Microbiol.* **31**, 2356–2360.

Rudd, R. J., and Trimarchi, C. V. (1980). Tissue culture technique for routine isolation of street strain rabies virus. *J. Clin. Microbiol.* **12**, 590–593.

Rudd, R. J., and Trimarchi, C. V. (1987). Comparison of sensitivity of BHK-21 and murine neuroblastoma cells in the isolation of a street strain rabies virus. *J. Clin. Microbiol.* **25**, 1456–1458.

Rudd, R. J., and Trimarchi, C. V. (1989). The development and evaluation of an *in vitro* virus isolation procedure as a replacement for the mouse inoculation test in rabies diagnosis. *J. Clin. Microbiol.* **27**, 2522–2528.

Rudd, R. J., and Trimarchi, C. V. (1997). Evans Blue counterstain in the rabies fluorescent antibody test. Abstracts of the Eighth Annual Rabies in the Americas Conference, November 2–6, Kingston, Ontario.

Sabouraud, A., Smith, J. S., Orciari, L. A., de Mattos, C., de Mattos, C., and Rohde, R. (1999). Typing of rabies virus isolates by DNA enzyme immunoassay, *J. Clin. Virol.* **12**, 9–19.

Saiki, R. K. (1989). The design and optimization of the PCR. In *PCR Technology: Principles and Applications for DNA Amplification*, H. A. Erlich (ed.), pp. 7–16. Stockton Press, New York.

Schaftenaar, W. (1998). Clinically silent rabies infection in (zoo) bats (Letter). *Vet. Rec.* **143**, 86–87.

Smith, J. S., Reid-Sanden, F. L., Roumillat, L. F., Trimarchi, C. V., Clark, K., Baer, G. M., and Winkler, W. G. (1986). Demonstration of antigen variation among rabies virus isolates by using monoclonal antibodies to nucleocapsid proteins. *J. Clin. Microbiol.* **24**, 573–580.

Smith, J. S. (1991). Rabies serology. In *The Natural History of Rabies*, G. M. Baer (ed.), 2nd ed., pp. 235–252. CRC Press, Boca Raton, FL.

Smith, J. S. (1995). Rabies virsus In *Manual of Clinical Microbiology*, P. R. Murray, E. J. Baron, M. A. Pfaller, F. C. Tenover, and P. H. Yolken (eds.), pp. 997–1003. ASM Press, Washington.

Smith, J. S., Fishbein, D. B., Rupprecht, C. E., and Clark, K. (1991). Unexplained rabies in three immigrants in the United States: A virologic investigation. *New Engl. J. Med.* **324**, 205–211.

Smith, J. S., Orciari, L. A., and Yager, P. A. (1995). Molecular epidemiology of rabies in the United States. *Semin. Virol.* **6**, 387–400.

Smith, J. S., Yager, P. A., and Baer, G. M. (1996). A rapid fluorescent focus inhibition test (RFFIT) for determining rabies virus neutralizing antibody. In *Laboratory Techniques in Rabies*, F. X. Meslin, M. M. Kaplan, and H. Koprowski (eds.), 4th ed., pp. 181–192. World Health Organization, Geneva.

Smith, J. S., Trimarchi, C. V. and Neill, S. U. (1996). *Rabies Testing Proficiency Forum: Avoiding Cross-Contamination*. Wisconsin State Laboratory of Hygeine, Madison.

Smith, J. S., and Orciari, L. (1997). The use of RT-PCR in the rabies diagnostic laboratory. The 8th Annual Rabies in the Americas Conference, Kingston, Ontario, Canada.

Smith, J. S. (2000). Quality control for fluorescent antibody tests for rabies virus. International Meeting on Research Advances and Rabies Control in the Americas, Lima, Peru.

Sugiyama, M., Yoshiki, R., Tatsuno, Y., Hiraga, S., Itoh, O., Gamoh, K., and Minamoto, N. (1997). A new competitive enzymer-linked immunosorbent assay demonstrates adequate immune levels to rabies virus in compulsorily vaccinated Japanese domestic dogs. *Clin. Diag. Lab. Immunol.* **4**, 727–730.

Surreau, P., Ravisse, P., and Rollin, P. E. (1991). Rabies diagnosis by animal inoculation, identification of Negri bodies, or ELISA. In *The Natural History of Rabies*, G. M. Baer (ed.), 2nd ed., pp. 203–217. CRC Press, Boca Raton, FL.

Tierkel, E. S., and Atanasiu, P. (1996). Rapid microscopic examination for Negeri bodies and preparation of specimens for biological tests. In *Laboratory Techniques in Rabies*, F. X. Meslin, M. M. Kaplan, and H. Koprowski, (eds.), 4th ed., pp. 55–65. World Health Organization, Geneva.

Tordo, N., Poch, O., Ermine, A., and Keith, G. (1986). Primary structure of leader RNA and nucleoprotein genes of the rabies genome: Segmented homology with VSV. *Nucleic Acids Res.* **14**, 2671–2673.

Tordo, N., Bourhy, H., and Sacramento, D. (1995). Polymerase chain reaction technology for rabies virus. In *The Polymerase Chain Reaction (PCR) for Human Viral Diagnosis*, J. P. Clewley (ed.), pp. 125–145. CRC Press, Boca Raton, FL.

Trimarchi, C. V., Rudd, R. J., and Abelseth, M. K. (1986). Experimentally induced rabies in four cats inoculated with a rabies virus isolated from a bat. *Am. J. Vet. Res.* **47**, 777–780.

Trimarchi, C. V., and Debbie, J. G. (1991). The fluorescent antibody in rabies. In *The Natural History of Rabies*, G. M. Baer (ed.), 2nd ed., pp. 219–233. CRC Press, Boca Raton, FL.

Trimarchi, C. V. (1994). 1993 summary of rabies in New York State. *The Rabies Reporter* **4**, 4–5.

Trimarchi, C. V., and Briggs, D. J. (1999). The diagnosis of rabies. In *Rabies: Guidelines for Professionals*, pp. 55–66. Veterinary Learning Systems. Trenton, NJ.

Trimarchi, C. V. (2000). Rabies In *Clinical Virology Manual,* S. Specter, R. Hodinka, and S. Young (eds.), pp. 335–338. ASM Press, Washington.

Umoh, J. V., and Blenden, D. C. (1983). Use of monoclonal antibodies in diagnosis of rabies virus infection and differentiation of rabies and rabies-related viruses. *J. Virol. Methods* **1**, 33–46.

Warner, C. K., Whitfield, S. G., Fekadu, M., and Ho, H. (1997). Procedures for reproducible detection of rabies virus antigen, mRNA and genome *in situ* in formalin fixed tissues. *J. Virol. Methods* **67**, 5–12.

Warner, C. K., Zaki, S. R., Shieh, W., Whitfield, S. G., Smith, J. S., Orciari, L. A., Shaddock, J. H., Niezgoda, M., Wright, C. W., Goldsmith, C. S., Sanderlin, D. W., Yager, P. A., and Rupprecht, C. E. (1999). Laboratory investigation of human deaths from vampire bat rabies in Peru. *Am. J. Trop. Med. Hyg.* **60**, 502–507.

Webster, L. T., and Dawson, J. R. (1935). Early diagnosis of rabies by mouse inoculation: Measurement of humoral immunity to rabies by mouse protection test. *Proc. Soc. Exp. Biol. Med.* **32**, 570–573.

Webster, W. A., and Casey, G. A. (1996). Virus isolation in neuroblastoma cell culture. In *Laboratory Techniques in Rabies*, F. X. Meslin, M. M. Kaplan, and H. Koprowski (eds.), 4th ed., pp. 96–104. Geneva, World Health Organization.

Willis, K., Tims, T., Schweitzer, K., Davis, R., and Briggs, D. (2000). A change in sampling methodology at the Kansas State University Rabies Diagnostic Laboratory. International Meeting on Research Advances and Rabies Control in the Americas, Lima, Peru.

Whitby, J. E., Heaton, P. R., Whitby, H. E., Osullivan, E., and Johnstone, P. (1997). Rapid detection of rabies and rabies-related viruses by RT-PCR and enzymer-linked immunosorbent assay. *J. Virol. Methods* **69**, 63–72.

Wiktor, T. J., and Clark, H. F. (1973). Application of the plaque assay technique to the study of rabies virus-neutralizing antibody interactions. *Ann. Microbiol (Paris)* **124**, 271–282.

Wiktor, T. J., Flamand, A., and Koprowski, H. (1980). Use of monoclonal antibodies in diagnosis of rabies virus infection and differentiation of rabies and rabies-related viruses. *J. Virol. Methods* **1**, 33–46.

Zaidman, G. W., and Billingsley, A. (1998). Corneal impression test for the diagnosis of acute rabies encephalitis. *Ophthalmology* **105**, 249–251.

10

Immunology

MONIQUE LAFON

Institut Pasteur, Unité de Neuro-immunologic Virale
75724 Paris Cedex 15
France

I. INTRODUCTION

Rabies is a unique neurologic infection that can be prevented by postexposure vaccination, at least when the vaccine is administrated to patients within a reasonable period of time after a rabies exposure. Thus vaccine efficiency can be conferred by immunization even after the virus enters the body and reaches the nervous system. Because of the immune privilege status of the nervous system and the ability of rabies virus to impair immune responsiveness in secondary lymphoid organs, it is intriguing to understand how immunization against rabies can prevent or limit virus progression toward and/or through the nervous system. In this chapter the mechanisms involved in specific immune responses, as well as the molecular basis of rabies vaccine protection, are discussed.

351

II. MOLECULAR COMPONENTS OF A SPECIFIC IMMUNE RESPONSE

After binding to major histocompatibility complex (MHC) molecules that are displayed at the surface of antigen-presenting cells (APCs), peptides derived from specific "foreign" antigens of invading pathogens or vaccines trigger an immune response against the invading pathogen. The CD4+ T-lymphocytes recognize foreign and vaccine-specific antigens once they have been processed through the MHC class II exogenous presentation pathway by specific cells, the APCs. Dendritic cells (DCs), macrophages, and B cells can process foreign antigens through the exogenous MHC class II pathway. They sample the extracellular environment for foreign antigens, process them intracellularly, and associate the digested antigen with MHC class II molecules. Once presented by the MHC, the peptides of the digested foreign antigen are recognized by T cells bearing the appropriate T-cell receptor (TCR) and CD4 molecule. Signaling via the TCR and CD4 molecule triggers activation of T cells and their differentiation into two functional subsets, the T-helper 1 (Th1) and T-helper 2 (Th2) cells. The distinction of the two subsets is based on the cytokines they secrete: Interferon-gamma (IFN-γ) is the signature cytokine for Th1 cells, whereas interleukin-4 (IL-4) is the signature cytokine for the Th2 cells. Generation of Th1 cells is under the control of IL-12 produced by macrophages and DCs. Th1 cells limit the proliferation of pathogens via IFN-γ production and provide help for antibody production by B-lymphocytes.

The CD8+ T cells, in contrast to CD4+ T cells, recognize foreign antigen that has been processed by the endogenous pathway of cells expressing MHC class I molecules. Infected cells export microorganism peptides embedded in the groove of MHC class I molecules to the cell surface. The peptide-charged infected cells activate T cells expressing the CD8 accessory surface molecules and the appropriate TCR. Activated CD8+ T-lymphocytes produce IFN-γ and kill the infected cells via cytotoxicity by means of perforin and granzyme release and/or Fas-mediated lysis. Maturation of the T cells takes place in the secondary lymphoid organs such as the lymph nodes and the spleen. APCs must migrate to these organs to induce an efficient immune response.

Tipping the balance of the CD4+ or CD8+ T-cell response to an antigen depends on the nature of the foreign or invading antigen. Live microorganisms trigger a CD8+ T-cell cytotoxic response, whereas recognition of an inert peptide or protein induces CD4+ T-cell recruitment. In particular, vaccines composed of live attenuated microorganisms trigger T-cell-mediated immunity that may be crucial in mediating protection against pathogens such as viruses that replicate in the cells. DNA vaccines and recombinant virus vaccines, which induce production of viral antigens by live cells, belong to the same category as live attenuated vaccines. Both vaccines generate mainly CD8+ T (cytotoxic) cells. In contrast, vaccines prepared with inactivated (killed) virus particles or portions (subunit) of

TABLE I

Comparative Analysis of Various Vaccine Formulations[a]

	Live attenuated vaccine	DNA vaccine	Recombinant vaccine	Killed vaccine
B cells	+++	++	++	+++
CD4+ T cells	+/− Th1	+++ Th1	+	+/− Th1
CD8+ T cells	+++	++	+++	−
MHC class	I and II	I and II	I and II	II

[a]From Seder and Hill (2000), reprinted with permission from *Nature*, Copyright 2000 Macmillan Magazines Limited.

virus particles that are sampled by the MHC class II APCs trigger CD4+ T-cell activation and the generation of a humoral (B-cell) immune response (Table I).

At present, rabies vaccines for humans and domestic animals are killed-virus vaccines containing full-sized intact proteins G, N, NS/P, M, and L of the virus (see Chap. 2). They are expected to trigger a CD4+ T-cell and a humoral B-cell response. The use of live-virus vaccines composed of an attenuated rabies virus strain or recombinant virus such as vaccinia that expresses the rabies virus G is restricted to wild animal immunization. This type of vaccine is expected to trigger an additional strong CD8+ T-cell response.

III. IMMUNE RESPONSES DURING RABIES VIRUS INFECTION

The native tropism of rabies virus is to infect the nervous system. The immune responses triggered during rabies virus infection are peculiar because of the status of the nervous system as an immunoprivileged site (Medawar, 1948; Barker and Billingham, 1977). The immunoprivilege is based mainly on the restriction of immune T-cell migration and the lack of professional APCs. In addition, to enforce this lack of immune efficacy, the pathogenic strains of rabies virus trigger an immunosuppressive state of the immune response in the periphery (spleen). As a result, there is a global subversion of the host immune defences by rabies virus. This can be seen as a successful, well-tailored adaptation of rabies virus to the host. One would expect that the host's natural capacity to fight such well-adapted virus is greatly limited.

A. Immune Privilege Status of the Central Nervous System

Rules that dictate immune function are subject to specialization of regional tissues. As well as mucosal tissues that develop a specific mucosal immune system, the "eyes/brain and nerves" can be regarded as having a distinctive regional immune system whose specific rules, designated by the term *immune privilege* or *immunoprivilege*, are not yet understood. The relative isolation of the central nervous system (CNS) from a normal immune response has long been thought to be due to the presence of several passive barriers [e.g., tight endothelium junctions of the blood–brain barrier (BBB) and absence of lymph ducts]. The BBB provides an almost complete block to the passage of antibodies and complement into the CNS (Miller, 1999). However, after selective injury of the CNS parenchyma, which can occur during an infection, proinflammatory cytokines and chemokines attract activated lymphocytes from the periphery that can pass through the BBB (Hickey *et al.*, 1991). Evidence that B cells enter the brain can be found during infection (Borna disease virus) or after intracerebral inoculation of antigen (Hatalski *et al.*, 1998a, 1998b; Knopf *et al.*, 1998). Once across the BBB, it seems that the capacity of the migrating activated T-lymphocytes to clear the infection from the CNS is restricted by at least three different factors:

1. Inefficient presentation of antigens (active downregulation of MHC class I and II molecules by live neurons and absence of professional APCs)

2. Apoptosis of activated lymphocytes by the Fas/FasL apoptosis mechanism

3. Immunosuppression of the T-cell response and Th1 cells in particular by immunosuppressive factors such as norepinephrine and vasoactive intestinal peptide

Expression of MHC class I molecules on neurons and expression of costimulatory molecules on brain cells and capillary endothelial cells are minimal, leading to anergy or lack of activation of T cells that can pass through the BBB. It has been proposed that electrically live neurons repress the expression of MHC class I molecules, leading to an absence of antigen presentation in a healthy CNS (Neumann *et al.*, 1995). Noninjured, live neurons downregulate the expression of MHC class I and class II molecules on glial cells as well as their own surfaces. In contrast, dying neurons allow the expression of MHC class I and class II molecules as well as β_2-microglobulin (Neumann *et al.*, 1996, 1997). This active control of MHC class I molecule expression makes infected neurons unable to present foreign antigens. The active control of MHC class I molecules can be exerted via ionic transfer or via secretion of soluble factors such as vasoactive intestinal peptide (VIP), neuropeptides (e.g., norepinephrine) (Frohman *et al.*, 1988a, 1988b), or neurotrophins (Thoenen, 1995; Lo, 1995; Neumann *et al.*, 1998).

After injury or stress, unrepressed parenchymal cells such as glial cells can become APCs because they can express MHC class II and molecular adhesion molecules. They also produce IL-12, which favors the development of a Th1-cell response. However, this activation is counteracted by activated astrocytes that are poor APCs and inhibit this production and favor a Th2-cell response (Aloisi, 2000). Thus there is an active dysregulation that counters the presentation of the foreign antigen in the Th1-cell pathway.

Development of a primary response against a pathogen requires that APCs migrate from the infected site into the secondary lymphoid organs. Glial cells are resident CNS cells that do not leave the CNS. In the case of a pathogen that is strictly restricted to the CNS parenchyma, even if glial cells present pathogen peptides, they cannot trigger a primary immune response against the pathogen because they do not reach the secondary lymphoid organs. However, activation of pathogen-specific lymphocytes can arise if pathogen peptides are picked up by the DCs. The DCs are professional APCs present in the meninges, the cerebrospinal fluid (CSF), and the choroid plexus (Fisher and Bielinsky, 1999; Fisher et al., 2000; Pashenkov et al., 2001). They are migratory cells that can leave the CNS via blood vessels and are routed through the secondary lymphoid organs such as cervical lymph nodes, where they allow a primary immune response to develop against pathogen antigens. The pathogen-specific activated lymphocytes can then migrate through the BBB and enter the CNS.

However, it is not clear yet whether the migratory activated cytotoxic lymphocytes can eliminate infected neuronal cells. Indeed, it has been proposed that activated lymphocytes bearing Fas molecules on their surface are subjected to death when encountering the Fas ligand (FasL) molecules expressed by CNS resident cells (Griffith et al., 1999; Flugel et al., 2000). Fas is a molecule of the tumor necrosis factor-alpha (TNF-α) family that contains a cytoplasm death domain. Its interaction with FasL triggers caspase activation (first caspase 8 and then caspase 3), driving the signal for death in the cell that bears Fas (Suda and Nagata, 1994; Nagata and Godstein, 1995; Bellgrau et al., 1995; Bellgrau and Duke, 1999). Resident CNS cells such as astrocytes and neurons express FasL (Bechmann et al., 1999). Fas is expressed on the surface of activated lymphocytes, which pass through the BBB. Thus activated lymphocytes should be triggered to death. It was proposed that Fas/FasL-mediated apoptosis could be a mechanism to limit the function of infiltrating lymphocytes in the CNS.

Moreover, endogenous immunosuppressive factors are secreted by glial cells, such as tumor growth factor-beta (TGF-β), VIP, α-melanocyte-stimulating hormone (α-MSH), and calcitonin gene–related peptide (CGRP) (Stanitz, 1994; Irani et al., 1997). It also has been proposed that inappropriate presentation by nonprofessional APCs may induce anergy rather than activation of T cells (Gold et al., 1996). At the present time, the efficiency of these mechanisms and the susceptibility of different subsets of lymphocytes (B cells, CD4+ T cells, or CD8+ T cells) to these immunosuppressive mechanisms are unknown and require further investigation. Altogether these data indicate that the CNS is a hostile environment in which to trigger an efficient immune response. This can be regarded as an adaptive mechanism leading to protection of nervous tissue and specialized cells such as neurons that have a limited potential for regeneration and whose function is a prerequisite for life.

Once lymphocytes have been activated in the periphery, either by injection of vaccine in the periphery or by filtration of virus antigens by professional migrating DCs from the CNS, a normal immune response can take place in the periphery (Cserr and Knopf, 1992). However, the efficiency of these lymphocytes might be annihilated because of the control of the Fas/FasL death pathway or immunosuppressive factors in the CNS.

B. Immunoreactivity of the CNS in Fatal Encephalitic Rabies

How does the CNS of the host maintain an immune privileged status in rabies? Perhaps the question can be answered, at least in part, with illustration of the following experiments that use the mouse as an animal model for rabies. Strains of rabies virus have been adapted to mouse CNS. Some virus strains such as the challenge virus standard (CVS) strain of fixed rabies virus cause a fatal infection of the CNS. After injection of CVS in the hindlimbs, progressive infection of the spinal cord and brain is accompanied by the production of the inflammatory cytokines IL-1, TNF-α, IL-6, and chemokines (e.g., MCP-1) (Marquette *et al.*, 1996; Camelo *et al.*, 2000). They attract lymphocytes that migrate through the BBB. However, the potency of migratory lymphocytes in clearing the infection is questionable because the course of rabies virus infection is similar in nude mice compared with their immunocompetent counterparts (*BALB/c* mice). Similar disease development in both the immunocompetent mouse and mice lacking T cells (nude mice) indicates that T cells are inefficient in controlling acute rabies virus encephalitis. This strongly suggests that the virus subverts the immune response and that T cells that infiltrate the CNS cannot control the infection. Thus the inefficiency of migrating T cells in controlling the infection could indicate that (1) T cells are non-rabies-specific, (2) they are anergic, or (3) they are destroyed by apoptosis shortly after they enter the CNS. The first possibility has not yet been addressed experimentally. The second possibility could result from the poor expression of MHC class II on glia in the infected animals that is observed during infection (Irwin *et al.*, 1999). The last possibility raises an intriguing consideration to explain the immune privileged status of the CNS. The fact that activated migratory lymphocytes encounter apoptosis is strongly supported by the observation that in the spinal cord of mice injected in the periphery, many nonneuronal cells are apoptotic. The apoptotic cells (TUNEL staining) correspond to CD3+ T cells. They could not be detected by day 9 postinfection (Camelo *et al.*, 2000). The presence of apoptotic CD3+ T cells is consistent with the destruction of activated T cells by the CNS environment, as observed in a CNS infection by Sindbis virus (Havert *et al.*, 2000). Thus the study of innate immunity in the CNS during rabies virus encephalitic infection indicates that the natural host defense is reduced and the immune privilege of the CNS is dramatically maintained.

C. Immune Unresponsiveness

In addition to the capacity of rabies virus to escape immune surveillance inside the CNS, it also can subvert the host immune response outside the CNS in the spleen. In contrast to infections such as measles virus or human immunodeficiency virus (HIV), in which immunosuppression results in the destruction of immune cell effectors, rabies virus–induced immunosuppression is a consequence of nervous system infection that induces neuroimmune deregulations.

Fatal encephalitis induced by pathogenic strains of rabies virus, including CVS or a "street" rabies virus, is accompanied by an immunodepression characterized by the impairment of the lymphocyte response and marked by a loss of cellular-mediated immunity (Wiktor *et al.*, 1977). This is concomitant with the unresponsiveness of spleen cells to lectin (ConA) stimulation *in vitro* (Hirai *et al.*, 1992; Perrin *et al.*, 1996; Camelo *et al.*, 2001). The decline in the lymphoproliferative response of splenocytes to an *in vitro* ConA stimulation but not to lipopolysaccharide (LPS) from the sixth day of infection is associated with a decrease in the number of splenocytes secreting IL-2, IFN-γ, and TNF-α (Th1 pattern) but not of the number secreting IL-4 (Th2 pattern). No quantitative modifications of the different spleen populations (CD4+ and CD8+ T cells, B cells, NK cells) were observed. The decrease in immune responsiveness depends on the pathogenicity of the strain. Abortive strains of rabies virus such as the Pasteur virus (PV) do not induce immunosuppression (Camelo *et al.*, 2001; Perrin *et al.*, 1996), suggesting that a certain threshold of dysfunction and/or inflammation of the nervous system is required. On the contrary, in the lymphoid cell depletion that characterizes rabies virus infection (Torres-Angel *et al.*, 1988), the immune suppression is not under the control of the hypothalamic–pituitary–adrenergic (HPA) axis because adrenalectomy, which interupts the production of corticosteroid hormones, does not modify the rabies virus–specific cytotoxic response (Wiktor *et al.*, 1985). Besides the contribution of the hormonal control of the immune response by the HPA axis, there is new evidence that the CNS control also can be exerted through a direct local delivery of neurotransmitters to peripheral immune organs by efferent nerves. Neurons deliver catecholamines locally to immune cells bearing the appropriate receptors, signaling them to secrete cytokines such as IL-6, TNF-α, or IL-10 that can perturb the immune response (Straub *et al.*, 1998). The precise mechanisms of catecholamine control in rabies remain to be elucidated. Neuronal immunosuppression induced by the viral stress of rabies virus infection can strengthen the subversion of the immune system by this CNS infection. It could represent an additional factor in the global unresponsiveness of the host to rabies.

The sequence of events that occurs during fatal encephalitis is illustrated schematically in Fig. 1. After the virus enters the nervous system by terminal nerve endings, neuromuscular junctions, and muscle spindles, it travels through the axons of connective neuronal networks. Rabies virus infects mainly neurons (Murphy *et al.*, 1973, Wunner, 1987). Infection triggers production of chemokines and inflammatory cytokines that attract activated lymphocytes to migrate through the BBB. However, these lymphocytes are not rabies virus–specific because they have not been activated in the periphery. Absence of activation in the periphery results in a scarcity of infected cells outside the CNS and absence of viral antigen that can be "seen" by professional APCs. Rabies virus strains causing encephalitis produce a noncytopathogenic infection that preserves the physical integrity of the neuron. Thus there is no antigen to be picked up by the APCs and delivered to the immune system. Absence of an immune response is strengthened by the capacity of the pathogenic strain of rabies virus to induce peripheral immunosuppression. As a consequence, the virus escapes the immune response and invades the entire nervous system.

D. Immunoreactivity in the CNS during Abortive Rabies

Valuable information has been garnered from various analyses of immune factors induced in the course of a nonfatal rabies virus infection to identify the

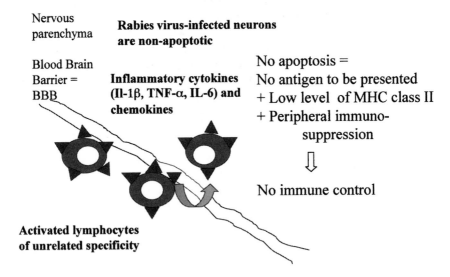

Fig. 1. CNS immune privilege is strongly maintained during encephalitic fatal rabies.

protective mechanisms against rabies virus CNS infection. Fixed laboratory strains of rabies virus that have been selected by serial passages in cell culture for their defined periods of growth have been particularly useful to study immunore-activity in the CNS during abortive rabies. Some virus strains such as PV or Evelyn-Rokitnicki-Abelseth (ERA) have conserved their neurotropism. However, when injected in the hindlimbs of mice, they were nonfatal and induced an irre-versible flaccid paralysis of the inoculated limbs (Smith, 1981; Weiland et al., 1992; Sugamata et al., 1992; Galelli et al., 2000). This aspect of the disease is characterized by the transient presence of rabies virus antigens in the CNS and enlargement of dorsal root ganglia adjacent to the inoculated limb. Development of paralysis depends on three linked events: (1) the levels of infection, (2) apop-tosis in the CNS, and (3) the progressive parenchymal infiltration of CD4+ and CD8+ T cells at the site of infection. It was demonstrated in immunosuppressed mice following cyclophosphamide treatment and in nude mice that when paraly-sis does not occur, it is replaced by a lethal rabies encephalitis. This indicates that the T-cell response is involved in the local paralysis and in the ultimate protec-tion. CD8+ T-depleted or the β_2-microglobulin knockout mice (which fail to express MHC class I molecules and as a result are deficient in the CD8+ T-cell response) do not develop paralysis but develop a severe lethal encephalitis (Hooper et al., 1998; Galelli et al., 2000). Apoptosis could be observed in the CNS of the mice. However, in contrast to virulent rabies virus infection (Jackson and Rossiter, 1997; Theerasurakarn and Ubol, 1998), apoptosis induced by the PV strain of rabies virus was not due to a direct deleterious effect of the virus. Instead, it appears to be due to a T-cell-dependent immune response triggered by the virus, as shown by the absence of apoptosis in the heavily infected CNS of nude mice. This indicates that development of paralysis is not due to a direct dele-terious effect of virus on neurons but is linked to an immunopathologic process involving CD8+ T cells. MHC class I molecules were found to be expressed in the CNS parenchyma during rabies virus infection (Irwin et al., 1999; Prosniak et al., 2001). MHC class I expression in rabies virus–infected CNS definitely involves neurons; thus it cannot be excluded that neurons die as a result of direct killing by CD8+ T cells. However, the mechanisms by which T cells mediate injury could result in release of the proinflammatory cytokines and chemokines that they secrete. IFN-γ is a potent activator of microglia, inducing upregulation of MHC class II expression, phagocytosis, and production of cytokines (Merrill and Benveniste, 1996). Cytokines may damage neural cells directly or act indi-rectly via activation of macrophages and microglial cells. These cells secrete factors toxic to oligodendrocytes, such as nitric oxide (NO) and TNF-α. NO was found to be produced in the brain during rabies virus infection (Hooper et al., 1995). Destruction of oligodendrocytes, the cells that produce the protective sheath of myelin around axons of neurons, may participate in neuronal death by deprivation of their protection. Apoptosis of infected neurons may have a physiologic role in protecting the CNS from the progression of infection and allowing contact between virus and immune components. It has been suggested that neuronal apoptosis could be a host defense mechanism to limit the propagation of the infection toward the CNS (Morimoto *et al.*, 1999).

In addition to the T-cell involvement, antibodies participate in protection against abortive strains (Hooper *et al.*, 1998). Antibodies collaborate with IFN-γ–dependent CNS inflammation to clear virus from the CNS. This is associated with strong expression of MHC class II molecules in the brain parenchyma (Irwin *et al.*, 1999). Altogether these findings suggest that B- and T-cell responses are efficient for protection in abortive rabies virus infection (Fig. 2). Infection of the CNS by an abortive strain of rabies virus induces apoptosis in neurons, upregulation of MHC class II antigens in nervous tissue, production of cytokines and chemokines, and infiltration of lymphocytes. Apoptosis is a T-cell-mediated process produced by the CD8+ T cells. Infection of the CNS is transient, and mice survive despite irreversible paralytic sequelae. In contrast to rabies virus infection with a pathogenic strain, where the immune response is completely switched off, an abortive infection of the nervous system actually is controlled by the immune response (Table II). Thus the strength of the immune privilege of the infected CNS depends on the pathogenicity of the strains. This strongly suggests that the capacity of the virus to subvert the host immune response depends on the nature of the virus.

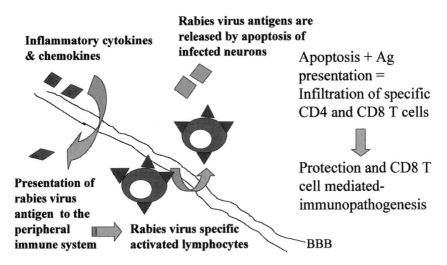

Fig. 2.   Relative CNS immune privilege in abortive rabies.

TABLE II

Rabies Virus Pathogenicity Correlates with the Ability of the Virus to Control the Host Immune Response[a]

	Encephalitic fatal rabies (CVS)	Abortive paralytic rabies (PV[b] or RV-194-2[c])
T-Lymphocytes are protective	No	Yes
T-Lymphocyte infiltration	Yes	Yes, mainly CD8+ T cells
Neuronal apoptosis and release of viral antigens	Sporadic	Wide spread
CNS associated antibodies	Undetectable	High
Inflammatory cytokines, chemokines	Yes	Yes (no IL-6)
Immunosuppression	Yes	No[d]
Immune privilege	Maintained	Decreased
Control of the virus infection	No	Yes
Survival of the animal	No	Yes
Virus cycle	Complete (virus reaches the brain)	Abortive (transient CNS infection); CD8+ T cell-mediated immunopathology is observed (paralysis)

[a] Virus inoculation was performed in the hindlimbs of the mice.
[b] From Galelli et al. (2000).
[c] From Irwin et al. (1999).
[d] From Camelo et al. (2000, 2001).

IV. IMMUNOLOGIC BASIS FOR POSTEXPOSURE VACCINATION EFFICIENCY

Comparison of the immunopathologic events that participate in virus clearance from the CNS helps to identify the survival factors necessary for protection. Survival is associated with a T-cell response, the production of antibodies, a high expression of MHC class II, and the presence of many apoptotic cells. A dual role is assigned to the CD8+ T cells: They participate in CNS clearance by controlling infection together with antibodies, and in contrast, they induce neuronal apoptosis, and thus initiate an imunopathologic reaction.

A. Protective Role of CD4 Lymphocytes

T lymphocytes play an important role in the immune defence against rabies virus. Demonstration that rabies virus is a T-cell-dependent antigen was established by experiments in T-lymphocyte-deficient mice, immunosuppressed, and reconstituted animals. In contrast to immunocompetent control animals, immunosuppressed mice were unable to mount an antibody response after rabies vaccination and resist a challenge of infectious virus (Turner, 1976; Mifune *et al.*, 1981). The use of immunosuppressive agents in mice confirms the protective role of T lymphocytes (Smith, 1981). Depletion of CD4+ T cells did not allow vaccinated mice to resist a peripheral challenge (Celis, 1990). Similarly, depletion of the CD4+ subset of T cells in the first 10 days of the infection resulted in fatal infection of mice (Perry and Lodmell, 1991) that were naturally resistant to a "street" rabies virus injected by the peripheral route (Lodmell, 1983).

B. Protective Role of Antibodies and B Lymphocytes

Virus-neutralizing antibodies under the control of T-helper cells play a critical role in immunoprotection. The glycoprotein (G) of rabies virus is responsible for the induction of virus-neutralizing antibodies. Its ability to mount a protective immune response depends on its structure. Soluble G, a glycoprotein lacking the 58 carboxy-terminal amino acids, elicited 15 times fewer neutralizing antibodies than the intact full-length G and failed to protect mice (Dietzschold *et al.*, 1983). Immunoglobulins of G isotype (IgGs), but not IgM, confer passive protection against rabies virus (Turner, 1978).

Antibodies against the N protein can be detected in human sera after immunization with inactivated rabies vaccines or after natural infection (Herzog *et al.*, 1992; Kasempimolporn *et al.*, 1991). These antibodies cannot neutralize the virus. Nevertheless, it has been proposed that they could confer protection in experimental rabies (Lodmell *et al.*, 1993). Their mode of action remains to be determined and could be linked either to their ability to block virus replication inside the cell as observed *in vitro* after antibodies were artificially injected into infected cells (Lafon and Lafage, 1987) or to their capacity to "neutralize" an unknown function of the free N protein (see Chap. 2).

A protective role of B cells as a source of virus-neutralizing antibodies was first suspected in rabies because the resistance of different strains of mice correlated with levels of neutralizing antibodies that they can develop against rabies virus. The high-antibody responders were resistant to peripheral virus challenge, whereas the low-antibody responders were susceptible (Templeton *et al.*, 1986). The second line of evidence that antibodies can protect against rabies virus infection came from B-lymphocyte depletion experiments using either anti-isotype antibody or B-cell-deficient mice. Depletion of B cells using anti-isotype antibodies that compromise the animal's capacity to mount an antibody response while leaving the T-cell response intact demonstrated that B cells play an essential role at least in the clearance of the attenuated high-egg-passage (HEP) strain of rabies virus (Miller *et al.*, 1978). Mice lacking B cells (J_{hD} knockout mice) develop a progressive disease when infected intranasally with an attenuated strain of rabies virus (CVS-F3), and they succumb to infection (Hooper *et al.*, 1998).

Antibody-mediated clearance of rabies virus from the CNS was demonstrated with a single monoclonal antibody (Dietzschold *et al.*, 1992; Dietzschold, 1993). It was shown that this particular antibody mediates complete clearance of virus from the CNS without the help of antibody-dependent cell-mediated cytotoxicity or complement-dependent lysis. This particular function is not shared with other neutralizing monoclonal antibodies. While the mechanisms involved remain unclear and specific transcytosis (mechanism of entry of antibody inside the target cell) cannot be excluded, the types and roles of antibodies involved in clearing neuronal infections need to be delineated. In particular, it will be of interest to precisely characterize the properties of antibodies that can cross the BBB. The BBB is impermeable to most antibodies. However, the blood barrier that surrounds nerves is less impermeable than the BBB (Moalem *et al.*, 1999), giving a chance for antibodies to clear the virus in the early steps of nerve infection. In addition, it is likely that a large fraction of the protective role of antibodies may operate before the virus enters the nervous system. Hence antibodies can neutralize rabies virus particles before they reach the nervous shield.

C. Role of CD8 Lymphocytes

Early studies indicate that mice vaccinated with a live attenuated strain of rabies virus vaccine (ERA) and to a lesser extent with inactivated vaccine produce cytotoxic T cells capable of lysing rabies virus–infected target cells (Wiktor *et al.*, 1977). In contrast, fully virulent viruses do not induce cytotoxic T cells (Wiktor *et al.*, 1985). Glycoprotein and N and NS/P protein are inducers of cytotoxic T cells (Wiktor *et al.*, 1984, Reddehase *et al.*, 1984, Celis, 1990, Larson *et al.*, 1991). However, a series of experiments designed to identify the immune system components involved in protection against rabies virus infection strongly suggested that cytotoxic T cells alone are not sufficient to confer protection against rabies virus. When mice were vaccinated with a mutated form of recombinant rabies virus G (expressed by a recombinant vaccinia virus containing a G gene that contains a leucine in position 8 instead of a proline) and compared with mice vaccinated with the nonmutated G, the mice did not develop neutralizing antibodies (Wiktor *et al.*, 1984), whereas they induced a similar CD8+ T-cell response (Celis, 1990). Mice vaccinated with the mutated G were not protected, indicating the importance of neutralizing antibodies. Moreover, depletion of CD8+ T cells has no effect on the resistance of mice to a street rabies virus or on the survival rate of vaccinated animals (Perry and Lodmell, 1991). The reconstitution of mice with a cytotoxic T-cell clone specific for the G induces protection only in the case of abortive rabies virus infection (ERA strain) (Kawano *et al.*, 1990). Since this is only observed with abortive rabies virus strains and not in encephalitic rabies virus infection, it can be concluded that CD8+ T cells probably are not primordial in immunoprotection.

D. How Rabies Vaccines Protect in Postexposure Treatment

The most important role of rabies vaccine is in the induction of a sustained antibody response with the help of CD4+ T-lymphocyte activation. Rabies is an exception because it is generally thought that cytotoxic T cells are more important to clear virus infection from tissues than antibodies. Diseases for which cytotoxic T cells play a major role in prevention are Thl-healing diseases (Garenne and Lafon, 1997). In contrast, rabies, for which antibodies are a major factor in controlling the propagation of the virus, belongs to the group of Th2-healing diseases (Garenne and Lafon, 1997). Moreover, activation of CD8+ T cells induces a pathologic reaction that is associated clinically with paralysis. This information probably should discourage the use of live vaccines, such as DNA vaccines or recombinant virus, as postexposure vaccines (Lodmell and Ewatts, 2001) because of the tremendous risk of mounting a strong deleterious CD8 response in the CNS. Nevertheless, these types of new-generation vaccines would be appropriate still for preexposure vaccination regimens because of the robustness of live immunization.

The inactivated postexposure vaccines that induce mainly B-cell activation with the help of CD4+ T cells (see Table I) are the most appropriate choice to preserve integrity of the CNS. Postexposure vaccines probably confer protection because they prime an immune response in the periphery in secondary organs. Activated lymphocytes, CD4+ cells, antibody-secreting plasmocytes, and possibly antibodies can migrate into the CNS parenchyma (Fig. 3). New investigations are necessary to understand exactly the sequence and nature of events that confer protection. Three important aspects of these events require future attention and better comprehension. The first one is to understand why apoptosis and the CNS suppressive environment are not efficient against CD4+ and T cells and B cells. The second is to understand whether some antibodies cross the endothelium of capillary vessels, and the third is to understand by what mechanisms antibodies and CD4+ T cells clear neuronal rabies virus infection.

V. CONCLUSIONS

It has been known for a long time that CNS viral infections are lethal because the CNS is an immune privileged site in which immune functions are restricted.

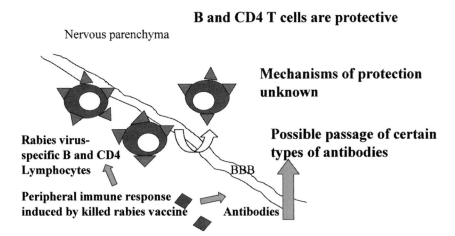

Fig. 3.   Immune responses triggered by a killed postexposure vaccine.

Moreover, some viruses have evolved powerful strategies that allow them to adapt the immune privilege and to escape from this local immune response. The rabies virus invades the nervous system by stealth and becomes invisible to the immune system after it enters the CNS because apoptosis of the infected neurons is not induced. Rabies virus antigens cannot be captured by professional APCs or trigger a primary immune response. This first step in immunosubversion is strengthened by peripheral immunosuppression mediated by the infection of the brain.

Despite these well-adapted viral strategies, rabies virus infections can be limited by humoral immunity (antibodies, B cells), suggesting that the virus only incompletely controls the immune response. This raises hopes for therapy. Today, with an increased understanding of the particular properties that rule the function of the regional immune system in the CNS, we can propose a biologic relevance and rationale for heuristic choices elaborated by former vaccine designers. On the other hand, the success of vaccination of patients after they have been infected, i.e., postexposure vaccination, or the use of serotherapy urges us to revisit how strict is the immune privilege and to investigate further the mechanisms that leave the immune B-cell response intact in immunoprivileged organs.

REFERENCES

Aloisi, F. (2000). Regulation of T-cell responses by CNS-antigen presenting cells: Different roles for microglia and astrocytes. *Immunol. Today* **21**, 141–147.

Barker, C. F., and Billingham, R. E. (1977). Immunologically privileged sites. *Adv. Immunol.* **25**, 1–54.

Bechmann, I., Mor, G., Nilsen, J., Eliza, M., Nitsch, R., and Naftolin, F. (1999). FasL is expressed in the normal rat and human brain: Evidence for the existence of an immunological brain barrier. *Glia* **27**, 62–74.

Bellgrau, D., Gold, D., Selawry, H., Moore, J., Franzusoff, A., and Duke, R. C. (1995). A role for CD95 ligand in preventing graft rejection. *Nature* **377**, 630–632.

Bellgrau, D., and Duke, R. C. (1999). Apoptosis and CD95 ligand in immune privileged sites. *Int. Rev. Immunol.* **18**, 547–562.

Camelo, S., Lafage, M., and Lafon, M. (2000). Absence of the p55Kd TNF-α receptor promotes survival in rabies virus acute encephalitis. *J. Neurovirol.* **6**, 507–518.

Camelo, S., Lafage, M., Galelli, A., and Lafon, M. (2001). A selective role for the p55Kd TNF-α receptor in immune unresponsiveness induced by an acute viral encephalitis. *J. Neuroimmunol.* **113**, 95–108.

Cserr, H. F., and Knopf, P. M. (1992). Cervical lymphatics, the blood–brain barrier and the immunoreactivity of the brain: A new view. *Immunol. Today* **13**, 507–512.

Celis, E., Rupprecht, C. E., and Plotkin, S. A. (1990). New and improved vaccines against rabies. In *New Generation Vaccines*, G. C. Woodrow and M. M. Levine (eds.), pp. 419–437. Dekker, New York.

Dietzschold, B., Wiktor, T. J., Wunner, W. H., and Varrichio, A. (1983). Chemical and immunological analysis of the rabies soluble glycoprotein. *Virology* **124**, 330–337.

Dietzschold, B., Kao, M., Zag, Y. M., Chen, Z. Y., Maul, G., Fu, Z. F., Rupprecht, C. E., and Koprowski, H. (1992). Delineation of putative mechanisms involved in antibody-mediated clearance of rabies virus from the central nervous system. Proc. *Natl. Acad. Sci. USA* **89**, 7252–7256.

Dietzschold, B. (1993). Antibody-mediated clearance of viruses from the mammalian central nervous system. *Trends Microbiol.* **1**, 63–66.

Fisher, H.-G., and Bielinski, A. K. (1999). Antigen presentation function of brain-derived dendritiform cells depends on astrocyte help. *Int. Immunol.* **11**, 1265–1272.

Fisher, H.-G., Bonifas, U., and Reichmann, G. (2000). Phenotype and functions of brain dentritic cells emerging during chronic infection of mice with *Toxoplasma gondii*. *J. Immunol.* **164**, 4826–4834.

Flugel, A., Schwaiger, F. W., and Neumann, H. (2000). Neuronal FasL induces cell death of encephalitogenic T-lymphocytes. *Brain Pathol.* **10**, 353–364.

Frohman, E. M., Vayuvegula, B., Gupta, S., and Van Den Noort, S. (1988a). Norepinephrine inhibits γ-interferon-induced histocompatibility class II (Ia) antigen expression on cultured astrocytes via β₂-adrenergic signal transduction mechanisms. *Proc. Natl. Acad. Sci. USA* **85**, 1292–1296.

Frohman, E. M., Frohman, T. C., Vayuvegula, B., Gupta, S., and Van Den Noort, S. (1988b). Vasoactive intestinal polypeptide inhibits the expression of the MHC class II antigens on astrocytes. *J. Neurol. Sci.* **88**, 339–346.

Galelli, A., Baloul, L., and Lafon, M. (2000). Abortive rabies virus central nervous infection is controlled by T-lymphocyte local recruitment and induction of apoptosis. *J. Neurovirol.* **6**, 359–372.

Garenne, M., and Lafon, M. (1997) Sexist diseases. *Perspect. Biol. Med.* **41**, 176–189.

Gold, R., Schmied, M., Tontsch, U., Hartung, H. P., Wekerle, H., Toyka, K. V., and Lassmann, H. (1996). Antigen presentation by astrocytes primes rat T-lymphocytes for apoptotic cell death: A model for T-cell apoptosis *in vivo*. *Brain* **119**, 651–659.

Griffith, T. S., Bruner, T., Fletcher, S. M., Green, D. R., and Derguson, T. A. (1999). Fas ligand–induced apoptosis as a mechanism of immune privilege. *Science* **270**, 1189–1192.

Hatalski, C. G., Hickey, W. F., and Lipkin, W. I. (1998a). Humoral immunity in the central nervous system following infection with Borna disease virus. *J. Neuroimmunol.* **90**, 128–136.

Hatalski, C. G., Hickey, W. F., and Lipkin, W. I. (1998b). Evolution of the immune response in the central nervous system following infection with Borna disease virus. *J. Neuroimmunol.* **90**, 137–142.

Havert, M. B., Schofield, B., Griffin, D., and Irani, D. N. (2000). Activation of divergent neuronal cell death pathways in different target cell populations during neuroadapted Sindbis virus infection of mice. *J. Virol.* **74**, 5352–5356.

Hickey, W. F., Hsu, B. L., and Kimura, H. (1991). T-lymphocyte entry into the central nervous system. *J. Neurosci. Res.* **28**, 254–260.

Hirai, K., Kawano, H., Mifune K., Fujii, H., Nishizono, A., Shichijo, A., and Mannen, K. (1992). Suppression of cell-mediated immunity by street rabies virus infection. *Microbiol. Immunol.* **36**, 1277–1290.

Hertzog, M., Lafage, M., Montano-Hirose, J. A., Scott-Algara D., and Lafon, M. (1992). Nucleocapsid specific T- and B-cell responses in humans after rabies vaccination. *Virus Res.* **24**, 77–89.

Hooper, D. C, Ohnishi, S. T., Kean, R., Numagami. Y., Dietzschold, B., and Koprowski, H. (1995). Local nitric oxide production in viral and autoimmune diseases of the nervous system. *Proc. Natl. Acad. Sci. USA* **92**, 5312–5316.

Hooper, D. C., Morimoto, K., Bette, M., Weihe, E., Koprowski, H., and Dietzschold, B. (1998). Collaboration of antibody and inflammation in clearance of rabies virus from the central nervous system. *J. Virol.* **72**, 3711–3719.

Irani, D. N., Lin, K., and Griffin, D. (1997). Regulation of brain-derived T cells during acute central nervous system inflammation. *J. Immunol.* **158**, 2318–2326.

Irwin, D. J., Wunner, W. I., Ertl, H., and Jackson, A. (1999). Basis of rabies virus neurovirulence in mice: Expression of major histocompatibility complex class I and class II mRNAs. *J. Neurovirol.* **5**, 485–494.

Jackson, A. C., and Rossiter, I. P. (1997). Apoptosis plays an important role in experimental rabies virus infection. *J. Virol.* **71**, 5603–5607.

Kasempimolporn, S., Hemachuda, T., Khawplod, P., and Manatsathit, S. (1991). Human immune response to rabies nucleocapsid and glycoproteins antigens. *Clin. Exp. Immunol.* **84**, 195–199.

Kawano, H. K., Mifune, K., Ohuchi, M., Mannen, K., Cho, S., Hiramatsu, K., and Schichijo, A. (1990). Protection against rabies in mice by a cytotoxic T-cell clone recognizing the glycoprotein of rabies virus. *J. Gen. Virol.* **71**, 281–287.

Knopf, P. M., Harling-Berg, C. J., Cserr, H. F., Basu, D., Sirulnick, E. J., Nolan, S. C., Park, J. T., Keir, G., Thompson, E. J., and Hickey, W. F. (1998). Antigen-dependent intrathecal antibody synthesis in the normal rat brain: Tissue entry and local retention of antigen-specific B cells. *J. Immunol.* **161**, 692–701.

Lafon, M., and Lafage, M. (1987). Antiviral activity of monoclonal antibodies specific for internal proteins of the rabies virus. *J. Gen. Virol.* **68**, 3113–3123.

Larson, J. K., Wunner, W. H., Otvos, L. J. R, and Ertl, H. C. J. (1991). Identification of an immunodominant epitope within the phosphoprotein of rabies virus that is recognized by both class I– and class II–restricted T cells. *J. Virol.* **65**, 5673–5679.

Lo, D. C. (1995). Neurotrophic factors and synaptic plasticity. *Neuron* **15**, 979–981.

Lodmell, D. L. (1983). Genetic control of resistance to street rabies virus in mice. *J. Exp. Med.* **157**, 451–490.

Lodmell, D. L., Esposito, J. J., and Ewalt, L. C. (1993). Rabies virus antinucleoprotein antibody protects against rabies virus challenge and replication *in vitro*. *J. Virol.* **67**, 6080–6086.

Lodmell, D. L., and Ewalt L. C. (2001). Postexposure DNA vaccination protects mice against rabies virus. *Vaccine* **19**, 2468–2473.

Marquette, C., Ceccaldi, P. E., Ban, E., Weber, P., Haour, F. and Tsiang, H. (1996). Induction of immunoreactive interleukin-1β and tumor necrosis factor-α in the brains of rabies virus–infected rats. *J. Neuroimmunol.* **68**, 45–51.

Medawar, P. B. (1948). Immunity to homologous grafted skin: III. The fate of skin homografts transplanted to the brain, to subcutaneous tissue, and to the anterior chamber of the eye. *Br. J. Exp. Pathol.* **29**, 58–69.

Merrill, J. E., and Benveniste, E. N. (1986). Cytokines in inflammatory brain lesions: Helpful and harmful. *Trends Neurosci.* **19**, 331–338.

Mifune, K., Takeuchi, E., Napiokowski, P. A., Yamada, A., and Sakamoto, K. (1981). Essential role of T-cells in the post-exposure prophylaxis of rabies in mice. *Microbiol. Immunol.* **25**, 895–904.

Miller, D. W. (1999). Immunobiology of the blood–brain barrier; *J. Neurovirol.* **5**, 570–578.

Miller, A., Morse, H. C., Winklestein, J., and Nathanson, N. (1978). The role of antibody in recovery from experimental rabies. Effect of depletion of B and T cells. *J. Immunol.* **121**, 321–326.

Moalem, G., Monsonego, A:, Shani, Y., Cohen, I. R., and Schwartz, M. (1999). Differential T-cell response in central and peripheral nerve injury: Connection with the immune privilege. *FASEB J.* **13**, 1207–1217.

Morimoto, K., Hooper, D. C., Spitsin, S., Koprowski, H., and Dietzschold, B. (1999). Pathogenicity of different rabies virus variants inversely correlates with apoptosis and rabies virus glycoprotein expression in infected primary neurons cultures. *J. Virol.* **73**, 510–518.

Murphy, F. A., Harrison, A. K., Winn, W. C., and Bauer, S. P. (1973). Comparative pathogenesis of rabies and rabies like viruses: Infection of the central nervous system and centrifugal spread of virus to peripheral tissues. *Lab. Invest.* **29**, 1–16.

Nagata, S., and Goldstein, P. (1995). The Fas death factor. *Science* **267**, 1449–1456.

Neumann, H., Cavalié, A., Jenne, D. E., and Wekerle, H. (1995). Induction of MHC class I genes in neurons. *Science* **269**, 549–552.

Neumann, H., Boucraut, J., Hahnel, C., Misgeld, T., and Wekerle, H. (1996). Neuronal control of MHC class II inductibility in rat astrocytes and microglia. *Eur. J. Neurosci.* **8**, 2582–2590.

Neumann, H., Schmidt, H., Cavalié, A., Jenne, D. E., and Wekerle, H. (1997). MHC class I expression in single neurons of the central nervous system: Differential regulation by interferon-α and tumor necrosis factory-γ. *J. Exp. Med.* **185**, 305–316.

Neumann, H., Misgeld, T., Matsumuro, K., and Wekerle, H. (1998). Neurotrophins inhibit class II inductibility of microglia. Involvement of the p75 receptor. *Proc. Natl. Acad. Sci. USA* **95**, 5779–5784.

Pashenkov, M., Huang, Y.-M., Kostulas, V., Haglund, M., Söderström, M., and Link, H. (2001). Two subsets of dendritic cells are present in human cerebrospinal fluid. *Brain* **124**, 480–492.

Perrin, P., Tino De Franco, M., Jallet, C., Fouque, F., Morgeaux, S., Tordo, N., and Colle, J.-F. (1996). The antigen-specific cell-mediated immune response in mice is suppressed by infection with pathogenic lyssaviruses. *Res. Virol.* **147**, 289–299.

Perry, L., and Lodmell, D. L. (1991). Role of CD4+ and CD8+ T cells in murine resistance to street rabies virus. *J. Virol.* **65**, 3429–3434.

Prosniak, M., Hooper, D. C., Dietzschold, B., and Koprowski, H. (2001). Effect of rabies virus infection on gene expression in mouse brain. *Proc. Natl. Acad. Sci. USA* **98**, 2758–2763.

Reddehase, M. J., Cox, J. H., and Koszinowski, U. H. (1984). Frequency analysis of cytolytic T-lymphocytes precursors (CTL-P) generated *in vivo* during lethal rabies infection of mice: II. Rabies virus genus specificity of CTL-P. *Eur. J. Immunol.* **14**, 1039–1043.

Seder, R. A., and Hill, A. V. S. (2000). Vaccines against intracellular infections requiring cellular immunity. *Nature* **406**, 793–798.

Smith, J. (1981). Mouse model for abortive rabies infection of the central nervous system. *Infect. Immun.* **31**, 297–308.

Stanitz, A. M. (1994). Neuronal factors modulating immunity. *Neuroimmunomodulation* **1**, 217–230.

Straub, R. H., Westermann, J., Schölmerich, J., and Falk, W. (1998). Dialogue between the CNS and the immune system in lymphoid organs. *Immunol. Today* **19**, 409–413.

Suda, T., and Nagata, S. (1994). Purification and characterization of the Fas/FasL that induces apoptosis. *J. Exp. Med.* **179**, 873–879.

Sugamata, M., Miyazawa, M., Mori, S., Spangrude, G. J., Ewalt, L. C., and Lodmell, D. L. (1992). Paralysis of street rabies virus–infected mice is dependent on T-lymphocytes. *J. Virol.* **66**, 1252–1260.

Templeton, J. W., Holmberg, C., Garber, T., and Sharp, M. (1986). Genetic control of serum neutralizing-antibody response to rabies vaccination and survival after a rabies challenge infection in mice. *J. Virol.* **59**, 98–102.

Thoenen, H. (1995). Neurotrophins and neuronal plasticity. *Science* **270**, 593–598.

Theerasurakarn, S., and Ubol, S. (1998). Apoptosis induction in brain during the fixed strain of rabies virus infection correlates with onset and severity of illness. *J. Neurovirol.* **4**, 407–414.

Torres-Anjel, M., Volz, D., Torres, M., Turk, M., and Tshikula, G. (1988). Failure to thrive, wasting syndrome and immunodeficiency in rabies: A hypophyseal/hypothalamic/thymic axis effect of rabies virus. *Rev. Infect. Dis.* **10**, 710–725.

Turner, G. S. (1976). Thymus-dependence of rabies vaccine. *J. Gen. Virol.* **33**, 535–538.

Turner, G. S. (1978). Immunoglobulin (IgG) and (IgM) antibody responses to rabies vaccine. *J. Gen. Virol.* **40**, 595–604.

Weiland, F., Cox, J. H., Meyer, S., Dahme, E., and Reddehase, M. J. (1992). Rabies virus neuritic paralysis: Immunopathogenesis of nonfatal paralytic rabies. *J. Virol.* **66**, 5096–5099.

Wiktor, T. J., Doherty, P. C., and Koprowski, H. (1977). *In vitro* evidence of cell-mediated immunity after exposure of mice to both live and inactivated rabies virus. *Proc. Natl. Acad. Sci. USA* **74**, 334–338.

Wiktor, T. J., Macfarlan, R. I., Reagan, K., Diertzschold, B., Curtis P., Wunner, W., Kieney, M.-P., Lathe, R., Lecocq, J. P., Mackett, M., Moss, B., and Koprowski, H. (1984). Protection from rabies by a vaccinia virus recombinant containing the rabies virus glycoprotein gene. *Proc. Natl. Acad. Sci. USA* **81**, 7194–7198.

Wiktor, T. J., Macfarlan, R. I., and Koprowski, H. (1985). Rabies virus pathogenicity. In *Rabies in the Tropics*, E. Kuwert, C. Mérieux, H. Koprowski, and K. Bögel (eds.), pp. 21–29. Springer-Verlag, New York.

Wunner, W. H. (1987). Rabies viruses: Pathogenesis and immunity. In *The Rhabdoviruses*, R. R. Wagner (ed.), pp. 361–426. Plenum Press, New York.

11

Vaccines

DEBORAH J. BRIGGS

College of Veterinary Medicine
Kansas State University
Manhattan, Kansas 66506

DAVID W. DREESEN

Lida Corporation
Winterville, Georgia 30683

WILLIAM H. WUNNER

The Wistar Institute
Philadelphia, PA 19104-4268

I. HUMAN RABIES VACCINES

A. Introduction

Human rabies vaccines have a long history beginning with the first antirabies treatment developed by Pasteur, Roux, and their colleagues in 1885 (Geison, 1990). During the first two decades after the Pasteur treatment, several other methods were used for rabies vaccine production, all of which used rabies virus–infected brain tissue as a source of antigen. All the rabies vaccines that immediately followed the original Pasteur treatment were produced and applied using the same theory of serial injections of increasingly virulent rabies virus–infected nerve tissue. In these early rabies vaccines, the virulence of the rabies virus was decreased in phases by heating the infected material for increasing amounts of time or temperatures. Finally, in the early 1900s, two important modifications were made in the production of rabies vaccines. Fermi and Semple introduced the use of phenol to chemically inactivate rabies virus–infected nerve tissue. Additionally, they used the same inactivated suspension for all injections. These two changes allowed tests of safety and potency to be conducted and a wider distribution of rabies vaccines because they could be distributed in vials for individual use. In 1973, the World Health Organization (WHO) recommended that Fermi-type rabies vaccines be discontinued because they contained residual, live, fixed rabies virus. Semple rabies vaccine is still used widely today in developing countries and differs from Fermi vaccines in that the rabies virus is inactivated by phenol or β-propiolactone (BPL) during production. Historically, nerve tissue rabies vaccines were prepared and administered at Pasteur Institutes initially established throughout the world to treat large numbers of patients exposed to rabid animals. The practice of treating exposed patients at a central location instead of at hospitals or medical clinics is still in effect today in most developing countries.

The presence of the myelin component of nervous tissue in Semple vaccine has resulted in severe neuroparalytic adverse reactions and even death in some recipients (Hemachuda *et al.*, 1987; Meslin and Kaplan, 1996). To overcome sensitivity reactions to myelin, Fuenzalida and Palacios (1955) developed a rabies vaccine in which newborn mice were infected intracerebrally with rabies virus and the brain material was harvested before the mice reached 9 days of age. This "suckling mouse brain" rabies vaccine is currently widely used throughout all of

Latin America and parts of Asia and Africa. Unpurified nerve tissue vaccines (NTVs) helped to prevent many deaths after exposure to rabid animals when they were first developed. Today, the production and administration of NTVs continue to be financially supported by the governments of many developing countries. NTVs are used mainly to provide postexposure treatment (PET) to the poorer segments of the population who cannot afford more expensive cell culture rabies vaccines. Hopefully, within the next 5 years, the use of inexpensive intradermal vaccination regimens will replace outdated, painful, and highly allergenic NTVs.

The first non-nervous tissue rabies vaccine, duck embryo vaccine (DEV), became available commercially in the United States in 1957, and the use of NTVs throughout North America declined continually. Although DEV produced significantly fewer reactions among rabies vaccines, 21 cases of severe neurologic complications (including 2 deaths) were reported out of a total of 595,000 recipients between 1958 and 1975, (Meslin and Kaplan, 1996). The first modern cell culture rabies vaccine, the human diploid cell vaccine (HDCV), was introduced into the United States in 1978. HDCV produced significantly higher immunogenicity and lower severe allergic reactions compared with previous rabies vaccines (Plotkin, 1980).

B. Global Administration of Human Rabies Vaccines

There are three types of rabies vaccines currently administered to humans throughout the world: (1) nerve tissue–derived vaccines, (2) high-quality cell-culture vaccines produced under stringent quality control and quality assurance standards, and (3) lower-quality cell-culture vaccines that do not adhere to federal drug administration regulations or national pharmacopeia standards in industrialized countries. A combined total of over 50 million doses, including all three types of rabies vaccines, are administered annually worldwide. Twenty million doses of the vaccines are still NTV (Haupt, 1999; Pan American Health Organization, 1999; WHO, 2000, in press). The number of doses of vaccine required per patient for one PET varies according to the type of rabies vaccine that is used. If an exposed patient receives NTV for PET, 7–15 doses are required. In the case of low-quality cell-culture vaccines, 5–10 doses are required, and if high-quality cell-culture vaccines are used, only 5 doses are required. In industrialized countries, only high-quality cell-culture rabies vaccines are licensed for use in humans, whereas most of the rabies vaccines administered in developing countries are either NTVs or lower-quality cell-culture rabies vaccines.

It is interesting to note that most of the administration of PET as well as most human deaths are reported from Asia, indicating that there is a tremendous lack of patient awareness and local availability of good-quality rabies vaccines in that region of the world. The true incidence of human rabies in African countries is presently unknown, although it is presumed to be grossly underreported (WHO, 1998). Most of the reported human fatalities in Asia and Africa occur as a result of bites inflicted by rabid dogs. In most developing countries of the world, rabies remains endemic in the canine population, and there are millions of unvaccinated stray or community-owned dogs living in close association with humans (Wandeler *et al.*, 1993; Barth, 1994; WHO, 1998). The incidence of rabies in humans has been reduced dramatically in developing countries that have adopted countrywide strategies to replace NTVs with cell-culture rabies vaccines and/or have implemented a successful canine vaccination and control program (Fishbein and Baer, 1988; Mitmoonpitak *et al.*, 1997). It is clear that both strategies are necessary to prevent human deaths from rabies.

C. Present Nerve Tissue Rabies Vaccines

NTVs are produced from the brain tissue of animals infected with a fixed strain of rabies virus. After harvesting the brain material, the virus is inactivated with phenol or BPL and then diluted to a final concentration of 2–5% of brain tissue. The shelf life of NTVs is short, usually 6 months or less, and the potency of these vaccines is often questionable, especially when they are not kept under adequate refrigeration temperatures. There are two NTVs presently used in developing countries throughout the world, Semple rabies vaccine produced from rabies virus–infected sheep or goat brain tissue and Fuenzalida–Palacios rabies vaccine produced from rabies virus–infected suckling mouse or rat brain tissue.

Semple rabies vaccine was developed in 1911 at the Central Research Institute in Kasauli, India, by Sir David Semple and continues to be the most widely used rabies vaccine in India, Pakistan, and some other developing countries in Asia and Africa. To prepare the vaccine, very young sheep are injected intracerebrally with a fixed strain of rabies virus originating from the original Pasteur strain. The sheep are euthanitized 6–7 days later when they begin to demonstrate clinical signs of rabies. Their brains are removed and homogenized in a solution containing the inactivating agent phenol or BPL. The solution is filtered to remove large particles and dispensed into vials. The final concentration of brain tissue in the vaccine preparation depends on the manufacturer but usually is 5%. Semple rabies vaccine is dispensed in volumes of 2 ml for children and 5 ml for adults. The number of doses required to treat one patient depends on the individual manufacturers and governmental recommendation but generally ranges between 7 and 15 doses. The shelf life of Semple rabies vaccine is approximately 6 months (Lépine *et al.*, 1973; Singh and Kumar, 1999). In addition to the fact that Semple rabies vaccine is extremely painful to receive, it also can cause severe neurologic adverse reactions (reported to range between 1 in 142 and 1 in 7000) due to the presence of myelinated tissue in the vaccine (Meslin and Kaplan, 1996). In addition, the injection of sheep brain–derived rabies vaccines significantly increases the potential for transmission of spongiform encephalopathies from infected sheep to humans (Martino, 1993; Arya, 1994).

To overcome the neurologic complications of the Semple vaccine, a rabies vaccine was developed in the brain tissue of newborn suckling mice because their brains are not yet myelinated (Fuenzalida and Palacios, 1955). Fuenzalida and Palacios first developed and produced the suckling mouse brain rabies (SMB) vaccine in Chile in 1963, and by 1965, it had become the only vaccine used in humans in Latin America.

SMB vaccine generally is prepared from fixed rabies virus strains originally isolated in Chile. Mice not older than 1 day are injected intracerebrally, and brain tissue is harvested approximately 4 days later. Rabies virus–infected brain tissue is diluted and inactivated with ultraviolet light or BPL. The final concentration of brain tissue in SMB vaccine depends on the manufacturer but usually is around 10%. The WHO recommends that all SMB vaccines have a potency of 1.3 International Units per dose (WHO, 1973). The vaccine generally is supplied in 1- to 2-ml doses, and the shelf life of 1 year can be extended if the suspension is lyophilized (Diaz, 1996). Although the adverse reactions associated with SMB vaccines are lower (1 in 8000) than with Semple rabies vaccine, the case mortality rate in affected patients who received SMB vaccine is higher (22%) than in affected patients who received Semple vaccine (4.8%) (Meslin and Kaplan, 1966; Nogueira, 1988).

In 2001, the WHO issued a resolution calling for the complete replacement of NTVs by 2006 with modern cell-culture rabies vaccines. In some developing countries, NTVs already have been replaced through the use of reduced-dosage intradermal regimens for PET (see Chap. 12). These intradermal PET schedules have proved to be an efficacious and cost-effective method to eliminate the use of poor-quality, allergenic NTVs (Chutivongse et al., 1990; Briggs et al., 2000).

D. Cell-Culture Rabies Vaccines

Rabies vaccines derived from cell culture are unquestionably far superior to NTVs. Cell-culture rabies vaccines are highly purified and therefore produce few severe allergic reactions. According to WHO recommendations, all cell-culture rabies vaccines must have a minimum potency of 2.5 IU per dose and induce high levels of rabies virus neutralizing antibody (Nicholson, 1996; WHO, 1992). Due to the higher potency and immunogenicity of cell-culture rabies vaccines, the number of doses required for PET was reduced from the 7–15 required for NTVs to 5 for the cell-culture vaccine. Very few patients who have received the modern cell-culture rabies vaccines after exposure have succumbed to rabies. A review of the case histories of the patients who died after treatment with cell-culture rabies vaccines indicates that they did not receive the complete WHO-recommended PET (Plotkin *et al.*, 1999).

The first highly successful cell-culture vaccine was produced in the 1960s in human diploid cells by Wiktor and colleagues at The Wistar Institute in Philadelphia (Wiktor *et al.*, 1969). Human diploid cell vaccine (HDCV) received international recognition when it was used successfully to treat humans exposed to severe wounds by rabid dogs and wolves in Iran (Bahmanyar *et al.*, 1976). HDCV is produced in human fibroblast cells using the Pitman–Moore strain of rabies virus originally isolated by Pasteur. It is purified and concentrated by ultracentrifugation and inactivated with BPL. HDCV changed the concept of rabies vaccination, and its proven record of safety and efficacy encouraged the use of preexposure prophylaxis (PEP) for patients at continual risk of exposure due to their vocation or hobby. HDCV was licensed for use in the United States in 1980 and has been in continual use for both pre- and postexposure rabies vaccination since that time. Due to the reduced vaccination regimens and apparent safety of HDCV, the Advisory Committee on Immunization Practices (ACIP) originally recommended routine boosters every 2 years for people at frequent risk of exposure to rabies (CDC, 1991). However, HDCV is not completely free from adverse reactions, and one report indicated that up to 10% of individuals previously vaccinated with HDCV developed severe immune-complex reactions after receiving boosters (Dreesen *et al.*, 1986). Therefore, in 1999, the ACIP changed its recommendation from routine boosters every 2 years to serologic evaluation for the presence of rabies virus neutralizing antibodies for individuals at continual or frequent risk of exposure to rabies. Routine booster doses of vaccine are administered only when rabies neutralizing antibody levels fall below 1:5 according to the ACIP (CDC, 1999) (see Chap. 12). Although HDCV produces high serologic titers, high production costs and low virus yields make this vaccine unaffordable in developing countries of the world, where the majority of human rabies deaths occur (Plotkin *et al.*, 1999).

In the 1980s, a second cell-culture vaccine, purified chick embryo cell rabies vaccine (PCECV), was developed by Barth and colleagues (Barth *et al.*, 1984). PCECV is propagated in primary chick fibroblast cells using the Flury LEP strain of rabies virus. The virus is inactivated by BPL and purified by zonal centrifugation. The production of PCECV on chick fibroblasts permits a very high yield of virus as compared with virus production on human diploid cells. PCECV is a highly purified rabies vaccine that also produces fewer severe adverse reactions than HDCV, including the immune-complex reactions after receiving boosters (Bijok, 1985). PCECV is used worldwide in both industrialized and developing countries.

A further reduction in the cost of rabies vaccines was provided by the introduction of production using continuous cell lines. Continuous cell lines originate from the spontaneous transformation of a diploid cell line into a heteroploid cell line and can be multiplied serially through an unlimited number of passages. Therefore, these cell lines can be potentially oncogenic. However, purification processes can be put in place to eliminate or at least reduce to a minimum acceptable level the amount of residual DNA in the vaccine (Perrin *et al.*, 1995). The most reliable human rabies vaccine produced from a continuous cell line is purified Vero cell rabies vaccine (PVRV) produced on Vero cells (vervet monkey origin). PVRV can be cultivated on microcarriers in large-scale biofermentors; thus large quantities of vaccine can be produced at a lower cost than HDCV. PVRV is inactivated by BPL and concentrated by ultracentrifugation. PVRV is used widely in developing countries, and although it is not licensed for use in North America, it is used extensively in Europe.

Another cell-culture vaccine licensed for use in the United States is "rabies vaccine adsorbed" (RVA). The RVA cell-culture vaccine was developed in the 1970s by the Michigan Department of Public Health by infecting fetal rhesus monkey kidney cells with the Kissling strain of rabies virus. RVA is purified by filtration, inactivated with β-propiolactone, and adjuvanted with aluminum phosphate (Barth and Franke, 1996).

Lower-quality cell-culture vaccines are beginning to be produced in developing countries as an alternative to NTVs. Since these vaccines do not adhere to strict regulations imposed by the U.S. Food and Drug Administration (FDA) or the European pharmacopeia, they are less expensive to produce. The two types of cell-culture vaccines currently being produced by local manufacturers in Latin America and Asia are the Vero cell rabies vaccine "copies" and primary hamster kidney cell rabies vaccines (PHKCVs). Millions of doses of PHKCV are administered to people exposed to rabid dogs throughout China and Russia.

E. Ensuring Vaccine Safety and Potency

All modern high-quality cell-culture vaccines for humans meet or exceed the published WHO standards (WHO, 1981, 1994). In addition, many individual countries have more stringent requirements that must be met prior to a rabies vaccine receiving licensure. Rabies vaccines for humans must have a potency of at least 2.5 IU per dose using the National Institutes of Health (NIH) test and must have data proving that they are totally inactivated prior to release. Major pharmaceutical companies producing high-quality cell-culture vaccines must have in-process controls to maintain their standard of vaccine production. Additionally, they are required to investigate any vaccine-related health problems that occur, including all severe allergic reactions and treatment failures reported to them.

II. RABIES VACCINES FOR DOMESTIC ANIMALS

A. Introduction

The widespread vaccination of domestic dogs has proved to be the most effective measure for the reduction of human rabies cases. Louis Pasteur initiated research into animal rabies vaccines in the early 1880s (Bunn, 1991) during his quest for a means to prevent rabies in humans. Virus obtained from a rabid dog was first passed serially in rabbits by intracerebral inoculation at specified time intervals. Dogs were then vaccinated at various time intervals and challenged with rabies virus. Although this method produced acceptable results, Pasteur found that by serial intracerebral inoculation of monkeys with the dog-origin virus the incubation period increased, whereas the virulence of the virus decreased. Pasteur demonstrated that dogs vaccinated by this regimen were resistant to subsequent challenge with virulent "street" (non-laboratory-propagated) rabies virus.

To improve on the safety of these early attempts to produce a rabies vaccine, in 1885 Pasteur partially inactivated the virus by desiccation (Bunn, 1991). In a review by Friedberger and Frohner (1904), it was reported that Hogyes, Protopopoff, and others conducted further studies to improve on the safety and efficacy of vaccines for dogs and to reduce the number of doses needed. In 1927, the First International Rabies Conference recommended that "fixed" virus for canine rabies vaccines be completely inactivated or attenuated so that they caused no disease in dogs vaccinated either subcutaneously (SC) or intramuscularly (IM) (Schoeing, 1930). For the next several decades, virtually all nerve-tissue-origin (NTO) vaccines were inactivated with phenol using the method described by Semple (Bunn, 1991). However, NTO killed vaccines for dogs and other animals often resulted in postvaccinal nervous system reactions that could result in the death of the vaccinated animals (Bunn, 1991). Better vaccines were needed.

To improve this situation, embryonated chicken eggs were used for serial passage of the Flury strain (a human rabies virus isolate) (Koprowski and Cox, 1948). The virus initially was passed 136 times in 1-day-old chicks. Vaccine produced from the 40th to the 50th chicken embryo passage was designated as *low-egg-passage* (LEP). While effective in dogs, the vaccine occasionally caused rabies in young pups, cats, and cattle (Bunn, 1991). To increase the safety of the vaccines in these species, the serial passages of the Flury strain were increased in embryonated eggs until the virus was found to be nonpathogenic for dogs when inoculated intracerebrally following the 205th passage (Koprowski *et al.*, 1954). This *high-egg-passage* (HEP) vaccine was safe for use in cats and cattle (by the IM route), as well as in dogs as young as 3 months of age.

B. Modified Live Virus Vaccines

The Flury and Kelev strains of rabies virus are used to produce chick-embryo-origin (CEO) modified live virus (MLV) rabies vaccines (Bijok, 1985; Arai *et al.*, 1991). The Street Alabama Dufferin (SAD) strain, which is adapted to hamster kidney tissue (Fenje, 1960), and the Evelyn–Rokitnicki–Abelseth (ERA) strain, which is grown on porcine kidney cells (Abelseth, 1964), are also used commonly to produce MLV rabies vaccines (Reculard, 1996). In addition, several other MLV vaccines have been produced over the years. These MLV rabies vaccines, especially those using the CEO, SAD, and ERA strains are still used extensively in Asia and Africa and parts of Europe and have been adapted for oral immunization of carnivores, including domestic dogs and cats (Blancou *et al.*, 1996). Potency tests for MLV rabies vaccines for animal use consist of measuring the titer of infectious virus in a sample from each filling lot. If the titer is not less than that proved efficacious in the species of animal for which the vaccine is intended, the vaccine is released for use (Sizaret, 1996).

Even though MLV rabies vaccines have been proved to be efficacious and of value in many parts of the world over the years, the use of inactivated (killed) cell-culture rabies vaccines is increasing in areas of the world where MLV vaccines are still in use. No MLV rabies vaccines are licensed for use in the United States.

C. Killed Cell-Culture Rabies Vaccines

The inactivated (killed) rabies vaccines require that the rabies virus be produced in high concentrations. This is accomplished initially by growing the virus (primarily the CVS-11, PM-NIL 2, and PV-BHK 21 strains) in the brain tissue of rabbits, baby hamster kidney (BHK) cells, SMB, guinea pig brain cells, CEO cells, Vero cells, or other substrates (Precausta *et al.*, 1991; Reculard, 1996). Neonatal mice are used for production of the vaccine strains because they lack the antigenic myelin that caused encephalomyelitis occasionally noted in animals vaccinated with earlier SMB, NTO killed rabies vaccines.

Various methods have been and are used to render the virus nonpathogenic to produce the inactivated rabies vaccines. These include, but are not limited to, BPL, ultraviolet (UV) light, and acetylethyleneimine and other amines. Phenol and formaldehyde are no longer recommended (Reculard, 1996). The most commonly used inactivating agent is BPL. Once inactivated, adjuvants are added to the vaccine to increase the immune response to the antigen. The most common adjuvants are aluminum hydroxide, aluminum phosphate, saponin (cattle vaccines), and rarely, oil adjuvants (Precausta, 1991). Much of the information on cell lines, inactivating methods, and adjuvants are proprietary and cannot be reported specifically for any one vaccine. The stability of these inactivated cell-culture rabies vaccines has allowed them to be combined with other vaccines and bacterins. The potency and safety of the inactivated rabies vaccines have proved to be quite good.

D. The NIH Test

In 1974, the National Institutes of Health (NIH) of the U. S. Department of Health and Human Services adopted a test to measure the potency of inactivated rabies vaccines (Seligmann, 1973). This was necessary because of the poor performance of the initially manufactured tissue-culture-origin vaccines (Bunn, 1991). The NIH potency test relies on exposure to one challenge virus strain, the challenge virus standard or CVS strain thought to be derived from the original Pasteur isolate (Baer, 1997). This test has some inherent bias when comparing vaccine efficacy against wild (street) virus strains as compared with the CVS strain (Wonderli, 1992; Baer, 1997). Although a number of other tests are used to measure vaccine potency throughout the World (WHO, 1984, 1994; Ferguson *et al.*, 1984; Perrin *et al.*, 1990; Rooijakkers *et al.*, 1996), the NIH test is considered the "gold standard" for measuring the ability of an inactivated vaccine to protect against virus challenge.

E. Postvaccinal Complications

Due to their higher antigenic mass and the use of adjuvants, the inactivated rabies vaccines have produced both local and systemic postvaccinal reactions. The most common nonneurologic reactions include soreness, lameness, and regional lymphadenopathy in the injected limb. Fever and anaphylaxis also have been reported (Greene *et al.*, 1998; Dreesen, 1999). Focal vasculitis and granulomas have been reported 3–6 months after vaccination (Greene *et al.*, 1998). Postvaccinal sarcomas may develop, especially in cats, months to years following vaccination (Dubielzig *et al.*, 1993; Kass *et al.*, 1998). These sarcomas are often aggressive and invasive. The new generation of vectored recombinant vaccines now appearing on the market, such as the avipoxvirus vaccine recently licensed or use for cats in the United States (a live recombinant rabies glycoprotein–canarypox–vectored vaccine), should produce few, if any, allergic or neoplastic reactions (Greene *et al.*, 1998). Recombinant vaccines for wildlife rabies control are discussed in Sect. III A.

F. WHO Report

The WHO's World Survey of Rabies (1998) reported that there are at least 27 countries or territories that reported producing animal rabies vaccines during 1998. Fourteen countries used cell cultures, 11 used neural tissues, and 10 used embryonated eggs to produce rabies vaccines. Seven countries produced more than one type of rabies vaccine. Both MLV and inactivated rabies vaccines are produced worldwide. Brazil is the major producer of NTO vaccines for animal use, followed by Bangladesh, Romania, Tunisia, and El Salvador. These five countries account for 99.8% of the 23.5 million doses of NTO rabies vaccine, primarily of SMB origin (Fuenzalida strain), reported produced in the year. This same 1998 survey reported that the United States produced approximately 54 million doses of rabies vaccines of tissue culture origin (TCO), which is 84% of all TCO animal rabies vaccines produced. Vietnam is reportedly the primary source of the embryonated-egg-origin rabies vaccines for animals, producing 88% of this vaccine worldwide. It should be noted here that Argentina, France, Germany, India, and a number of other countries that presumably produce animal rabies vaccines did not contribute to the WHO (1998) report.

G. Rabies Vaccines in Latin America

During the 2-year period 1998–1999, the availability of rabies vaccines for dogs and cats in Latin America increased by 10.7%, and the total doses of vaccine administered for these species rose by 3.1% (Pan American Health Oranization/World Health Organization, 2001). Vaccine coverage increased from 2.2% in Brazil to 36.7% in the southern cone (Argentina, Chile, Paraguay, and Uruguay). However, there was a 16.3% decline in the Andean area (Bolivia, Columbia, Ecuador, Peru, and Venezuela) and a 6.8% decline in Central America. This same report indicates that in the Andean area, 67% of the canine population was vaccinated; the southern cone, 14.7%; Brazil, 85%; Central America, 38%; Mexico, 88%; and Latin Caribbean, 41%. The WHO recommends that 70% of dogs in a population should be effectively immunized to prevent an epidemic of canine rabies (Coleman, 1996). There were 3600 cases of canine rabies laboratory-confirmed in all of Latin America during 1998 and 2500 during 1999. During these same periods, cattle accounted for 3298 and 3225 cases and other domestic animals accounted for 575 and 593 cases, respectively.

H. Rabies Vaccines in the United States

Many rabies vaccines are currently marketed in the United States for use in domestic animals. One vaccine (the oral recombinant vaccinia–rabies glycoprotein virus vaccine) is licensed for restricted use in wildlife. As stated earlier, there are no MLV (attenuated) rabies vaccines for use in the United States. All currently licensed killed rabies vaccines intended for use in carnivores must protect 22 of 25 or 26 of 30 (or a statistically equivalent number) animals from an intramuscular challenge with a rabies virus for 90 days after challenge, and 80% of controls must die from the virus challenge (9 CFR 1, 2000). Alternative virus challenge requirements have been outlined when the test animals are of a species other than carnivores (9 CFR 1, 2000). The U.S. Department of Agriculture (USDA), Animal and Plant Health Inspection Service (APHIS), Center for Veterinary Biologics, has jurisdiction over licensure of rabies vaccines in the United States. The National Association of State Public Health Veterinarians (NASPHV) publishes annually the Compendium of Animal Rabies Prevention and Control (Compendium, 2001) in the *Journal of the American Veterinary Medical Association* and in the *Morbidity and Mortality Weekly Reports* (see http://www.cdc.gov/mmwr/). This compendium is a basis for animal rabies programs, and the NASPHV issues it as recommendations. Some states (i.e., Georgia) and various cities and counties adopt the recommendations in the compendium as regulations for animal rabies control and prevention.

I. Rabies Vaccines

The compendium for 2001 shows that there are 11 monovalent rabies vaccines licensed for dogs, 12 for cats, 1 for ferrets, 3 for horses, 4 for cattle, and 5 for sheep. Various rabies inactivated vaccines are combined with other biologicals for use in cats and horses (7 and 2 vaccines, respectively). In 2000, a new generation of vaccines was licensed for use in cats. These are the live recombinant rabies glycoprotein–canarypox–vectored vaccines, either monovalent or in combination (see Sect. IIIA2).

The inactivated vaccines of tissue origin should be used in animals at 3 months of age or older and then again 1 year later. This minimum age precludes maternal antibody blockage and recognizes the immature immune system's often poor response (Greene *et al.*, 1998). Depending on the vaccine, the animal species, and at times, local regulations, the animals should be vaccinated annually or triennially thereafter (Compendium, 2001). Again, depending on the vaccine and the species, the vaccine is administered either IM or SC, whereas some vaccines can be administered either way. The minimum age for vaccination is 8 weeks of age for the newly licensed vectored vaccines.

From an epidemiologic viewpoint, the effectiveness of canine rabies prevention and control programs can be measured by comparing reports of rabies in dogs with reports of increases in cat rabies during the recent raccoon rabies epidemic in the middle Atlantic and northeastern United States (Krebs *et al.*, 1997;

Hanlon *et al.*, 1998). This increase in rabies cases in cats, while dog rabies cases remained substantially unchanged, reflects the vaccine status of the two populations as well as the number of feral animals in the two populations (Eng and Fishbein, 1990; Petronek, 1998; Dreesen, 1999). In one of these reports, we learn that less than half (43%) of the rabies cases confirmed in the United States were of owned pets, whereas 84% of rabid dogs were pets (Eng and Fishbein, 1990). Of 54 respondents in the 1994 survey of state and community health officials, 74% stated that canine rabies vaccination was required by state law, whereas only 52% stated that cat vaccination was state law (Johnson and Walden, 1996). The need for cat vaccination and feral population control cannot be overemphasized (Dreesen, 1999). In fact, in the 1995 survey, over-the-counter sales of rabies vaccines were permitted in 22 states, and at that time, vaccination of wolf hybrids was permitted in 14 states; however, in all but 2 of these 14 states the owner was required to sign a liability statement. Fourteen states did not address the wolf-hybrid issue (Johnson and Walden, 1996).

J. Ferrets and Wolf Hybrids

In 1998, after extensive studies at the Centers for Disease Control and Prevention (CDC) (Niezgoda *et al.*, 1997), a rabies vaccine for ferrets was approved by the USDA APHIS. The guidelines for this rabies vaccine state that the ferret should be treated in a similar manner as a dog or cat with regard to vaccination and postexposure management (Compendium, 2001).

Vaccination of wolf hybrids with canine rabies vaccine is still a matter of considerable debate. The USDA APHIS is currently receiving and reviewing data on rabies vaccination of wolf hybrids. In a meeting of taxonomists in 1996, it was concluded that rabies vaccines for dogs *probably* would protect wolves and their hybrids because they are genetically virtually indistinct from the domestic dog (Dreesen, 1999). At least one well-documented case of rabies has occurred in a properly vaccinated wolf hybrid (Jay *et al.*, 1994). This animal was vaccinated with a 3-year vaccine at 4 months of age and received other vaccines and bacterins and an antihelminic on the same day. Six months later the animal was found with a dead skunk in its mouth. Within 3 weeks, the animal developed signs suggestive of rabies, was euthanitized, and rabies was confirmed in laboratory tests. Currently, in 2001, there are no licensed rabies vaccines for wolf hybrids.

K. Rabies Virus Variants of Wildlife Animals in the United States

Using genetic typing, distinctive patterns of nucleotide substitution are identified by direct sequencing of amplified genomic material using polymerase chain reaction (PCR) technology (Smith *et al.*, 1993; Tordo, 1996). These new and more sophisticated techniques have provided evidence of specific differences in rabies viruses within and between animal species in various geographic areas of the world (see Chap. 3). Various virus relationships such as genotypes or strains of rabies virus are noted and determined by nucleotide sequence homology. There are at least five strains of skunk rabies virus in the United States, as well as multiple strains of bat rabies viruses. Raccoon, dog, and cat rabies infections are caused by identifiable strains of the virus in the United States, as are several strains in various fox species. The strains of the virus occurring in dogs in the United States can be differentiated from those occurring elsewhere in the world. Even though rabies viruses differ within and between various animal species, it appears from epidemiologic evidence that regardless of the virus strain, a properly administered rabies vaccine given to an immunocompetant animal is capable of protecting the animal from rabies virus infection.

L. Postexposure Prophylaxis (PEP) for Domestic Animals

An animal should be immunized approximately 1 month after the primary vaccination when the peak antibody titer is reached (Compendium, 2001). Thus an animal is considered immunized if the primary vaccination was administered at least 30 days previously and the follow-up vaccinations have been administered as recommended by the vaccine package insert carrying the appropriate information and/or the compendium (2001). The NASPHV (Compendium, 2001) recommends that unvaccinated dogs, cats, and ferrets exposed to a known or suspected rabid animal should be euthanitized immediately. If not euthanitized, the animal should be placed in strict quarantine for 6 months and vaccinated 1 month prior to release. Animals with expired rabies vaccinations should be evaluated on a case-by-case basis. Currently, vaccinated dogs, cats, and ferrets should be revaccinated immediately following rabies exposure and kept under control and observation for 45 days. Vaccinated livestock exposed to rabies should be revaccinated and observed for 45 days (Compendium, 2001). If not vaccinated previously, food animals should be slaughtered within 7 days with disposal of tissues in the exposed area. If not slaughtered within this time period, the animal should be observed closely for 6 months.

As mentioned previously, the compendium (2001) is issued as recommendations only. Some states do not adhere strictly to the recommendations. The Texas Health and Safety Code originally followed the previously noted recommendations for animals exposed to rabies (Clark *et al.*, 1996). However, in 1988, the code was amended; unvaccinated domestic animals exposed to a rabid animal were to be euthanitized *or* vaccinated immediately after exposure, kept in isolation for 90 days, and given booster vaccinations in the third and eighth weeks of isolation. This regimen was based loosely on recommendations for humans exposed to rabies virus. A retrospective study found that 99.7% of 713 unvaccinated animals did not develop rabies during the 1979–1987 period when the recommendations of the NASPHV was followed (Clark *et al.*, 1996). Two PEP failures (0.3%) were reported. For the period 1988–1994, after the Texas code was amended to allow PEP for unvaccinated animals exposed to rabies, 629 of 632 animals (99.5%) that received the PEP booster vaccinations did not die of rabies. There was no statistical difference between the two regimens under conditions followed in Texas. In a follow-up study for the years 1995–1998, only 4 of 830 (0.5%) domestic animals that received the PEP protocol as recommended during the preceding 7-year period developed clinical rabies (Wilson *et al.*, 2001). The authors concluded that this is an effective PEP protocol and "has been proven to be effective for the control of rabies in animals." This alternative method of PEP in the handling of unvaccinated domestic animals exposed to rabies, as practiced in Texas, has not been endorsed by the NASPHV (Compendium, 2001).

III. THE NEXT GENERATION OF RABIES VACCINES

For the past two decades, investigators have been searching for alternative immunizing vectors that have all the advantages of virus replicating agents for total stimulation of the immune response in animals and humans without the undesirable side effects that are sometimes associated with the killed or modified live rabies virus vaccines. The present high-quality cell-culture rabies vaccines for humans are virtually 100% efficacious when they are used in accordance with the present ACIP or WHO recommendations for pre- or postexposure vaccination. One could say that there is little need to develop a more efficacious human rabies vaccine. However, improvements certainly can be made to the present human rabies vaccines. For example, less expensive rabies vaccines are desperately needed in developing countries to replace the present NTVs. It is unrealistic to imagine that the expensive vaccines and vaccination protocols currently used in industrialized countries will be able to be implemented widely in developing countries. Therefore, new-generation rabies vaccines must be developed that are inexpensive enough to vaccinate millions of people at risk in canine rabies–endemic countries. One of the possibilities for the next generation of human rabies vaccines to meet this specific need, which has been investigated in humans, is the nonreplicating recombinant canarypox virus that expresses the rabies virus glycoprotein as the key immunogenic component (Cadoz *et al.*, 1992). Live canarypox virus that expresses the rabies glycoprotein already has been licensed as a combination-type vaccine for use in cats (Compendium, 2001). Ease of production in high titer and induction of a full range of immune responses are among the many advantages that poxviruses have as a vector for vaccination in humans. Another vaccine vector that has potential and is currently being investigated for human vaccination is the replication-defective human adenovirus recombinant expressing the rabies glycoprotein (Xiang *et al.*, 1996). Using a different approach, another possibility is to apply DNA vaccine technology to develop a rabies vaccine that could be mass produced inexpensively and contain more than one antigenic component to protect individuals not only against rabies but also against other rabies-like viruses (i.e., Mokola, Duvenhage, and Lagos bat viruses) (see Chap. 2). Currently, this technology is being explored in nonhuman primates with the objective of developing a rabies DNA vaccine for humans because it is possible that it would provide additional protection to persons at risk of exposure to rabies in areas where rabies-related viruses also have been identified (Bahloul *et al.*, 1998; Lodmell *et al.*, 1998; Lodmell and Ewalt, 2001). Another possibility currently being investigated is the expression of the rabies virus glycoprotein in plants (McGarvey *et al.*, 1995; Yusibov *et al.*, 1997). These and other candidate vaccine vector systems are being developed as possible next-generation rabies vaccines for protection of humans and wildlife animals. Some of the next-generation rabies vaccines and vaccine vector systems under development are described more fully below.

Finally, the lengthy vaccination schedules associated with PET in humans for rabies are a deterrent for many people in developing countries who cannot afford to travel several times to distant antirabies centers to receive treatment. A rabies vaccine that would provide protection from a challenge without the cost involved in traveling five or more times to a clinic for a postexposure regimen would be tremendously advantageous in both developing and industrialized countries.

A. Oral Rabies Vaccines for Wildlife

1. SAG-1 and SAG-2 Modified Live Rabies Virus Vaccines

The first attempts to vaccinate free-ranging animals that act as vectors for the spread of rabies virus among wildlife species began in the 1970s in Europe (Aubert *et al.*, 1984). Following many field trials in several European countries using intense baiting methods and baits that were filled with the SAD strain of rabies virus, the disease began to disappear from major parts of those countries where the trials were conducted (Pastoret *et al.*, 1987; Irsara *et al.*, 1990). The vaccinal baits were ladened with the traditional rabies virus vaccine strains (SAD–Berne and the attenuated SAD–B19), but these live-virus vaccines unfortunately contained some residual pathogenicity for a variety of rodents in the field (Artois *et al.*, 1992). This lead to the development of rabies vaccine strains that were based on low-virulence variants of the SAD strain that could be isolated from the parental strain using an appropriate monoclonal antibody. The variants that were selected from the SAD–Berne strain, based on their resistance to neutralization by the epitope-specific monoclonal antibody that recognizes arginine 333, had a serine instead of arginine in position 333 of the envelope glycoprotein. The phenotype of the variant viruses was, as expected from previous findings with the ERA and CVS strains, slightly pathogenic in suckling mice but avirulent (nonpathogenic) in adult mice by all routes of inoculation (Dietzschold *et al.*, 1983; Coulon *et al.*, 1983; Seif *et al.*, 1985; Leblois and Flamand, 1988; Tuffereau *et al.*, 1989). The two rabies virus variants that were derived from the SAD–Berne virus were designated the SAG-1 and SAG-2 (SAD-Avirulent-Gif) vaccines (LeBlois *et al.*, 1990; Coulon *et al.*, 1992; Lafay *et al.*, 1994). In the SAG-1 virus vaccine, a single nucleotide mutation in codon 333 produces the serine substitution, and in SAG-2, a double mutation in the same position codes for glutamine, both substituting for arginine 333 in the viral surface glycoprotein of the parental SAD–Berne strain. SAG-1 is considered safe for wildlife vaccines and has been used extensively in rabies vaccination field trials to control rabies in fox populations in Europe with no evidence of reverting to the parental phenotype (Aubert *et al.*, 1994; Artois *et al.*, 1997). SAG-2, on the other hand, is genetically more stable because it would have to undergo two mutations rather than one to revert to the virulent parental strain. SAG-2 also has been tested, by the oral route, in various nontarget as well as potential target species with no side effects and is considered safe (Fekadu *et al.*, 1996; Bingham *et al.*, 1997).

2. Live Recombinant Poxvirus-Vectored Vaccines

In the early 1980s, soon after the rabies virus glycoprotein gene was cloned and its sequence was determined, efforts were initiated to produce what has become the first heterologous recombinant virus vaccine for use in oral vaccination of wildlife against rabies (Kieny *et al.*, 1984; Wiktor *et al.*, 1984). This recombinant rabies vaccine was developed at a time when the vaccinal baits containing the traditional rabies virus vaccine strains (SAD–Berne and the attenuated SAD-B19), which were being used for immunization of free-ranging foxes in Europe, were raising serious concerns about their safety for certain wildlife species (Winkler *et al.*, 1976; Attois *et al.*, 1992). It therefore was essential, from a safety perspective, to develop a vaccine that could be used in baits, would be rabies virus–free, and still would induce full protection against a rabies virus challenge in animals that were vaccinated subcutaneously or by scarification with the vaccine. It also was to be equally effective as an oral vaccine. Fortunately, this was achieved with vaccinia virus (Copenhagen strain) as a virus vector in which the glycoprotein gene of the ERA strain of rabies virus was inserted into the thymidine kinase region of the vaccinia virus (VV) genome (Kieny *et al.*, 1984; Wiktor *et al.*, 1984). The vaccinia–rabies glycoprotein (VRG) recombinant virus was tested initially in laboratory animals, first by injecting the recombinant vaccine subcutaneously and later by administering the vaccine orally to laboratory mice. In both cases, virus-neutralizing antibodies (VNAs) were induced rapidly, and the animals were protected against a lethal rabies virus challenge (Wiktor *et al.*, 1984; Rupprecht *et al.*, 1988). Then, in a series of vaccine trials that followed in the United States and Europe, the safety and efficacy of the VRG virus vaccine administered parenterally or orally to a broad range of over 40 different families of animals, including the anticipated target species, the raccoon (*Procyon lotor*), was evaluated. These trials were conducted with major concerns for the release of multiple doses of the vaccine in baits and the unknown effects on nontarget wildlife populations, the possible long-term genetic and thermal stability of the vaccine vector, and the multiple public health implications. Nevertheless, the vaccine trials demonstrated that the recombinant VRG virus vaccine was capable of inducing high titers of VNAs and of protecting animals from rabies virus (Wiktor *et al.*, 1985; Rupprecht *et al.*, 1986; Brochier *et al.*, 1990, 1991, 1995; Demettre *et al.*, 1992). After comparing various immunization routes (i.e., by intramuscular, buccal scarification, and oral) under different experimental protocols, the proof of principal therefore was established that the VRG virus vaccine is safe and efficacious to administer as an oral rabies vaccine to wildlife. Soon, other poxviruses, including the orthopoxvirus of raccoon (Esposito *et al.*, 1992) and avianpox viruses, such as the fowlpox (Taylor *et al.*, 1988) and canarypox (Taylor *et al.*, 1991; Cadoz *et al.*, 1992) viruses, as well as different strains of VV, were investigated as possible alternative virus vectors for expression of rabies virus antigens. Some of these developments, which also underline the importance of the rabies nucleoprotein in protection (Fekadu *et al.*, 1992; Fujii *et al.*, 1994; Hooper *et al.*, 1994), could well become the live recombinant rabies vaccines of the next generation, if not for oral use, as a vaccine for parenteral immunization. In 1995, the VRG virus vaccine (RABORAL V-RG) was licensed by the USDA APHIS for restricted use in oral immunization of raccoons and is now available commercially.

3. Live Recombinant Adenovirus-Vectored Vaccines

Initial interest in the development of an oral adenovirus-vectored rabies vaccine stemmed from the long-time use of nonattenuated adenoviruses as oral vaccines against respiratory infection (Chaloner-Larsson *et al.*, 1986). To use the adenovirus as an expression vector, the rabies glycoprotein gene was inserted into the replication-nonessential E3 locus of the human adenovirus type 5 genome, and this was tested orally in several animal species, including mice, dogs, foxes, and skunks (Prevec *et al.*, 1990; Charlton *et al.*, 1992). With a growing interest in the use of adenoviruses to express the rabies glycoprotein and possibly the nucleoprotein for gene therapy as well as vaccination, the adenovirus-vectored vaccines clearly have moved into the realm of possible next-generation vaccines (Xiang *et al.*, 1996; Wang *et al.*, 1997). The more recently developed adenovirus vectors, of human serotypes 2 and 5, have been made replication-defective by the deletion of essential genes from the E1 locus that are required for the initiation of viral replication. The E3 gene locus is also deleted to downregulate expression of major histocompatibility complex antigens and protect the adenovirus-infected cells from T-cell-mediated destruction (Wold and Gooding, 1991; Yang *et al.*, 1994). Interestingly, the adenovirus recombinant expressing the rabies glycoprotein, given subcutaneously (parenteral immunization) to mice during the neonatal period or at several weeks of age, induces an immune response to rabies virus even in the presence of maternally transferred immunity to rabies virus (Wang *et al.*, 1997). This promotes the possibility of vaccinating the young animals during the early postnatal period. A recent report also demonstrates for the first time that the recombinant adenovirus expressing the rabies virus glycoprotein is capable of inducing high titers of antirabies VNA in dogs previously immunized with rabies vaccine (Tims *et al.*, 2000). The levels of VNA induced in these dogs following the booster immunization with the recombinant adenovirus are reported to be higher than the levels that can be achieved with the conventional vaccines, suggesting that the recombinant adenovirus rabies vaccine is capable of inducing a strong anamnestic response in dogs. It remains to be confirmed experimentally whether the recombinant adenovirus rabies vaccine will be efficacious in dogs immunized prior to 3 months of age (Tims *et al.*, 2000).

4. Oral Rabies Vaccines Derived from Plants

In the last two decades, plants have become prospects in the vaccine development process for effective, inexpensive, and safe production and delivery of vaccines (Yusibov *et al.*, 1999; Koprowski and Yusibov, 2001; Streatfield *et al.*, 2001). Plant viruses, such as tobacco mosaic virus (TMV) and tomato bushy stunt virus, serving as vectors for expression of foreign antigens in plants, have provided prototypes of plant-derived, genetically manufactured vaccines produced in tomatoes and tobacco leaves (McGarvey *et al.*, 1995; Yusibov *et al.*, 1997). To capitalize on the advantages of plants and plant crops for protein expression, particularly the tobacco plant, which include their suitability as hosts for plant virus–vectored protein expression and their considerable biomass for protein production, plant virus–based expression vectors will be the focus of much interest (Yusibov *et al.*, 1999). First it was necessary to show that vaccine antigens are expressed in a form that is immunogenic for mice immunized intramuscularly (Yusibov *et al.*, 1997). Then it followed that mice that were immunized orally (by gastric intubation or by feeding on antigen-producing spinach leaves) or parenterally (by intraperitoneal injection) with the plant-derived rabies-specific antigen could be protected from a lethal rabies virus challenge (Modelska *et al.*, 1998). These new approaches are promising and much needed to address the concerns of cost, safety, and accessibility of vector-produced proteins and vaccines for the future control of rabies. The many advantages of plant production systems in obtaining large amounts of products from transgenically or virally infected plants have been noted by several laboratories and commercial companies devoted to producing antibodies, antigens, and other medically important proteins (Yusibov and Koprowski, 1998).

B. Nucleic Acid (DNA)–Based Rabies Vaccines

DNA-based vaccines were developed initially as a rather simple (a basic plasmid preparation) yet versatile approach to the induction of immune responses when injected directly into the host compared with conventional vaccines (Donnelly *et al.*, 1994). Most significantly, they provide an efficient way to induce a cytolytic CD8+ T-cell response against an antigen in addition to VNA and CD4+ cells. The CD8+ T-cell response is an important aspect of the immune response that often fails to be evoked by recombinant antigens and synthetic peptides, either alone or in conventional inactivated vaccines (Germain, 1994; reviewed in Donnelly *et al.*, 1997). Protection against rabies, as in many other viral diseases, is mediated by neutralizing antibodies and/or T-lymphocytes, i.e., CD4+ T-helper (Th) cells and CD8+ cytotoxic T-lymphocytes (CTLs). Fortunately, the DNA vaccine strategy provides the required induction of cytolytic CD8+ cells (Donnelly *et al.*, 1997). Unfortunately, delivery of the DNA to the target cells where it can induce the complete immune response tends to be inefficient.

The first demonstration that a plasmid vector carrying a rabies virus antigen could immunize and protect animals against rabies virus challenge was accomplished with a plasmid carrying the rabies glycoprotein (ERA strain) gene (Xiang *et al.*, 1994). The rabies DNA vaccine stimulated a specific immune response, including antibodies, Th-cells, and CTLs. Various studies that followed addressed different aspects that might influence the efficacy of rabies DNA vaccines, including the effects of cytokines and certain parameters of the expression vector that are likely to play a role in DNA vaccine efficacy. One of these studies focused on the viral promoter (a regulatory element in the plasmid) in DNA vaccines to give a broader tissue specificity and greater strength of inducing transcription in the transfected target cell (Xiang *et al.*, 1995). The study showed that when the cytomegalovirus (CMV) promoter was used to replace the simian virus 40 (SV40) promoter, it made little difference to the rabies glycoprotein expression following intramuscular inoculation, whereas the two promoters showed a significant difference in their ability to express the rabies glycoprotein *in vitro*. In both cases, DNA vaccination induced immunity to rabies virus that was extraordinarily longlasting. Other studies by the same investigators examined the expressive effects of different cytokines on the immune system when coinoculated with a rabies DNA vaccine that expresses the rabies glycoprotein (Xiang and Ertl, 1995; Xiang *et al.*, 1997). Interestingly, expression of the granulocyte–macrophage colony-stimulation factor (GM-CSF) had the effect of enhancing the Th-cell and B-cell response to the rabies virus glycoprotein, presumably by triggering activation of local dendritic cells that present antigen to T cells. However, the anti-glycoprotein antibody response was transient in the presence of coexpressed GM-CSF and was sustained less well compared with the antibody response to the plasmid expressing the rabies virus glycoprotein alone (Xiang and Ertl, 1995). In contrast, when plasmid DNA expressing interferon-gamma (IFN-γ) was coinoculated with the plasmid expressing the rabies virus glycoprotein, the effect of the IFN-γ was dependent on the promoter in the plasmid that controls expression. Surprisingly, the effect of the promoter controlling IFN-γ expression was to elicit a rather weak Th-cell response and antibody response to rabies virus glycoprotein.

To exploit the potential versatility of DNA-based vaccines for rabies and address another important aspect of immune protection against rabies viruses, the ability of a DNA vaccine to protect against different lyssavirus genotypes simultaneously was investigated. The possibility that a multivalent vaccine of at least two viral antigens would protect against more than one lyssavirus genotype was tested (Bahloul *et al.*, 1998). The glycoprotein from the rabies virus (genotype 1) and the glycoprotein from Mokola virus (genotype 3) were expressed individually (by two separate plasmids) or as a chimeric protein (by one plasmid). The chimeric glycoprotein gene encoded the amino-terminal part of the Mokola virus glycoprotein and the carboxy-terminal part of the rabies virus (PV strain) glycoprotein. All three DNA vaccines were fully immunoprotective against a lethal rabies virus challenge in mice, inducing a range of antigen-specific and nonspecific immune responses following intramuscular injection. The cross-reactivity studies were impressive in that the DNA expressing the rabies virus glycoprotein showed cross-reactivity against Duvenhage virus (genotype 4), European bat lyssaviruses 1 and 2 (genotypes 5 and 6, respectively), and the homologous rabies virus (genotype 1). The Mokola virus glycoprotein showed cross-reactivity against Lagos bat virus (genotype 2) as well as Mokola virus (genotype 3), and the chimeric glycoprotein showed cross-reactivity against all genotypes except genotype 4, which was weakly neutralized (Bahloul *et al.*, 1998).

Different routes of DNA immunization have proved useful to elicit immune responses that are protective in a variety of experimental models (Donnelly *et al.*, 1994; Xiang *et al.*, 1995; Ray *et al.*, 1997; Lodmell *et al.*, 1998a,b; Perrin *et al.*, 2000). But not all routes are equally effective for induction of rabies VNA in all animal models (Lodmell *et al.*, 1998b). These include intramuscular, intradermal, and direct intracellular epidermal delivery of plasmid DNA-coated gold microparticles via a handheld gene gun. The gene gun permits a more simple and rapid delivery of DNA in comparison with a typical needle injection, and more importantly, the gene gun is thought to propel the DNA-coated beads through the plasma membrane of cells. Consequently, cells are transfected directly without invoking a cellular internalization mechanism (Lodmell *et al.*, 1998a). Because DNA vaccines do not contain a protein component (other than what they express), the host does not mount an immune response to the vaccine booster immunization after receiving the primary immunization. A booster immunization with the gene gun elicits a strong anamnestic response and protection from rabies virus challenge (Lodmell *et al.*, 1998b). Rabies VNA titers are boosted dramatically when animals are vaccinated with DNA by the gene gun, and the fact that this was demonstrated successfully in nonhuman primates bodes well for the preexposure immunization of humans using rabies DNA vaccine coated on beads propelled by the gene gun.

One notable problem with rabies DNA vaccines is the delayed onset of the rabies VNA response following DNA immunizations. Consequently, to be successful in rabies PET, DNA immunization systems and strategies will need to be modified to accelerate the VNA response (Lodmell *et al.*, 2001). Several methods for optimization of DNA vaccine expression and improved vaccine immunogenicity have been investigated, but few have actually accelerated the onset of antibody production. These include the use of adjuvents, delivery of the DNA in liposomes, and adding immunostimulatory sequences into the DNA backbone to enhance antibody responses (Sato *et al.*, 1996; Jones *et al.*, 1997; Roman *et al.*, 1997; Chen *et al.*, 1998). One approach that does appear to accelerate the onset of rabies VNA production involved the strategy of combining several sites in which to vaccinate with the use of different vaccination techniques and multiple booster immunizations (Lodmell and Ewalt, 2001). A site for DNA vaccine injection that has produced a much stronger antibody response than intramuscular injection in quadriceps or an intradermal injection into abdominal skin is the ear pinna (Forg *et al.*, 1998). This was confirmed with the rabies DNA vaccine. After primary immunization with the rabies DNA vaccine given intradermally in the ear pinna of mice, via gene gun vaccination, rabies VNAs were detected 7 days after vaccination, which is a significant improvement over mice that received vaccine in only one anatomic site (Lodmell and Ewalt, 2001). In a postexposure model, the rabies DNA vaccine given in two or more sites and in multiple doses was as effective as the HDVC vaccinations given in the same intervals and frequency. Thus rabies DNA vaccines have considerable promise for human rabies PET and, at some point in the future, perhaps with further DNA vaccine development, are worth pursuing.

REFERENCES

Abelseth, M. K. (1964). Propagation of rabies virus in pig kidney cell culture. *Can. Vet. J.* **5**, 84–86.
Arai, Y. T., Ogata, T., and Oya, A. (1991). Studies on Japanese-produced chick embryo cell culture rabies vaccines. *Am. J. Trop. Med. Hyg.* **44**, 131–134.

Artois, M., Cliquet, F., Barrat, J., and Schumacher, C. L. (1997). Effectiveness of SAG1 oral vaccine for the long-term protection of red foxes (*Vulpes vulpes*) against rabies. *Vet. Rec.* **140**, 57–59.

Artois, M., Guittre, C., Thomas, I., Leblois, H., Brochier, B., and Barrat, J. (1992). Potential pathogenicity for rodents of vaccines intended for oral vaccination against rabies: A comparison. *Vaccine* **10**, 524–528.

Arya, S. C. (1994). Transmissible spongiform encephalopathies and sheep-brain-derived rabies vaccines. *Biologicals* **22**, 73.

Aubert, M. F. A., Masson, E., Artois, M., and Barrat, J. (1994). Oral wildlife rabies vaccination field trials in Europe, with recent emphasis on France. *Cur. Top. Microbiol. Immunol.* **187**, 219–243.

Baer, G. M. (1997). Evaluation of an animal rabies vaccine by use of two types of potency tests. *Am. J. Vet. Res.* **58**, 837–840.

Bahloul, C., Jacob, Y., Tordo, N., and Perrin, P. (1998). DNA-based immunization for exploring the enlargement of immunological cross-reactivity against the lyssaviruses. *Vaccine* **16**, 417–425.

Bahmanyar, M., Fayaz, A., Nour-Salehi, S., Mohammadi, M., and Koprowski, H. (1976). Successful protection of humans exposed to rabies infection: Post-exposure treatment with the new human diploid cell rabies vaccine and antirabies serum. *JAMA* **236**, 2751–2754.

Barth, R. K. (1994). Rabies in animals. *J. Gen. Med.* **6**, 4.

Barth, R., and Franke, V. (1996). Retal rhesus monkey lung diploid cell vaccine for humans. In *Laboratory Techniques in Rabies*, F.-X. Meslin, M. M. Kaplan, and H. Koprowski (eds.), 4th ed., pp. 297–300. World Health Organization, Geneva.

Barth, R., Gruschkau, H., Bijok, U., Hifenhaus, J., Hinz, J., Milcke, L., Mosier, H., Jaeger. O., Ronneberger, H., and Weinmann, E. (1984). A new inactivated tissue culture rabies vaccine for use in man: Evaluation of PCEC vaccine by laboratory tests. *J. Biol. Standard* **12**, 29–46.

Bijok, U. (1985). Purified chick embryo cell (PCEC) rabies vaccine: A review of the clinical development. In *Improvements in Rabies Postexposure Treatment*, I. Vodopija, K. G. Nicholson, S. Smerdel, and U. Bijok (eds.), pp. 103–111. Zagreb Institute of Public Health.

Bingham, J., Schumacher, C. L., Aubert, M. F. A., Hill, F. W. G., and Aubert, A. (1997). Innocuity studies of SAG-2 oral rabies vaccine in various Zimbabwean wild non-target species. *Vaccine* **15**, 937–943.

Blancou, J., and Meslin, F.-X. (1996). Modified live-virus rabies vaccination for oral immunizations of carnivores. In *Laboratory Techniques in Rabies*, F.-X. Meslin, M. M. Kaplan, and H. Koprowski (eds.), 4th ed., pp. 324–337. World Health Organization, Geneva.

Briggs, D. J., Banzhoff, A., Nicolay, U., Sirikwin, S., Dumavibhat, B., Tongswas, S., and Wasi, C. (2000). Antibody response of patients after postexposure rabies vaccination with small intradermal doses of purified chick embryo cell vaccine or purified vero cell rabies vaccine. *Bull. WHO* **78**, 693–698.

Brochier, B., Costy, F., and Pastoret, P.-P. (1995). Elimination of fox rabies from Belgium using a recombinant vaccinia–rabies glycoprotein vaccine: An update. *Vet. Mcrobiol.* **46**, 269–279.

Brochier, B., Kieny, M. P., Costy, F., Coppens, P., Bauduin, B., Lecocq, J. P., Languet, B., Chappuis, G., Desmettre, P., Afiademanyo, K., Libois, R., and Pastoret, P.-P. (1991). Large-scale eradication of rabies using recombinant vaccinia–rabies vaccine. *Nature* **354**, 520–522.

Brochier, B., Thomas, I., Bauduin, B., Leveau, T., Pastoret, P.-P., Languet, B., Chappuis, B., Desmettre, P., Blancou, J., and Artois, M. (1990). Use of vaccinia–rabies recombinant virus for the oral vaccination of foxes against rabies. *Vaccine* **8**, 101–104.

Bunn, T. O. (1991). Canine and feline rabies vaccines, past and present. In *The Natural History of Rabies*, G. M. Baer (ed.), 2d ed., pp. 415–425. CRC Press, Boca Raton, FL.

Cadoz, M., Strady, A., Meignier, B., Taylor, J., Tartaglia, J., Paoletti, E., and Plotkin, S. (1992). Immunisation with canarypox virus expressing rabies glycoprotein. *Lancet* **339**, 1429–1432.

CDC (1991). Human rabies prevention — United States, 1991: Recommendations of the Advisory Committee on Immunization Practices (ACIP). *Morbid. Mortal. Weekly Rep.* **40**, (RR-3), 1–14.

CDC (1999). Human rabies prevention — United States, 1999: Recommendations of the Advisory Committee on Immunization Practices (ACIP). *Morbid. Mortal. Weekly Rep.* **48**, (RR-1), 1–21.

Chaloner-Larsson, G., Contreras, G., Furesz, J., Boucher, D. W., Krepps, D., Humphreys, G. R., and Mohanna, S. M. (1986). Immunization of Canadian Armed Forces personnel with live types 4 and 7 adenovirus vaccines. *Can. J. Public Health* **77**, 367–370.

Charlton, K. M., Artois, M., Prevec, L., Campbell, J. B., Casey, G. A., Wandeler, A. I., and Armstrong, J. (1992). Oral rabies vaccination of skunks and foxes with a recombinant human adenovirus vaccine. *Arch. Virol.* **123**, 169–179.

Chen, S. C., Jones, D. H., Fynan, E. F., Farrar, G. H., Clegg, J. C., Greenberg, H. B., and Herrmann, J. E. (1998). Protective immunity induced by oral immunization with a rotavirus DNA vaccine encapsulated in microparticles. *J. Virol.* **72**, 5757–5761.

Chutivongse, S., Wilde, H., Supich, C., Baer, G. M., and Fishbein, D. B. (1990). Postexposure prophylaxis for rabies with antiserum and intradermal vaccination. *Lancet* **335**, 896–898.

Clark, K. A., and Wilson, P. J. (1996). Postexposure rabies prophylaxis and preexposure vaccination failure in domestic animals. *J. Am. Vet. Med. Assoc.* **208**, 1827–1830.

Coleman, P. G., and Dye, C. (1996). Immunization coverage required to prevent outbreaks of dog rabies. *Vaccine* **14**, 185–186.

Compendium of animal rabies vaccines, 2001. (2001). *J. Am. Vet. Med. Assoc.* **218**, 26–31.

Coulon, P., Lafay, F., Leblois, H., Tuffereau, C., Artois, M., Blancou, J., Benmansour, A., and Flamand, A. (1992). The SAG: A new attenuated oral rabies vaccine. In *Wildlife Rabies Control*, K. Bögel, F.-X. Meslin, and M. Kaplan (eds.), pp. 105–111. Wells Medical, Kent.

Coulon, P., Rollin, P. E., and Flamand, A. (1983). Molecular basis of rabies virus virulence: II. Identification of a site on the CVS glycoprotein associated with virulence. *J. Gen. Virol.* **64**, 693–696.

Desmettre, P., Languet, B., Chappuis, G., Brochier, B., Thomas, I., Lecocq, J.-P., Kieny, M.-P., Blancou, J., Aubert, M., Artois, M., and Pastoret, P.-P. (1990). Use of vaccinia rabies recombinant for oral vaccination of wildlife. *Vet. Microbiol.* **23**, 227–232.

Diaz, A. M. (1996). Suckling-mouse brain vaccine. In *Laboratory Techniques in Rabies*, F.-X. Meslin, M. M. Kaplan, and H. Koprowski (eds.), 4th ed., pp. 243–250. World Health Organization, Geneva.

Dietzschold, B., Wunner, W. H., Wiktor, T. J., Lopes, A. D., Lafon, M., Smith, C. L., and Koprowski, H. (1983). Characterization of an antigenic determinant of the glycoprotein that correlates with pathogenicity of rabies virus. *Proc. Natl. Acad. Sci. USA* **80**, 70–74.

Donnelly, J. J., Ulmer, J. B., and Liu, M. A. (1994). Immunization with DNA. *J. Immunol. Methods* **176**, 145–152.

Donnelly, J. J., Ulmer, J. B., Shiver, J. W., and Liu, M. A. (1997). DNA vaccines. *Ann. Rev. Immunol.* **15**, 617–648.

Dreesen, D. W. (1999). Preexposure rabies immunization. In *Rabies: Guidelines for Medical Professionals*, pp. 36–43. Veterinary Learning Systems, Trenton, NJ.

Dreesen, D. W., Bernard, K. W., Parker, R. A., Deutsch, A. J., and Brown, J. (1986). Immune complex–like disease in 23 persons following a booster dose of rabies human diploid cell vaccine. *Vaccine* **4**, 45–49.

Dubielzig, R. R., Hawkins, K. L., and Miller, P. C. (1993). Mycoplastic sarcoma originating at the site of rabies vaccination in a cat. *J. Vet. Diag. Invest.* **5**, 637–638.

Eng, T. R., and Fishbein, D. B. (1990). Epidemiologic factors, clinical findings, and vaccination status of rabies in cats and dogs in the United States in 1988. *J. Am. Vet. Med. Assoc.* **197**, 875–878.

Esposito, J. J., Knight, J. C., Shaddock, J. H., Novembre, F. J., and Baer, G. M. (1988). Successful oral rabies vaccination of raccoons with raccoon poxvirus recombinants expressing rabies virus glycoprotein. *Virology* **165**, 313–316.

Fekadu, M., Nesby, S. L., Shaddock, J. H., Schumacher, C. L., Linhart, S. B., and Sanderlin, D. W. (1996). Immunogenicity, efficacy, and safety of an oral rabies vaccine (SAG-2) in dogs. *Vaccine* **14**, 465–468.

Fedadu, M., Sumner, J. W., Shaddock, J. H., Sanderlin, D. W., and Baer, G. M. (1992). Sickness and recovery of dogs challenged with a street rabies virus after vaccination with a vaccinia virus recombinant expressing rabies virus N protein. *J. Virol.* **66**, 2601–2604.

Fenji, P. (1960). Propagation of rabies virus in a culture of hamster kidney cells, *Can. J. Microbiol.* **6**, 479–483.

Ferguson, M., Seagrott, V., and Schild, G. C. (1984). A collaborative study on the use of single immunodiffusion for the assay of rabies glycoprotein. *J. Biol. Standard* **12**, 283–294.

Fishbein, D. B., and Baer. G. M. (1988). Animal rabies: Implications for diagnosis and human treatment. *Ann. Intern. Med.* **109**, 935–937.

Forg, P., von Hoegen, P., Dalemans, W., and Schirrmacher, V. (1998). Superiority of the ear pinna over muscle tissue as site for DNA vaccination. *Gene Ther.* **5**, 789–797.

Friedberger, E., and Frohner, E. (1904). *Friedberger and Frohner's Veterinary Pathology*, Vol. 1, 4th ed., Hurst and Blackett, London.

Fuenzalida, E., and Palacios, R. (1955). Un método mejorado en la preparaciün de la vacuna antirábica [An improved method for preparation of rabies vaccine] *Bol. Inst. Bacteriol. Chile* **8**, 3–10.

Fujii, H., Takita-Sonoda, Y., Mifune, K., Hirai, K., Nishizono, A., and Mannen, K. (1994). Protective efficacy in mice of post-exposure vaccination with vaccinia virus recombinant expressing either rabies virus glycoprotein or nucleoprotein. *J. Gen. Virol.* **75**, 1339–1344.

Geison, G. L. (1990). Pasteur, Roux, and rabies: Scientific versus clinical mentalities. *J. Hist. Med.* **45**, 341–365.

Germain, R. N. (1994). MHC-dependent antigen processing and peptide presentation: Providing ligands for lymphocyte activation. *Cell* **76**, 287–299.

Greene, C. E., and Dreesen, D. W. (1998). Rabies. In *Infectious Diseases of the Dog and Cat*, C. E. Greene (ed.), 2nd ed., pp. 114–126. W. B. Saunders, Philadelphia.

Hanlon, C. A., and Rupprecht, C. E. (1998). The reemergence of rabies. In *Emerging Infections*, W. M. Schield, D. Armstrong, and J. M. Hughes, (eds.), pp. 59–80. ASM Press, Washington.

Haupt, W. (1999). Rabies — Risk of exposure and current trends in prevention of human cases. *Vaccine.* **17**, 1742–1749.

Hemachudha, T., Griffin, D. E., Giffels, J. J., Johnson, R. T., Moser, A. B., and Phanuphak, P. (1987). Myelin basic protein as an encephalitogen in encephalomyelitis and polyneuritis following rabies vaccination. *New Engl. J. Med.* **316**, 369–373.

Hendrick, M. J., Shafer, F. S., Goldschmidt, M. H., Haviland, J. C., Schelling, S. H., Engler, S. J., and Gliatto, J. M. (1994). Comparison of fibrosarcomas that developed at vaccination sites and at non-vaccination sites in cats: 239 cases (1991–1992). *J. Am. Vet. Med. Assoc.* **205**, 1425–1429.

Hooper, D. C., Pierard, I., Modelska, A., Otvos, L., Jr., Fu, Z. F., Koprowski, H., and Dietzschold, B. (1994). Rabies ribonucleocapsid as an oral immunogen and immunological enhancer. *Proc. Natl. Acad. Sci. USA* **91**, 10908–10912.

Irsara, A. Bressan, G., and Mutinelli, F. (1990). Sylvatic rabies in Italy: Epidemiology. *J. Vet. Med.* **B37**, 53–63.

Jay, M. T., Reilly, K. F., DeBess, E. E., Haynes, E. H., Bader, D. R., and Barrett, L. R. (1994). Rabies in a vaccinated wolf-dog hybrid. *J. Am. Vet. Med. Assoc.* **205**, 1729–1732.

Johnson, W. B., and Walden, M. B. (1996). Results of a national survey of rabies control procedures. *J. Am. Vet. Med. Assoc.* **208**, 1667–1672.

Jones, D. H., Corris, S., McDonald, S., Clegg, J. C., and Farrar, G. H. (1997). Poly(DL-lactide-CO-glycolide)–encapsulated plasmid DNA elicits systemic and mucosal antibody responses to encoded protein after oral administration. *Vaccine* **15**, 814–817.

Kass, P. H., Barnes, W. G., Spangler, W. L., Chomel, B. B., and Culbertson, M. R. (1993). Epidemiologic evidence for casual relation between vaccination and fibrosarcoma tumorigenisis in cats. *J. Am. Vet. Med. Assoc.* **203**, 396–405.

Kieny, M.-P., Lathe, R., Drillien, R., Spehner, D., Skory, S., Schmitt, D., Wiktor, T., Koprowski, H., and Lecocq, J. P. (1984). Expression of rabies virus glycoprotein from a recombinant vaccinia virus. *Nature* **312**, 163–166.

Koprowski, H., and Cox, H. R. (1948). Studies on chick embryo adapted rabies virus: I. Culture characteristics and pathogenicity. *J. Immunol.* **60**, 533–536.

Koprowski, H., Black, J., and Nelson, D. J. (1954). Studies on chick-embryo-adapted rabies virus: VI. Further changes in pathogenic properties following prolonged cultivation in the developing chick embryo. *J Immunol.* **72**, 94–97.

Koprowski, H., and Yusibov, V. (2001). The green revolution: Plants as heterologous expression vectors. *Vaccine* **19**, 2735–2741.

Krebs, J. W., Rupprecht, C. E., and Childs, J. E. (1997). Rabies surveillance in the United States during 1996. *J. Am. Vet. Med. Assoc.* **211**, 1525–1539.

Lafay, F., Benejean, J., Tuffereau, C., Flamand, A., and Coulon, P. (1994). Vaccination against rabies: Construction and characterization of SAG2, a double avirulent derivative of SAD$_{Berne}$. *Vaccine* **12**, 317–320.

Leblois, J., and Flamand, A. (1988). Studies on pathogenicity in mice of rabies virus strains used for oral vaccination of foxes in Europe. In *Vaccination to Control Rabies in Foxes*, P. P. Pastoret, B. Brochier, I. Thomas, and J. Blancou (eds.), pp. 101–104. Commission of the European Communities, Luxumbourg.

LeBlois, H., Tuffereau, C., Blancou, J., Artois, M., Aubert, A., and Flamand, A. (1990). Oral immunization of foxes with avirulent rabies virus mutants. *Vet. Microbiol.* **23**, 259–266.

Lépine, P., Atanasiu, P., Gamet, A., and Vialat, C. (1973). Phenolized, freeze-dried sheep brain vaccine: B. Method used at the Pasteur Institute, Paris. In *Laboratory Techniques in Rabies*, M. M. Kaplan and H. Koprowski (eds.), 3d ed., pp. 223–233. World Health Organization, Geneva.

Lodmell, D. L., and Ewalt, L. C. (2001). Post-exposure DNA vaccination protects mice against rabies virus. *Vaccine* **19**, 2468–2473.

Lodmell, D. L., Ray, N. B., and Ewalt, L. C. (1998a). Gene gun particle-mediated vaccination with plasmid DNA confers protective immunity against rabies virus infection. *Vaccine* **16**, 115–118.

Lodmell, D. L., Ray, N. B., Parnell, M. J., Ewalt, L. C., Hanlon, C. A., Shaddock, J. H., Sanderlin, D. S., and Rupprecht, C. E. (1998b). DNA immunization protects nonhuman primates against rabies virus. *Nature Med.* **4**, 949–952.

Martino, A. D. (1993). Transmissible spongiform encephalopathies and the safety of naturally derived biologicals. *Biologicals* **21**, 61–66.

McGarvey, P. B., Hammond, J., Denelt, M. M., Hooper, D. C., Fu, Z. Z., Dietzschold, B., Koprowski, H., and Michaels, F. H. (1995). Expression of the rabies virus glycoprotein in transgenic tomatoes. *Biotechnology* **13**, 1484–1487.

Meslin, F. X., and Kaplan, M. M. (1973). General considerations in the production and use of brain-tissue and purified chicken-embryo rabies vaccines for human use. In *Laboratory techniques in rabies*, F.-X. Meslin, M. M. Kaplan, and H. Koprowski (eds.), 4th ed., pp. 204–212. World Health Organization, Geneva.

Mitmoonpitak, C., Wilde, H., and Tepsumetanon, W. (1997). Current status of animal rabies in Thailand. *J. Vet. Med. Sci.* **59**, 457–460.

Modelska, A., Dietzschold, B., Sleysh, N., Fu, Z. F., Steplewski, K., Hooper, D. C., Koprowski, H., and Yusibov, V. (1998). Immunization against rabies with plant-derived antigen. *Proc. Natl. Acad. Sci. USA* **95**, 2481–2485.

Nicholson, K. G. (1996). Cell-culture vaccines for human use: general considerations. In *Laboratory Techniques in Rabies*, F.-X. Meslin, M. M. Kaplan, and H. Koprowski (eds.), 4th ed., pp. 271–279. World Health Organization, Geneva.

Niezgoda, M., Briggs, D. J., Shaddock, J. H., *et al.* (1997). Pathogenesis of experimentally induced rabies in the domestic ferret. *Am. J. Vet. Res.* **58**, 1327–1331.

Nogueira, Y. L. (1998). Adverse effect versus quality control of the Fuenzalida–Palacios antirabies vaccine. *Rev. Inst. Med. Trap. São Paulo* **40**, 295–299.

Pan American Health Organization/World Health Organization (1999). XI Inter-American Meeting, at the Ministerial Level, on Animal Health: Regional program for the elimination of human rabies transmitted by dogs in the Americas: Analysis of progress 1990–1998. Washington, DC, April 13–15, 1999. World Health Organization, Geneva.

Pan American Health Organization/World Health Organization (2001). XI Inter-American Meeting, at the Ministerial Level, on Health and Agriculture: Report of the VIII meeting of directors of national rabies control programs in Latin America (REDIPRA), São Paulo, Brazil, May 2–4, 2001. World Health Organization, Geneva.

Pastore, P. P., Frisch, R., Blancou, J., Wolff, F., Brochier, B., and Schneider, L. G. (1987). Campagne internationale de vaccination antirabique du renard par voie orale menée au grand-duché de Luxembourg, en Belgique et an France. *Ann. Med. Vet.* **131**, 441–447.

Perrin, P., Jacob, Y., Aquilar-Sétien, A., Loza-Rubio, E., Jallet, C., Desmézières, E., Aubert, M., Cliquet, F., and Tordo, N. (2000). Immunization of dogs with a DNA vaccine induces protection against rabies virus. *Vaccine* **18**, 479–486.

Perrin, P., Madhusudana, S., Gontier-Jallet, C., Petres, S., Tordo, N., and Merten, O.-W. (1995). An experimental rabies vaccine produced with a new BHK-21 suspension cell culture process: Use of serum-free medium and perfusion-reactor system. *Vaccine* **13**, 1244–1250.

Perrin P., Morgeaux, S., and Sureau, P. (1990). *In vitro* rabies vaccine potency appraisal by ELISA: Advantages of the immunocapture method with neutralizing anti-glycoprotein monoclonal antibody. *Biologicals* **18**, 321–330.

Petronek, G. J. (1998). Free roaming and feral cats: Their impact on wildlife and human beings. *J. Am. Vet. Med. Assoc.* **212**, 218–226.

Plotkin, S. A. (1980). Rabies vaccine prepared in human cell cultures: Progress and perspectives. *Rev. Infect. Dis.* **2**, 433–448.

Plotkin, S.A., Rupprecht, C. R., and Koprowski, H. (1999). Rabies vaccine. In *Vaccines*, S. A. Plotkin and W. A. Orenstein, (eds.), 3d ed., pp. 743–766. W. B. Saunders, Philadelphia.

Precausta, P., and Soulebot, J.-P. (1991). Vaccines for domestic animals In *The Natural History of Rabies*, G. M. Baer, (ed.), 2d ed., pp. 445–459. CRC Press, Boca Raton, FL.

Prevec, L., Campbell, J. B., Christie, B., Belbeck, L., and Graham, F. L. (1990). A recombinant human adenovirus vaccine against rabies. *J. Infect. Dis.* **161**, 27–30.

Ray, N. B., Ewalt, L. C., and Lodmell, D. L. (1997). Nanogram quantities of plasmid DNA encoding the rabies virus glycoprotein protect mice against lethal rabies virus infection. *Vaccine* **15**, 892–895.

Reculard, P. (1996). Cell-culture vaccines for veterinary use. In *Laboratory Techniques in Rabies*, (F.-X. Meslin, M. M. Kaplan, and H. Koprowski (eds.), 4th ed., pp. 314–323. World Health Organization, Geneva.

Roman, M., Martin-Orozco, E., Goodman, J. S., Nguyen, M. D., Sato, Y., Ronaghy, A., Kornbluth, R. S., Richman, D. D., Carson, D. A., and Raz, E. (1997). Immunostimulatory DNA sequences junction as T helper-1-promoting adjuvents. *Nature Med.* **3**, 839–854.

Rooijakkers, E. J., Uittenbogaard, J. P., Groen, J., and Osterhous, A. D. (1996). Rabies vaccine potency control: Comparison of ELISA systems for antigenicity testing. *J. Virol. Methods* **58**, 111–119.

Rupprecht, C. E., Hamir, A. N., Johnston, D. H., and Koprowski, H. (1988). Efficacy of vaccinia–rabies glycoprotein recombinant virus vaccine in raccoons (*Procyon lotor*). *Rev. Infect. Dis.* **10** (Suppl. 4), S803–809.

Rupprecht, C. E., Wiktor, T. J., Johnston, D. H., Hamir, A. N., Dietzschold, B., Wunner, W. H., Glickman, L. T., and Koprowski, H. (1986). Oral immunization and protection of raccoons (*Procyon lotor*) with a vaccinia–rabies glycoprotein recombinant virus vaccine. *Proc. Natl. Acad Sci. USA* **83**, 7947–7950.

Sato, Y., Roman, M., Tighe, G., Lee, D., Corr, M., Nguyen, M. D., Silverman, G. J., Lotz, M., Carosn, D. A., and Raz, E. (1996). Immunostimulatory DNA sequences necessary for effective intradermal gene immunization. *Science* **273**, 352–354.

Schoenig, H. W. (1930). Experimental studies with killed canine rabies vaccine. *J. Am. Vet. Med. Assoc.* **76**, 25–27.

Seif, I., Coulon, P., Rollin, P. E., and Flamand, A. (1985). Rabies virus virulence: Effect on pathogenicity and sequence characterization of mutations affecting antigenic site III of the glycoprotein. *J. Virol.* **53**, 926–935.

Seligmann, E. B., Jr. (1973). Potency tests requirements of the United States National Institutes of Health (NIH). In *Laboratory Techniques in Rabies*, M. M. Kaplan and H. Koprowski, (eds.), 3d ed., pp. 279–289. World Health Organization, Geneva.

Singh, S., and Kumar. T. A. (1999). Rabies vaccines: An overview. *J. Assoc. Prevent. Rabies India* **1**, 14–20.

Sizaret, P. (1996). General considerations in testing the safety and potency of rabies vaccines. In *Laboratory Techniques in Rabies*, F.-X. Meslin, M. M. Kaplan, and H. Koprowski (eds.), 4th ed., pp. 355–359. World Health Organization, Geneva.

Smith, J. S., and Seidel, H. D. (1993). Rabies: A new look at an old disease. *Prog. Med. Virol.* **40**. 82–106.

Streatfield, S. J., Jilka, J. M., Hood, E. E., Turner, D. D., Bailey, M. R., Mayor, J. M., Woodward, S. L., Beifuss, K. K., Horn, M. E., Delaney, D. E., Tizard, I. R., and Howard, J. A. (2001). Plant-based vaccines: Unique advantages. *Vaccine* **19**, 2742–2748.

Taylor, J., Trimarchi, C., Weinberg, R., Languet, B., Guillemin, F., Desmettre, P., and Paoletti, E. (1991). Efficacy studies on a canarypox–rabies recombinant virus. *Vaccine* **9**, 190–193.

Taylor, J., Weinberg, R, Languet, B., Desmettre, P., and Paoletti, E. (1988). Recombinant fowlpox virus inducing protective immunity in non-avian species. *Vaccine* **6**, 497–503.

Tims, T., Briggs, D. J., Davis, R. D., Moore, S. M., Xiang, Z., Ertl, H. C. J., and Fu, Z. F. (2000). Adult dogs receiving a rabies booster dose with a recombinant adenovirus expressing rabies virus glycoprotein develop high titer of neutralizing antibodies. *Vaccine* **18**, 2804–2807.

Title 9, Part 113.209, *Code of Federal Regulations* (2000). Rabies vaccine, killed virus, pp. 602–604. U. S. Government Printing Office, Washington.

Tordo, N. (1996). Characteristics and molecular biology of the rabies virus. In *Laboratory Techniques in Rabies*, F.-X. Meslin, M. M. Kaplan, and H. Koprowski (eds.), 4th ed., pp. 28–51. World Health Organization, Geneva.

Tuffereau, C., Leblois, H., Bennejean, J., Coulon, P., Lafay, F., and Flamand, A. (1989). Arginine or lysine in position 333 of ERA and CVS glycoprotein is necessary for rabies virulence in adult mice. *Virology* **172**, 206–212.

Wandeler, A. I., Matter, H. C., Kappeler, A., and Budde, A. (1993). The ecology of dogs and canine rabies: A selective review. *Rev. Sci. Technol. Off. Int. Epiz.* **12**, 51–71.

Wanderlie, P. S. (1992). An improved method for the *in vivo* efficacy testing of rabies vaccine in mice. Ph.D. thesis, University of Georgia, Athens, GA.

Wang, Y., Xiang, Z., Pasquini, S., Ertl, H. C. J. (1997). The use of an E1-deleted, replicative-defective adenovirus recombinant expressing the rabies virus glycoprotein for early vaccination of mice against rabies virus. *J. Virol.* **71**, 3677–3683.

Wiktor, T. J., Macfarlan, R. I., Dietzschold, B., Rupprecht, C., and Wunner, W. H. (1985). Immunogenic properties of vaccinia recombinant virus expressing the rabies glycoprotein. *Ann. Inst. Pasteur Virol.* **136E**, 405–411.

Wiktor, T. J., Macfarlan, R. I., Reagan, K. J., Dietzschold, B., Curtis, P. J., Wunner, W. H., Kieny, M.-P., Lathe, R., Lecocq, J. P., Mackett, M., Moss, B., and Koprowski, H. (1984). Protection from rabies by a vaccinia recombinant containing the rabies virus glycoprotein gene. *Proc. Natl. Acad. Sci. USA* **81**, 7194–7198.

Wiktor, T. J., Sokol, F., Kuwert, E., and Koprowski, H. (1969). Immunogenicity of concentrated and purified rabies vaccine of tissue culture origin. *Proc. Soc. Exp. Biol. Med.* **131**, 799–805.

Wilson, P. J., and Clark, K. A. (2001). Postexposure rabies prophylaxis protocol for domestic animals and epidemiologic characteristics of rabies vaccination failures in Texas: 1995–1999. *J. Am. Vet. Med. Assoc.* **218**, 522–525.

Winkler, W. G., Shaddock, J. H., and Williams, L. W. (1976). Oral rabies vaccine: Evaluation of its infectivity I three species of rodents. *Am. J. Epidemiol.* **104**, 294–298.

Wold, W. S. M., and Gooding, L. R. (1991). Region E3 of adenovirus: A cassette of genes involved in host immunosurveillance and virus–cell interactions. *Virology* **184**, 1–8.

World Health Organization Expert Committee on Rabies (1973). Sixth report. WHO Technical Report Series No. 523. WHO, Geneva.

World Health Organization Expert Committee on Biological Standardization (1981). Thirty-First Report. Requirements for Rabies Vaccine for Human Use. WHO Technical Report Series No. 658. WHO, Geneva.

World Health Organization Expert Committee on Rabies (1984). Seventh Report. WHO Technical Report Series No. 709. WHO, Geneva.

World Health Organization Expert Committee on Rabies (1992). Eighth Report. WHO Technical Report Series No. 824. WHO, Geneva.

World Health Organization Expert Committee on Biological Standardization (1994). Forty-Third Report. WHO Technical Report Series No. 840. WHO, Geneva.

World Health Organization. (1998). Report of visits to South Africa, Zimbabwe, Mozambique, Malawi, Zambia from 30 September to 9 November 1997 and Uganda and Tanzania from 24 November to 15 December 1997 in relation to rabies. ZDI/98.5. WHO, Geneva.

World Health Organization (2000). World survey of rabies for the year 1998. No. 34. WHO/CDS/CSR/APH/99.6. WHO, Geneva.

Xiang, Z. Q., and Ertl, H. C. J. (1995). Manipulation of the immune response to a plasmid-encoded viral antigen by coinoculation with plasmids expressing cytokines. *Immunity* **2**, 129–135.

Xiang, Z. Q., He, Z., Wang, Y., and Ertl, H. C. J. (1997). The effect of interferon-γ on genetic immunization. *Vaccine* **15**, 896–898.

Xiang, Z. Q., Spitalnik, S., Cheng, J., Erikson, J., Wojczyk, B., and Ertl, H. C. J. (1995). Immune responses to nucleic acid vaccines to rabies virus. *Virology* **209**, 569–579.

Xiang, Z. Q., Spitalnik, S., Tran, M., Wunner, W. H., Cheng, J., and Ertl, H. C. J. (1994). Vaccination with a plasmid vector carrying the rabies virus glycoprotein gene induces protective immunity against rabies virus. *Virology* **199**, 132–140.

Xiang, Z. Q., Yang, Y., Wilson, J. M., and Ertl, H. C. J. (1996). A replication-defective human adenovirus recombinant serves as a highly efficacious vaccine carrier. *Virology* **219**, 220–227.

Yang, Y., Ertl., H. C. J., and Wilson, J. M. (1994). MHC class I–restricted cytotoxic T-lymphocytes to viral antigens destroy hepatocytes in mice infected with E1-deleted recombinant adenoviruses. *Immunity* **1**, 433–442.

Yusibov, V., and Koprowski, H. (1998). Plants as vectors for biomedical products. *J. Med. Food* **1**, 5–12.

Yusibov, V., Modelska, A, Steplewski, K., Agadjanyan, M., Weiner, D., Hooper, D. C., and Koprowski, H. (1997). Antigens produced in plants by infection with chimeric plant viruses immunize against rabies virus and HIV-1. *Proc. Natl. Acad. Sci. USA* **94**, 5784–5788.

Yusibov, V., Shivprasad, S., Turpen, T. H., Dawson, W., Koprowski, H. (1999). Plant viral vectors based on tobamoviruses. *Curr. Topics Microbiol. Immunol.* **240**, 81–94.

Zoonoses control. (1997). *WHO Weekly Epidemiol. Rec.* **35**, 266–267.

12

Public Health Management of Humans at Risk

DEBORAH J. BRIGGS

College of Veterinary Medicine
Kansas State University
Manhattan, Kansas 66506

I. INTRODUCTION

Rabies vaccines and postexposure treatment (PET) have improved dramatically since Pasteur and his colleagues administered the first rabies vaccine on July 6, 1885. On that day, Joseph Meister, who had been bitten 14 times by a rabid

401

dog 60 hours earlier, began a painful series of injections containing increasingly virulent rabies virus–infected rabbit spinal cord (Pasteur, 1885). The fact that Joseph Meister survived both the exposure to the rabid dog and the virulent live rabies virus in the last doses of vaccine suspension was the first indication that PET could provide protection from almost certain death after an exposure to a rabid animal. Rabies is unique in that unlike many other diseases that infect human beings, most people have some basic knowledge about the clinical symptoms that accompany the disease. This is probably due to a combination of contributing factors, including the horrific nature of the disease, the almost certain fatal outcome once infected, and Hollywood's portrayal of the clinical manifestations of rabies. Even though the fear associated with rabies causes many people in North America and Europe to seek PET unnecessarily, in many developing countries of the world, tens of thousands of human rabies deaths occur annually due to failure to seek appropriate PET.

In as much as the first human rabies vaccine was administered after exposure rather than as a preventative measure prior to exposure to a rabid animal, this revolutionary approach was perhaps successful due to the relatively long incubation period that often occurs in rabies. In fact, in most cases, administration of PET within a reasonable amount of time after exposure will allow the immune system to mount a sufficient immune response to provide protection before the virus can invade the nervous system and kill the host it has infected. Indeed, the success of Pasteur's treatment and subsequent crude nerve tissue rabies vaccines followed by more purified and highly potent second-generation cell-culture rabies vaccines for PET generally have discouraged the promotion and use of preexposure vaccination programs in regions of the world where canine rabies is endemic and where preexposure prophylactic rabies vaccination could save many lives (Bernard et al., 1991).

Despite the development and production of modern cell-culture vaccines, some developing countries still endorse the use of poor-quality nerve tissue vaccines in exposed patients that come to public antirabies clinics for PET (Haupt, 1999). There are two nerve tissue vaccines that are still being produced in large quantities and administered to humans in developing countries today: the Semple vaccine and the Fuenzalida–Palacios vaccine (see Chap. 11). Semple vaccine, developed in 1911 by Dr. David Semple and used mainly in Asia and Africa, is produced from rabies virus–infected sheep, goats, or rabbits and uses a phenolized method to partially or totally inactivate the rabies virus (Vodopija et al., 1991). The problem with Semple vaccine is that deaths occur that are attributed to neurologic complications associated with the presence of myelinated tissue in the vaccine (Hemachudha et al., 1987). Neurologic complications have been reported in as many as 1 in 120 to 1 in 400 recipients of Semple vaccine (Hemachudha et al., 1987; Swaddiwudhipong et al., 1987). Today, Semple vaccine produced in sheep brain is made by at least 9 government-supported manufacturing sites in India. Since Semple vaccine is less expensive to produce than cell-culture vaccines, it is the vaccine chosen by the government to be supplied free of charge to public antirabies clinics for administration to approximately 2 million patients throughout India annually (Dutta *et al.*, 1999; John, 1997). Semple vaccine is also produced and distributed in other developing countries in Asia and Africa (Plotkin *et al.*, 1999).

Fuenzalida–Palacios rabies vaccine, first developed in Chili in 1955, is produced from rabies virus–infected suckling mouse brain tissue because substantial myelination occurs in the brain during postnatal development. This vaccine, which was developed to overcome the neurologic complications associated with the Semple vaccine, is still distributed widely throughout South America and parts of Latin America today (Fuenzalida *et al.*, 1964).

In most of the geographic regions where Semple and Fuenzalida–Palacios vaccines are used commonly, canine rabies is also endemic (Plotkin *et al.*, 1999). The presence of canine rabies and the concurrent administration of low-quality nerve tissue vaccine are the major reasons for the large number of human rabies deaths reported from these regions, especially in Asia (Parviz *et al.*, 1998). In North America and Europe, endemic canine rabies has been eliminated through mandatory vaccination programs, licensing policies, and dog control regulations (Hanlon *et al.*, 1999). Many countries in South America also have made tremendous progress in the elimination of canine rabies through government-sponsored vaccination and eradication programs (PAHO, 1999). The elimination of canine rabies throughout South America most certainly will continue to reduce the incidence of human rabies on that continent. However, similar programs are not yet feasible in Asian countries, where a significant percentage of the population belongs to Buddhist or other religious organizations that abhor the killing of animals. In addition, the lack of government resources in Asian and African countries severely limits the necessary financial support required for massive canine vaccination programs. Therefore, no major progress in the elimination of canine rabies in Asia and Africa has been made to date (Bhanganda *et al.*, 1993).

The public health threat of rabies is not only a problem for developing countries where canine rabies is endemic. In the few rabies-free regions of the world, new or previously identified rabies virus serotypes can be introduced indirectly through the importation or migration of infected animals from rabies-endemic countries. One such example was reported recently in Australia, where a previously unknown lyssavirus was identified in Australian fruit bats (Fraser *et al.*, 1996; Gerrard, 1997; Halpin *et al.*, 1999). The virus has been named *Australian bat lyssavirus* (ABLV) and is classified as a genotype 7 lyssavirus. ABLV has infected and caused the death of at least two humans with classic rabies symptoms (Hanna *et al.*, 2000). If it is true that ABLV actually entered Australia recently, rather than being present but undetected prior to the documented human deaths, the route through which the virus entered the continent is unknown. It is possible that one or more fruit bats infected with ABLV migrated to Australia from a rabies-endemic area, thus introducing the previously unrecognized lyssavirus into Australia.

In North America, where domestic animal rabies is well controlled, rabies in wildlife species continues to be a problem and results in many domestic animal and human exposures annually (Krebs *et al.*, 2000). In South America, where great progress is being made toward elimination of canine rabies, vampire bat rabies remains a difficult problem to overcome (Lopez *et al.*, 1992). Until such time as rabies is eliminated in the canine and wildlife populations of the world, public health management of humans at risk of exposure to rabies must depend on PET or preexposure prophylaxis rabies vaccination.

II. PREEXPOSURE VACCINATION

Preexposure vaccination as a prophylaxis should be offered to people who are at increased risk of exposure to rabies due to their vocation, hobby, or other activities (CDC, 1999a; WHO, 1992). Individuals at increased risk include, but are not limited to, rabies research and diagnostic laboratory workers, veterinarians, animal control workers, spelunkers, and people who handle wild animals (Table I). Preexposure vaccination also should be offered to international travelers visiting regions of the world where canine rabies is enzootic and immediate access to the appropriate biological is limited, difficult, or impossible to obtain (Hatz *et al.*, 1995). In addition, the administration of preexposure vaccination should be considered for some populations at risk in developing countries, especially children, where canine rabies is enzootic, dog bites are frequent, rabies immune globulin (RIG) is unavailable, and/or travel to antirabies treatment centers may be inconvenient (Sabchareon *et al.*, 1998).

Preexposure vaccination is beneficial for the following reasons: (1) the need for RIG is eliminated, (2) PET vaccine regimen is reduced from five to two doses, (3) protection against rabies is possible if PET is delayed, (4) protection against inadvertent exposure to rabies is possible, and (5) the cost of PET is reduced.

Preexposure vaccination for prophylaxis simplifies PET in persons subsequently exposed to rabies by reducing the required number of vaccine doses from five to two and by eliminating the need for RIG. The purpose of RIG is to provide passive immunity against rabies virus by neutralizing (inactivating) virus that could have been inoculated into the wound at the time of exposure until the body can produce its own anti-rabies virus neutralizing antibodies (RVNA). RIG must not be administered as part of the regimen for PET following preexposure vaccination because it may dampen the immune response in individuals who have received preexposure vaccination. RIG is not required, moreover, because once the immune

TABLE I

Risk Assessment for Preexposure Vaccination[a]

Risk category	Nature of risk	Typical populations	Preexposure recommendations
Continuous	Virus present continuously, often in high concentrations; specific exposures likely to go unrecognized; bite, nonbite, or aerosol exposure	Rabies research laboratory workers[b]; rabies biologics production workers	Primary course; serologic testing every 6 months; booster vaccination if antibody titer is below acceptable level[c]
Frequent	Exposure usually episodic, with source recognized, but exposure also might be unrecognized; bite, nonbite, or aerosol exposure	Rabies diagnostic laboratory workers[b], spelunkers, veterinarians and staff, and animal control and wildlife workers in rabies-enzootic areas	Primary course; serologic testing every 2 years; booster vaccination if antibody titer is below acceptable level[c]
Infrequent (greater than population at large)	Exposure nearly always episodic, with source recognized; bite or nonbite exposure	Veterinarians and animal control workers in areas with low rabies rates, veterinary students, travelers visiting areas where rabies enzootic and immediate access to appropriate medical care including biological is limited	Primary course; no serologic testing or booster vaccination
Rare (population at large)	Exposure always episodic, with source recognized; bite or nonbite exposure	U.S. population[d] at large, including persons in rabies-epizootic areas	No vaccination necessary

[a]From CDC (1999). Human rabies prevention — United States, 1999. Recommendations of the Advisory Committee on Immunization Practices (ACIP). *Morbid. Mortal. Weekly Rep.* **48** (RR-l), 6.

[b]Judgment of relative risk and extra monitoring of vaccination status of laboratory workers are the responsibility of the laboratory supervisor.

[c]Minimum acceptable antibody level is complete virus neutralization at a 1:5 serum dilution by the rapid fluorescent focus inhibition test. A booster dose should be administered if the titer falls below this level.

[d]These recommendations are applicable to the general population in all developed countries.

system has been primed in preexposure vaccination, an anamnestic response will occur immediately after the booster series (PET) is initiated (Fishbein *et al.*, 1986; Bernard *et al.*, 1987).

Preexposure vaccination also may provide additional protection if a delay in treatment occurs or if incorrect medical advice is given during travel, as has occurred with travelers in remote areas (Krause *et al.*, 1999; Arguin *et al.*, 2000). Additionally, preexposure vaccination most certainly protects against inadvertent exposures. This is evident when one considers that no one residing in the United States who received preexposure vaccination with a modern cell-culture vaccine has contracted rabies (Noah *et al.*, 1998). Last, the cost of PET is reduced in individuals who have received preexposure vaccination. For example, although five doses of vaccine are still required (three doses for the primary series and two doses for the booster), the cost savings for RIG alone is considerable (Murray *et al.*, 2000).

A. Intramuscular Preexposure Vaccination

Human diploid cell rabies vaccine (HDCV), purified chick embryo cell vaccine (PCECV), and rabies vaccine absorbed (RVA) are licensed for intramuscular (IM) preexposure vaccination by the Food and Drug Administration (FDA) (see Chap. 11). HDCV, PCECV, and RVA should be administered as 1.0 ml per dose. Although purified Vero cell rabies vaccine (PVRV) and purified duck embryo cell rabies vaccine (PDEV) are not licensed by the FDA, they are licensed for IM preexposure use in other countries outside North America. PVRV is administered as a 0.5-ml IM dose, and PDEV is administered as a 1.0-ml IM dose. The preexposure IM vaccination regimen consists of the administration of three doses of vaccine. One dose is given on each of days 0, 7, and either day 21 or day 28 (Table II). There is no need to conduct serologic testing immediately after preexposure vaccination in healthy individuals because clinical studies have demonstrated excellent immune responses to all vaccines (CDC, 1999a).

B. Intradermal Preexposure Vaccination

The intradermal (ID) preexposure vaccination schedule is identical to the IM preexposure schedule. That is, one dose of vaccine is administered ID in the area over the deltoid on days 0, 7, and either day 21 or 28. HDCV for ID use is packaged as a single dose of lyophilized vaccine and is equipped with a disposable syringe. When the ID vaccine is injected correctly, a bleb or papule is evident on the skin. If this does not occur due to improper injection or leakage, a second injection should be administered into the other arm (CDC, 1999a). Currently, there is no human rabies vaccine packaged and sold as a multidose vial; vaccine packaged and licensed for IM use is not licensed for ID use. Therefore, it is

TABLE II

Preexposure Vaccination

Vaccination	Route of administration	Regimen
Primary[a]	Intramuscular (HDCV,[d] PCECV,[e] RVA,[f] or PVR[g]) Intradermal (HDCV)	1.0 ml into the deltoid on days 0 and 7 and either 21 or 28 0.1 ml on days 0 and 7 and either 21 or 28
Routine	Intramuscular (HDCV, PCECV, RVA, or PVRV)	1.0 ml into the deltoid on day 0
Booster[b]	Intradermal (HDCV)	0.1 ml into the deltoid on day 0
Booster after exposure[c]	Intramuscular (HDCV, PCECV, RVA, or PVRV)	1.0 ml into the deltoid on day 0

[a]Administered to previously unvaccinated person.

[b]Administered as a routine procedure to maintain a measurable serologic titer.

[c]Administered after an exposure to a known or suspected rabid animal.

[d]Human diploid cell rabies vaccine.

[e]Purified chick embryo cell rabies vaccine.

[f]Rabies vaccine adsorbed.

[g]Purified Vero cell rabies vaccine.

recommended that a 1.0-ml IM vaccine should not be used as a multidose vial for ID injection. Contamination could occur when rabies vaccines that do not contain a preservative are injected multiple times to withdraw 0.1 ml for several ID injections. In addition, the use of a nonapproved syringe for ID vaccination could result in vaccine being left in the hub of the syringe, leakage, and inadequate injection (Fishbein et al., 1987).

In a retrospective study comparing the longevity of serologic titers after ID and IM administration of HDCV, measurable serologic titers did not last as long in recipients of ID HDCV (Briggs et al., 1992). In this study, titers measured at 2 years after vaccination indicated that only 7% of recipients of IM HDCV had a titer below 1:5, the serologic level recognized by Advisory Committee on Immunization Practices (ACIP) as being adequate, whereas 26% of recipients of ID HDCV had a titer below 1:5. In a cost-benefit analysis, the cost-benefit scenario is greater for IM preexposure vaccination when the costs of serologic testing to determine RVNA levels and additional boosters required to maintain an adequate titer after ID vaccination are taken into consideration (Murray et al., 2000).

If the antimalarial chloroquine phosphate is being administered during rabies preexposure vaccination, the IM rather than the ID mode of administration should be used. This recommendation was made after a Peace Corp Volunteer died of rabies despite having completed a full ID preexposure series 6 months previously (CDC, 1983). Further studies confirmed a reduced RVNA response when chloroquine was administered concurrently with HDCV (Bernard et al., 1985; Pappaioanou et al., 1986). The effect of other antimalarial drugs on rabies vaccination has not been investigated fully. Two preliminary reports on the investigation of mefloquine administration and concurrent rabies vaccination indicate that the reduction in RVNA response may not be as dramatic as has been reported with chloroquine (Foster et al., 1999; Lau, 1999). However, further studies need to be conducted prior to changing the current recommendations that preclude the use of ID preexposure vaccination while taking antimalarial medications. Persons traveling to rabies-endemic countries where malaria is present who choose to have the ID route of administration should complete the entire preexposure vaccination prior to initiation of antimalarial prophylaxis. If this is impossible, then the preexposure series should be completed using the IM mode of administration.

C. Routine Booster Doses of Rabies Vaccine

Persons at frequent or constant risk of rabies exposure (see Table I) should have their serum tested routinely for the presence of RVNA (CDC, 1999a). The time between serologic tests depends on the category of risk associated with the situation. For example, rabies researchers and vaccine production workers should have serologic testing conducted every 6 months. If serum levels of RVNA fall below 1:5 (according to the ACIP guidelines) or 0.5 IU/ml [according to World Health Organization (WHO) guidelines], one booster dose of vaccine should be administered (CDC, 1999a; WHO, 1992). Routine booster vaccination can be administered either IM or ID. For persons at frequent risk of exposure, serologic testing should be conducted every 2 years. Again, if levels fall below 1:5 (ACIP) or 0.5 IU/ml (WHO), one routine booster dose should be administered. Routine booster doses of rabies vaccine should not be administered unless serum levels fall below the ACIP- or WHO-recognized levels.

D. Preexposure Vaccination in Immunosuppressed Patients

In one preexposure clinical study using the IM regimen conducted in 13 children infected with HIV-1, the geometric mean titers (GMTs) were significantly lower in HIV-infected patients than in uninfected children (Thisyakorn et al., 2000). Total cell counts conducted on HIV-infected and uninfected children indicated that the average CD4+ count was 16.54% in HIV-infected children and 31.14% in uninfected children. The RVNA values in children with CD4+ counts of less than 15% were significantly lower on days 14, 21, 28, 60, 180, and 360 after vaccination. Four of the children with CD4+ counts of less than 15% did not develop any antibody response after vaccination. This study and one other clinical study in HIV-infected patients who received a five-dose PET series (Deshpande *et al.*, 2000) indicate that immunosuppressed patients with low CD4+ counts either do not produce or produce low levels of RVNA after rabies vaccination. Therefore, persons with depressed immune systems should avoid circumstances that would require preexposure vaccination. If this is impossible, preexposure should be administered IM, and serologic testing should be conducted 2 weeks after completion of the series to confirm that the patient has responded immunologically to the vaccine (CDC, 1999a). If no RVNA can be detected after the third dose of vaccine, the patient may have a very low CD4+ count and be unable to respond immunologically to antigen presentation. In this case, patients should be counseled as to the potential lack of protection from exposure to rabies and encouraged to avoid activities where rabies exposure is a risk.

III. POSTEXPOSURE TREATMENT

A. Rabies Exposure

The WHO has categorized exposures according to their severity (Table III). An exposure to rabies occurs when rabies virus may enter the body of a human or animal through an open cut or wound or mucous membrane. Since rabies virus cannot enter the body through intact or unbroken skin, simply being in the same area or room or touching the fur of a rabid animal does not constitute an exposure to rabies. Every potential exposure to rabies should be evaluated on a case-by-case basis. Factors that need to be considered when investigating a potential exposure include the epidemiology of rabies in the area, the species of animal involved, the type of contact between the suspected rabid animal and victim (provoked or unprovoked), and the anatomic location and severity of exposure (Moore *et al.*, 2000). Most often exposures occur through bite wounds, although some nonbite exposures also may require PET. Moreover, bite wounds by small animals such as bats may be so minor as not to be detected (CDC, 1998b).

Nonbite exposures sometimes are difficult to evaluate when compared with bite wounds that cause obvious tissue damage (Moran *et al.*, 2000). Nonbite exposures include the contamination of abrasions or existing open wounds through virus-infected saliva or neural tissue. Aerosol transmission of rabies has been documented four times in humans (Conomy *et al.*, 1977; Constantine, 1962; Winkler *et al.*, 1973). However, it is extremely rare to contract rabies through aerosol transmission, and this is only likely to occur when large quantities of rabies virus are inhaled directly. Two of the four reported cases of aerosol transmission were documented laboratory exposures, and two cases occurred after exposure to millions of Mexican free-tailed bats in the Frio Cave in Texas. All four victims likely were exposed to large amounts of rabies virus in a confined

TABLE III

World Health Organization Postexposure Prophylaxis Recommendations[a]

Category	Type of contact with a suspected or confirmed rabid domestic or wild[b] animal or animal unavailable for observation	Recommended treatment
I	Touching or feeding of animals Licks on intact skin	None, if reliable case history is available
II	Nibbling of uncovered skin Minor scratches or abrasions without bleeding Licks on broken skin	Administer vaccine immediately[c] Stop treatment if animal remains healthy throughout an observation period of 10 days or if animal is killed humanely and found to be negative for rabies by appropriate laboratory techniques
III	Single or multiple transdermal bites or scratches Contamination of mucous membrane with saliva (i.e. licks)	Administer rabies immuno-globulin and vaccine immediately[c] Stop treatment if animal remains healthy throughout an observation period[d] of 10 days or if animal is killed humanely and found to be negative for rabies by appropriate laboratory techniques

[a]From WHO Expert Committee on Rabies (1992). Eighth report. World Health Organization Technical Report 824, p. 55. WHO, Geneva.

[b]Exposure to rodents, rabbits, and hares seldom, if ever, requires specific antirabies treatment.

[c]If an apparently healthy dog or cat in or from a low-risk area is placed under observation, the situation may warrant delaying initiation of treatment.

[d]This observation period applies only to dogs and cats. Except in the case of threatened or endangered species, other domestic and wild animals suspected as rabid should be killed humanely and their tissues examined using appropriate laboratory techniques.

area. Exposure to a single or even multiple rabid animals in an open space does not constitute an aerosol exposure to rabies virus.

Although scratches (that break the skin) inflicted by a rabid animal are a low risk, they should be considered an exposure to rabies (CDC, 1999a). Virus could be present on the claws of a rabid animal if the claws were contaminated with infected saliva or neural tissue.

There have been eight reported cases of human-to-human transmission of rabies through direct corneal transplants from patients who died of an encephalitic disease later confirmed or suspected to be rabies (Javadi *et al.*, 1996). Due to the rabies fatalities associated with corneal grafts, strict guidelines are now in place to prevent further cases by transmission through transplantation of human tissues.

Although virus has been isolated from tears and saliva of infected humans (Sureau *et al.*, 1991), infection through direct human-to-human transmission is extremely rare. Six anecdotal reports of human-to-human transmission have been recorded (Helmick *et al.*, 1987). Two non-laboratory-confirmed cases were reported to have occurred in Ethiopia (Fekadu *et al.*, 1996). The only known exposure for the two patients in Ethiopia was to family members who subsequently died of rabies. One was exposed through a kiss and the other through a bite. Medical staff that administer routine health care to rabies-infected patients need not receive PET unless they have had a direct exposure to the saliva of a rabid patient into an open skin lesion or mucous membrane. Recommendations for evaluating the exposure of medical staff caring for a rabies patient have been published (Remington *et al.*, 1985). The recommendations include educating personnel as to the risks and definition of an exposure, using questionaires to determine the extent and type of contact, and administering PET only to persons who have had percutaneous or mucous membrane contact with saliva, respiratory secretions, corneas (tears), and/or cerebrospinal fluid.

In North America, a healthy dog, cat, or ferret that inflicts a bite can be observed for 10 days (National Association of State Public Health Veterinarians, 2001). If the dog or cat remains healthy for 10 days after the exposure, the animal can be presumed not to have been shedding rabies virus at the time of the exposure. The observation period of 10 days is based on historical evidence that a dog or cat infected with a variant of rabies virus from North America would demonstrate clinical signs of rabies infection within 10 days of virus being present in saliva. Recent studies investigating the shedding period of several North American variants of rabies virus in ferrets have confirmed that ferrets similarly can be observed for 10 days (Neizgoda *et al.*, 1997, 1998).

In regions where rabies is present in wildlife, bites inflicted by wild animals known to harbor rabies virus should be considered an exposure (Chomel, 1999). If possible, a wild animal that has inflicted a wound should be caught and tested immediately at a reliable diagnostic laboratory to determine if it is positive for rabies virus infection. If the animal is confirmed positive for rabies or is unavailable for testing, PET should be initiated as soon as possible (Trimarchi *et al.*, 1999). In North America, there are many species of terrestrial wildlife that transmit rabies, including raccoons, skunks, foxes, and coyotes. However, bat-associated variants of rabies virus are confirmed most often to be the cause of human rabies deaths in the United States (Noah *et al.*, 1998). Twenty-two (78%) of the 37 human rabies cases that have occurred in the United States between 1990 and

1998 have been attributed to a bat-associated variant of rabies virus (Noah *et al.*, 1998; CDC, 1997, 1998a, b). Although an unrecognized bat bite is the most likely explanation for these deaths, to date, a definitive history of a bat bite was established for only one of these cases. Guidelines for evaluation of bat rabies exposures are defined by the ACIP (CDC, 1999a). Direct contact between a bat and a human should be considered an exposure unless the exposed person can be sure that a bite, scratch, or exposure to a mucous membrane did not occur. PET also should be considered when a bat is found in the same room as a sleeping or incapacitated person or an unattended child and the bat is unavailable for testing. If a person is in the same room or vicinity as a bat and is confident that he or she has not been in physical contact with the bat, then this should not be considered to be an exposure to rabies. If bats are present in an attic or other rooms in a house occupied by humans, the bats should be removed humanely from the house and preventative measures taken to prevent their return. One method to remove bats without physically coming in contact with them is to seal all entrances into the dwelling after the bats have vacated the premises. This can be accomplished most successfully by placing small-mesh netting over the access points into and out of the building. Bats can exit freely and climb down the netting to escape but are unable to find their way back up through the netting into the dwelling again.

Other circumstances that might occur but do not constitute an exposure include contact with a domestic pet that has taken food or water from the same bowl as a wild animal; contact with blood, urine, or feces; petting the fur of a rabid animal; or an accidental needle stick containing a killed animal rabies vaccine.

B. Wound Treatment and HRIG/ERIG

Proper wound cleansing procedures are the first line of defense against rabies virus infection and should be initiated as soon as possible after exposure. All wounds should be cleansed thoroughly with soap and water and, if possible, irrigated with a virucidal agent such as povidone–iodine solution (Hatchett, 1991). Experimental evidence indicates that washing a wound helps to reduce rabies virus infection by eliminating or inactivating viral particles that may have been inoculated into the tissue at the time of the exposure (Dean *et al.*, 1963; Kaplan *et al.*, 1962). In addition, tetanus prophylaxis and antibacterial treatment (although antibiotics are not administered routinely, they are almost always indicated for high-risk wounds) also should be initiated for all animal bites that cause tissue damage (Fleisher, 1999). Primary closure of wounds by suturing should be avoided if possible. However, cosmetic factors should be taken into account, particularly with facial wounds. If surgical manipulation is unavoidable, RIG (diluted with saline if the volume is not sufficient to inject into all wounds) should be infiltrated prior to surgical closure (Wilde, 1997).

In order to implement immediate passive immunization in previously unvaccinated persons, PET always should include the administration of RIG. RIG should be injected around the wound of every category III exposure (see Table III). RIG provides passive immunity until the immune system of a vaccinated individual produces its own RVNA or active immunity. In clinical trials, RVNA was detectable from 7–10 days after immunization (Lang et al., 1998a). In the event that RIG was not administered when PET was initiated, it can be given up to 7 days after the first dose of vaccine, after which time it is presumed that RVNA (active immunity) is present. RIG is produced in both humans (HRIG) and equines (ERIG), although HRIG is the only product licensed for use in North America. HRIG should be infiltrated around the wound at a volume of 20 IU/kg of body weight (Table IV). The protocol for administration of ERIG is identical to that for HRIG with the exception that 40 IU/kg should be administered around the wound. If the volume of RIG is too small to infiltrate all open wounds, it should be diluted in physiologic buffered saline prior to injection. If it is not anatomically feasible to infiltrate the entire amount of RIG around the wound site, the remainder should be injected IM at a site distant from the vaccine injection site. In clinical trials, the administration of RIG slightly decreased the active production of RVNA (Khawplod et al., 1996; Lang et al., 1998b). Therefore, no more than the recommended amount should be administered.

C. Vaccine Administration

PET consists of five doses of cell-culture vaccine; one dose is given on each of days 0, 3, 7, 14, and 28. As mentioned earlier, one dose of RIG is administered at the time of the first injection of vaccine (see Table IV). All vaccine is administered IM in the deltoid area in adults. In children, the vaccine can be administered in the anterolateral thigh area. It is unacceptable to administer vaccine in the gluteal area because this may lead to lower antibody levels and failure of PET (Fishbein, 1988).

D. Postexposure Treatment for Previously Vaccinated Persons

Persons who have received preexposure immunization or PET with a cell-culture vaccine should receive two IM boosters, one each on days 0 and 3. Recently, a study was conducted on veterinary students, who previously had received preexposure immunization, to determine the immune response after one booster (on day 0) versus two boosters (one each on days 0 and 3). In this study, there was no significant difference in the GMT 1 week after the respective boosters (Briggs et al., 2001). In another study, similar findings were reported after a single dose of

TABLE IV

Rabies Postexposure Prophylaxis Schedule — United States, 1999[a]

Vaccination status	Treatment	Regimen[b]
Not previously vaccinated	Wound cleansing	All PETs should begin with immediate thorough cleansing of all wounds with soap and water. If available, a virucidal agent such as a povidone–iodine solution should be used to irrigate the wounds.
	RIG	Administer 20 IU/kg of body weight (HRIG). If anatomically feasible, the full dose should be infiltrated around the wound(s), and any remaining volume should be administered IM at an anatomic site distant from vaccine administration. Also, RIG should not be administered in the same syringe as vaccine. Because RIG might partially suppress active production of antibody, no more than the recommended dose should be given
	Vaccine	HDCV, RVA, or PCEC, 1.0 ml, IM (deltoid area[c]), one each on days 0^d, 3, 7, 14, and 28.
Previously vaccinated[e]	Wound cleansing	All PETs should begin with immediate thorough cleansing of all wounds with soap Water. If available, a virucidal agent such as a povidone–iodine solution should be used to irrigate the wounds.
	RIG	RIG should *not* be administered.
	Vaccine	HDCV, RVA, or PCECV 1.0 ml, IM (deltoid area[c]), one each on days 0^d and 3.

[a] From CDC (1999). Human rabies prevention — United States, 1999. Recommendations of the Advisory Committee on Immunization Practices (ACIP). *Morbid. Mortal. Weekly Rep.* **48**, (RR-1), 12.

[b] These regimens are applicable for all age groups, including children.

[c] The deltoid area is the only acceptable site of vaccination for adults and older children. For younger children, the outer aspect of the thigh may be used. Vaccine should never be administered in the gluteal area.

[d] Day 0 is the day the first dose of vaccine is administered.

[e] Any person with a history of preexposure vaccination with HDCV, RVA, or PCECV; prior postexposure prophylaxis with HDCV, RVA, or PCECV; or previous vaccination with any other type of rabies vaccine and a documented history of antibody response to the prior vaccination.

cell-culture vaccine was administered to previously immunized persons (Vodopija *et al.*, 1997). However, for the present time, the current recommendations, which state that two booster doses of vaccine should be administered to previously vaccinated persons, should be followed in the event of a known exposure to a rabid animal (CDC, 1999a; WHO, 1992).

It could be detrimental to administer RIG to persons previously immunized with a rabies cell-culture vaccine because RIG can lower the anamnestic response to booster doses of rabies vaccine. Additionally, a complete PET regime, including RIG, should be administered to persons previously vaccinated with low-quality rabies vaccines (i.e., other than a modern cell-culture vaccine) unless a serologic test confirming the presence of RVNA was conducted prior to the exposure (see Table IV).

E. Postexposure Treatment in Immunosuppressed Patients

Of the more than 30 million adults living with HIV/AIDS, 95% are located in developing countries where canine rabies is endemic (Report on the Global HIV/AIDS Epidemic, 1999). In many of these countries, the availability of modern cell-culture rabies vaccines and RIG is limited or completely absent. There has been at least one documented human case of rabies in a patient infected with HIV (Adle-Biassette *et al.*, 1996). The victim was diagnosed in France but was bitten previously by a dog in Mali and did not undergo a complete regimen of PET. In one study investigating PET in HIV-infected patients, the immunologic response was demonstrated to be correlated with the CD4+ count (Table V) (Deshpande *et al.*, 2000). In this study, patients with CD4+ counts below $400/mm^3$ either did not produce any detectable RVNA or had very low levels of RVNA after five doses of a highly potent cell-culture vaccine. Similar findings were reported in children who had received a three-dose preexposure regimen using HDCV (Thisyakorn, 2000). In this case, children with CD4+ counts that were less than 15% of normal had GMTs below 0.5 IU/ml, the antibody level considered by the WHO to be an adequate immune response after vaccination. These reports indicate that the most appropriate PET for immunocompromised patients is prompt and thorough wound care using soap and water and an antivirucidal agent followed by the appropriate dose of RIG. All patients with category II and III exposures should receive RIG as well as the full five-dose PET vaccination regimen (see Tables III and IV).

F. Alternate Reduced Postexposure Treatment Regimes

There are three reduced-dose vaccine regimens regularly used for PET and recommended by the WHO for use in developing countries, where the cost of the

TABLE V

Immune Response of HIV-Infected Patients after Receiving Five Doses of PCECV[a]

Group	Day after first dose of vaccine[b]	Geometric mean Titer (IU/ml)	Percent of patients with antibody titers above 0.5 IU/ml[c]
Control[d]	0	< 0.05	0
(n = 18)	14	7.8	100
	30	12.2	100
	37	17.1	100
Asymptomatic[e]	0	< 0.05	0
(n = 29)	14	1.1	64
	30	2.0	89
	37	2.9	76
Symptomatic[f]	0	< 0.05	0
	14	0.3	25
	30	0.4	42
	37	0.6	57

[a] From Deshpande *et al.* (2000).

[b] Five doses of IM PCECV were administered, one each on days 0, 3, 7, 14, and 30.

[c] 0.5 IU/ml is considered to be an adequate response after vaccination (CDC, 1999a).

[d] Uninfected with HIV.

[e] HIV-infected with no evident clinical symptoms.

[f] HIV-infected and demonstrating obvious clinical symptoms of disease.

five-dose IM PET is prohibitive (WHO, 1997). These alternate regimes are named after the number of doses of vaccine administered on each day of the PET schedule. One of the reduced regimens, known as the *2-1-1 schedule*, was developed for IM PET (Vodopija *et al.*, 1988). In this regimen, subjects are vaccinated IM at two sites on day 0 (one injection is given in the right deltoid and one in the left deltoid), one site on day 7, and one site on day 21. On days 7 and 21, injections are administered in alternate deltoids. This schedule is approved for use with HDCV, PCECV, PVRV, and PDEV.

Two reduced schedules involving the use of ID PET have been recommended for use in developing countries by the WHO. Since there are no rabies cell-culture vaccines containing a preservative currently licensed for multidose purposes, all PET schedules that use ID regimens use vaccine packaged and licensed for IM use only. Therefore, in order to avoid contamination due to numerous needle sticks in the same vial to remove several ID doses of rabies vaccine, the WHO recommends that all vaccine be used or discarded within 6 hours of reconstitution. This means that when ID PET regimens are used, multiple individuals must be vaccinated on the same day using the same vial. Therefore, the ID PET schedules are limited for use in large antirabies treatment centers where many patients are treated on a daily basis. The first reduced ID PET vaccination regimen was developed at the Thai Red Cross and requires 0.1 ml of vaccine to be injected at eight sites on day 0 (not given on day 3), four sites on day 7 (not given on day 14), and one site on days 28 and 90 (Warrell *et al.*, 1985). This regimen is named the *8-0-4-0-1-1* schedule in conjunction with the number of doses and days on which the vaccine is administered. The number of vials of vaccine required for the 8-0-4-0-1-1 schedule is reduced from the five vials required in the traditional Essen schedule (1 ml administered on days 0, 3, 7, 14, and 28) to less than two vials. In addition, one less office visit is required. A second two-site ID schedule was developed by the Thai Red Cross and has become known as the *Thai Red Cross* or *2-2-2-0-1-1 ID schedule*. In this schedule, vaccine is injected at two sites on days 0, 3, and 7 and at one site on days 28 and 90. HDCV, PVRV and PCECV have WHO approval using the 2-2-2-0-1-1 regimen (Briggs *et al.*, 2000; Chutivongse *et al.*, 1990; WHO, 2001).

G. Pregnancy

Pregnancy is not a contraindication to PET after exposure to a known rabid animal (Varner *et al.*, 1982). In three retrospective studies conducted in Thailand and India, there were no reported fetal abnormalities associated with rabies vaccination (Chutivongse *et al.*, 1989, 1995; Sudarshan *et al.*, 1999). In one of the studies conducted on 202 pregnant women in Thailand, complete follow-up was available for 190 patients (Chutivongse *et al.*, 1995). Spontaneous abortions occurred in 8 (4.2%) of the women, a rate that was reported to be similar to that reported in the general Thai population. Of the 8 abortions, 3 occurred within 24 hours, 4 between days 3 and 7, and 1 on day 14 after the dog bite. It was concluded that the 8 abortions were caused by trauma from the attack rather than from the rabies vaccine. In another retrospective study conducted on 29 pregnant women in India, 25 were available for follow-up during pregnancy and after birth (Sudarshan *et al.*, 1999). In this report, no congenital deformities occurred, and no abortions were reported. Antibody titers were above 0.5 IU/ml in all women tested at 14 days after vaccination was initiated, and antibody was detected in 6 of the babies tested. None of the women available for follow-up at 1 year after treatment has died of rabies.

IV. TRAVEL TO DEVELOPING COUNTRIES

Preexposure vaccination should be offered to adventure travelers as well as government, health, and religious officials spending extended periods of time in remote areas of developing countries where canine rabies is endemic. In one report, 1.3% of travelers spending an average of 17 days in Thailand experienced a dog bite, 8.9% were licked by a dog, and 0.5% required PET (Phanuphak *et al.*, 1994). In another survey, the estimated number of dog bites that occurred in missionaries and long-term residents was 18.2 per 1000 persons (Bjorvatn *et al.*, 1980). Another report has indicated that PET in Peace Corps Volunteers was 550 times higher than in the general population of the United States (Bernard *et al.*, 1991). In the human rabies cases confirmed in the United States between 1980 and 1996, 12% were associated with a canine variant of rabies found outside the United States (Noah *et al.*, 1998). None of these patients received a complete PET series. Rabies deaths also have been reported in other victims in other countries when the correct PET was not administered, usually after an exposure to a rabid dog (Fescharek *et al.*, 1991). Other human rabies deaths have been reported despite reportedly "correct" PET treatment, but on closer evaluation, the WHO/ACIP prescribed recommendations were not followed (Wasi *et al.*, 1997). One such case was reported from South Africa in which HRIG and HDCV were administered appropriately, but the HDCV was injected into the gluteal area rather than the upper deltoid (Shill *et al.*, 1987).

In a study evaluating the management of animal bites among 67 long-term residents in the tropics, 51% of dog bite victims who should have received a complete PET did not receive any PET, and 19% received insufficient PET (Hatz *et al.*, 1995). Twenty-eight percent of the victims were children, of whom 85% did not receive PET or PET was incomplete. No RIG was administered in 10 patients with category III exposures, and 41% did not consider the possibility of rabies exposure when bitten. Additionally, 40% of the bites were unprovoked.

Medical treatment can be complicated and/or frustrating for foreigners to obtain in developing countries. Additionally, RIG and/or potent cell-culture rabies vaccines may not be available. In these circumstances, preexposure vaccination would add an additional margin of safety until appropriate medical facilities could be reached. However, travelers should not omit or delay obtaining the appropriate PET and should obtain medical advice as soon as possible. Delaying or neglecting PET could result in infection and the development of clinical rabies. At least one case of rabies has been reported in a Peace Corps Volunteer who had received ID preexposure vaccination but did not seek PET after being bitten by a dog (Bernard *et al.*, 1985). The lack of protection in this case probably was due to the ID route of vaccination and the fact that the volunteer was taking chloroquine as a prophylactic measure against malaria, which has been demonstrated to reduce antibody response to rabies vaccination (Pappaioanou *et al.*, 1986). Travelers receiving preexposure rabies vaccination concurrently with antimalarial drugs should receive the vaccine via the IM route, not the ID route (see Sect. IIB).

V. ADVERSE REACTIONS TO CELL-CULTURE VACCINES

Both local and systemic reactions have been recorded in clinical trials after the administration of cell-culture vaccines (Burridge *et al.*, 1982; Dreesen *et al.*, 1989; Jaiiaroensup *et al.*, 1998). The local reactions included pain, erythema, redness, swelling, warmth, itching, pruritus at the injection site, skin discoloration, induration, rash, and lymphadenopathy. Systemic reactions included fever, headache, influenza-like symptoms, regional lymphadenopathy, malaise, myalagia, nausea, mild edema of extremity, joint and back pain, dizziness, hives, and rash.

Allergic reactions associated with the administration of booster doses of HDCV have been reported to occur more frequently than with other cell-culture vaccines. In one study, 10% of veterinary students who received a booster dose of HDCV reported an immune-complex-like disease (Dreesen *et al.*, 1986). The disease consisted primarily of urticaria, macular rash, angioedema, and arthralgia. All the students recovered without sequelae. In another study, 3% of subjects who received a booster dose of HDCV developed generalized urticaria or wheezing within 1 day of receiving a booster, and 3% developed urticaria within 6–14 days of the booster (Fishbein *et al.*, 1993). The major cause of the immune-complex reactions has been linked to the production of IgE antibodies against β-propiolactone–altered human serum albumin in the production process of HDCV (Swanson *et al.*, 1987). β-Propiolactone is the inactivating agent, and human serum albumin is used as a stabilizer in the production of HDCV. These reactions have been treated successfully with antihistamines, epinephrine, and steroids (Plotkin *et al.*, 1999).

VI. INTERCHANGEABILITY OF VACCINES

It may be necessary to interchange vaccines during PET due to the unavailability of vaccine or the occurrence of adverse reactions. In the United States, a recent study indicated that an anamnestic response occurred when persons vaccinated previously with HDCV were subsequently boosted with PCECV, thus indicating that the vaccines were interchangeable (Briggs *et al.*, 2001). Interchangeability of modern cell-culture rabies vaccine has been practiced for many years in countries such as the Philippines, Thailand, and Sri Lanka without reported vaccine failures (WHO/CSR/APH, 2001). Generally, however, it is recommended that the same vaccine be used throughout preexposure vaccination and PET. If this is impossible, the vaccination regimen should be completed with a WHO-recommended vaccine (WHO, 1992). To date, there have been no immunogenicity studies investigating the interchange of IM versus ID in vaccination series. Therefore, this practice should be the exception, and serologic testing is highly recommended in such patients.

VII. LARGE-SCALE HUMAN EXPOSURES

An animal in an interactive display (i.e., a petting zoo, fair, school, or other public event) that contracts rabies potentially can expose dozens or even hundreds of people to rabies during a short period of time. One investigation of 22 large-scale human exposure incident indicated that between 16,000 and 40,000 PETs occur every year as a result of numerous people being exposed to presumed or confirmed rabid animals in a public setting (Rotz *et al.*, 1998). These types of exposures usually involve a companion animal (CDC, 1999b). Large-scale PET also has resulted from the consumption of unpasteurized milk from confirmed rabid cows (CDC, 1999c). Pasteurization of milk to be consumed by humans would eliminate the potential for exposure to rabies from a rabid cow. Vaccination should be strongly considered for animals that will have contact with the public. In addition, handling of wildlife for school displays should not be attempted by unvaccinated, unlicensed personnel.

VIII. RABIES VACCINATION OF ANIMALS

The implementation of vaccination programs in the 1940s virtually eliminated canine rabies in North America (see Chap. 4). A review of the incidence of dog rabies in the United States in 1988 indicates that 57% of confirmed rabid dogs were less than 1 year of age, 84% were considered to be pets, and 85% were from a rural environment (Eng *et al.*, 1990). The dogs confirmed rabid had a question-able, unknown, or no vaccination history. It is an important statistic to bear in mind that dog bites are the 12th most common cause of injuries in North America and pose a human health risk for contracting rabies (Heath *et al.*, 1998). Wounds inflicted by domestic animals should be washed promptly and thoroughly (see Sect. IVB), and medical attention should be sought immediately. The administra-tion of PET will depend on the ability to locate and confine the animal, the health and vaccination status of the animal, and whether wildlife or domestic animal rabies is present in the area. All these issues should be evaluated by medical personnel prior to implementing PET.

In the United States, cats are the most frequently diagnosed rabid domestic animal (Krebs *et al.*, 2000). The majority of documented cases of cat rabies occurred as a result of spillover from the raccoon epizootic in the eastern United States. The reason that more cats than dogs are diagnosed rabid is most likely due to the fact that there are fewer vaccination and leash laws for cats, and therefore, fewer cats are vaccinated and confined by their owners.

In order to prevent human exposures, stray or unwanted animals should be removed from human contact. All domestic animals should be vaccinated, and proof of current vaccination should be maintained in a safe and accessible place for verification in case of exposure. Vaccination of domestic pets will protect the animals from contracting rabies, thus reducing the number of human exposures and PETs required. In addition, animals on display at public events where human interaction is possible should be vaccinated.

Oral vaccination programs for wild animals generally are limited to one target species in rabies-endemic or -epizootic areas (Hanlon *et al.*, 1999). Contact with a wild animal should be considered a potential exposure to rabies, and medical advice should be sought. Contact with wild animals by an unvaccinated, unqualified person should be avoided.

IX. POSTEXPOSURE TREATMENT IN DEVELOPING COUNTRIES

The highest number of human rabies cases occurs in developing countries located in the tropics, where canine rabies is endemic (King *et al.*, 1993). Reduction of canine rabies in these countries would cause a significant reduction in the number of human fatalities attributed to exposures to rabid dogs. The WHO recommends vaccination of 70% of the canine population in order to prevent outbreaks of rabies (WHO, 1987). According to data presented in one report, vaccination of 70% of the canine population would prevent 96.5% of all major outbreaks of rabies (Coleman *et al.*, 1996). However, without governmental support for such extensive canine vaccination programs, it is unlikely that human rabies deaths can be reduced by this method. Therefore, human rabies must be eliminated through increased PETs and preexposure prophylaxis where possible.

Most patients receiving PET at antirabies clinics (ARCs) in developing countries receive nerve tissue vaccine because they cannot afford higher-priced tissue culture vaccines. Due to the pain and neuroparalytic complications associated with administration of Semple vaccine, the complete series of 10–14 injections in the abdomen is rarely completed (Fig. 1) (Shankar *et al.*, 2000). Some of the problems associated with rural patients coming to one ARC in India included delay of PET due to the distance of the ARC from the site of the exposure, proper first aid measures not undertaken immediately following animal bites, suturing of class III exposures without prior administration of RIG, unavailability of nerve tissue or cell-culture vaccine in rural areas, lack of awareness of the primary treating physician as to proper PET, and nonreporting of human rabies cases (Reddy *et al.*, 2000).

Thirty thousand human deaths are reported in India annually, more than in any other country in the world (WHO, 2000). Accurate mortality figures of the total number of human rabies deaths worldwide are not available due to insufficient data partly because rabies is not a reportable disease in many countries. In countries that report large numbers of deaths due to rabies, canine rabies is the main source of infection, and many victims of dog bites still receive crude nerve tissue

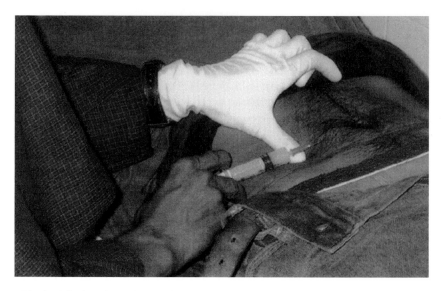

Fig. 1.   Injection of Semple nerve tissue rabies vaccine subcutaneously into the abdominal wall of a patient bitten by a potentially rabid dog. Postexposure treatment consists of at least 10 injections of Semple vaccine. Adults receive 5 ml per injection, and children receive 2 ml per injection.

vaccine. For example, in India, two-thirds of the approximately 3 million patients who receive PET every year are given Semple vaccine (Dutta *et al.*, 1999; John, 1997). Replacing nerve tissue rabies vaccines, i.e., Semple vaccine, with cell-culture rabies vaccines would without a doubt prevent unnecessary neurologic disability and save thousands of human lives every year. However, the replacement of low-cost, poor-quality nerve tissue vaccines with more expensive, highly purified, and highly potent cell-culture rabies vaccines is currently impossible in many developing countries where canine rabies is endemic due to insufficient governmental funding, a lack of awareness of the problem, and inadequate support from the appropriate medical authorities. The introduction of reduced PET vaccination regimes using cell-culture rabies vaccines would lower the cost of PET in developing countries, thus allowing more patients access to high-quality, effective rabies vaccines. However, increasing the availability of cell-culture rabies vaccines is only part of the solution required to reduce the incidence of human rabies. In addition, there is a need to increase the availability of highly purified RIG (or a suitable alternative) to fill the demand for passive immune protection, as recommended by the WHO, and a critical need to eliminate canine rabies through effective vaccination programs.

Finally, although rabies is one of the oldest diseases known to humanity and is virtually 100% preventable, the reasons why tens of thousands of people continue to die unnecessarily every year should be evaluated. Although a few human fatalities may be reported due to a deviation from the recommended PET regimen, most deaths occur due to a failure to seek PET, the unavailability of rabies vaccines in rabies-endemic areas, or because an exposed person received a poor-quality nerve tissue rabies vaccine. Some of these problems can be overcome when a greater awareness of the impact of human rabies is brought to the attention of the governments of developing countries. However, it will take the combined efforts of governmental health officials in rabies-endemic countries, the WHO, vaccine manufacturers, and rabies researchers to significantly reduce or eliminate the incidence of human rabies in the future.

REFERENCES

Adle-Biassette, H., Bourhy, H., Gisselbrecht, M., Chretien, F., Wingertsmann, L., Baudrimont, M., Rotivel, Y., Godeau, B., and Gray, F. (1996). Rabies encephalitis in a patient with AIDS: A clinicopathological study. *Acta. Neuropathol.* **92**, 415–420.

Arguin, P. M., Krebs, J. W., Mandel, E., Guzi, T., and Childs, J. E. (2000). Survey of rabies preexposure and postexposure among missionary personnel stationed outside the United States. *J. Travel Med.* **7**, 10–14.

Bernard, K. W., and Fishbein, D. B. (1991). Pre-exposure rabies prophylaxis for travellers: Are the benefits worth the cost? *Vaccine* **9**, 833–836.

Bernard, K. W., Fishbein, D. B., Miller, K. D., Parker, R. A., Waterman, S., Sumner, J. W., Feid, F. L., Johnson, B. K., Rollins, A. J., Oster, C. N., Schonberger, L. B., Baer, G. M., and Winkler, W. G. (1985). Pre-exposure rabies immunization with human diploid cell vaccine: Decreased antibody responses in persons immunized in developing countries. *Am. J. Trop. Med. Hyg.* **34**, 633–647.

Bernard, K. W., Mallonee, J., Wright, J. C., Reid, F. L., Makintubee, S., Parker, R. A., Dwyer, D. M., and Winkler, W. G. (1987). Preexposure immunization with intradermal human diploid cell rabies vaccine. *JAMA* **257**, 1059–1063.

Bhanganada, K., Wilde, H., Sakolsataydorn, P., and Oonsombat, P. (1993). Dog-bite injuries at a Bangkok teaching hospital. *Acta Tropica* **55**, 249–255.

Bjorvatn, B., and Gundersen, S. G. (1980). Rabies exposure among Norwegian missionaries working abroad. *Scand. J. Infect. Dis.* **12**, 257–264.

Briggs, D. J., Banzhoff, A., Nicolay, U., Sirikwin, S., Dumavibhat, B., Tongswas, S., and Wasi, C. (2000). Antibody response of patients after postexposure rabies vaccination with small intradermal doses of purified chick embryo cell vaccine or purified vero cell rabies vaccine. *Bull. WHO* **78**, 693–698.

Briggs, D. J., Dreesen, D. W., Nicolay, U., Chin, J. E., Davis, R., Gordon, C., and Banzhoff, A. (2001). Purified chick embryo cell culture rabies vaccine: Interchangeability with human diploid cell culture rabies vaccine and comparison of a one-dose versus two-dose post-exposure booster regimen for previously immunized persons. *Vaccine* **19**, 1055–1060.

Briggs, D. J., and Schwenke, J. R. (1992). Longevity of rabies antibody titre in recipients of human diploid cell rabies vaccine. *Vaccine* **10**, 125–129.

Burridge, M. J., Gaer, G. M., Sumner, J. W., and Sussman, O. (1982). Intradermal immunization with human diploid cell rabies vaccine. *JAMA* **248**, 1611–1614.

CDC (1983). Human rabies — Kenya. *Morbid. Mortal. Weekly Rep.* **32**, 494–495.

CDC (1997). Human rabies — Montana and Washington. *Morbid. Mortal. Weekly Rep.* **46**, 770–774.

CDC (1998a). Human rabies — Texas and New Jersey. *Morbid. Mortal. Weekly Rep.* **47**, 1–5.

CDC (1998b). Human rabies — Virginia, 1998. *Morbid. Mortal. Weekly Rep.* **48**, 95–97.

CDC (1999a). Human rabies prevention — United States, 1999. Recommendations of the Advisory Committee on Immunization Practices (ACIP). *Morbid. Mortal. Weekly Rep.* **48** (RR-1), 1–21.

CDC (1999b). Public health response to a potentially rabid bear cub — Iowa, 1999. *Morbid. Mortal. Weekly Rep.* **48**, 971–973.

CDC (1999c). Mass treatment of humans who drank unpasteurized milk from rabid cows — Massachusetts, 1996–1998. *Morbid. Mortal. Weekly Rep.* **48**, 228–229.

Chomel, B. B. (1999). Rabies exposure and clinical disease in animals. In *Rabies: Guidelines for Medical Professionals*, pp. 20–26. Veterinary Learning Systems, Trenton, NJ.

Chutivongse, S., and Wilde, H. (1989). Postexposure rabies vaccination during pregnancy: Experience with 21 patients. *Vaccine* **7**, 546–548.

Chutivongse, S., Wilde, H., Benjavongkulchai, M., Chomchey, P., and Punthawong, S. (1995). Postexposure rabies vaccination during pregnancy: Effect on 202 women and their infants. *Clin. Infect. Dis.* **20**, 818–820.

Chutivongse, S., Wilde, H., Supich, C., Baer, G. M., and Fishbein, D. B. (1990). Postexposure prophylaxis for rabies with antiserum and intradermal vaccination. *Lancet* **335**, 896–898.

Coleman, P. G., and Dye, C. (1996). Immunization coverage required to prevent outbreaks of dog rabies. *Vaccine* **14**, 85–186.

Conomy, J. P., Leibovitz, A., McCombs, W., and Stinson, J. (1977). Airborne rabies encephalitis: Demonstration of rabies virus in the human central nervous system. *Neurology* **27**, 67–69.

Constantine, D. G. (1962). Rabies transmission by nonbite route. *Public Health Rep.* **77**, 287–289.

Dean, D. J., and Baer, G. M. (1963). Studies on the local treatment of rabies-infected wounds. *Bull. WHO* **28**, 477–486.

Deshpande, A., Briggs, D. J., and Banzhoff, A. (2000). Investigation of immune resonse to purified chick embryo cell tissue culture rabies vaccine (PCECV) in HIV infected individuals using a simulated post-exposure regimen. XIII International AIDS Conference, Durban, South Africa, July 2000, pp. 163–167.

Dreesen, D. W., Bernard, K. W., Parker, R. A., Deutsch, A. J., and Brown, J. (1986). Immune complex–like disease in 23 persons following a booster dose of rabies human diploid cell vaccine. *Vaccine* **4**, 45–49.

Dreesen, D. W., Fishbein, D. B., Kemp, D. T., and Brown, J. (1989). Two-year comparative trial on the immunogenicity and adverse effects of purified chick embryo cell rabies vaccine for pre-exposure immunization. *Vaccine* **7**, 397–400.

Dutta, A. K., and Kanwal, S. K. (1999). Rabies and its prevention *J. Assoc. Prevent. Control Rabies India* **1**, 5–13.

Eng, T. R., and Fishbein, D. B. (1990). National study group on rabies: Epidemiologic factors, clinical findings and vaccination status of rabies in cats and dogs in the United States in 1988. *J. Am. Vet. Med. Assoc.* **197**, 201–209.

Fekadu, M., Endeshaw, T., Alemu, W., Bogale, Y., Teshager, T., and Olson J. G. (1996). Possible human-to-human transmission of rabies in Ethiopia. *Ethiop. Med. J.* **34**, 123–127.

Fescharek, R., Schwarz, S., Quast, U., Gandhi, N., and Karkhanis, S. (1991). Postexposure rabies prophylaxis: When the guidelines are not respected. *Vaccine* **9**, 868–872.

Fishbein, D. B., Bernard, K., W., Miller, K. D., Van der Vlugt, T., Gaines, C. E., Bell, J. T., Sumner, J. W., Reid, F. L., Parker, R. A., Horman, J. T., Pinsky, P. F., Schonberger, L. B., Baer, G. M., and Winkler, W. G. (1986). The early kinetics of the neutralizing antibody response after booster immunizations with human diploid cell rabies vaccine. *Am. J. Trop. Med. Hyg.* **35**, 663–670.

Fishbein, D. B., Pacer, R. E., Holmes, D. F., Ley, A. B., Yager, P., and Tong, T. C. (1987). Rabies pre-exposure prophylaxis with human diploid cell rabies vaccine: A dose–response study. *J. Infect. Dis.* **156**, 50–55.

Fishbein, D. B., Sawyer, L. A., Reid Sanden, F. L., and Weir, E. H. (1988). Administration of human diploid-cell rabies vaccine in the gluteal area. *New Engl. J. Med.* **318**, 124–125.

Fishbein, D. B., Yenne, K. M., Dreesen, D. W., Teplis, C. F., Mehta, N., and Briggs, D. J. (1993). Risk factors for systemic hypersensitivity reactions after booster vaccinations with human diploid cell rabies vaccine: A nationwide prospective study. *Vaccine* **11**, 1390–1394.

Fleisher, G. R. (1999). The management of bite wounds. *New Engl. J. Med.* **340**, 138.

Foster, R., and Briggs, D. J. (1999). Pre-exposure immune response of persons receiving purified chick embryo cell vaccine while receiving the anti-malarial drug mefloquine (Abstract). X International Meeting for the Advancement of the Investigation and Control of Rabies in the Americas Meeting, San Diego, CA.

Fraser, G. C., Hooper, P. T., Lunt, R. A., Gould, A. R., Gleeson, L. J., Hyatt, A. D., Russell, G. M., and Kattenbelt, J. A. (1996). Encephalitis caused by a *Lyssavirus* in fruit bats in Australia. *Emerg. Infect. Dis.* **2**, 327–331.

Fuenzalida, E., Palacios, R., and Borgono, J. M. (1964). Anti-rabies antibody response in man to vaccine made from infected suckling-mouse brains. *Bull. WHO* **30**, 431–436.

Gerrard, J. (1997). Fatal encephalitis and meningitis at the Gold Coast Hospital, 1980–1996. *Commun. Dis. Intell.* **6**, 32–33.

Halpin, K., Young, P. L., Field, H., and Mackenzie, J. S. (1999). Newly discovered viruses of flying foxes. *Vet. Microbiol.* **16**, 83–87.

Hanlon, C. A., Childs, J. E., and Nettles, V. F. (1999). Article III: Rabies in wildlife. *J. Am. Vet. Med. Assoc.* **215**, 1612–1617.

Hanna, J. N., Camey, I. K., and Smith, G. A. (2000). Australian bat lyssavirus infection: A second human case, with a long incubation period. *Med. J. Aust.* **172**, 597–599.

Hatchett, R. P. (1991). Rabies: The disease and the value of intensive care treatment. *Intensive Care Nurs.* **7**, 53–60.

Hatz, C. F., Bidaus, J. M., Eichenberger, K., Mikulics, U., and Junghanss, T. (1995). Circumstances and management of 72 animal bites among long-term residents in the tropics. *Vaccine* **13**, 811–815.

Haupt, W. (1999). Rabies — Risk of exposure and current trends in prevention of human cases. *Vaccine* **17**, 1742–1749.

Heath, S. E., and Chomel, B. B. (1998). Risk factors, prevention and prophylaxis of dog bites for disaster response personnel in the United States. *Prehosp. Disaster Med.* **13**, 133–136.

Helmick, C. G., Tauxe, R. V., and Vernon, A. A. (1987). Is there a risk to contacts of patients with rabies? *Rev. Infect. Dis.* **9**, 511–517.

Hemachudha, T., Griffin, D. E., Giffels, J. J., Johnson, R. T., Moser, A. B., and Phanuphak, P. (1987). Myelin basic protein as an encephalitogen in encephalomyelitis and polyneuritis following rabies vaccination. *New Engl. J. Med.* **316**, 369–373.

Jaiiaroensup, W., Lanag, J., Thipkong, P., Wimalaratne, O., Samranwataya, P., Saikasem, A., Chareonwai, S., Yenmuang, W., Prakongsri, S., Sitprija, V., and Wilde, H. (1998). Safety and efficacy of purified Vero cell rabies vaccine given intramuscularly and intradermally: Results of a prospective randomized trial. *Vaccine* **16**, 1559–1562.

Javadi, M. A., Fayaz, A., Mirdehghan, S. A., and Ainollahi, B. (1996). Transmission of rabies by corneal graft. *Cornea* **15**, 431–433.

John, T. J. (1997). An ethical dilemma in rabies immunisation. *Vaccine* **15**, S12–S15.

Kaplan, M. M., Cohen, D., Koprowski, H., Dean, D., and Ferrigan, L. (1962). Studies on the local treatment of wounds for the prevention of rabies. *Bull. WHO* **26**, 765–775.

Khawplod, P., Wilde, H., Chomchey, P., Benjavongkulchai, M., Yenmuang, W., Chaiyabutr, N., and Sitprija, V. (1996). What is an acceptable delay in rabies immune globulin administration when vaccine alone had been given previously? *Vaccine* **14**, 389–391.

King. A. A., and Turner, G. S. (1993). Rabies: A review. *J. Comp. Pathol.* **108**, 1–39.

Krause, E., Grundmann, H., and Hatz, C. (1999). Pretravel advice neglects rabies risk for travelers to tropical countries. *J. Travel Med.* **6**, 163–167.

Krebs, J. W., Rupprecht, C. R., and Childs, J. E. (2000). Rabies surveillance in the United States during 1999. *J. Am. Vet. Med. Assoc.* **217**, 1799–1811.

Lang, J., Gravenstein, S., Briggs, D., Miller, B., Froeshle, J., Dukes, C. Le Mener, V., and Lutsch, C. (1998a). Evaluation of the safety and immunogenicity of a new, heat-treated human rabies immune globulin using a sham, post-exposure prophylaxis of rabies. *Biologicals* **26**, 7–15.

Lang, J., Simanjuntak, G. H., Soerjosembodo, S., Koesharyono, C., and the MAS054 Clinical Investigator Group (1998b). Suppressant effect of human or equine rabies immunoglobulins on the immunogenicity of post-exposure rabies vaccination under the 2-1-1 regimen: A field trial in Indonesia. *Bull. WHO* **76**, 491–495.

Lau, J. (1999). Intradermal rabies vaccination and current use of mefloquine. *J. Travel Med.* **6**, 140–141.

Lopez, A. R., Miranda, P. P., Tejada, E. V., and Fishbein, D. B. (1992). Outbreak of human rabies in the Peruvian jungle. *Lancet* **339**, 408–411.

Moore, D. A., Sischo, W. M., Hunter, A., and Miles, T. (2000). Animal bite epidemiology and surveillance for rabies postexposure prophylaxis. *JAMA* **217**, 190–194.

Moran, G. J., Talan, D. A., Mower, W., Newdow, M. Ong, S., Nakase, J. Y., Pinner, R. W., and Childs, J. E. (2000). Appropriateness of rabies postexposure prophylaxis treatment for animal exposures. *JAMA* **284**, 1001–1007.

Murray, K. O., and Arguin, P. M. (2000). Decision-based evaluation of recommendations for preexposure rabies vaccination. *J. Am. Vet. Med. Assoc.* **216**, 188–191.

National Association of State Public Health Veterinarians. (2001). Compendium of animal rabies, prevention and control, 2001. *J. Am. Vet. Med. Assoc.* **218**, 26–31.

Neizgoda, M., Briggs, D. J., Shaddock, J., Dreesen, D. W., and Rupprecht, C. E. (1997). Rabies pathogenesis in the domestic ferret. *Am. J. Vet. Res.* **58**, 1327–1331.

Niezgoda, M., Briggs, D. J., Shaddock, J., and Rupprecht. C. (1998). Viral excretion in domestic ferrets (*Mustela putorius furo*) inoculated with a raccoon rabies isolate. *Am. J. Vet. Res.* **59**, 1629–1632.

Noah, D. L., Drenzek, C. L., Smith, J. S., Krebs, J. W., Orciari, L., Shaddock, J., Sanderlin, D., Whitfield, S., Fekadu, M., Olson, J. G., Rupprecht, C. R., and Childs, J. E. (1998). Epidemiology of human rabies in the United States, 1980 to 1996. *Ann. Intern. Med.* **128**, 922–929.

Pan American Health Organization/World Health Organization. (1999). XI Inter-American Meeting, at the Ministerial Level, on Animal Health. Regional Program for the Elimination of Human Rabies Transmitted by Dogs in the Americas: Analysis of Progress 1990–1998. Washington, DC.

Pappaioanou, M., Fishbeinn, D. B., Dreesen, D. W., Schwartz, I. K., Campbell, G. H., Sumner, J. W., Patchen, L. C., and Brown, W. J. (1986). Antibody response to preexposure human diploid-cell rabies vaccine given concurrently with chloroquine. *New Engl. J. Med.* **314**, 280–284.

Parviz, S., Luby, S., and Wilde, H. (1998). Postexposure treatment of rabies in Pakistan. *Clin. Infect. Dis.* **27**, 751–756.

Pasteur, L. (1885). Méthode pour prévenir la rage après morsure. *C. R. Acad. Sci. (Paris)* **101**, 765–774.

Phanuphak, P., Ubolyam, S., and Sirivichayakul, S. (1994). Should travellers in rabies endemic areas receive pre-exposure rabies immunization? *Ann. Med. Interne (Paris).* **145**, 167–176.

Plotkin, S. A., Rupprecht, C. R., and Koprowski, H. (1999). Rabies vaccine. In *Vaccines*, S. A. Plotkin and W. A. Orenstein (eds.), 3rd ed., pp. 743–766. W. B. Saunders, Philadelphia.

Reddy, A. V., and Sampath, G. (2000). Post exposure treatment: Some experiences. *J. Assoc. Prevent. Control Rabies India.* **1**, 33–35.

Remington, P. A., Shope, T., and Andrews, J. (1985). A recommended approach to the evaluation of human rabies exposure in an acute-care hospital. *JAMA* **254**, 67–69.

Report on the Global HIV/AIDS Epidemic, June 1998. (1999). World Health Association and Joint United Nations Programme on HIV/AIDS.

Rotz, L. D., Hensley, J. A., Rupprecht, C. E., and Childs, J. E., (1998). Large-scale human exposures to rabid or presumed rabid animals in the United States: 22 cases (1990–1996). *J. Am. Vet. Med. Assoc.* **212**, 1198–1200.

Sabchareon, A., Chantavanich, P., Pasuralertsakul, S., Pojjaroen-Anant, C., Prarinyanupharb, V., Attanath, P., Singhasivanon, V., Buppodom, W., and Lang, J. (1998). Persistence of antibodies in children after intradermal or intramuscular administration of preexposure primary and booster immunizations with purified Vero cell rabies vaccine. *Pediatr. Infect. Dis. J.* **17**, 1001–1007.

Shankar, S. K., Madhusudana, S. N., and Satyanarayana, S. H. (2000). Pathological morbidity following Semple type antirabies vaccine in India and why we need to replace it. *J. Assoc. Prevent. Control Rabies India* **1** (2), 15–20.

Shill, M., Baynes, R. D., and Miller, S. D. (1987). Fatal rabies encephalitis despite appropriate post-exposure prophylaxis. *New Engl. J. Med.* **316**, 1257–1258.

Sudarshan, M. K., Madhusudana, S. N., and Mahendra, B. J. (1999). Post-exposure prophylaxis with purified Vero cell rabies vaccine during pregnancy: Safety and immunogenicity. *J. Commun. Dis.* **31**, 229–236.

Sureau, P., Ravisse, P., and Rollin, R. E. (1991). Rabies diagnosis by animal inoculation, identification of Negri bodies, or ELISA. In *The Natural History of Rabies*, G. M. Baer, (end.), 2nd ed., pp. 204–217. CRC Press, Boca Raton, FL.

Swaddiwudhipong, W., Prayoonwiwat, N., Kunasol, P., and Choomkasien, P. (1987). A high incidence of neurological complications following Semple anti-rabies vaccine. *SE Asian J. Trop. Med. Public Health* **18**, 526–531.

Swanson, M. C., Rosanoff, E., Gurwith, M., Deitch, M., Schnurrenberger, P., and Reed, C. E. (1987). IgE and IgG antibodies to β-propiolactone and human serum albumin associated with urticarial reactions to rabies vaccine. *J. Infect. Dis.* **155**, 909–913.

Thisyakorn, U., Pancharoen, C., Ruxrungtham, K., Ubolyam, S., Khawplod, P., Tantawichien, T., Phanuphak, P., and, Wilde, H. (2000). Safety and immunogenicity of preexposure rabies vaccination in children infected with human immunodeficiency virus type 1. *Clin. Infect. Dis.* **30**, 218.

Trimarchi, C. V., and Briggs, D. J. (1999). The diagnosis of rabies. In *Rabies: Guidelines for Medical Professionals*, pp. 55–66. Veterinary Learning Systems, Trenton, NJ.

Varner, M. W., and McGuinness, G. A. (1982). Rabies vaccination in pregnancy. *Am. J. Obstet. Gynecol.* **143**, 717–718.

Vodopija, I., and Clark, H. F. (1991). Human vaccination against rabies. In *The Natural History of Rabies*, G. M. Baer (ed.), 2nd ed., pp. 571–595. CRC Press, Boca Raton, FL.

Vodopija, R., Lafon, M., Baklaic, Z., Ljubicic, M., Svjetlicic, M., and Vodopija, I. (1997). Persistence of humoral immunity to rabies 1100 days after immunization and effect of a single booster dose of rabies vaccine. *Vaccine* **5**, 571–574.

Vodopija, R., Sureau, P., Smerdel, S., Lafon M., Baklaic, Z., Ljubicic, M., and Svjetlicic, M. (1988). Interaction of rabies vaccine with human rabies immunoglobulin and reliability of a 2-1-1 schedule application for postexposure treatment. *Vaccine* **6**, 283–286.

Warrell, M. J., Nicholson, K. G., Warrell, D. A., Suntharasamai, P., Chanthavanich, P., Viravan, C., Sinhaseni, A., Cheiwbamroongkiat, M., Pouradier-Duteil, X., Xueref, C., Phangfung, R., and Udomsakdi, D. (1985). Economical multiple-site intradermal immunization with human diploid-cell-strain vaccine is effective for post-exposure rabies prophylaxis. *Lancet* **i**, 1059–1062.

Wasi, C., Chaiprasithikul, P., Thongcharoen, P., Choomkasien, P., and Sirikawin, S. (1997). Progress and achievement of rabies control in Thailand. *Vaccine* **15**, S7–S11.

Wilde, H. (1997). Rabies, 1996, *Int. J. Infect. Dis.* **1**, 135–142.

Winkler, W. G., Fashinell, T. R., Leffingwell, L., Howard, P., and Conomy, J. P. (1973). Airborne rabies transmission in a laboratory worker. *JAMA* **226**, 1219–1222.

World Health Organization (1992). World Health Organization expert committee on rabies: Eighth report. WHO Technical Report Series 824. WHO, Geneva.

World Health Organization (1987). Guidelines for Dog Rabies Control. VPH/83.43 Rev. 1. WHO, Geneva.

World Health Organization (1997). World Health Organization Recommendations on Rabies Post-Exposure Treatment and the Correct Technique of Intradermal Immunization against Rabies. WHO/EMC/ZOO96.6. WHO, Geneva.

World Health Organization (2000). World Survey of Rabies for the Year 1998. No. 34, WHO/CDS/CSR/APH/99.6. WHO, Geneva.

World Health Organization (2001). Intradermal Application of Rabies Vaccines: Report of a WHO Consultation. Bangkok, Thailand 5–6 June 2000. WHO/CDS/CDSRAPH/2000.05. WHO, Geneva.

13

Control of Dog Rabies

KONRAD BÖGEL

Veterinary Public Health Division of Communicable Diseases
World Health Organization
CH-1211 Geneva 19
Switzerland

I. Introduction
II. History
    A. Early Knowledge of Epidemiology and Control
    B. Development of National Services and Programs
    C. Mass Vaccination and Dog Control
    D. Limits of Stray-Dog Control
    E. End of the Myth of Stray-Dog Elimination in Developing Countries
III. Dog Accessibility: A New Term in Canine Rabies Control
IV. Present Approaches to Dog Rabies Control
V. Significance of Public Awareness and Interdisciplinary Collaboration
VI. Research on Oral Vaccination
VII. Summary
    References

I. INTRODUCTION

Despite all efforts and success stories, rabies is still rampant in large areas of the world, particularly in developing countries. In this chapter, attention will focus on new scientific developments with respect to dog ecology, handling of the stray-dog problem, oral vaccination techniques, cost-effectiveness of control operations, and historical reports on links between wolves and dogs in rabies epidemics and the predominant factor of public awareness. Reports on canine rabies-elimination programs are readily available from the World Health Organization (WHO) and Pan American Health Organization (PAHO) (WHO, 1984a, 1997; *Pasteur et la Rage*, 1985; Meslin *et al.*, 2000).

429

II. HISTORY

A. Early Knowledge of Epidemiology and Control

Reservoirs of rabies viruses in dogs appear to be distinct from those in other species. Apparently, the fox virus, being well adapted to its principal host, has hardly been seen to establish doublets or even triplets of consecutive cases in dogs (WHO, 1976; Aubert and Duchene, 1996). However, little is known about the ease of virus transmission from wolves and jackals to dogs with consecutive chains of infection and vice versa. Facing this uncertainty, genuine dog rabies with or without involvement of a secondary host species is assumed wherever dog-to-dog transmission occurs as a regular feature of an epidemic.

Records and guidelines on hunting by "packs of hounds" hand down to our generation a rather particular experience. Dogs for hunting were kept well supervised. During hunting, exposure to rabies occurred in large groups at one time. "Textbooks" on hunting, though not concerned with health services, appear to be an almost forgotten source of information on rabies. However, they might have been crucial in the development of official schemes of dog rabies control. These early books were written by and for high aristocratic and even royal circles. A publication from 1573 on hunting by packs of hounds points to rabies transmission from foxes to dogs and compares this as being "like from wolves" (Du Fouilloux, 1573; Tombal, 1985). Salnove in 1655 describes wolf and dog as the most susceptible species for rabies, the disease being transmitted by bite and breath (Tombal, 1985). From observation of exposed packs of hounds, it was known at that time that the incubation period generally is 6 weeks, that the disease occurs in a silent or furious form (d'Youville, 1788), and that animals die within 9 days of the onset of symptoms (Du Fouilloux, 1573). Records refer to killing of rabid and bitten animals. Killing of the whole pack of exposed "hounds" was early practice (Du Fouilloux, 1573; Salnove, 1655). Advice also was given to separate and observe contact animals. As early as 1788, a 1-year quarantine was suggested for dogs under observation, since in 1763 a dog was reported to have developed rabies symptoms about "13 moons" (about 12 months) after it had been bitten by a rabid animal (d'Youville, 1788).

Another source is the experience gained in urban areas. Without going back to Greek and Roman history, we may look at practices in cities in earlier centuries. Protected by high town walls and controlled entrances, cities represented circumscribed epidemiologic entities. This facilitated prevention and control. I own an original copy of a public notice of the City of Bologna, Italy, dated June 11, 1829. This notice informs the citizens that "yesterday a dog entered the town through Portal Galliera and has bitten a number of persons, because it was either naturally ferocious or carrying rabies. The persons bitten have already been cared for by a physician, and we may now only hope that the terrible hypothesis of rabies may not become true. We have also well-founded suspicion that the dog has bitten other dogs without the knowledge of their owners...." The orders then given describe in detail the following measures: (1) in-house confinement of all dogs in such a way that nobody can be bitten when entering the premises, (2) leashing of dogs when outside (otherwise considered as stray or ownerless animals), (3) killing by police of all dogs found outside houses, even if wearing collars, (4) immediate reporting of all dog bites with all circumstances for further public health measures, (5) reporting by dog owners in case their dog is bitten or shows lesions, and (6) validity of the order until further notice. In fact, this order comprises the "classical" measures of urban rabies control. Obligatory muzzling of dogs was added in European countries toward the end of the nineteenth century (Meslin *et al.*, 2000).

B. Development of National Services and Programs

The "classical" measures just described proved very effective at the community level. However, for countrywide rabies elimination, a well-functioning veterinary or health system was required with comprehensive legislation and adequate infrastructure. In a systematic manner, governments had to ensure notification and observation of cases, tracing back and forward, killing of animals infected or suspected to be infected, official observation of contacts and movement/contact restriction (confinement, leashing, muzzling), removal of freely roaming dogs, and quarantine in international transfer. The preconditions for such a control system evolved in Europe during the nineteenth century when national services of "veterinary police" began to cope with rabies and other major epidemic diseases in domestic animals. Scandinavian countries were reported to be rabies-free toward the end of the nineteenth century. Countries of central and western Europe followed early in the twentieth century, with some episodes of resurgence during and following World War I and World War II (WHO, 1984a; Meslin *et al.*, 2000). Early in the twentieth century, international institutions began to play a leading role in rabies surveillance, research, and control. Forerunners were the "global" network of Pasteur Institutes and the Pan American Sanitary Bureau, then the Health Organization of the League of Nations, the International Office of Epizootics, and eventually the World Health Organization (WHO) with its Expert Committee on Rabies (Bögel and Blajan, 1985).

C. Mass Vaccination and Dog Control

Results in Europe of countrywide rabies elimination by the classic procedure were so convincing that some governments (e.g., Germany and Austria) prohibited vaccination against rabies up to the 1970s. It was feared that immune dogs might mask the actual spread of the virus. In fact, first reports on mass vaccination from Japan were, after all, not very convincing. It took Japan from 1921–1957 to completely eliminate rabies (Meslin *et al.*, 2000). The success of large-scale vaccination in Hungary prior to and during the World War II became known internationally with considerable delay (Manninger, 1968). Meanwhile, excellent results of mass vaccination and rigorous stray-dog control were reported from Malaysia by Wells (1957). In 1973, the WHO Expert Committee on Rabies strongly recommended compulsory dog vaccination in combination with rigorous stray-dog control (WHO, 1973). Destruction of the superfluous stray-dog population, even by shooting and poisoning, became a basic element of rabies control, particularly in developing countries. Hong Kong reported being free of rabies in 1956, the Province of Taiwan, China, in 1961, Portugal in 1961, Uruguay 1983, and except single cases along the national borders, Zimbabwe in 1961, Uganda in 1961, and Israel about 1969 (WHO 1984a; Meslin *et al.*, 2000). In the 1970s, veterinary services of a number of countries purchased guns and ammunition for dog control or used special devices for the application of strychnine. However, at this time, programs were imposed on the communities by force. Certain communities, particularly animal protectionists and mass media, raised their voices because methods of mass destruction of dogs largely were inhumane and dangerous for people. Modified strategies evolved (Bögel *et al.*, 1982).

In 1984 the WHO Expert Committee on Rabies looked at dog control in a wider ecologic and social context (WHO, 1948b): capturing and killing dogs in a humane manner, but shooting and poisoning only in emergencies. Habitat control, including community education, reproduction control, and management techniques became new areas supported by the WHO policies of primary health care and community participation (WHO, 1984b). The WHO and the World Society for the Protection of Animals developed jointly the *Guidelines for Dog Population Management* (WHO–WSPA, 1990), which provide advice on legislation and techniques and a new definition of stray dogs.

Of course, the combination of vaccination and dog control underwent adaptation to national and local conditions. In areas with relatively few unsupervised dogs, removal of freely roaming and unvaccinated animals had its impact more on responsible dog ownership than on the size of dog populations. The first attempt, exploiting the psychological effect of stray-dog control as an adjunct to vaccination, might have been the immunization program in two areas of the United States in 1948, where dog rabies was brought to an abrupt end (Tierkel, 1950). Applied over the whole United States with its vast territories, canine rabies dropped from about 5000 cases in 1953 to less than 300 in 1968, and the residual cases related to rabies reservoirs in wildlife. In a similar way, remaining foci of infection were eliminated in Europe: in Italy in 1971, Greece in 1979, and Yugoslavia about 1982 (WHO, 1984a).

Mass vaccination combined with classic means of dog control also became the policy of choice wherever rabies was reintroduced in rabies-free areas, perhaps with the exception of the Guam outbreak in 1967, where poisoned baits where placed overnight to control strays. Outbreaks in Malaga, Spain, in 1975, Laredo, Texas, in 1976, Hong Kong in 1983, Belgium in 1961, French Somalia in 1962, Malaysia in 1966 and 1970, and the United Kingdom in 1969 and 1970 are referred to by the WHO (1984a). About 17 episodes of canine rabies imported into France between 1965 and 1995 were critically reviewed by Aubert and Duchene (1996).

D. Limits of Stray-Dog Control

Evidence of the limits of dog removal was reported from a number of developing countries. In Asia and South America, but also in urban and semiurban areas of Africa, 30% or even up to 60% of dogs were believed to be "strays," which cannot be vaccinated. However, 70% of a dog population needs to be immunized to stop rabies (WHO, 1984b). Under such conditions, countries mobilized enormous resources to cope with the stray-dog problem. However, almost none of the programs succeeded, and reports on rabies elimination became rare (WHO, 1984a; Meslin et al., 2000). Yet proponents of stray-dog removal claimed that the decrease by about 70% of human cases in South America was due in part to dog decimation and that similar results in Asian and African countries would fully justify the policy. Rabies persisted, however, in all these places, so a causal correlation between rabies decrease and stray-dog control must be questioned (Meslin et al., 2000). First of all, the decrease in human cases must be ascribed to dog vaccination but partially also to improved surveillance, postexposure treatment, and awareness as well as social changes. Decrease in rabies incidence in animals may well correlate with a regression of stray-dog populations, but the latter may not be due to stray-dog removal. Conditions in a European city of 1 million inhabitants may serve as an example: About 6000 dogs were removed annually over 15 years, and the disappearance of stray dogs was thought to be the result. Population biologists showed, however, that removal of 5% of a population having an annual turnover of 30–40% strengthens rather than reduces such a population. In such campaigns, predominantly weak, sick, and less productive animals are captured so that more shelter and food are left to the productive population segment and health risks are reduced (WHO–WSPA, 1990). The decrease in freely roaming dogs in cities was explained by socioeconomic changes in the human population and an increase in traffic.

National policies had to be examined critically. First, economic analyses indicated that a program of dog rabies elimination by intensive vaccination campaigns is cheaper than the perpetuation of semieffective measures, which are very expensive (Motschwiller, 1998; Bögel and Meslin, 1990). Second, the procedure of dog catching and killing instead of vaccination appears erroneous in the epidemiologic context. Removing an animal leaves behind a gap and increases territorial movement and contact rates, whereas vaccinating and releasing the dog in its habitat creates a barrier to virus transmission.

E. End of the Myth of Stray-Dog Elimination in Developing Countries

About 1980 WHO experts began to complain that much knowledge had accrued on fox ecology from WHO-coordinated research, but almost nothing was known about the dynamics of dog populations. Failures of dog rabies control simply might have been due to policies ignoring basic mechanisms of population biology. In order to overcome scientific shortcomings, three research projects were initiated by the WHO with United Nations Development Program (UNDP) support in Sri Lanka, Tunisia, and Ecuador in 1984, primarily coordinated by F. Meslin (Meslin et al., 2000), A. Wandeler (Wandeler and Budde, 1993), and G. Beran and M. Frith (1998). Under different sociocultural conditions, the studies addressed the following questions: What are the ecologic factors that determine segments of dog populations, and how can these segments be defined? What is the population turnover, and what is its importance for control measures? What constitutes dog population management from an ecologic and ethical point of view?

The results changed views drastically (WHO, 1988). In fact, not more than 4–6% of the dog population could be seized annually, even in situations of an upsurge of human and animal rabies cases. In one year, extreme efforts were made in the Guayaquil project, and about 24% of the estimated dog population was removed. No significant effect on population size and rabies incidence was noted (WHO, 1988). An annual turnover of 30–40% of the dog population was shown to be quite "normal" in the countries involved in the WHO project. Under such conditions, dog populations exert such pressure for survival that this compensates almost immediately and continuously for removed animals. Studies carried out by WHO-associated teams in Morocco, Zambia, and Turkey corroborate these results (Meslin et al., 2000).

With the erroneous value of destroyed dogs in mind, the number of dogs eliminated should be contrasted with the quantity of dogs immunized, e.g., 32 million dogs vaccinated versus 800,000 dogs removed in South America in 1997, or 180,000 dogs vaccinated versus about 30,000 removed annually in Tunisia, or 196,000 dogs eliminated in Chile over 2 years, an equivalent of about one-fourth of the number of dogs vaccinated (Meslin et al., 2000). As impressive as such figures might appear to a control manager, they point only to the use of resources for a very expensive procedure of dog capture and euthanasia, on the one hand, and inadequate vaccination coverage, on the other, apart from the continuing costs of human postexposure treatment and epidemiologic surveillance/diagnosis.

III. DOG ACCESSIBILITY: A NEW TERM IN CANINE RABIES CONTROL

Rather accidentally, *dog accessibility* became a key condition and term in canine rabies control. WHO experts define this term as the percentage of dogs in a given population that can be caught by a person without special effort (Bögel and Joshi, 1990; Schumacher and Meslin, 1998). Nothing better than this new term signifies the changes in rabies control policies, and this is best explained by the event in 1986 that led to its introduction (Bögel and Joshi, 1990). A WHO Intercountry Training Course on Dog Population Management had just finished. The participants had left Nepal with new knowledge on ecologic approaches to dog control, the conclusions of the meeting in mind: "Dog populations are more heterogeneous than free-living wild animals," and "removal of all stray dogs (estimated 40–60% of the dog population) was necessary for successful rabies control."

The day following the departure of the experts and trainees, the WHO secretary of the meeting, who planned to spend a quiet day of writing in Kathmandu, was perplexed to see virtually all dogs in the streets adorned with painted marks on their foreheads and a yellow flower collar. Even the "stray dogs" on the heap of kitchen waste near the hotel wore these marks. It seemed as if the dogs of Kathmandu had waited until departure of the WHO experts, just to fool them. It was October 31, the holy day *kukor puja*, devoted to the dog. Families gave food to dogs at home or on the street and worshipped them with the ceremonial signs. The WHO secretary, now retired and writing this chapter, immediately hired a rickshaw and counted dogs with or without ceremonial marks or household association. The term of *dog accessibility* was born. A 3-day study in Kathmandu and two other nearby townships followed. The total expenses (for transportation) did not exceed US$25 for this large-scale field trial on dog accessibility. Even the assistant to the principal investigator (his wife) served voluntarily with great pleasure. Walking through the streets in a nonsystematic manner, the accessibility of dogs by foreigners and individual reference persons was recorded as well as their household associations. Interviewing people clarified the status of nonaccessible dogs. They were either aggressive, defending their premises in the absence of their family, or fugitive, mostly because their home was further away or even on another street. Children led the "investigation team" to all the places where dogs outside the premises took a rest and shelter from the sun and heat. In general, all dogs were known to the people (Bögel and Joshi, 1990).

Result: A surprisingly high percentage (86–97%) of dogs was found accessible and amenable by at least one "reference person" and to be associated with a "reference household."

Based on these findings, an intensive vaccination program was carried out in 1989 in the town of Lalitpur. This campaign was carefully prepared based on principles of community participation, taking advantage of the experience gained in the WHO project in Guayaquil, Ecuador (WHO, 1984) but without any dog removal in mind. The project consisted of comprehensive planning using the management tools described by WHO (1984a); intensive public education by loud-speaker hailing, banners, posters, leaflets, radio and television broadcasts, newspaper articles, participation of schoolteachers, presentation of a WHO videofilm on canine rabies, and so on; a survey of 755 households on awareness, willingness to cooperate, and associated dogs; dog ecology study, including marking and recapture of vaccinated dogs to estimate the total dog population and the proportion of dogs vaccinated; and vaccine application by six teams at fixed vaccination points, two clean-up teams subsequently going house to house in areas of inadequate vaccination coverage.

Result: 8400 dogs received vaccine, and these accounted for 68% of the total dog population (Bögel and Joshi, 1990).

From then on, the accessibility of dogs became the most important condition and factor overlying other definitions of dog segments (see Sect. IV). The study area in Nepal was too small for data on the course of the epidemic. In Lalitpur, single human cases occurred at intervals of years. However, in Lima, Peru, and its harbor, i.e., under totally different sociocultural conditions, the health impact of swift mass vaccination of dogs was demonstrated. This vaccination experiment was implemented by the French Mission Bioforce in collaboration with Peruvian authorities, and data on the course and end of a serious rabies epidemic became available about the time of the Nepal experiment (Lombard *et al.*, 1989). Within 1 month, 273,000 dogs, including as many stray dogs as possible, and 54,000 cats were vaccinated by 110 teams. The size of the total dog population was determined by an internationally recommended procedure. Under test were the management procedure, the efficacy of the inactivated vaccine used, the persistence of antibody in immunized animals, and the overall impact on the epidemic. Rabies disappeared for a number of years. The campaign reached 65% of the estimated dog population in addition to the 12.7% that had been vaccinated already before by private veterinarians and official vaccination centers. Thus the total vaccination coverage reached 77.7%. Two years later, rabies antibody still could be demonstrated in 89% of the immunized dogs.

Another example of swift mass vaccination of 35,000 dogs and associated research has been reported from the Philippines (WHO, 1994) for an area of extremely high dog density, the human–dog ratio being 3.8:1. Applying the WHO/EPI cluster survey technique, a vaccination coverage of 72.5% was determined. However, the dog marking and visual recapture survey resulted only in 47.4% vaccination coverage, the difference possibly being due to rapid loss of marks before evaluation.

IV. PRESENT APPROACHES TO DOG RABIES CONTROL

In 1992, the WHO Expert Committee on Rabies examined with extreme care all scientific data on the controversial issue of stray-dog decimation and reached the following conclusion:

> On the basis of the results obtained so far in these studies, the Committee recommended drastic changes in rabies control policies as compared with those previously adopted and practised by most national authorities and communities. There is no evidence that removal of dogs has ever had a significant impact on dog population densities or the spread of rabies. The population turnover of dogs may be so high that even the highest recorded removal rates (about 15% of the dog population) are easily compensated for by increased survival rates. In addition, dog removal may be unacceptable to local communities. Therefore, this approach should not be used in large-scale control programmes unless ecological and socio-cultural studies show it to be feasible [WHO, 1992a].

Unfortunately, the new policy, even today, has not yet found its way to the planners and managers in many countries. Obsolete programs, which place so much nonsubstantiated emphasis on dog removal, continue even today, although they fail with respect to their original zerotarget for dog rabies. Wrong advice and advisers persist along with these programs, still working with faulty assumptions made up to the 1970s (WHO Expert Committee, 1973), even up to 1984, although with some modification (WHO Expert Committee, 1984).

As a consequence, many national programs in South America, Asia, and Africa with the original aim of eliminating dog rabies converted silently to control operations that resulted in a somewhat reduced incidence of rabies and exposure. In these countries, vaccination covers hardly 40% of the dog population (Meslin *et al.*, 2000). The experience may be summed up as: *The dream of dog population reduction attracts lax vaccination to form an ineffective, if not dishonest, combination.*

In order to facilitate legislation and a practical approach, these definitions of segments of dog populations (WHO and WSPA, 1990; WHO, 1993) were adopted by the WHO Expert Committee on Rabies and brought in line with the new findings (WHO, 1992a):

Restricted or supervised dogs: Fully dependent on their owners and fully restricted or supervised; *accessible.*

Family dogs: Fully dependent on their owners, but their movements are only partially restricted; *accessible.*

Neighborhood or community dogs: Partially dependent on humans and partially restricted or unrestricted in movements; *accessible.*

Feral dogs: Independent and unrestricted, having no referral household or person, often in packs and not wanted by people, *nonaccessible*.

Owned dogs: Ecologically irrelevant term, which should be used only in connection with administrative measures exerted on them, e.g., licensing, tax, movement restrictions, or vaccination. Dogs of this group have reference person(s) or household(s) and belong to one of the preceding categories of restricted, family, or neighborhood dogs; *accessible*.

Stray dogs: Ecologically irrelevant term, which should be used only to define a dog that is not in compliance with local rabies control regulations, e.g., not vaccinated, on leash, confined, or supervised. It can belong to various categories of dogs described earlier and may just be freely roaming part of the day or night, or it may be lost, abandoned, or feral; accessible or nonaccessible.

For mass vaccination programs, the differentiation between accessible and nonaccessible dogs is significant.

The dog vaccination programs and research projects under WHO auspices led to a vast collection of results and recommendations. The experience is reflected in a number of publications and guidelines. Although varying between and within countries, some major conclusions of worldwide application can be drawn (Meslin, 2000; WHO, 1998):

- Contrary to what local officers in most countries perceived, a relatively small proportion of animals is actually found without a reference person or household. Most of the dogs caught and eliminated would be accessible in well-organized programs.

- Mass elimination of freely roaming and unsupervised dogs is likely to be counterproductive to community participation and should not be undertaken prior to thorough ecologic and sociocultural investigation. Vaccination and release of caught animals may be of greater significance in rabies control.

- The size of the dog population generally is underestimated, so the proportion of vaccinated dogs is overestimated. For seized dogs, this error might even be larger. Only recommended methods of dog population measurement should be used.

- In general, permanent vaccination centers reach a low proportion of the owned and accessible dogs. With mobile vaccination centers operating in areas of a diameter as small as a few hundred meters, between 40% and 85% of the dog population could be reached. In order to maintain a desired immunization level, there is need of regular vaccination campaigns at annual or biannual intervals in addition to continuing vaccination services at centers for young and introduced dogs.

- In countries where freely roaming and unsupervised dogs are rare, the threat of stray-dog elimination remains an adjunct of compulsory vaccination in order to foster responsible dog ownership.

However, is this really the very end of the myth of dog elimination in canine rabies control? It seems, at least, that in some countries dog accessibility may fall short of critical levels. Although being an exception rather than the rule, further research should clarify whether low accessibility is more an expression of human behavior toward dogs and disease control or really a peculiarity of the dogs in a particular environment, e.g., in Yemen (Meslin, personal communication, 2000) and areas of Turkey (WHO, 1992b). New techniques, such as oral dog vaccination (see Sect. VI) also may help overcome this problem.

V. SIGNIFICANCE OF PUBLIC AWARENESS AND INTERDISCIPLINARY COLLABORATION

Rabies has been notable since ancient times for its peculiarities of exposure and disease, which are unique. It is only communicable disease for which the moment of infection is known and associated with a fearful accident, namely, the unexpected bite by a furious animal. Subsequent stages are not less dramatic: incertitude during a long period of incubation and certainty of a horrible death once symptoms develop. This sequence of events associates rabies with an incomparable public awareness, and in return, this is an important prerequisite for its control. Signs in dogs and wildlife are in addition so pathognomic that an outbreak could hardly be missed. People in endemic or freshly invaded areas of high incidence generally are well aware of risks. They take all kinds of protective measures, including personal defence, as seen in African villages: persons walking within the village with a stick, e.g., on the way to school, to check attacking dogs. Stray dogs are killed and others are subject to movement and contact restrictions.

As much as fear and awareness of rabies contribute to its control, as deplorable is the warning awareness in areas that have been free of the disease for some years. From a first, undetected case in an imported dog, long incubation periods permit the virus to spread in erratic patterns before it is detected and brought under control. The index case noted may well be a human case. However, at least professionals in animal and human health should be trained to detect freshly introduced rabies promptly. Services should inform the population at risk. In fact, the sequence of events has to pass through a line of detection filters in most outbreaks. In the case of dog rabies, these point of suspicion are as follows: (1) the owner of the dog who notices unusual symptoms, or (2) the veterinarian to whom the sick animal may be presented, or (3) a bitten person if the circumstances of the bite are unusual, or (4) the physician when a patient reports an unusual dog bite and seeks treatment. Despite all these detection points, lack of awareness still takes its toll. The following example of a human rabies case in Spain (WHO Collaborating Center, 1978–1980) should be taken as a warning for dog owners and professionals in rabies-free areas and countries: The victim was a physician bitten by his own dog, thus representing the preceding key individuals all in one person. Even more tragic, the victim, being a physician and dog owner, was not informed of a fresh episode of imported dog rabies that had occurred about 80 km from his place of residence and was subject to rigorous measure by the Ministry of Agriculture.

This raises the question of interdisciplinary collaboration, which calls for permanent challenge not only with respect to epidemiologic surveillance but also with respect to cost-effectiveness of all the measures taken in prevention and control. Some aspects were mentioned earlier (Bögel and Meslin, 1990; Motschwiller, 1988). A review with pertinent recommendations is included in Annex 4 of the WHO Expert Committee Report (1992a).

VI. RESEARCH ON ORAL VACCINATION

The WHO began to coordinate research on oral rabies immunization in dogs in about 1985. Major problems of dog vaccination in developing countries called for a solution (see Sect. IIE). Canine rabies reservoirs were responsible worldwide for 99% of human deaths due to rabies and for 90% of postexposure treatment. Referring to this situation, a first WHO consultation on oral vaccination of dogs against rabies was organized in 1988 (WHO, 1988b). Results of laboratory studies in Europe and Africa and of a field trial in China were the starting points of international research over more than 10 years ago. The WHO, with the participation of the International Office of Epizootic (OIE) in Paris, entrusted the studies mainly to its network of WHO collaborating centers. The conditions differed markedly from those encountered in oral immunization of foxes in that 10 times more vaccine virus was shown to be needed to immunize a dog. Unfortunately, this high dose carries increased risks to animals that could inadvertently take up a bait containing vaccine virus. Moreover, oral vaccine is not given to dogs far outside in nature but close or even inside human habitation. This leads to even more stringent requirements for oral dog vaccine and its application. On the other hand, oral dog vaccination offers great advantages over parenteral vaccination. Dogs need not to be caught and the bait could be handed over to the owners, who may give the bait under conditions familiar to the animal.

WHO consultations have concentrated on major aspects: potential areas for application and basic data on bait composition and acceptance (WHO, 1992b), safety testing in target and nontarget species (WHO, 1993), dog ecology including accessibility (WHO, 1994), progress review and regulatory requirements

(WHO, 1994), safety studies and requirements including vaccinia–recombinant rabies vaccine (WHO, 1998), and overall review and guidelines for research and field application (Schumacher and Meslin, 1998). Whereas most of the field studies so far have been carried out with placebo baits, some limited field trials have already been carried out with vaccine virus. Vaccine type studies are mainly those examined and used for rabies control in wildlife: (1) modified-live rabies viruses (MLV), such as SAD strains (B-19, Berne, P5/88), SAG strains (double mutants of SAD), and ERA strain, and (2) recombinant live viruses (RLV), such as vaccinia–rabies glycoprotein (VRG) recombinant virus, human adenovirus-5 recombinants, and rabbitpox–rabies glycoprotein (RPRG) recombinant virus (see Chap. 11).

A table summarizing results with these vaccine candidates was published by WHO (1998). This research in target and nontarget species led to increasing confidence in this technique, although the relatively high amount of virus required and low rate of seroconversion still call for considerable improvement.

VII. SUMMARY

Movement restriction of dogs, killing of rabid and bitten dogs, separation and observation of possibly exposed dogs, and removal of stray dogs remain the classic means of control that have led to the elimination of canine rabies in European countries in the nineteenth and the first half of the twentieth century. Between 1950 and about 1975, vaccine application in combination with destruction of stray dogs permitted a number of countries, including developing countries, to eliminate canine rabies virus. The combination of vaccination with classic control measures is still the method of choice in locations where dog rabies is introduced in a rabies-free area or country. In order to cope with a high proportion of freely roaming and unsupervised dogs, the policy of mass destruction of dogs was adopted widely in the world. However, over the years, this proved to be ineffective, with hardly more than 4% of the total dog population being removed per year. This removal rate is almost immediately compensated for by the survival pressure of other dogs, which generally are nonvaccinated. The WHO gave advice to change such policies and apply methods that aim at higher dog accessibility. With few exceptions, 70–80% of dogs could, in fact, be vaccinated under conditions prevailing in developing countries. WHO-coordinated research may bring about oral dog rabies vaccination as an adjunct to parenteral mass vaccination. This may facilitate rabies control where dogs are difficult to vaccinate by injection, should such conditions become apparent. Global eradication of rabies from its canine reservoir thus may become a realistic goal. Prospective analyses show that dog rabies elimination or even eradication is feasible and more economic than the maintenance of expensive services for human postexposure treatment, in addition to those for surveillance and inadequate control of rabies in dogs.

REFERENCES

Aubert, M., and Duchene, M. J. (1996). L'importation en France de carnivores domestiques en incubation de rage de 1968 à 1995. *BEMRAF* **26** (2), 1–8.

Beran, G., and Frith, M. (1988). Domestic animal rabies control: An overview. *Rev. Infect. Dis.* **10**, 672–677.

Bögel, K., and Blajan, L. (1985). Coopération internationale et controle de la rage. In *Pasteur et la Rage*, pp. 235S–240S. Information Technique des Services Vétérinaires, Ministére de Agriculture, Paris.

Bögel, K., Andral, L., Beran, G., Schneider, L.G., and Wandeler, A. (1982). Dog rabies elimination: A trend analysis and program proposal prepared by a WHO working group. *Int. J. Zoon.* **9** (2), 97–112.

Bögel, K., and Joshi, D. D. (1990). Accessibility of dog populations for rabies control in Kathmand, Nepal. *Bull. WHO* **68**, 611–617.

Bögel, K., and Meslin, F.-X. (1990). Economics of human and canine rabies elimination: Guidelines for program orientation. *Bull. WHO* **68**, 281–291.

d'Youville (1788). *Traité de Vérnerie*; cited in Tombal (1985).

Du Fouilloux (1573). *Traité de Vénerie*; re-edidet by Roger Dacosta 1979; cited in Tombal (1985).

Lombard, M., Chappuis, G., Chomel, B., and de Beublain, T. D. (1989). Three years of epidemiological and serological results after a dog rabies vaccination campaign in Lima, Peru. In *WHO–Kovalenko All Union Institute-Merieux Foundation Report of the Workshop on Rabies Control in Asian Countries, Samarkand*, Foundation Marcel Merieux (ed.), pp. 67–76. Lyon.

Manninger, R. (1968). Rabies in Hungary during the past forty years. *Mag. Allotor. Lap.* **23**, 5–13.

Meslin, F.-X., Fishbein, D. B., and Matter, H. C. (1994). Rationale and prospects for dog rabies elimination in developing countries. In *Lyssavirus*, C. E. Rupprecht, B. Dietzschold, and H. Koprowski (eds.), pp. 1–26. Springer-Verlag, Berlin.

Meslin, F.-X., Miies, M. A., and Gemmell, M. A. (2000–2001). Zoonoses control in dogs. In *Dogs, Zoonoses and Public Health*, C. Macpherson, F.-X. Meslin, and A. Wandeler (eds.). CAB International, London (in press).

Motschwiller, E. (1988). Epidemiological and ecological aspects of dog rabies and its control in countries of the third world [German]. Inaugural dissertation, Verterinary Faculty, University of Munich, Germany.

Pasteur et la Rage (1985). Information Technique des Services Vétérinaires, Ministére de Agriculture, Paris.

Salnove, R. (1655). *La Vénerie Royale*; cited in Tombal (1985).

Schumacher, C. L., and Meslin, F.-X. (1998). Guidelines for Research on Oral Rabies Vaccines. Working Document to WHO Consultation on Field Application of Oral Vaccines for Dogs. WHO, Geneva.

Tierkel, E. S., Graves, L. M., Tuggle, H. G., and Wandley, S. L. (1950). Effective control of an outbreak of rabies in Memphis and Shelby County, Tennessee. *Am. J. Public Health* **40**, 1084–1088.

Tombal, A. (1985). La Rage, la Chasse et la Foret. In *Pasteur et la Rage*, pp. 37–40. Information Technique des Services Vétérinaires, Ministère de Agriculture, Paris.

Wandeler, A. I., Matter, H. C., Kappeler, A., and Budde, A. (1993). The ecology of dogs and canine rabies: A selective review. *Rev. Sci. Tech. OIE* **12**, 51–71.

Wells, C. W. (1957). Rabies control in Malaya, August 1952–October 1956. *Bull. WHO* **17**, 1025–1029.

World Health Organization (1973). Sixth Report of the WHO Expert Committee on Rabies. Technical Report Series No. 523. WHO, Geneva.

World Health Organization (1976). Report of Consultations on the WHO/FAO coordinated Research Programme on Wildlife Rabies in Europe. Document WHO/VPH/76.2. WHO, Geneva.

World Health Organization (1984a). *Guidelines for Dog Rabies Control*, K. Bögel (ed.). Document VPH/83.43. WHO, Geneva.

World Health Organization (1984b). Seventh Report of the WHO Expert Committee on Rabies. Technical Report Series No. 709. WHO, Geneva.

World Health Organization (1988). Report of a WHO Consultation on Dog Ecology Studies Related to Rabies Control. Document WHO/Rab.Res./88.25. WHO, Geneva.

World Health Organization (1992a). Eigth Report of the WHO Expert Committee on Rabies. Technical Report Series No. 824. WHO, Geneva.

World Health Organization (1992b). Third Consultation on Oral Immunisation of Dogs against Rabies. Document WHO/Rab.Res./92.38. WHO, Geneva.

World Health Organizations (1993). Report of the 4th Consultation on Oral Immunisation of Dogs against Rabies. Document WHO/Rab.Res./93.42. WHO, Geneva.

World Health Organization (1994). Report of the 5th Consultation on Oral Immunisation of Dogs against Rabies. Document WHO/Rab.Res./94.45. WHO, Geneva.

World Health Organization (1997). World Survey of Rabies No. 33. Document WSR. WHO, Geneva.

World Health Organization (1998). Oral Immunisation of Dogs against Rabies: Report of the 6th Consultation. Document WHO/EMC/ZDI/98.13. WHO, Geneva.

World Health Organization Collaborating Center, Tübingen (1978–1980). *Rabies Bulletin Europe*, Quarterly Reports, Tübingen, Germany.

World Health Organization–World Society for the Protection of Animals (1990). Guidelines for Dog Population Management. WHO Document Zoon/90.165. WHO, Geneva.

14

Rabies Control in Wildlife

DAVID H. JOHNSTON

Johnston Biotech
Sarnia, Ontario N7V 3B5
Canada

ROWLAND R. TINLINE

Queen's GIS Laboratory
Queen's University
Kingston, Ontario K7L 3N6
Canada

I. THE CONCEPT OF CONTROLLING RABIES IN WILDLIFE

Since the early observations of Jenner and Pasteur, pioneers in the concept of vaccination, scientists have been fascinated with the idea of using a modified disease organism to generate immunity against that disease. From the early successes have evolved today's vaccines for both humans and domestic animals, and it was only a natural progression of this idea that vaccination of wild animals might be considered to further remove the threat of rabies. In 1966, this led the World Health Organization (WHO) Expert Committee on Rabies to call for research into the possible rabies vaccination of free-ranging wild animals (WHO, 1966). Carnivores, particularly dogs, have transmitted rabies since early recorded history, and there was then a call for control not only in dogs but also in other wild canids such as foxes. But how to vaccinate a wild animal? Carnivores, as the scientific order *Carnivora* implies, gain their principal nutrition by eating flesh, and the fact that rabies transmission by this group is by biting provided a possible mode of delivery for the vaccine as well. Oral vaccination had long been the goal of pharmaceutical enterprise, but to carry this approach to wildlife seemed insurmountable. One of the first researchers, George Baer, tried to orally vaccinate foxes with the existing injectable rabies vaccines LEP and HEP (see Chap. 11), and he showed that the concept of oral rabies vaccination was possible (Baer, 1988). Winkler (1992) carried the injectable concept to the field with a trap mechanism that would inject the animal that triggered the trap, but large-scale field application by this method quickly was seen to be impracticable. Baits containing poisons had long been used by humans to kill predators. Would it be possible to incorporate a vaccine in place of poison within a bait? Many prototype baits were first field tested by ground and aerial distribution in small-scale field trials without an oral vaccine while those vaccines were being developed (Black and Lawson, 1970; Baer *et al.*, 1971; Johnston, 1975; Linhart *et al.*, 1997). Instead of using an actual vaccine, chemical fluorochrome markers such as calcein, rhodamine, or tetracycline were put into the baits to test the feasibility of reaching the high percentage of animals necessary to vaccinate a large, wild population of rabies vectors (Linhart and Kennelly, 1967; Linhart *et al.*, 1997; Ellenton and Johnston, 1979; Wandeler *et al.*, 1975). This early work, without actual vaccine in the baits, showed that the concept of mass baiting of a wild species, in this case the red fox (*Vulpes vulpes*), was feasible and lead to the first wild release of an oral vaccine in chicken head baits in Switzerland in 1977 (Steck *et al.*, 1982; Winkler, 1992). These early beginnings provided a glimmer of hope that a vaccination system for wildlife could be developed but also showed the need for the integration of a wide range of technical resources to implement large-scale oral rabies vaccination programs (ORVPs). The scientific and technical evolution that followed this impetus by the WHO Expert Committee on Rabies has been one of the broadest-based endeavors in modern medicine (Bögel *et al.*, 1992). Over 30 specialities can be listed as contributing to the ORV endeavors that have developed since.

Figure 1 illustrates the many interrelated steps that have been followed in establishing a program for rabies control in wild carnivores ranging from the diagnosis of rabies in wild species to the development of a management team to carry out the program, monitor its success, and handle all related aspects of funding, licensing, liability, and public relations. Each of these steps are described below.

II. CHIROPTERAN RABIES CONTROL

The question of rabies control in *Chiroptera* requires techniques different from the oral vaccination approach for terrestrial carnivores outlined in Fig. 1. The use of anticoagulants to reduce vampire bat (*Desmodus rotundus*) populations feeding on cattle has proved successful in limiting vampire bat infection (Arellano-Sota, 1988). These techniques are quite labor-intensive, requiring contact either with the bat, bat roosts, or the bitten animals, principally cattle. The control of rabies in insectivorous bats, especially *Eptesicus fuscus*, the big brown bat, and *Lasionycteris noctivagans*, the silver haired bat, which are major sources of human exposure and deaths, will tax the ingenuity of scientists long into the future (Messenger *et al.*, 2002) (see Chap. 5).

III. INITIATION OF WILDLIFE RABIES CONTROL PROGRAMS

The initiation of wildlife rabies control programs has been stimulated by impending epizootics but also precipitated by unexpected happenings. In Canada, it is curious that the site of the first recorded human death from wildlife rabies in 1819 also was the site of the origin of the Canadian wildlife rabies control program in 1967. The Duke of Richmond, Governor-in-Chief of British North America, died at Richmond, Ontario, in 1819 from the bite of a rabid fox (Jackson, 1994), and in 1967, also at Richmond, 4-year-old Donna Featherstone died of rabies contracted from the bite of a stray cat. It was her death that precipitated public demand for the Province of Ontario to mount a well-funded control program against fox rabies, which had been epizootic in the Province since 1954 (Johnston and Beauregard, 1969). That program still has government support after 34 years and has been successful in nearly eliminating arctic fox-strain rabies from the province (MacInnis *et al.*, 2001). The benefits now apparent from this investment have far outweighed the cost. A similar series of events involving two human deaths from a coyote-associated (*Canis latrans*) strain of rabies in Texas stimulated the initiation of the Texas Oral Rabies Vaccination Program, chronicled by Finley (1998).

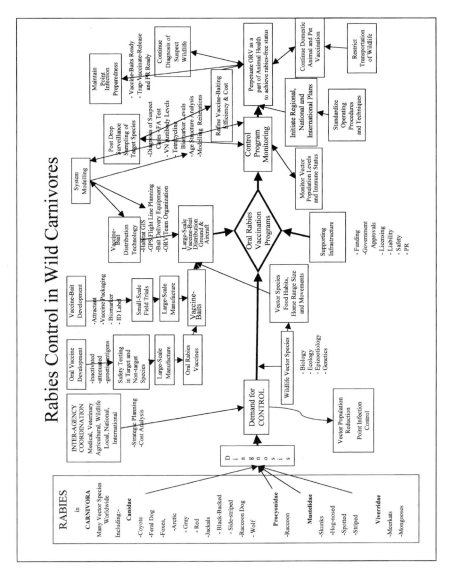

Fig. 1. Rabies control in wild carnivores.

The initiation of wildlife rabies control, as it has evolved today, requires the careful integration of a complex series of events and disciplines. It presents an opportunity for all areas of science and technology, from fur trappers to virologists and pilots to politicians, to come together in a cooperative effort to control a virus that is harmful to animals and humans alike. To be effective, all components of a wildlife control system must function together as a coherent system (McGuill *et al.*, 1997; Nunan, 1999). Modification or omission of any component of the control system may alter the efficiency and outcome of the whole control program, sometimes deleteriously (Stöhr and Meslin, 1996).

The time dimension is important with regard to both the initiation and continuation of a control program if rabies-free status is to be achieved and maintained in an area. In the past, rabies epizootics have flourished in the absence of timely control efforts or appropriate technology. Even when appropriate control technologies are at hand today, lack of political will often has wasted precious time, allowing epizootics to gain hold and advance into virgin animal populations. Disrupted programs can exacerbate existing ecologic and epidemiologic conditions and prolong epizootics (Müller, 1997). Conversely, timely, efficient programs have proved effective in halting advancing epizootic fronts, and it is apparent that the field of wildlife rabies control technology has developed to the point where wildlife rabies epizootics in several species and jurisdictions can be controlled, if not eradicated.

IV. DIAGNOSIS OF SUSPECT WILDLIFE

Paramount to the initiation of any ORVP is a delineation of the problem in wildlife: the diagnosis of suspect cases (see Chap. 9), identification of the strains of rabies virus that are isolated (see Chap. 3), the species involved (see Chap. 5), and where in the local ecology and epizootiology these species fit in relation to humans, pets, and domestic animals. A comprehensive and continuing diagnostic system is a control imperative if wildlife rabies is to be controlled and eventually eradicated.

V. ANIMAL POPULATION REDUCTION: THE FIRST CALL FOR CONTROL

With any nuisance animal problem, the first human response is often "shoot the offender." Animal population reduction is a control method that immediately suggests itself when an epizootic arises, but this approach largely has been unsuccessful in eliminating rabies in a wild endemic situation. However, population reduction may have its place as a component of control technology when applied to a newly established point focus of infection springing up in a naive population.

Point infection control (PIC) has been successful in limiting the spread of a new focus of raccoon-strain rabies that appeared in Ontario in 1999 after moving across the St. Lawrence River from adjacent New York State (Rosatte *et al.*, 2001b).

VI. VECTOR SPECIES BIOLOGY, EPIDEMIOLOGY, AND GENETICS

Before wildlife rabies control can be initiated confidently, the epidemiology of the existing rabies situation should be understood as fully as possible. This requires the submission and diagnosis of rabies-suspect animals, both domestic and wild. In the past, the extent of epizootics in wildlife often has become apparent only after domestic animal diagnosis has been expanded to include wild species (Andral and Joubert, 1975; Rupprecht *et al.*, 1995). While the principal wildlife vectors in an epizootic usually are readily apparent, the role of secondary vectors in perpetuating the outbreak may not be well understood but can prove crucial. Examples of secondary vector importance include the role of striped skunks (*Mephitis mephitis*) in maintaining the arctic variant of rabies virus in eastern North America, particularly Ontario (Tinline, 1988; MacInnes *et al.*, 2001). Skunks are known to be long-term incubators of this strain (Charlton *et al.*, 1988) and can pose a source of viral reintroduction to the principal vector, the red fox, once populations rebound beyond the threshold necessary to support an epizootic (Voigt *et al.*, 1985). Similarly, in the raccoon-strain (*Procyon lotor*) epizootics currently advancing in the northeastern United States (Maine, Massachusetts, New Hampshire, New York, Ohio, and Vermont) and Canada (Ontario, Quebec and New Brunswick), the skunk is an important wildlife vector, second only to the raccoon, and its role in maintaining this strain during interepizootic troughs in the raccoon population remains to be fully evaluated (Childs *et al.*, 2000). Also, the role of foxes, red and gray (*Urocyon cinereoargenteus*), is not without comment. While the raccoon is the principal wildlife vector in terms of incidence in this epizootic, foxes are also diagnosed within the epizootic areas, and in a few cases, rabid foxes have appeared up to 100 km ahead of the raccoon front, suggesting a hypothesis of how long jumps in the front are possible because red foxes, in particular, are capable of long dispersal movements (Rosatte, 2001a). In attempting to control rabies in wildlife, it is therefore important to understand the ecologic relationship among the potential wildlife hosts, particularly if oral vaccination is proposed as a control method. During the development of ORV, there has been much research into the viral genetics of wild rabies strains and attenuated and recombinant vaccine strains (see Chap. 3). The genotypic variation in target mammalian populations responding to these antigens also needs understanding if we are to clarify the long-term impact of ORV control on a population. In Ontario, for example, it is known that there was a shift in the population genotypes in red foxes following the invasion of arctic fox–strain rabies from arctic Canada in the 1950s. The red fox population, noted for its overt coat color genotypes ranging through nine color phases from cherry red to silver, changed in composition (Butler, 1951; Lloyd, 1980). The homozygous cherry red genotype disappeared from southern Ontario after the initial epizootic, but the exact genetic-related reasons remain unclear. With current genetic mapping technology, it will be possible to monitor changes in the genetic composition of vector species as well as the infecting viruses before, during, and after epizootics (Lin *et al.*, 1972; Wandeler *et al.*, 1994; Nadin-Davis *et al.*, 1996).

VII. TRANSPORTATION OF WILDLIFE

The mode of introduction of a point outbreak is not always known, but as with many other disease organisms, it is becoming clear that translocation by humans, either intentional or unintentional, often is the origin of infected wildlife, e.g., raccoon (Nettles *et al.*, 1979; Jenkins *et al.*, 1988; Rosatte and MacInnes, 1989), coyote (CDC, 1995), and bat (Rupprecht *et al.*, 1995; Messenger *et al.*, 2002). Therefore, jurisdictions are encouraged to implement stronger legislation regulating the importation, distribution, and relocation of wildlife (CDC, 2001a).

VIII. ORAL RABIES VACCINE DEVELOPMENT

The development of rabies vaccines for oral administration to wildlife has been complex (see Chap. 11). It involves a host of considerations, including efficacy testing in the target vector species first by intramuscular and then by oral routes. As with the release of any new biologically active agent, whether vaccine, antibiotic, or pesticide, there is concern for safety. The release of a pesticide molecule, engineered in a laboratory, is under direct human control when released, and further release can be limited even though it may persist in the biologic web (e.g., DDT), whereas an organism capable of reproduction, such as a live-virus vaccine, has the potential for amplification and divergence in nature. Safety testing in animals, including humans, that may contact the vaccine bait in the field is therefore a prime consideration, and therein lies the quest for an ideal wildlife vaccine (Fekadu *et al.*, 1991; Charlton *et al.*, 1992; Hu *et al.*, 1997; Masson *et al.*, 1997; Tims *et al.*, 2000; Wandeler, 2000; CDC, 2001b).

IX. VACCINE BAIT DEVELOPMENT

Virtually any material thought attractive to a target species has been tested as a potential bait to carry the oral vaccine. These are reported in a comprehensive review by Linhart et al. (1997). In addition to the safety of the rabies vaccine antigen itself, safety of the entire bait materials is important. The bait is both a chemically and physically complex object that will be released unretrievably into the environment, and therefore, the safety of all bait constituents and their freedom from pathogens must be ensured. The release of a prion-bearing component could have far-reaching complications in large-scale free wild release (Charlton, 1984; CDC, 2000). As a physical object, a bait can cause deleterious consequences. Heavy, hard baits may become lethal projectiles when dropped from the air; sharp-cornered vaccine packages may become lodged in the throat of ingesting animals if gulped.

Two main types of rabies vaccine baits are currently in use in large-scale ORV programs in North America. These are the Raboral V-RG Bait manufactured by Merial, Inc., Athens, Georgia (Merial, 1999), containing the vaccinia–rabies glycoprotein recombinant vaccine (V-RG) (Rupprecht et al., 1986), which is inserted into a fishmeal polymer cube (Hanlon et al., 1998) manufactured by Bait-Tek, Inc., Orange, Texas. The second bait is the Ontario Bait, containing either the live attenuated ERA vaccine (Lawson and Bachmann, 2001), (manufactured by Artemis Technologies, Inc., Guelph, Ontario, Canada), or the same Merial V-RG vaccine used in the Raboral V-RG Bait (Bachmann et al., 1990; Rosatte et al., 1992; MacInnes et al., 2001). These baits all contain tetracycline as a biomarker. There are many other recent bait developments and ORV programs for the various carnivore species listed in Fig. 1 (Perry et al., 1988; Nyberg et al., 1992; Creekmore et al., 1994; Svrcek et al., 1995; Brochier et al., 1996; Follman et al., 1996; Matter et al., 1998; Bingham et al., 1999; Hammami et al., 1999; Masson et al., 1999; Bruyere et al., 2000).

X. BIOMARKERS

Biomarker chemicals biologically bound to an animal's tissues can be incorporated into baits as a means of tracking the fate of a bait. Many biomarker chemicals have been investigated and rejected for various reasons, e.g., incompatibility due to toxicity, taste aversion, short detection half-life in tissues, or cost. An ideal biomarker should be homogeneous with the vaccine but not impair vaccine efficacy and should be detectable for months or years following bait ingestion by an animal. To date, an ideal marker that is compatible with vaccine, long lasting, inexpensive, and safe has not been developed. Tetracyclines, the common antibiotics, have been used for their propensity to chelate with hydroxyapatite during bone mineralization, forming a long-term mark in bones and teeth (Linhart et al., 1967). They have proved useful in verifying not only bait contact but also primary and booster vaccine bait ingestion regimens from counts of fluorescent lines in tooth dentin (Fig. 2A). When yearly biomark ingestion lines are correlated with the age of the animal from cementum growth zones and virus-neutralizing antibody (VNA) levels, they can indicate the duration of detectable immune levels of VNA and the anamnestic response from yearly booster bait regimens (Figs. 2*B* and 3) (Lawson and Bachmann, 1997; Vrzal and Matouch, 1996; Johnston *et al.*, 1999). When an area is baited, all animals that eat baits will be "tagged" with the biomark, and this has proved useful for tracking animal dispersal from a baited area (e.g., movement of red foxes, coyotes, and raccoons across the St. Lawrence River between Ontario and New York State) (L. L. Bigler, personal communication). However, tetracyclines can be found in wildlife at low levels derived from agricultural sources, usually less than 5% (Nunan *et al.*, 1994). This has proved complicating in some programs (Linhart *et al.*, 1997), but if specimens of the target species are examined for ambient levels prior to baiting, this can be taken into account (Hanlon *et al.*, 1993; Fearneyhough *et al.*, 1998). Microscope filter combinations that help differentiate tetracycline bait biomarks from naturally occurring fluorescent artifacts in teeth (e.g., collagen autofluorescence; see Fig. 2) are described by Johnston *et al.* (1999). There is, however, a need for unique, long-lasting marker materials that can be used in combination with tetracycline to produce unique lifelong biomarks in teeth. Such biomarkers will further help to monitor the portion of a population that has received exposure to a vaccine and to determine, in the absence of declining VNA evidence, when to rebait the area (see Fig. 3). Specimens (heads) submitted for routine rabies diagnosis also can be used to establish the sex-age structure of the infected vector populations (Moore, 1966; Johnston and Beauregard, 1969) and may be of particular value for post-ORV monitoring of biomarkers in animals that have dispersed from the baited area.

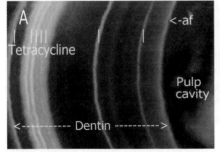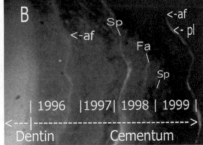

Fig. 2.   Sections of carnivore teeth showing yellow fluorescent lines from the ingestion of rabies vaccine baits containing tetracycline as a biomarker (undecalcified cross sections, ultraviolet fluorescence; ×100). (*A*) Coyote canine tooth with seven daily tetracycline lines from vaccine baits (E. Oertli and M. G. Fearneyhough, Texas Department of Health). (*B*) Canine tooth from 4-year-old raccoon with yearly tetracycline lines in cementum (G. Nohrenberg, USDA, APHIS, Wildlife Services). Sp, spring baits 1998 and 1999; Fa, fall bait 1998; af, autofluorescent collagen; pl, periodontal ligament. *(Photo by Carl Hansen.)*

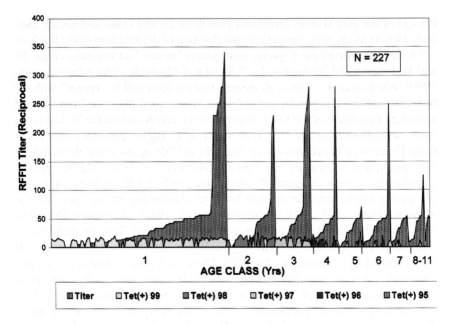

Fig. 3.   1999 South Texas coyote population. Individual profiles of rabies virus-neutralizing anti-body RFFIT titers (J. Morrill, DOD Food and Diagnostic Laboratory) and vaccine bait tetracycline biomarks by year class (E. Oertli and M. G. Fearneyhough, Texas Department of Health).

XI. ORV INITIATION

In any area where ORV treatment is contemplated, it is imperative that the biology and epidemiology of the local wildlife rabies vector populations be understood before treatment is initiated. In most areas, there usually are general ecologic studies and inventories of the principal wildlife species that will help establish baseline information on population levels and their interaction with domestic animals and humans. Also, if the success of the ORV program is to be evaluated after treatment, specimens of the target species should be tested before treatment to establish "control" levels of existing VNA (Bigler *et al.*, 1983; Rosatte *et al.*, 1984; Hanlon *et al.*, 1989; Hill *et al.*, 1992) and biomarker levels (Hanlon *et al.*, 1993; Nunan *et al.*, 1994; Fearneyhough *et al.*, 1998) in the population.

It should be remembered that ORV is a total system and not just a medicament of the sort we use in human medicine to cure an ill. ORV is a system that must attain vaccine efficacy in a particular species, but also of equal importance are the biology and population dynamics of that species and the interactions within the ecosystem in which it lives and reproduces following treatment (Müller, 1997). Programs that consider only dropping baits and disregard the results in the vector populations may later encounter untoward complications. Wild populations are constantly changing in composition and density, particularly during and after a rabies epizootic (Childs *et al.*, 2000). Rebounding populations following the suppression of rabies as a major mortality factor may create other problems. While the natural intervention of other mortality factors, e.g., pathogens such as distemper, ultimately will limit the population, further human intervention, such as the use of reproductive inhibitor technology, may be considered (Kreeger, 1997). Rabies control in wildlife is an ongoing scenario and one in which monitoring and follow-up are mandatory if rabies control and a rabies-free status are to be achieved and maintained. This requires continued public and governmental support, particularly during interepizootic lows.

XII. IMPORTANCE OF THE HOME RANGE OF VECTOR SPECIES IN BAIT DISTRIBUTION

The concept of oral vaccination is basically the same as parenteral vaccination, one immunizing dose per individual. Therefore, under wild conditions, we must place the bait within the home range of the target animal. If we could rely on each member of a wild species only taking one bait, there would be no problem, but unfortunately, this is not the case. Some workers have suggested that we must know the density of the target species in order to determine how many baits to drop, but this is not the case either because there are many other species or "things" that consume baits. For example, autumn leaf fall or crop harvest may obliterate baits in woods and fields, insects may make baits unpalatable, or wet marshy areas and river valleys baited for raccoons may easily "consume" baits if they do not float. Therefore, at present, the only way to decide on the parameters of bait density and distribution pattern for a particular area is by empirical experimentation. Fortunately, there are now many experimental ORV programs from which to draw experience, but each geographic area and vector species possess unique factors that can modify ORV results. During the bait-available period immediately after the baits are dropped, every individual of a vector species moves within a delineated home range of a specific size. If the baits are not placed within that bait-available home range, the individual will not encounter a bait and have the opportunity for vaccination. Bait distribution patterns therefore should be established that provide enough baits per home range to ensure vaccination of that individual in the presence of bait-eating competitors. Conversely, if too many baits are dropped, the baiting system is not efficient, and baits are wasted that could be applied elsewhere. Another related factor is the variability in home-range size between sex and age classes in the population. Depending on the time of year, adults usually have larger home ranges than young animals, and yet the young are usually the largest cohort in a carnivore population (Windberg, 1988). The bait distribution parameters therefore should be tailored to reach this cohort provided the bait drop is after the young are immunocompetent (Lawson *et al.*, 1997; Müller *et al.*, 2001). If baiting criteria are not scaled to accommodate their smaller home ranges, then in summer a proportion of these animals will be missed, and some will reappear as unvaccinated adults in later years. In establishing the home-range parameters of a species, we can refer to existing studies for general information, but radiotelemetry studies of vector species home ranges are needed during the baiting periods throughout the year for different ORV areas. Most bait uptake studies have shown that more than 50% of baits are consumed by 1 week and more than 80% by 2 weeks (Johnston *et al.*, 1982; Linhart *et al.*, 1997). Therefore, the extent of the target animal's movements inside its home range is critical to bait uptake during this short period. If the home range is small and movement is limited, e.g., the movement of female raccoons during the spring perinatal period, distribution patterns with widely spaced lines may miss many individuals that would be covered by the larger home ranges later in the year. Home-range size and movement information from telemetry studies during the bait-available period can be incorporated into simulation models and GIS flight-planning programs to further enhance bait distribution success (Tinline *et al.*, 1999; Hauschildt *et al.*, 2001).

XIII. LARGE-SCALE VACCINE BAIT DISTRIBUTION TECHNOLOGY

During the past 30 years, development of vaccine bait distribution technology has progressed from hand-dropped test baits to systems in many countries capable of air dropping thousands of baits per day (Johnston *et al.*, 1975, 1982; Steck *et al.*, 1982; MacInnes *et al.*, 1992; Müller *et al.*, 1993; Fearneyhough *et al.*, 1998; Robbins, 1998; Hauschildt *et al.*, 2001). There are three principal aspects to bait delivery: (1) ground versus airborne distribution, (2) automation of airborne bait delivery systems, and (3) organization of the bait delivery team. Ground distribution includes placing baits by hand or throwing baits along roadways from moving vehicles. Airborne distribution ranges from hand baiting by helicopter to automated dropping systems with fixed-wing aircraft. The decision to use a particular method depends largely on the scale of the operation, budget considerations, target species, and the need for locational accuracy to select habitats and avoid nontarget areas. For small areas, hand baiting is the most efficient for locational accuracy. In practice, hand baiting has been useful for urban areas and specific habitat types. To cover large areas uniformly, airborne delivery by helicopter or fixed-wing aircraft is most feasible. The decision to use helicopters or fixed-wing aircraft depends on the scale of the operation, the local land use (suburban or rural), targeted habitat baiting versus uniform distribution, the required operating characteristics of the delivery platform (range, load, operating speed, and cost per hour), and the need for computerized baiting control machinery to automate the dropping process. Compare, for example, the operating characteristics of the Ontario Ministry of Natural Resources (OMNR) Twin Otter, the fixed-wing aircraft used most often in the large-scale ORV programs in North America, with the Ministry's Bell 206Ll helicopter (Table I). The Twin Otter has a potential range of 5 hours. The Bell 206Ll has a potential range of 3 hours. In Ontario, the "slim" bait (23 g) is dropped at 20 baits per square kilometer along flight lines 2 km apart (Rosatte *et al.*, 1998; MacInnes, 2001). Thus, in 1 hour of continuous operation, the Twin Otter delivers 40 baits per kilometer over 270 km, a total of 10,800 baits; the Bell 207Ll helicopter, on the other hand, will deliver only 7200 baits. Considering only the difference in operating costs, the delivery cost per baits is about US$0.90 per bait for either aircraft. The important difference, however, is that the helicopter's effective operating time is only slightly over 1 hour per flight due to the need for frequent reloading and extra ferry time to and from the drop zone. In comparison, the Twin Otter can operate for 3–4 hours. Hence ferrying time using a helicopter is approximately three times more than with a Twin Otter. Depending on the size and shape of the baited area and the location of the airport, estimates indicate that this extra ferry time can increase the delivery cost per bait by up to 50%. Also, the bait machinery needed to handle current baits (20–30 g) is too large and heavy to install in the Bell helicopter. These comparisons make clear the need for smaller, lighter, but efficient baits and bait dropping machinery that can be used in helicopters and smaller aircraft.

The use of global positioning systems (GPS) in navigation technology in the 1990s has greatly enhanced aircraft baiting operations. Typical GPS equipment

TABLE I

Comparison of Flight Parameters and Costs between the deHavilland Twin Otter Fixed-Wing Aircraft and the Bell 206Ll Helicopter

	Twin otter	Bell 206Ll
Maximum flight duration	5 hr	3 hr
Payload for 2 hours (includes fuel and pilot)	1671 kg	440 kg
Weight of bait machinery	272 kg	na
Effective load for 2-hour flight including bait machinery and 3 crew at 180 lb (82 kg) each	1153 kg	194 kg
Maximum bait load for 2-hour flight (23 g Ontario bait)	50,130	8435
Typical operating speed	270 km/hr	180 km/hr
Cost per hour (including pilot and fuel, external rates)	US$970	US$630
Baits dropped per hour at 20 baits per km^2	10,800	7200
Area baited per hour at 20 baits per km^2	540 km^2	360 km^2

provides 24-hour, all-weather location accuracy to within 100 m. This allows air-craft to follow preprogrammed flight lines. Also, aircraft ground speed can be cal-culated easily, which allows the navigator to set the speed of the baiting machine to the prescribed target drop rate per kilometer with an accuracy of ($\pm 5\%$). When millions of baits are being dropped, larger percentage errors in distribution preci-sion can be costly. In addition to using GPS, Ontario has developed the FPLAN software to preplan flight routes, upload waypoints to the GPS navigation system, and track results after the drop. The FPLAN software has been used successfully in a number of large-scale ORV programs in North America (Hauschildt *et al.*, 2001).

The last element of flight planning is organization of the ground and flight crew team. A typical large-scale control operation uses three Twin Otters and requires a team to handle refueling, reloading, and flight crew changes every 2–3 hours, up to four times per day, for a program of several days. A typical flight crew consists of a pilot, a navigator, and two to four crew members to operate the baiting machine. Each flight will drop 20,000–30,000 baits, and this requires a substantial crew for ground-related operations, radio watch, and flight-planning logistics. Operations are weather-dependent because all low-level flying, for safety reasons, is visual (VFR) and requires clear visibility of the terrain. Large-scale operations are expensive, and most areas in North American have made extensive use of inter-ested volunteers as crew. Because of the need to coordinate a team of 30–60 per-sonnel, Texas and Ontario cooperated to add crew-management database software to the flight-control software FPLAN described earlier.

XIV. POSTDROP SURVEILLANCE OF TARGET SPECIES

While serum VNA titers are normally used in laboratory experiments to verify vaccine efficacy, for technical reasons, they often fail to indicate the true immune status of a wild population under treatment. This is due to several factors, in par-ticular to the unknown time period between vaccine bait ingestion and serum sampling. If taken too soon, seroconversion may not have occurred; if taken too late, the antibody titer may have decayed below detectable levels even though the animal has established immune memory and is resistant.

The incorporation of a chemical biomarker in the bait along with the vaccine can give additional evidence of vaccine bait contact. If no marker except the vaccine is present in the bait and VNA samples are negative, there is no way to verify that the oral vaccine baiting system is working, i.e., if animals are not finding the baits, not eating the baits, or the vaccine itself is not producing immunity. Also, in a success-ful ORV system without a marker, if rabies cases drop to zero and VNA also declines over time, there is no way to verify the proportion of the vector population that may still have immunity or at what point rebaiting is necessary to maintain a greater than

50% level of protection against reinvasion. For these reasons, some form of marker is needed in a vaccine bait. While an ideal marker has yet to be developed, marker molecules, such as the tetracyclines, that are mineralized directly into the hard tissues during growth can provide a lifelong history of the animals' vaccine bait regimen. The dentin of a young Texas coyote (see Fig. 2A) shows the tetracycline biomarks from the primary vaccine bait regimen from bait contacted during a 2-month period following a bait drop in January 1999. The cementum of a 4-year-old Ohio raccoon with three tetracycline lines from bait ingestions over 2 years (see Fig. 2B) indicates that this animal had contact with a priming vaccine bait in the spring of 1998, followed by two booster vaccine baits in the fall of 1998 and the spring of 1999. Figure 3 illustrates the complex profiles of vaccine bait history that have evolved in the South Texas coyote population during a 5-year ORV program. The population is made up of 1- to 11-year-old animals (see Fig. 3, age classes 1–11), with animals in the first year class (0–1 years) comprising nearly 50% of the population sample. Some animals in each year class are tetracycline biomark (+), indicating vaccine bait contact, but did not show detectable VNA (cutoff dilution > 1:5), and others show titers of more than 1:50. There are several possible explanations for the lower titers comprising part of the wild population profile in contrast with those seen in controlled laboratory experiments: (1) The animal may have eaten a bait, be biomark (+), but not have effectively contacted the oral vaccine and developed detectable VNA (see Chap. 5); (2) the animal may have contacted the vaccine, be biomarked (which takes < 24 hours), but be VNA (−) because the serum sample was taken before detectable antibody formation (2–3 weeks) [e.g., the biomark (+), VNA (−) animals in year class 1 of Fig. 3], or (3) the animal may have contacted the vaccine, be biomark (+), but the circulating VNA may have decayed to an undetectable level even though the animal may still have immune memory [e.g., the biomark (+), VNA (−), animals in year classes 2 and 3]. Unfortunately, there is no way to challenge the immunity of this category of animal, as can be done under laboratory control. Even if the animal were captured and challenged in captivity, the associated stress undoubtedly would compromise the experiment. In 5- to 11-year-old animals (year classes 5–11), there is a noticeable number of VNA (+), biomark (−) animals. This is related to slower growth and lack of mineralization of the tetracycline into the tooth cementum of older animals (Johnston *et al.*, 1999). The ultraviolet–fluorescent lines in the cementum of older animals generally are thinner and more difficult to detect (Johnston *et al.*, 1997) (see Fig. 2B).

XV. VACCINE BAITING COSTS

Rabies vaccine baiting over large areas is expensive (Uhaa *et al.*, 1992; Meltzer, 1996; Kreindel *et al.*, 1998; Selhorst *et al.*, 2000). Justifying large costs for novel methods has been difficult for local governments because results were uncertain until recently. However, when compared with the continuing cost of rabies control and continuing human risk from a rabies endemic fed by wildlife reservoirs, in the 1970s several countries opted to develop the oral vaccination idea even though it was highly experimental. Currently, other jurisdictions, with the portent of an invading epizootic, have opted for ORV, and they have been successful in preventing the establishment of an enzootic state. Initial successes in North America where ORV barriers have held for at least 1 year against raccoon-strain rabies include parts of Florida (Olson *et al.*, 2000), Massachusetts (Robbins *et al.*, 1998), New Jersey (Roscoe *et al.*, 1998), New York (Bigler *et al.*, 2001), and Ohio (Smith *et al.*, 1999), and also against the canine-coyote strain in Texas (Fearneyhough *et al.*, 1998). The blocking of raccoon-strain rabies from entering Ontario is still underway (spring 2001), and success is at present uncertain (Rosatte *et al.*, 2001a).

XVI. VACCINE BAITING EFFICIENCY AND COST REDUCTION

ORV is a relatively inefficient method of vaccinating an animal rabies vector (i.e., many vaccine doses are required per animal vaccinated versus one dose per animal by parenteral injection). Therefore, with limited budgets for rabies control, efficient use of vaccine baits is imperative for the operating agency. In many early programs when funds were limited and efficient bait distribution parameters unknown, programs deployed too few baits, too thinly, with too few bait drops from year to year, and the results often were disappointing (Stöhr *et al.*, 1996). Attempts to compare failed and successful programs have been extremely difficult due to the many variables in baiting parameters that must be applied in different areas with different vector species and different "bait-eating" competitors (Linhart *et al.*, 1997). Variables affecting baiting success include the geographic area to be baited, target species and target species density, bait-eating competitor density, habitat variability, year-to-year climate and phenologic changes, time of year, crop rotation, harvest time and leaf fall, the vaccine-bait parameters themselves (including bait type, vaccine type, biomarker type and concentration, bait density, and the distribution criteria, i.e., ground versus air, habitat-oriented versus uniform baiting flight lines), and the variability in postdrop sampling and lack of standardized sampling analyses.

Results to date indicate that for a vaccine baiting system to be successful in limiting rabies spread and at the same time to be efficient, the following criteria must be met:

1. To become immune, an individual animal of the target species needs to consume only one bait containing an efficacious vaccine (i.e., a vaccine with > 90 % seroconversion efficiency, see Chap. 11).

2. For an individual animal to eat only one baits, the bait must be dropped within its active home range during the bait-available period. Bait dropped

outside this home range, no matter how many, are of no value. Also, enough baits must be dropped within the home range so that at least one bait is found by the target individual before all the baits are eaten by other competitors.

3. The target vector population is able to resist continuing a rabies epizootic if approximately 50–70% of the population finds a vaccine bait, becomes immune, and maintains that immunity for an extended period (Voigt *et al.*, 1985; Tischendorf *et al.*, 1998).

4. A cost-efficient program will achieve the 70% population bait consumption level using only an average of one bait per individual of the target species.

XVII. BAITING SUCCESS GUIDELINES

A. Improving Efficiency and Reducing Cost

By assessing the baiting parameters of some successful programs, the following guidelines are being developed and refined using three variables from post-drop surveillance results: (1) the age of the animal, (2) the VNA level, and (3) the count of tetracycline biomarks in teeth (see Figs. 2 and 3) (Table II). More comparative data are needed from ongoing programs to refine this method, but it has the potential to improve baiting efficiency.

TABLE II

Baiting Success Guidelines Derived from Counts of Tetracycline Biomarks in Teeth of Carnivore Vector Species

Species (location)	Sample (n) (year class)	Tetracycline biomark (%+)	Median (range) biomarks/(+) animal	Baiting success guideline (type)
Coyote (TX)[a]	111 (1st yr class)	78	4.1 (1–11)	BSG, type 1
Raccoon (NY)[b]	207 (all yr classes)	73	2.0 (1–9)	BSG, type 2
Raccoon (OH)[c]	22 (1st yr class)[d]	76	1.5 (1–6)	BSG, type 2
Red Fox (ON)[e]	210 (all yr classes)	70	2.8 (1–28)	BSG, type 2
Gray Fox (TX)[a]	50(1st yr class)	46	1.4 (1–5)	BSG, type 3

[a] E. Oertli and M. G. Fearneyhough, Texas Department of Health.

[b] Bigler and Lein (2001).

[c] G. Nohrenberg, USDA, APHIS, Wildlife Services.

[d] Limited test sample.

[e] Johnston and Voigt (1982).

Tetracycline biomarker positivity rate (the presence of tetracycline fluorescence in bones or teeth) indicates baiting success, but by itself it does not indicate baiting efficiency if overbaiting is occurring (i.e., more than one bait per animal). However, when coupled with the total biomark count per animal, it can indicate baiting efficiency. It can show if baits are being distributed uniformly (i.e., are some animals getting too many baits, while others do not get any). The number of baits contacted per target animal is determined from counts of tetracycline bait ingestion lines in teeth by ultraviolet–fluorescence microscopy (Johnston *et al.*, 1999) (see Fig. 2*A*). Specimens up to 1 year old give the best count of biomarks because of their rapid tooth growth, which separates bait ingestion lines more clearly than in older animals (see Fig. 2*B*).

B. Guidelines

The following baiting success guidelines (BSG) should help improve bait distribution efficiency and success. They are based on ORV programs where biomark counts are available and on some that have shown, in addition to a high rate of biomark positivity, an associated decline in rabies incidence in the treated populations (see Table II). The important variables to be modified are (1) bait density (baits per square mile) and (2) bait flight-line interval [the spacing (km)] between adjacent baiting flight lines (Tinline *et al.*, 1999).

1. *Type 1: high percentage of biomark (+) and high number of biomarks per animal. For any target species*: If tetracycline (+) is greater than 80% but less than 100% and median biomark count is greater than 2.0–3.0, then too many baits are being dropped but not enough bait flight lines are being used to spread the baits more uniformly over vector home ranges. Therefore, reduce bait density slightly but increase the number of bait lines (i.e., decrease bait flight line interval).

2. *Type 2: Low percentage of biomark (+) but high number of biomarks per animal. For any target species*: If tetracycline (+) is less than 80% but median biomark count is greater than 1.5–2.0, then enough baits are being dropped but not enough bait flight lines are being used to spread the baits more uniformly. Therefore, maintain bait density but increase number of bait flight lines (i.e., decrease bait flight-line interval).

3. *Type 3: Low percentage of biomark (+) and low number of biomarks per animal. For any target species*: If tetracycline (+) is less than 70% and median biomark count is less than 1.5, then not enough baits are being dropped and not enough bait flight lines are being used to spread the baits more uniformly. Therefore, increase bait density and increase the number of bait flight lines (i.e., decrease bait flight-line interval).

The degree of increase or decrease needed in baiting parameters derived from these guidelines is, at this point, empirical. Input from other successful programs is needed. A potential increase in program funding immediately enters into the equation when changes to ORVP baiting parameters are proposed. This need not necessarily be the case if some animals are getting too many baits while others receive none. Slight changes in bait density and flight-line interval can accomplish better distribution with little effect on budget. The AIRBAIT software program (D. H. Johnston, unpublished) has been used to calculate ORVP costs and efficiencies using various combinations of baiting variables, including size of drop zone, bait density and cost, bait line interval, aircraft type, and cost of fuel, to determine the most efficient baiting compromise for a given budget. The Texas ORVP example (see Table II) is one of the few cases where actual overbaiting of a vector population (coyotes) may be occurring. Conversely, using virtually the same baiting parameters, gray foxes were underbaited, probably due to their smaller home range compared with coyotes (Winberg, 1988).

XVIII. MODELING

Mathematical modeling has played a number of roles in the development of vaccination programs. Early deterministic models of the dynamics of fox rabies in Europe (Anderson, 1981; Smith and Harris, 1991) looked at the proportion of the target population that must be vaccinated to achieve herd immunity and therefore stop the spread of rabies. In the United States, Coyne (1989) also used a series of coupled differential equations to investigate the relative merits of culling and/or vaccination. The overall conclusion from this research was that a vaccination or a combination of vaccination and culling would be necessary to control rabies if it got established in the host population. These models, however, were highly simplified representations of reality and did not examine the potential impact that spatial behaviors such as territoriality, dispersal, and daily interaction would have on the patterns of spread and the persistence of the disease. Other groups began to develop spatial and stochastic models of spread (Voigt *et al.*, 1985; Murray *et al.*, 1986; Smith and Harris, 1991). In stochastic models, animal behaviors (dispersal, litter size, breeding success, incubation period, and contact rate) at any given time are determined from a random draw from probability distributions representing those behaviors. Thus, unlike deterministic models, every run of a stochastic model would produce slightly different results. Therefore, many runs were required to assess the variance of the output. Despite this inconvenience, these models became powerful tools for understanding the impact that small changes in input variables have on output variables. This sensitivity testing allowed modelers to develop a better understanding of the range of conditions under which a variable was important in the spread of rabies and when it was not.

For example, in Ontario, field experiments with air-dropped oral vaccine bait delivery systems (MacInnes and Johnston, 1975) suggested that uptake was on the order of 74%. Laboratory experiments, however, indicated that perhaps only 80% of animals eating a bait would seroconvert (Lawson and Bachmann, 1997). Taken together, these results indicated that only 50–60% of animals would have immune titers, a level just on the border between eradication and persistence noted in Anderson's 1981 paper. Using the Ontario fox rabies model (Voigt *et al.*, 1985), we were able to determine that immunity levels of 50–60% would eradicate fox rabies in areas where it is dominant and cyclic if the vaccination program were started in a year representing a trough of rabies incidence and continued for at least 6 years (Tinline, 1988). In essence, rabies would defeat itself by culling many susceptibles from the population, thereby increasing the bait-to-vector ratio and thus the probability of baiting success and vaccination. Therefore, eastern Ontario was chosen as the initial trial area in the fall of 1989 because it had a strong 3- to 4-year cycle of fox rabies, and it had peaked in the previous year. The success of this campaign has been described by MacInnes (2001). A similar modeling approach is now being developed for raccoon and skunk rabies in Ontario (Broadfoot *et al.*, 2001).

During the past decade, many others have explored the power of simulation models to answer questions such as (1) when to stop a vaccination campaign and what is the best control strategy, if rabies reappears (Thulke *et al.*, 2000), (2) optimal bait delivery strategies (Tinline *et al.*, 1999; Selhorst *et al.*, 2000), and (3) the impact of other control methods such as contraception (Kreeger *et al.*, 1997; Suppo *et al.*, 2000). In comparison with field experiments, simulation models are inexpensive, fast, pose no physical danger, and most important, allow controlled experimentation. The major disadvantage of these models is that they are based on "expert opinion" and limited data from field experiments and inherit the vagaries of both sources. Paradoxically, this disadvantage is also a major advantage. Simulation models force researchers to make explicit their assumptions and operating rules and, in doing so, force them to state clearly what is known and not known about the many variables in vector ecology. This, in turn, lays out clear directions for further field research and may, in many cases, represent the major gain from the exercise of modeling.

XIX. PROGRAM PERPETUATION

The outcome of successful programs has resulted in a curious conundrum. If there is no rabies there is no perceived need for control and therefore no public demand for funds to perpetuate a state of preparedness. It should be realized, therefore, that control of wildlife rabies, like control of any other communicable disease, will require ongoing programs. Support from the public and government must be continuous for rabies control in wildlife to succeed, at least in the short term (5–10 years), until more experience is gained with ORVP. In addition, all levels of government should initiate and enforce legislation curbing the translocation of wildlife, particularly across state boundaries and now, under North American Free Trade Agreement (NAFTA), across international boundaries (CDC, 2001a). Unintentional translocation of wildlife by natural dispersal or human conveyance will occur despite all efforts. Therefore, a state of perpetual preparedness should be maintained to be ready for reinvasion of a resident rabies-free vector population. Major plans are now in the offing to coordinated rabies control in the United States and Canada. The National Working Group on Rabies Prevention and Control has made recommendations for rabies control in wildlife in the United States (Hanlon *et al.*, 1999), and the International Regional Rabies Control Committee (United States–Canada) has outlined plans to coordinate control between the United States and Canada against the raccoon epizootic now underway in eastern North America. These programs should help coordinate regional efforts, stabilize funding, and encourage the initiation of standard operating procedures and techniques to establish wildlife rabies control as an integral component of the animal and human health system.

REFERENCES

Anderson, R. M., Jackson, H. C., May, R. M., and Smith, M. (1981). Population dynamics of fox rabies in Europe. *Nature* **289**, 765–771.

Andral, L., and Joubert, L. (1975). Epidemiologie et prophylaxie écologues de la rage. *Med. Mal. Infect.* **5**, 183–189.

Arellano-Sota, C. (1988). Biology, ecology and control of the vampire bat. *Rev. Infect. Dis.* **10** (Suppl. 4), S615–S619.

Bachmann, P., Bramwell, R. N., Fraser, S. J., Gilmore, D. H., Johnston, D. H., Lawson, K. F., MacInnes, C. D., Matejka, F. O., Miles, H. E., Pedde, M. A., and Voigt, D. R. (1990). Wild carnivore acceptance of baits for delivery of liquid rabies vaccine. *J. Wildlife Dis.* **26**, 486–501.

Baer, G. M., Abelseth, M. K., and Debbie, J. G. (1971). Oral vaccination of foxes against rabies. *Am. J. Epidemiol.* **93**, 487–490.

Baer, G. M. (1988). Oral rabies vaccination: An overview. *Rev. Infect. Dis.* **10** (Suppl. 4), S644–S648.

Bigler, L. L., and Lein, D. H. (2001). Wildlife rabies vaccination program — St. Lawrence region. USAHA Conference, Harrington, DE.

Bigler, W. J., Hoff, G. L., Smith, J. S., McLean, R. G., Trevino, H. A., and Ingwersen, J. (1983). Persistence of rabies antibody in free-ranging raccoons. *J. Infect. Dis.* **148**, 610.

Bingham, J., Schumacher, C. L., Hill, F. W., and Aubert, A. (1999). Efficacy of SAG-2 oral rabies vaccine in two species of jackal (*Canis adustus and Canis mesomelas*). *Vaccine* **17**, 551–558.

Black, J. G., and Lawson, K. F. (1970). Sylvatic rabies studies in the silver fox (*Vulpes vulpes*): Susceptibility and immune response. *Can. J. Comp. Med.* **34**, 309–311.

Bögel, K., Meslin, F.-X., and Kaplan, M. (1992). *Wildlife Rabies Control: Proceedings of the Internation WHO Symposium 1990, Geneva.* Wells Medical, Royal Tunbridge Wells, England.

Broadfoot, J. D., Rosatte, R. C., and O'Leary, D. T. (2001). Raccoon and skunk population models for urban disease control planning in Ontario, Canada. *Ecol. App.* **11**, 295–303.

Brochier, B, Aubert, M. F., Pastoret, P. P., Masson, E., Schon, J., Lombard, M., Chappuis, G., Languet, B., and Desmettre, P. (1996). Field use of a vaccinia–rabies recombinant vaccine for the control of sylvatic rabies in Europe and North America. *Rev. Sci. Technol.* **15**, 947–970.

Bruyère, V., Vuillaume, P., Cliquet, F., and Aubert, M. (2000). Oral rabies vaccination of foxes with one or two delayed distributions of SAG2 baits during the spring.*Vet. Res.* **31**, 339–345.

Butler, L. (1951). Population sizes and colour phase genetics of the coloured fox in Quebec. *Can. J. Zool.* **29**, 24–41.

Centers for Disease Control and Prevention (1995). Translocation of coyote rabies — Florida, 1994. *Morbid. Mortal. Weekly Rep.* **44**, 580–587.

Centers for Disease Control and Prevention (2000). Notice to readers: Public Health Service recommendations for the use of vaccines manufactured with bovine-derived materials. *Morbid. Mortal. Weekly Rep.* **49**, 1137–1138.

Centers for Disease Control and Prevention (2001a). Compendium of animal rabies prevention and control, 2001. National Association of State Public Health Veterinarians, Inc. *Morbid. Mortal. Weekly Rep.* **50** (RR-08), 1–9.

Centers for Disease Control (2001b). Vaccinia (smallpox) vaccine recommendations of the Advisory Committee on Immunization Practices. *Morbid. Mortal. Weekly Rep.* **50** (RR-10), 1–25.

Charlton, K. M. (1984). Rabies: Spongiform lesions in the brain. *Acta Neuropathol. (Berl.)* **63**, 198–202.

Charlton, K. M., Webster, W. A., Casey, G. A., and Rupprecht, C. E. (1988). Skunk rabies. *Rev. Infect. Dis.* **10** (Suppl. 4), S626–S628.

Charlton, K. M., Artois, M., Prevec, L., Campbell, J. B., Casey, G. A., Wandeler, A. I., and Armstrong, J. (1992). Oral rabies vaccination of skunks and foxes with a recombinant human adenovirus vaccine. *Arch. Virol.* **123**, 169–179.

Childs, J. E., Curns, A. T., Dey, M. E., Real, L. A., Feinstein, L., Bjørnstad, O. N., and Krebs, J. W. (2000). Predicting the local dynamics of epizootic rabies among raccoons in the United States. *Proc. Natl. Acad. Sci. USA* **97**, 13666–13671.

Coyne, M. J., Smith, G., and McAllister, F. E. (1989). Mathematical model for the population biology of rabies in raccoons in the mid-Atlantic states. *Am. J. Vet. Res.* **12**, 2148–2154.

Creekmore, T. E., Linhart, S. B., Corn, J. L., Whitney, M. D., Snyder, B. D., and Nettles, V. F. (1994). Field evaluation of baits and baiting strategies for delivering oral vaccine to mongooses in Antigua, West Indies. *J. Wildlife Dis.* **30**, 497–505.

Ellenton, J. A., and Johnston, D. H. (1979). Oral biomarkers of calciferous tissues in carnivores. In *Transactions of the 1975 Eastern Coyote Workshop*, pp. 60–67. New Haven, CT.

Farry, S. C., Henke, S. E., Beasom, S. L., and Fearneyhough, M. G. (1998). Efficacy of bait distributional strategies to deliver canine rabies vaccines to coyotes in southern Texas. *J. Wildlife Dis.* **34**, 23–32.

Fearneyhough, M. G., Wilson, P. J., Clark, K. A., Smith, D. R., Johnston, D. H., Hicks, B. N., and Moore, G. M. (1998). Results of an oral rabies vaccination program for coyotes. *J. Am Vet. Med. Assoc.* **212**, 498–502.

Fekadu, M., Shaddock, J. H., Sumner, J. W., Sanderlin, D. W., Knight, J. C., Esposito, J. J., and Baer, G. M. (1991). Oral vaccination of skunks with raccoon poxvirus recombinants expressing the rabies glycoprotein or the nucleoprotein. *J. Wildlife Dis.* **27**, 681–684.

Finley, D. (1998). *Mad Dogs: New Rabies Plague.* Texas A&M University Press, College Station, TX.

Follmann, E. H., Ritter, D. G., and Baer, G. M. (1996). Evaluation of the safety of two attenuated oral rabies vaccines, SAG1 and SAG2, in six Arctic mammals. *Vaccine* **14**, 270–273.

Hammami, S., Schumacher, C., Cliquet, F., Tlatli, A., Aubert, A., and Aubert, M. (1999). Vaccination of Tunisian dogs with the lyophilised SAG2 oral rabies vaccine incorporated into the DBL2 dog bait. *Vet. Res.* **130**, 607–613.

Hanlon, C. L., Hayes, D. E., Hamir, A. N., Snyder, D. E., Jenkins, S. R., Hable, C. P., and Rupprecht, C. E. (1989). Proposed field evaluation of a rabies recombinant vaccine for raccoons (*Procyon lotor*): Site selection, target species characteristics, and placebo baiting trials. *J. Wildlife Dis.* **25**, 555–567.

Hanlon, C. A., Buchanan, J. R., Nelson, E., Niu, H. S., Diehl, D., and Rupprecht, C. E. (1993). A vaccinia-vectored rabies vaccine field trial: Ante- and post-moretem biomarkers. *Rev. Sci. Technol.* **12**, 99–107.

Hanlon, C. A., Niezgoda, M., Hamir, A. N., Schumacher, C., Koprowski, H., and Rupprecht, C. E. (1998). First North American field release of a vaccinia–rabies glycoprotein recombinant virus. *J. Wildlife Dis.* **34**, 228–239.

Hanlon, C. A., Childs, J. E., Nettles, V. F., and the National Working Group on Rabies Prevention and Control (1999). Recommendations of a national working group on prevention and control of rabies in the United States: III. Rabies in wildlife. *J. Am. Vet. Med. Assoc.* **215**, 1612–1619.

Hauschildt, P., Tinline, R. R., and Ball, D. G. A., (2001). Outfoxing rabies in Ontario. *GPS World*, May 2001, 34–39.

Hill, R. E., Jr., Beran, G. W., and Clark, W. R. (1992). Demonstration of rabies virus–specific antibody in the sera of free-ranging Iowa raccoons (*Procyon lotor*). *J. Wildlife Dis.* **28**, 377–385.

Hu, L., Ngichabe, C., Trimarchi, C. V., Esposito, J. J., and Scott, F. W. (1997). Raccoon poxvirus live recombinant feline panleukopenia virus VP2 and rabies virus glycoprotein bivalent vaccine. *Vaccine* **15**, 1466–1472.

Jackson, A. C. (1994). The fatal illness of the Fourth Duke of Richmond in Canada: Rabies. *Ann. R. Coll. Phys. Surg. Can.* **27**, 40–41.

Jenkins, S. R., Perry, B. D., and Winkler, W. G. (1988). Ecology and epidemiology of raccoon rabies. *Rev. Infect. Dis.* **10** (Suppl. 4), S620–S625.

Johnston, D. H., and Beauregard, M. (1969). Rabies epidemiology in Ontario. *Bull. Wildlife Dis. Assoc.* **5**, 357–370.

Johnston, D. H. (1975). The Principles of Wild Carnivore Baiting with Oral Rabies Vaccines. WHO Consultation on Oral Vaccination of Foxes, Frankfurt am Main, Item 5, Document 7. WHO, Geneva.

Johnston, D. H., and Voigt, D. R. (1982). A baiting system for the oral rabies vaccination of wild foxes and skunks. *Comp. Immunol. Microbiol. Infect. Dis.* **5**, 185–186.

Johnston, D. H., Fearneyhough, M. G., Hicks, B. N., and Moore, G. M. (1997). L'influence de l'âge de la population sur le succès apparent des essais de vaccination orale antirabique utilisant de la tétracycline comme marqueur. Colloque International sur la Rage, pp. 5–12. Institut Pasteur, Paris.

Johnston, D. H., Joachim, D. G., Bachmann, P., Kardong, K. V., Stewart, R. E. A., Dix, L. M., Strickland, M. A., and Watt, I. D. (1999). Aging furbearers using tooth structure and biomarkers. In *Wild Furbearer Management and Conservation in North America*, M. Novak, J. A. Baker, M. E. Obbard, and B. Malloch (eds.), CD Edition, pp. 228–243. Ontario Fur Managers Federation, Sault Ste Marie, Ontario.

Kreeger, T. J. (1997). *Contraception in Wildlife Management*. Technical Bulletin No. 1853, U.S. Department of Agriculture, Animal and Plant Health Inspection Service, Washington.

Kreindel, S. M., McGuill, M., Meltzer, M., Rupprecht, C., and DeMaria, A. (1998). The cost of rabies postexposure prophylaxis: One state's experience. *Public Health Rep.* **113**, 247–251.

Lawson, K. F., Chiu, H., Crosgrey, S. J., Matson, M., Casey, G. A., and Campbell, J. B. (1997). Duration of immunity in foxes vaccinated orally with ERA vaccine in a bait. *Can. J. Vet. Res.* **61**, 39–42.

Lawson, K. F., and Bachmann, P. (2001). Stability of attenuated live virus rabies vaccine in baits targeted to wild foxes under operational conditions. *Can. Vet. J.* **42**, 368–374.

Lin, C. C., Johnston, D. H., and Ramsden, R. O. (1972). Polymorphism and quinacrine fluorescence karotypes of red fox (*Vulpes vulpes*). *Can. J. Genet. Cytol.* **14**, 573–580.

Linhart, S. B., and Kennelly, J. J. (1967). Fluorescent bone labeling of coyotes with demethylchlortetracycline. *J. Wildlife Manag.* **31**, 317–321.

Linhart, S. B., Kappeler, A., and Windberg, L. (1997). A review of baits and bait delivery systems for free-ranging carnivores and ungulates. In *Contraception in Wildlife Management*, T. J. Kreeger (ed.), pp. 69–132. Technical Bulletin No. 1853, U.S. Department of Agriculture, Animal and Plant Health Inspection Service, Washington.

Lloyd, H. G. (1980). *The Red Fox*. B.T. Batsford, London.

MacInnes, C. D., and Johnston, D. H. (1975). *Ontario Fish and Wildlife Review* **14**, 17–20.

MacInnes, C. D., Johnston, D. H., Bachmann, P., Pond, B. A., Fielding, C. A., Nunan, C. P., Ayers, N. R., Voigt, D. R., Lawson, K. F., and Tinline, R. R. (1992). Design considerations for large-scale aerial distribution of rabies vaccine-baits in Ontario. In *Wildlife Rabies Control*, K. Bögel, F.-X. Meslin, and M. Kaplan (eds.), pp.160–167. Wells Medical, Kent, England.

MacInnes, C. D., Smith, S. M., Tinline, R. R., Ayers, N. R., Bachmann, P., Ball, D. G. A., Caulder, L. A., Crosgrey, S. J., Fielding, C., Hauschildt, P., Honig, J. M., Johnston, D. H., Lawson, K. F., Nunan, C. P., Pedde, M. A., Pond, B., Stewart, R. B., and Voigt, D. R. (2001). Elimination of rabies from red foxes in eastern Ontario. *J. Wildlife Dis.* **37**, 119–132.

Masson, E., Aubert, M. F., and Rotivel, Y. (1997). Human contamination by baits for vaccinating foxes against rabies in France. *Santé Publique* **9**, 297–313.

Masson, E., Bruyère-Masson, V., Vuillaume, P., Lemoyne, S., and Aubert, M. (1999). Rabies oral vaccination of foxes during the summer with the VRG vaccine bait. *Vet. Res.* **30**, 595–605.

Matter, H. C., Schumacher, C. L., Kharmachi, H., Hammami, S., Tlatli, A., Jemli, J., Mrabet, L., Meslin, F.-X., Aubert, M. F., Neuenschwander, B. E., and Hicheri, K. E. (1998). Field evaluation of two bait delivery systems for the oral immunization of dogs against rabies in Tunisia. *Vaccine* **16**, 657–665.

McGuill, M. W., Kreindel, S. M., DeMaria, A., and Rupprecht, C. E. (1997). Knowledge and attitudes of residents in two areas of Massachusetts about rabies and an oral vaccination program in wildlife. *J. Am. Vet. Med. Assoc.* **211**, 305–309.

Meltzer, M. I. (1996). Assessing the cost and benefits of an oral vaccine for raccoon rabies: A possible model. *Emerg. Infect. Dis.* **2**, 343–349.

Merial, Inc. (1999). *Control of Raccoon Rabies Using Merial's Raboral V-RG Vaccine*. Merial Inc., Athens, GA.

Messenger, S. L., Rupprecht, C. E., and Smith, J. S. (2002). Bats, emerging virus infections, and the rabies paradigm. In *Bat Ecology*, T. H. Kunz and M. B. Fenton (eds.). University of Chicago Press, Chicago.

Moore, K. L. (1966). The sex chromatin of various animals. In *The Sex Chromatin*, K. L. Moore (ed.), pp. 23–27. W. B. Saunders, Philadelphia.

Müller, T. F., Stöhr, K., Teuffert, J., and Stöhr, P. (1993). Erfahrungen mit der Flügzeugausbringung von Ködern zur oralen Immunisierung der Füchse gegen Tollwut in Ostdeutschland. *Dtsch. Tierarztl. Wochenschr.* **100**, 203–207.

Müller, T. F., Schuster, P., Vos, A. C., Selhorst, T., Wenzel, U. D., and Neubert, A. M. (2001). Effect of maternal immunity on the immune response of young foxes to oral vaccination with SAD B19. *Am. J. Vet. Res.* (in press).

Müller, W. W. (1997). Where do we stand with oral vaccination of foxes against rabies in Europe? *Arch. Virol. Suppl.* **13**, 83–94.

Murray, J. D., Stanley, A. A., and Brown, D. L. On the spatial spread of rabies among foxes. (1986). *Proc. R. Soc. Lond. [B]* **229**, 111–150.

Nadin-Davis, S. A., Huang, W., and Wandeler, A. I. (1996). The design of strain-specific polymerase chain reactions for discrimination of the raccoon rabies virus strain from indigenous rabies viruses of Ontario. *J. Virol. Methods* **57**, 1–14.

Nettles, V. F., Shaddock, J. H., Sikes, R. K., and Reyes, C. R. (1979). Rabies in translocated raccoons. *Am. J. Public Health* **69**, 601–602.

Nunan, C. P., MacInnes, C. D., Bachmann, P.; Johnston, D. H., and Watt, I. D. (1994). Background prevalence of tetracycline-like fluorescence in teeth of free ranging red foxes (*Vulpes vulpes*:), striped skunks (*Mephitis mephitis*) and raccoons (*Procyon lotor*) in Ontario, Canada. *J. Wildlife Dis.* **30**, 112–114.

Nunan, C. P. (1999). Legalities, insurance and liabilities in rabies control programs: What rabies researchers should know (Abstract). 10th Annual Rabies in the Americas Meeting, San Diego, CA.

Nyberg, M., Kulonen, K., Neuvonen, E., Ek-Kommonen, C., Nuorgam, M., and Westerling, B. (1992). An epidemic of sylvatic rabies in Finland — Descriptive epidemiology and results of oral vaccination. *Acta Vet. Stand.* **33**, 43–57.

Olson, C. A., Mitchell, K. D., and Werner, P. A. (2000). Bait ingestion by free-ranging raccoons and nontarget species in an oral rabies vaccine field trial in Florida. *J. Wildlife Dis.* **36**, 734–743.

Perry, B. D., Brooks, R., Foggin, C. M., Bleakley, J., Johnston, D. H., and Hill, F. W. (1988). A baiting system suitable for the delivery of oral rabies vaccine to dog populations in Zimbabwe. *Vet. Rec.* **123**, 76–79.

Robbins, A. H., Borden, M. D., Windmiller, B. S., Niezgoda, M., Marcus, L. C., O'Brien, S. M., Kreindel, S. M., McGuill, M. W., DeMaria, A., Rupprecht, C. E., and Rowell, S. (1998). Prevention of the spread of rabies to wildlife by oral vaccination of raccoons in Massachusetts. *J. Am. Vet. Med. Assoc.* **213**, 1407–1412.

Rosatte, R. C., and Gunson, J. R. (1984). Presence of neutralizing antibodies to rabies virus in striped skunks from areas free of skunk rabies in Alberta. *J. Wildlife Dis.* **20**, 171–176.

Rosatte, R. C., and MacInnes, C. D. (1989). Relocation of city raccoons. In *9th Great Plains Wildlife Damage Control Workshop Proceedings*, A. J. Bjugstad, D. W. Uresk, and R. H. Hamre (eds.), pp. 87–92. USDA Forest Service General Technical Report RM-171. Great Plains Agricultural Council Publication 127.

Rosatte, R. C., Power, M. J., and MacInnes, C. D. (1992). Trap-vaccinate-release and oral vaccination techniques for the control of rabies in foxes, skunks and raccoons in urban settings. In *Wildlife Rabies Control*, K. Bögel, F.-X. Meslin, and M. Kaplan (eds.), pp. 175–179. Wells Medical, Royal Tunbridge Wells, Kent, England.

Rosatte, R. C. (2001a). Long distance movement by a coyote and a red fox in Ontario: Implications for disease-spread. *Can. Field Nat.* (in press).

Rosatte, R. C., Donovan, D., Allan, M., Howes, L., Silver, A., Bennett, K., MacInnes, C., Davies, C., Wandeler, A., and Radford, B. (200lb). Emergency response to raccoon rabies introduction in Ontario. *J. Wildlife Dis.* **37**, 265–279.

Roscoe, D. E., Holste, W. C., Sorhage, F. E., Campbell, C., Niezgoda, M., Buchannan, R., Diehl, D., Niu, H. S., and Rupprecht, C. E. (1998). Efficacy of an oral vaccinia–rabies glycoprotein recombinant vaccine in controlling epidemic raccoon rabies in New Jersey. *J. Wildlife Dis.* **34**, 752–763.

Rupprecht, C. E., Wiktor, T. J., Johnston, D. H., Hamir, A. N., Dietzschold, B., Wunner, W. H., Glickman, L., and Koprowski, H. (1986). Oral immunization and protection of raccoons (*Procyon lotor*) with a vaccinia–rabies glycoprotein recombinant virus vaccine. *Proc. Natl. Acad. Sci. USA* **83**, 7947–7950.

Rupprecht, C. E., Smith, J. S., Fekadu, M., and Childs, J. E. (1995). The ascension of wildlife rabies: A cause for public health concern or intervention? *Emerg. Infect. Dis.* **1**, 107–114.

Selhorst, T., Thulke, H. H., and Muller, T. (2000). Threshold analysis of cost-efficient oral vaccination strategies against rabies in fox populations. *Proc. Soc. Vet. Epidemiol. Prevent. Med.* **2000**, 71–84.

Smith, G. C., and Harris, S. (1991). Rabies in urban foxes in Britain: The use of a spatial stochastic simulation model to examine the pattern of spread and evaluate the efficacy of different control regimes. *Philos. Trans. R. Soc. Lond. [B]* **334**, 459–479.

Smith, K. A., Krogwold, R., Smith, F., Hale, R., Collart, M., and Craig, C. (1999). The Ohio ORV Program (Abstract). 10th Annual Rabies in the Americas Meeting, San Diego, CA.

Steck, F., Wandeler, A., Bichsel, P., Capt, S., and Schneider, L. (1982). Oral immunisation of foxes against rabies. A field study. *Zentralbl. Veterinärmed.* **29**, 372–396.

Stöhr, K., and Meslin, F.-X. (1996). Progress and setbacks in the oral immunisation of foxes against rabies in Europe. *Vet. Rec.* **13**, 32–35.

Suppo, C., Nauline, J., Langlais, M., and Artois, M. (2000). A modeling approach to vaccination and contraception programmes for rabies control in fox populations. *Proc. R. Soc. Lond. [B]* **267**, 1575–1582.

Svrcek, S., Durove, A., Ondrejka, R., Zavadova, J., Suliova, J., Benisek, Z., Vrtiak, O. J., Feketeova, J., and Madar, M. (1995). Immunogenic and antigenic activity of an experimental oral rabies vaccine prepared from the strain Vnukovo-32/107. *Vet. Med. (Praha)* **40**, 87–96.

Thulke, H., Tischendorf, L., Staubach, C., Shelhorst, T., Jeltsch, F., Goretzki, J., Müller, T., Schluter, H., and Wissel, C. (2000). The spatiotemporal dynamics of a post-vaccination resurgence of rabies in foxes and emergency vaccination planning. *Prevent. Vet. Med.* **47**, 1–21.

Tims, T., Briggs, D. J., Davis, R. D., Moore, S. M., Xiang, Z., Ertl, H. C., and Fu, Z. F. (2000). Adult dogs receiving a rabies booster dose with a recombinant adenovirus expressing rabies virus glycoprotein develop high titers of neutralizing antibodies. *Vaccine* **18**, 2804–2807.

Tinline, R. R. (1988). Persistance of rabies in wildlife. In *Rabies*, J. B. Campbell and K. M. Charlton (eds.), pp. 301–322. Kluwer Academic, Boston.

Tinline, R. R., Ball, D. G. A., Nunan, C. P., and Venodrai, T. (1999). The impact of flight line spacing and baiting density on the uptake of oral rabies vaccine via aerial distribution (Abstract). 10th Annual Rabies in the Americas Meeting, San Diego, CA.

Tischendorf, L., Thulke, H., Staubach, C., Müller, M. S., Jeltsch, F., Goretzki, J., Shelhorst, T., Muller, T., Schlüter, H., and Wissel, C. (1998). Chance and risk of controlling rabies in large-scale and long-term immunized fox populations. *Proc. R. Soc. Lond. [B]* **265**, 839–846.

Uhaa, I. J., Dato, V. M., Sorhage, F. E., Beckley, J. W., Roscoe, D. E., Gorsky, R. D., and Fishbein, D. B. (1992). Benefits and costs of using an orally absorbed vaccine to control rabies in raccoons. *J. Am. Vet. Med. Assoc.* **15**, 201, 1873–1882.

Voigt, D. R., Tinline, R. R., and Broekhoven, L. H. (1985). Spatial simulation model for rabies control. In *Population Dynamics of Rabies in Wildlife*, P. J. Bacon (ed.), pp. 311–349. Academic Press, London.

Vrzal, V., and Matouch, O. (1996). Annual testing of immunity in foxes after oral rabies immunization. *Vet. Med. (Praha)* **4**, 107–111.

Wandeler, A. I., Pfotenhauer, P., and Stocker, C. (1975). Uber die Verwendung von Ködern zu biologischen Untersuchungen an Füchsen. *Rev. Suisse Zool.* **82**, 335–348.

Wandeler, A. I., Nadin-Davis, S. A., Tinline, R. R., and Rupprecht, C. E. (1994). Rabies epizootiology: An ecological and evolutionary perspective. *Curr. Top. Microbiol. Immunol.* **186**, 297–324.

Wandeler, A. I. (2000). Oral immunization against rabies: afterthoughts and foresight. *Schweiz. Arch. Tierheilk.* **142**, 455–462.

Windberg, L. A., (1988). Management implications of coyote spacing patterns in southern Texas. *J. Wildlife Manag.* **52**, 632–640.

Winkler, W. G., (1992). A review of the development of the oral vaccination technique for immunizing wildlife against rabies. In *Wildlife Rabies Control*, K. Bögel, F.-X. Meslin, and M. Kaplan (eds.), pp. 82–96. Wells Medical, Royal Tunbridge Wells, Kent, England.

World Health Organization (1966). WHO Expert Committee on Rabies. Fifth Report. WHO Technical Report Series 321. WHO, Geneva.

15

Future Developments and Challenges

ALAN C. JACKSON

Departments of Medicine (Neurology) and Microbiology and Immunology
Queen's University
Kingston, Ontario K7L 3N6
Canada

I. INTRODUCTION

At the dawn of the new millennium, rabies continues to be an important public health problem, as it was in antiquity. Although our knowledge about many aspects of the disease has increased greatly over the past several decades, the impact of reducing the incidence of human rabies cases has been restricted largely to developed countries. The road to effective control of rabies in the world remains long with many obstacles. Even in developed countries, rabies virus has shown an ability to reemerge and affect new animal hosts and threaten the health of humans, and it is likely that this trend will continue in the future. Costs associated with rabies prevention alone have been estimated as possibly more than 1 billion per year in the United States (Fishbein and Robinson, 1993). Unfortunately, economic investment for rabies control in developing countries has been limited in the past, but hopefully, this will soon change. Future developments in our understanding of rabies and management approaches will be considered in this final chapter.

473

II. PATHOGENSIS

Studies on the pathogenesis of rabies have focused predominantly on rodent models using fixed rabies virus strains and often have employed unnatural routes of inoculation. Although these experimental models are much more convenient and less expensive than more natural models, it is uncertain how what is learned from these studies also applies to natural rabies. Improved experimental models, including studies with "street" rabies virus strains in bats, skunks, dogs, and other vectors, likely will be developed in the future, although there is not yet a trend in this direction. Our understanding of many aspects of the pathogenesis is incomplete, and many questions remain unanswered. For example, the precise steps that take place during the long incubation period in rabies, including the exact cell types infected and molecular events, have not yet been elucidated. Polymerase chain reaction *in situ* hybridization technology has been available for a few years (Nuovo, 1997), but this technique has not yet been applied to studies of rabies pathogenesis. The virtual absence of rabies researchers using natural animal models probably accounts for the lack of progress in this area, which will be an important area for future development.

The bases for neuronal dysfunction in rabies are still not well understood, and the significance of neuronal cell death by apoptosis or other mechanisms in natural disease needs to be clarified. We do not have a good understanding of how rabies encephalitis results in the characteristic behavioral changes in rabies vectors, which is an essential step for transmission of the virus to new hosts. The basis for the species specificity of rabies virus strains is not understood at either the biologic or molecular level. Future research efforts hopefully will clarify many of these unanswered questions about rabies pathogenesis, and this information may be helpful in the development of new therapies (see Sect. V). Hopefully, sufficient resources, including funds and appropriate biohazard containment facilities, will become available in the future to expand studies in appropriate animal models.

III. EPIDEMIOLOGY AND MOLECULAR EPIDEMIOLOGY

Canine rabies has remained uncontrolled in many developing countries, particularly in Asia and Africa, resulting in the vast majority of the 30,000 reported human deaths per year (World Health Organization, 2000). Reported human cases of rabies probably are only the "tip of the iceberg," and the actual number of human cases worldwide is likely much higher (Meslin *et al.*, 1994). Sadly, children are frequently the victims of rabies, and 30–50% of reported cases of rabies occur in children under 15 years of age. Although there has been an important reduction in the number of human and dog cases of rabies in Latin America during the 1990s that is likely largely due to the strategy of mass vaccination of dogs (Pan American

Health Organization/World Health Organization, 1999, 2001), there has not been a significant decline in the number of cases worldwide in recent years. Rabies also has the ability to reemerge, which has occurred recently in insectivorous bats in the United States and in both frugivorous and insectivorous bats in Australia, resulting in sporadic human deaths and a persisting threat to humans (Noah *et al.*, 1998; Hanna *et al.*, 2000; McColl *et al.*, 2000). Over the last 50 years, a raccoon rabies epizootic has spread north to involve much of the eastern United States and recently has entered Canada (Wandeler *et al.*, 2000). Undoubtedly, rabies will reemerge in new host species in the future. Because the problem has not been studied thoroughly, we have only an incomplete understanding of the importance and epidemiology of a variety of *Lyssavirus* strains in Africa and other parts of the world. It is likely that new strains will be identified in the future. Currently, the importance of noncanine strains of rabies virus in the developing world is obscured by a large canine rabies problem and inadequate diagnostic evaluations.

IV. PREVENTION OF HUMAN RABIES AND CONTROL OF ANIMAL RABIES

Rabies prevention strategies include those directed at humans and those directed at the main animal vectors. Modern cell-culture vaccines for humans are safe and highly effective, but they are expensive and, consequently, out of reach for many people in developing countries. Nerve tissue vaccines regrettably are still used most frequently in many developing countries (Haupt, 1999), and they are associated with serious neurologic complications due to autoimmune disease. A resolution was passed at the 4th International Symposium on Rabies Control in Asia, held in Hanoi, Vietnam, in March 2001, to eliminate the use of nerve tissue vaccines in Asia by the year 2006 (D. J. Briggs, personal communication; World Health Organization, 2001). The future challenge is to produce modern rabies vaccines much more cheaply and thereby make them accessible to a much greater segment of the world's population. Already, more economical multisite intradermal immunization protocols have been developed that require much smaller quantities of vaccine than needed when given intramuscularly (Warrell and Warrell, 2000). Widespread preexposure rabies immunization of children in developing countries where canine rabies is endemic and rabies immune globulin is expensive or unavailable is an ambitious and expensive prospect. However, this is a viable option until dog rabies becomes controlled. The large number of patients with human immunodeficiency virus (HIV) infection and low CD4+ T-lymphocyte counts worldwide poses a challenge for effective postexposure rabies prophylaxis (Jaijaroensup *et al.*, 1999), and this is a particularly important problem in Asia and Africa.

The world production of human rabies immune globulin and equine rabies immune globulin is currently limited, and economic factors significantly restrict the use of these products (Haupt, 1999). The development of neutralizing human monoclonal antibodies against rabies virus for therapeutic use is currently underway (Champion *et al.*, 2000) and may provide an alternative for passive immunization of humans at risk after exposures.

Bat bites may result in trivial injuries (Jackson and Fenton, 2001), and it has become clear that they are not recognized in some cases. In the United States and Canada, there is an ongoing threat of unrecognized bites from insectivorous bats, and likely many human cases occur in situations where postexposure rabies prophylaxis would not be considered even under current revised rabies prevention guidelines in the United States (Centers for Disease Control and Prevention, 1999). Short of immunizing an entire population that has a relatively low risk of developing rabies, it is difficult to conceive what scientific advances would allow effective rabies prevention in the future for sporadic human cases due to unrecognized bat bites. The potential approach of using transgenic edible plants that code for the rabies virus glycoprotein as vaccines for both humans and animals (Yusibov *et al.*, 1997; Modelska *et al.*, 1998) is a novel idea and potentially could provide a means of immunizing an entire population, particularly in countries where rabies is endemic.

About half the world's population lives in areas where canine rabies is endemic, resulting in a threat of human exposures (Meslin *et al.*, 1994). Approaches that have been successful in controlling rabies in developed countries have not been applied successfully in developing countries for a variety of reasons, including high costs, lack of adequate infrastructure for management of dog rabies, widespread prevalence of feral dogs, and cultural and religious objections to various animal control measures. Appropriate education of the population and health care professionals is essential; many human deaths occur in developing countries because victims of dog bites do not seek medical treatment. Acquisition of modern biologicals for postexposure prophylaxis of human rabies is needed in developing countries. Rabies is 11th in global mortality from infectious diseases (Haupt, 1999) and currently accounts for about 1% of the global mortality due to infectious diseases (Meslin *et al.*, 1994). Because of the costs involved and the high prevalence of other infectious diseases that pose an even greater threat to humans, rabies is unlikely to receive the attention it requires for the development of a concerted effort for rabies control and elimination in the near future. Oral vaccination of dogs may offer the best promise for the control of rabies in many developing countries in which rabies is endemic (World Health Organization, 1998a,1998b). A strong global effort is needed for the elimination of canine rabies. In the long term, this approach likely would be cost-effective, but it would take several years before the cost savings would be realized from reductions in human postexposure prophylaxis.

Approaches for rabies control in wildlife using oral rabies vaccine programs have been very successful, particularly for rabies in Europe, Ontario, and Texas (Fearneyhough *et al.*, 1998; Hanlon *et al.*, 1999; MacInnes *et al.*, 2001). Campaigns for the control of raccoon rabies are much younger in their development, and their success cannot yet be evaluated fully (Hanlon *et al.*, 1999; Rosatte *et al.*, 2001). However, these programs are costly, and they must be repeated on a regular basis until disease is eradicated. Hopefully, there will be greater emphasis in the future on assessing the reason why particular programs either succeed or fail. Local population dynamics and spatial spread of rabies and other infectious diseases must be understood and overlaid on efforts to assess the long-term success of expensive interventions (Childs *et al.*, 2000; Dobson, 2000). In the future we can expect that geographic information systems and epidemiologic modeling will be used more widely to develop spatially explicit models in order to help refine and guide oral rabies vaccine distribution strategies as well as to aid in the development of contingency plans for targeting breaks in vaccine zones. Current approaches for the prevention of rabies in cattle transmitted by vampire bats using anticoagulants (Linhart *et al.*, 1972; Thompson *et al.*, 1972) have shown moderate success. However, the technical difficulties in delivering a vaccine to insectivorous bats in the field seem almost insurmountable based on our current knowledge.

V. DIAGNOSIS AND THERAPY OF HUMAN DISEASE

An improved understanding of the pathogenesis of rabies may lead to novel approaches to the therapy of the human disease. New antiviral agents and/or immunotherapies may be developed that have efficacy in established rabies. Despite future therapeutic advances that may occur, it is unlikely that neurologic outcomes will be good if the diagnosis is not made until late in the course of the disease. Rabies diagnosis is particularly difficult when there is no history of an animal exposure. Astute clinical practitioners always will be essential, even if there are improved diagnostic investigations (e.g., imaging and sensitive assays on body fluids, including saliva and cerebrospinal fluid) that allow confirmation of a diagnosis of rabies much earlier than is presently possible. Combinations of therapies may be more effective than single agents, similar to the current situation in antiretroviral therapy of HIV infection (Freedberg *et al.*, 2001). Although there is currently evidence of at least three rabies virus receptors (see Chap. 7), the relative importance of these receptors and possibly other unidentified receptors in the pathogenesis of the disease remains unclear. An improved understanding of the role and importance of rabies receptors may be useful in the design of new therapies for rabies. Novel neuroprotective therapies also may be developed that will be applicable to many viral infections of the nervous system as well as noninfectious neurologic diseases.

VI. SUMMARY

In summary, there are many challenges to control and eliminate rabies in animals and prevent human disease. A strong commitment from the governments of many countries is essential for this to be accomplished. Cooperation and adequate support of both the human health and veterinary sectors are necessary. Although costs are high, a long-term economic benefit can be anticipated, as well as a reduction in human suffering with a large impact on children in developing countries.

REFERENCES

Centers for Disease Control and Prevention (1999). Human rabies prevention — United States, 1999: Recommendations of the Advisory Committee on Immunization Practices (ACIP). *Morbid. Mortal. Weekly Rep.* **48** (RR-l), 1–21.

Champion, J. M., Kean, R. B., Rupprecht, C. E., Notkins, A. L., Koprowski, H., Dietzschold, B., and Hooper, D. C. (2000). The development of monoclonal human rabies virus–neutralizing antibodies as a substitute for pooled human immune globulin in the prophylactic treatment of rabies virus exposure. *J. Immunol. Methods* **235**, 81–90.

Childs, J. E., Curns, A. T., Dey, M. E., Real, L. A., Feinstein, L., Bjornstad, O. N., and Krebs, J. W. (2000). Predicting the local dynamics of epizootic rabies among raccoons in the United States. *Proc. Natl. Acad. Sci. USA* **97**, 13666–13671.

Dobson, A. (2000). Raccoon rabies in space and time. *Proc. Natl. Acad. Sci. USA* **97**, 14041–14043.

Fearneyhough, M. G., Wilson, P. J., Clark, K. A., Smith, D. R., Johnston, D. H., Hicks, B. N., and Moore, G. M. (1998). Results of an oral rabies vaccination program for coyotes. *J. Am. Vet. Med. Assoc.* **212**, 498–502.

Fishbein, D. B., and Robinson, L. E. (1993). Rabies. *New Engl. J. Med.* **329**, 1632–1638.

Freedberg, K. A., Losina, E., Weinstein, M. C., Paltiel, A. D., Cohen, C. J., Seage, G. R., Craven, D. E., Zhang, H., Kimmel, A. D., and Goldie, S. J. (2001). The cost-effectiveness of combination antiretroviral therapy for HIV disease. *New Engl. J. Med.* **344**, 824–831.

Hanlon, C. A., Childs, J. E., and Nettles, V. F. (1999). Article III: Rabies in wildlife. The National Working Group on Rabies Prevention and Control. *J. Am. Vet. Med. Assoc.* **215**, 1612–1619.

Hanna, J. N., Carney, I. K., Smith, G. A., Tannenberg, A. E. G., Deverill, J. E., Botha, J. A., Serafin, I. L., Harrower, B. J., Fitzpatrick, P. F., and Searle, J. W. (2000). Australian bat lyssavius infection: A second human case, with a long incubation period. *Med. J. Aust.* **172**, 597–599.

Haupt, W. (1999). Rabies: Risk of exposure and current trends in prevention of human cases. *Vaccine* **17**, 1742–1749.

Jackson, A. C., and Fenton, M. B. (2001). Human rabies and bat bites (Letter). *Lancet* **357**, 1714.

Jaijaroensup, W., Tantawichien, T., Khawplod, P., Tepsumethanon, S., and Wilde, H. (1999). Postexposure rabies vaccination in patients infected with human immunodeficiency virus. *Clin. Infect. Dis.* **28**, 913–914.

Linhart, S. B., Flores Crespo, R., and Mitchell, G. C. (1972). Control of vampire bats by means of an anticoagulant (Spanish). *Bol. Oficina. Sanit. Panama* **73**, 100–109.

MacInnes, C. D., Smith, S. M., Tinline,. R. R., Ayers, N. R., Bachmann, P., Ball, D. G., Calder, L. A., Crosgrey, S. J., Fielding, C., Hauschildt, P., Honig, J. M., Johnston, D. H., Lawson, K. F., Nunan, C. P., Pedde, M. A., Pond, B., Stewart, R. B., and Voigt, D. R. (2001). Elimination of rabies from red foxes in eastern Ontario. *J. Wildlife Dis.* **37**, 119–132.

McColl, K. A., Tordo, N., and Aguilar Setien, A. A. (2000). Bat lyssavirus infections. *Rev. Sci. Tech. Off. Int. Epiz.* **19**, 177–196.

Meslin, F.-X., Fishbein, D. B., and Matter, H. C. (1994). Rationale and prospects for rabies elimination in developing countries. In *Current Topics in Microbiology and Immunology*, Vol. 187: *Lyssaviruses*, C. E. Rupprecht, B. Dietzschold, and H. Koprowski (eds.), pp. 1–26. Springer-Verlag, Berlin.

Modelska, A., Dietzschold, B., Sleysh, N., Fu, Z. F., Steplewski, K., Hooper, D. C., Koprowski, H., and Yusibov, V. (1998). Immunization against rabies with plant-derived antigen. *Proc. Natl. Acad. Sci. USA* **95**, 2481–2485.

Noah, D. L., Drenzek, C. L., Smith, J. S., Krebs, J. W., Orciari, L., Shaddock, J., Sanderlin, D., Whitfield, S., Fekadu, M., Olson, J. G., Rupprecht, C. E., and Childs, J. E. (1998). Epidemiology of human rabies in the United States, 1980 to 1996. *Ann. Intern. Med.* **128**, 922–930.

Nuovo, G. J. (1997). *PCR in Situ Hybridization: Protocols and Applications*. Lippincott-Raven, Philadelphia.

Pan American Health Organization/World Health Organization (1999). XI Inter-American Meeting, at the Ministerial Level, on Animal Health: Report of the VII Meeting of Directors of National Rabies Control Programs, Puerto Vallarta, Mexico, December 12–14, 1998. World Health Organization, Geneva.

Pan American Health Organization/World Health Organization (2001). XII Inter-American Meeting, at the Ministerial Level, on Health and Agriculture: Report of the VIII Meeting of Directors of National Rabies Control Programs in Latin America (REDIPRA), São Paulo, Brazil, May 2–4, 2001. World Health Organization, Geneva.

Rosatte, R., Donovan, D., Allan, M., Howes, L. A., Silver, A., Bennett, K., MacInnes, C., Davies, C., Wandeler, A., and Radford, B. (2001). Emergency response to raccoon rabies introduction into Ontario. *J. Wildlife Dis.* **37**, 265–279.

Thompson, R. D., Mitchell, G. C., and Burns, R. J. (1972). Vampire bat control by systemic treatment of livestock with an anticoagulant. *Science* **177**, 806–808.

Wandeler, A. I., Rosatte, R. C., Williams, D., Lee, T. K., Gensheimer, K. F., Montero, J. T., Trimarchi, C. V., Morse, D. L., Eidson, M., Smith, P. F., Hunter, J. L., Smith, K. A., Johnson, R. H., Jenkins, S. R., and Berryman, C. (2000). Update: Raccoon rabies epizootic — United States and Canada, 1999. *Morbid. Mortal. Weekly Rep.* **49**, 31–35.

Warrell, M. J., and Warrell, D. A. (2000). Intradermal postexposure rabies vaccine regimens (Letter). *Clin. Infect. Dis.* **31**, 844–845.

World Health Organization (1998a). Oral Immunization of Dogs against Rabies: Report of the Sixth WHO Consultation Organized with the Participation of the Office International des Epizooties (OIE), Geneva, Switzerland, July 24–25, 1995. WHO/EMC/ZDI/98.13, pp. 1–28. World Health Organization, Geneva.

World Health Organization (1998b). Field Application of Oral Rabies Vaccines for Dogs: Report of a WHO Consultation Organized with the Participation of the Office International des Epizooties (OIE), Geneva, Switzerland, July 20–22, 1998. WHO/EMC/ZDI/98.15, pp. 1–22. World Health Organization, Geneva.

World Health Organization (2000). World Survey of Rabies No. 34 for the Year 1998. World Health Organization, Geneva.

World Health Organization (2001). Report of the 4th International Symposium on Rabies Control in Asia. Organized by the Merieux Foundation with the Cosponsorship of the World Health Organization. Hanoi, Vietnam, March 5–9, 2001 (in press). World Health Organization, Geneva.

Yusibov, V., Modelska, A., Steplewski, K., Agadjanyan, M., Weiner, D., Hooper, D. C., and Koprowski, H. (1997). Antigens produced in plants by infection with chimeric plant viruses immunize against rabies virus and HIV-1. *Proc. Natl. Acad. Sci. USA* **94**, 5784–5788.

Index